W0228048

Monographs on Pathology of Laboratory Animals

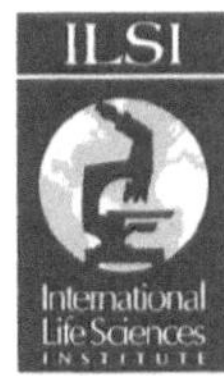

Sponsored by the International Life Sciences Institute

The following volumes have appeared so far

Endocrine System
1983. 346 figures. XV, 366 pages. ISBN 3-540-11677-X

Respiratory System
1985. 279 figures. XV, 240 pages. ISBN 3-540-13521-9

Digestive System
1985. 352 figures. XVIII, 386 pages. ISBN 3-540-15815-4

Urinary System
1986. 362 figures. XVIII, 405 pages. ISBN 3-540-16591-6

Genital System
1987. 340 figures. XVII, 304 pages. ISBN 3-540-17604-7

Nervous System
1988. 242 figures. XVI, 233 pages. ISBN 3-540-19416-9

Integument and Mammary Glands
1989.468 figures. XI, 347 pages. ISBN 3-540-51025-7

Hemopoietic System
1990. 351 figures. XVIII, 336 pages. ISBN 3-540-52212-3

Cardiovascular and Musculoskeletal Systems
1991. 390 figures. XVII, 312 pages. ISBN 3-540-53876-3

Eye and Ear
1991. 141 figures. XIII, 170 pages. ISBN 3-540-54044-X

Nonhuman Primates I
1993.235 figures. XIII, 221 pages. ISBN 3-540-56465-9
0-944398-15-4

Nonhuman Primates II
1993. 264 figures. XVI, 248 pages. ISBN 3-540-56527-2
0-944398-16-2

2nd editions to follow

Respiratory System
1996. 382 figures. Approx. 440 pages. ISBN 3-540-60383-2
0-944398-69-3

T.C. Jones C.C. Capen U. Mohr (Eds.)

Endocrine System

Second Edition

Completely Revised and Updated
with 521 Figures and 37 Tables

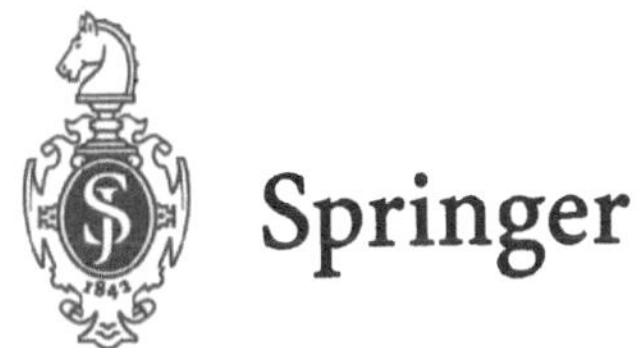

Springer

Thomas Carlyle Jones, D.V.M., D.Sc.
Professor of Comparative Pathology
Emeritus, Harvard Medical School
ILSI Research Foundation
1126 Sixteenth Street, N.W., Washington, DC 20036, USA

Charles C. Capen, D.V.M., Ph.D.
Professor of Veterinary Pathobiology and Chairman,
Department of Veterinary Biosciences, Professor of Endocrinology,
Department of Internal Medicine, College of Medicine,
The Ohio State University, 1925 Coffey Road,
Columbus, OH 43210-1093, USA

Ulrich Mohr, M.D.
Professor of Experimental Pathology
Medizinische Hochschule Hannover
Institut für Experimentelle Pathologie
Konstanty-Gutschow-Strasse 8
30625 Hannover, Germany

Distribution rights for North America, Canada, and Mexico by
International Life Sciences Institute (ILSI)
1126 Sixteenth Street NW, Washington, DC 20036, USA

2nd Edition
ISBN 978-3-642-64649-2 ISBN 978-3-642-60996-1 (eBook)
DOI 10.1007/978-3-642-60996-1

1st Edition

Library of Congress Cataloging-in-Publication Data. Endocrine system/T.C. Jones, C.C. Capen, U. Mohr eds. – 2nd ed. p. cm. – (Monographs on pathology of laboratory animals) Includes bibliographical references (p.) and index. ISBN 3-540-59477-9 1. Laboratory animals–Diseases. 2. Veterinary endocrinology. 3. Endocrine glands–Diseases. 4. Rodents–Diseases. 5. Rodents as laboratory animals. 6. Pathology, Comparative. I. Jones, Thomas Carlyle. II. Capen, Charles C. III. Mohr, U. (Ulrich) IV. Series. SF996.5.E5 1995 616.4'027–dc20. 95-31393

Typesetting: Best-set Typesetter Ltd., Hong Kong

SPIN: 10128517 25/3133/SPS – 5 4 3 2 1 0 – Printed on acid-free paper

Foreword to the Second Edition

The International Life Sciences Institute (ILSI) is a nonprofit, worldwide foundation established in 1978 to advance the understanding of scientific issues relating to nutrition, food safety, toxicology, risk assessment, and the environment. By bringing together scientists from academia, government, industry, and the public sector, ILSI seeks a balanced approach to solving problems of common concern for the well-being of the general public. This volume is the first of the Second Edition of *Monographs on Pathology of Laboratory Animals*. The series is designed to facilitate communication among those involved in the safety testing of foods, drugs, and chemicals. The complete set covers cardiovascular, musculoskeletal, digestive, endocrine, genital, hemopoietic, nervous, respiratory and urinary systems, eye and ear, integument and mammary glands, and nonhuman primates. The series is intended for use by pathologists, toxicologists, and others concerned with evaluating toxicity and carcinogenicity studies. ILSI is committed to supporting programs to harmonize toxicologic testing, to advance a more uniform interpretation of bioassay results worldwide, to promote a common understanding of lesion classifications, and to encourage wide discussion of these topics among scientists. Scientific understanding and cooperation will be improved worldwide through the series and this international project.

ILSI accomplishes its work through its branches and institutes. ILSI's branches currently include Argentina, Australasia, Brazil, Europe, Japan, Korea, Mexico, North America, Southeast Asia, and Thailand, and a focal point in China. The ILSI Health and Environmental Sciences Institute focuses on global environmental issues. ILSI Research Foundation includes the ILSI Allergy and Immunology Institute, ILSI Human Nutrition Institute, ILSI Pathology and Toxicology Institute, and ILSI Risk Science Institute.

Alex Malaspina
President
International Life Sciences Institute

Preface to the Second Edition

Approximately 10 years have elapsed since the first volume of the International Life Sciences Institute (ILSI) Monographs on Pathology of Laboratory Animals, Endocrine System was completed. New information of interest to pathologists has developed at a rather remarkable pace during the intervening years. Exceptional progress has been made in the routine identification of cell products in endocrine cells. A better understanding has developed of the mechanisms involved in cell metabolism, particularly involving toxins and carcinogens. Clear concepts have developed concerning the significance of some pathologic lesions in the endocrine system and their relation to human health and risk assessment. Standardized nomenclature has developed significantly during the 10-year period since the first volume and is being utilized on an international basis. This has resulted in significant improvement in communication of pathologic data to regulatory agencies and in scientific publications worldwide. This monograph series and others sponsored by ILSI have produced a significant effect on improved communications and the international acceptance of standardized nomenclature.

In this second edition, new formats have been used where more appropriate for the subjects to be covered. In many cases, the format used in the first edition still is useful. It is still necessary to recognize the morphologic features of pathologic lesions in order to identify them precisely, an essential step toward development of new insights into pathogenetic mechanisms and their use in decisions eventually applicable to public health.

The role of the hypothalamus in the control of the endocrine system has been increasingly appreciated. Methods useful to pathologists will continue to develop and be applied to the pathologic lesions of the hypothalamus to understand their effect on the rest of the endocrine system. Approaches to evaluate possible xenobiotic-induced changes in the hypothalamus are presented in this edition.

We are very grateful to the dedicated scientists from lands all around the world who have contributed to this volume. The authors are named in the list of contributors in the frontispiece of this volume, in the table of contents, and at the heading of each individual manuscript. The members of the editorial board are listed in the frontpiece. They are particularly to be thanked for their efforts in identifying authors and for the scientific review of individual manuscripts. The editors are especially grateful for the steadfast support of Dr. Alex Malaspina and to members of the ILSI staff and others who have helped in so many ways. We particularly wish to mention Ms. Sherri Lopez, Associate Editor and Manager of the Pathology and Toxicology Institute; Ms. Sharon Weiss, formerly the Associate Director of the Pathology and Toxicology Institute; as well as Ms. Frances DeLuca, Executive Assistant, Pathology and Toxicology Institute and Research Foundation.

We are grateful to Prof. Dr. Dietrich Goetze, Ms. Barbara Montenbruck, and others on the staff of Springer-Verlag for the quality of the finished book.

August 1995

T.C. Jones
C.C. Capen
U. Mohr

Contents

Contributors

Francesca Abramo, D.V.M.
Research Assistant, University of Pisa, Pisa, Italy

Annamaria Baiocco, D.V.M.
Research Assistant, University of Bern, Bern, Switzerland

Stephen W. Barthold, D.V.M., Ph.D.
Professor of Comparative Medicine, Yale University School of Medicine, New Haven, Connecticut, USA

Gilberto E. Bestetti, D.V.M.
Professor of Animal Pathology, University of Bern, Bern, Switzerland

Gary A. Boorman, D.V.M., M.S., Ph.D.
Chief, Pathology Branch, National Institute of Environmental Health Sciences, Research Triangle Park, North Carolina, USA

Claude E. Boujon, D.V.M.
Research Assistant, University of Bern, Bern, Switzerland

Alexander M. Cameron, D.V.M., Ph.D.
R.W. Johnson, Pharmaceutical Research Institute, Spring House, Pennsylvania, USA

Charles C. Capen, D.V.M, Ph.D.
Professor of Veterinary Pathobiology and Chairman, Department of Veterinary Biosciences, Professor of Endocrinology, Department of Internal Medicine, College of Medicine, The Ohio State University, 1925 Coffey Road, Columbus, Ohio, USA

William W. Carlton, D.V.M., Ph.D.
Leslie Morton Hutchings Distinguished Professor of Veterinary Pathology, Emeritus Purdue University, West Lafayette, Indiana, USA

James W. Crissman, D.V.M., Ph.D.
The Dow Chemical Company, Midland, Michigan, USA

Ronald A. DeLellis, M.D.
Professor of Pathology, Tufts University School of Medicine, Boston, Massachusetts, USA

Michael R. Elwell, D.V.M., Ph.D.
National Institute of Environmental Health Sciences, Research Triangle Park, North Carolina, USA

Heinrich Ernst, D.V.M.
Fraunhofer Institute of Toxicology and Aerosol Research, Hannover, Germany

Judith Fetters
System Analyst, National Center for Toxicological Research, Jefferson, Arkansas, USA

J.K. Frenkel, M.D., Ph.D.
Professor Emeritus, University of Kansas, Adjunct Professor, University of New Mexico, Santa Fe, New Mexico, USA

Charles H. Frith, D.V.M., Ph.D.
Consultant, Toxicology Pathology Associates, Little Rock, Arkansas, USA

Paul-Georg Germann, D.V.M.
Institute for Pathology and Toxicology, Byk Gulden, Hamburg, Germany

Dawn G. Goodman, V.M.D.
PATHCO, Inc., Ijamsville, Maryland, USA

Christian L. Gries, D.V.M., Ph.D.
Department of Toxicology and Pathology, Eli Lilly and Company, Greenfield, Indiana, USA

Corinne Guillaume-Gentil, Ph.D.
Research Assistant, University of Geneva, Geneva, Switzerland

James E. Heath, D.V.M.
Senior Pathologist, Southern Research Institute, Birmingham, Alabama, USA

Bernard Jeanrenaud, M.D.
Professor of Medicine, University of Geneva, Geneva, Switzerland

Kenji Kamino, M.D.
Hannover Medical School, Hannover, Germany

Michal Karasek, M.D., Ph.D.
Professor, Medical University, Lodz, Poland

Eberhard Karbe, Dr.med.vet., Ph.D.
Professor, Bayer AG, Wuppertal, Germany

Birgit Kittel, Dr.med.vet.
BASF AG, Abt. Toxikologie, Ludwigshafen, Germany

Adalbert Koestner, D.V.M., Ph.D.
Professor and Chair, Emeritus, Department of Veterinary Biosciences, The Ohio State University, Columbus, Ohio, USA

Kalman Kovacs, M.D., Ph.D., D.Sc, FRCP(C), FCAP, FRC(Path)
Professor of Pathology, St. Michael's Hospital, Toronto, Canada

Georg J. Krinke, MVDr., C.Sc., FVH Path.
Head of Experimental Pathology, CIBA GEIGY AG, Crop Protection, Basel, Switzerland

Christian Landes, Dr.med.vet., FTA Path.
Senior Pathologist, Deputy Head of Toxicological Pathology, CIBA-GEIGY Ltd, Crop Protection, Basel, Switzerland

Loic E. Longeart, D.V.M.
Group Leader, Pathology Department, Pfizer Centre de Recherche, Amboise, France

R. Yoshiyuki Osamura, M.D.
Professor of Pathology, School of Medicine Tokai University, Kanagawa, Japan

Miklós Palkovits, M.D., D.Sc., Ph.D.
Professor of Anatomy, First Department of Anatomy, Semmelweis University Medical School, Budapest, Hungary, and Laboratory of Cell Biology, National Institute of Mental Health, Bethesda, Maryland, USA

George A. Parker, D.V.M.
Mountainside, New Jersey, USA

James F. Reindel, D.V.M., Ph.D.
Staff Pathologist/Senior Research Associate, Parke-Davis Pharmaceutical Research Division, Warner-Lambert Co, Ann Arbor, Michigan, USA

Russel J. Reiter, Ph.D., D.Med.
Professor, The University of Texas Health Science Center, San Antonio, Texas, USA

Gerd K. Reznik, D.V.M., Ph.D.
Director, Institute for Pathology and Toxicology, BYK Gulden, Hamburg, Germany

Françoise Rohner-Jeanrenaud, Ph.D.
Research Associate, University of Geneva, Geneva, Switzerland

Giovanni L. Rossi, M.D.
Professor of Experimental Pathology, University of Bern, Bern, Switzerland

George E. Sandusky, Jr., D.V.M., Ph.D.
Lilly Research Laboratories, Greenfield, Indiana, USA

Hironobu Sasano, M.D.
Tohoku University School of Medicine, Sendai, Japan

Bernard Sass, V.M.D.(†)
Pathologist, Registry of Experimental Cancers, National Institutes of Health, Bethesda, Maryland, USA

Winslow D. Sheldon, D.V.M.
National Center for Toxicological Research, Pathology Associates, Inc., Jefferson, Arkansas, USA

Henk A. Solleveld, D.V.M., Ph.D.
Director, Morphologic Pathology and General Toxicology, SmithKline Beecham Pharmaceuticals, King of Prussia, Pennsylvania, USA

Lucia Stefaneanu, Ph.D.
Assistant Professor of Pathology, St. Michael's Hospital, University of Toronto, Toronto, Canada

John D. Strandberg, D.V.M., Ph.D.
Director, Division of Comparative Medicine, Johns Hopkins University School of Medicine, Baltimore, Maryland, USA

Shozo Takayama, M.D.
Vice Director, Cancer Institute, Tokyo, Japan

Arthur S. Tischler, M.D.
Professor of Pathology, Tufts University School of Medicine, Boston, Massachusetts, USA

Glen C. Todd, V.M.D., Ph.D.
Research Advisor, Retired, Crawfordsville, Indiana, USA

Hiroyuki Tsuda, M.D., Ph.D.
Chief, Chemotherapy Division, National Cancer Center Research Institute, Tokyo, Japan

Marion G. Valerio, D.V.M.
Rhone Poulenc Rorer, Collegeville, Pennsylvania, USA

John T. Yarrington, D.V.M., Ph.D.
Pathologist, Battelle Memorial Institute, Columbus, Ohio, USA

Frantisek Zak, M.D., Ph.D., FMH(Path.)
Associate Professor of Pathology, Consultant in Toxicological Pathology and Pathology of Tropical Diseases, CIBA-GEIGY AG, Basel, Switzerland

Pituitary

Functional and Pathologic Interrelationships of the Pituitary Gland and Hypothalamus in Animals

Charles C. Capen

Introduction

Concepts of Endocrinology

In the discussions to follow, statements are made which refer in general terms to the hypothalamus and the pituitary in most vertebrate species, including man. Examples are presented of pathologic alterations which have been studied in one or more species. In many instances, the biologic effects of a lesion in an endocrine organ of the living rat, mouse, or hamster are unknown. Knowledge of other species may be of value in this instance to predict the kind of biologic behavior which should be looked for in a laboratory rodent with a specific endocrine lesion. Specific differences in biologic behavior, frequency of occurrence, and other features will be discussed in the sections that are directed toward individual lesions in laboratory rodents.

Endocrine glands, such as the pituitary, are collections of specialized cells that synthesize, store, and release their secretions directly into the bloodstream. Since they lack a duct system, they are often referred to as ductless glands of internal secretion. They are interposed as sensing or signaling organs to detect changes in constituents of the extracellular fluid compartment (Fig. 1).

The secretory products of specialized endocrine cells are released into the extracellular fluids and transported via the blood to influence the rates of existing chemical reactions in populations of target cells in other tissues of the body. Target cells and other cells in the body are concerned with the degradation of hormones either by proteases on the cell surface, by lysosomal enzymes within the cell, or by conjugation with glucuronic acid or sulfate and excretion in the bile or urine (Fig. 1). Endocrine glands working in concert with the nervous system are concerned with the integration and coordination of a wide variety of physiologic activities involved in maintaining a constant internal environment.

The hormones secreted by the adenohypophysis are polypeptides, which share the following characteristics: (a) the primary site of action is at the plasma membrane of target cells (Fig. 2); (b) receptor proteins for the hormone are a part of the plasma membrane of target cells; (c) they are water soluble; (d) they have a short half-life in blood (usually measured in terms of minutes); and (e) they lack specific plasma-binding proteins.

Hormone Synthesis and Secretion

Endocrine cells concerned with the production of polypeptide hormones, such as in the adenohypophysis, have a well-developed endoplasmic reticulum with many attached ribosomes for

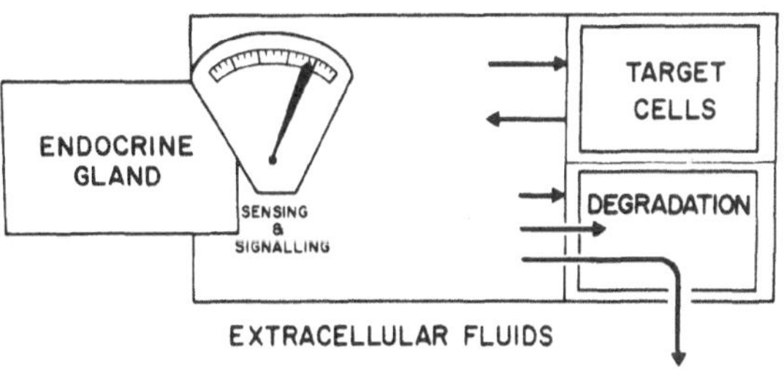

Fig. 1. Schematic representation of the endocrine system. Endocrine glands are interposed as sensing and signaling devices to detect changes in constituents of the extracellular fluid compartment. Hormones interact with specific target cells in the body to elicit a biologic response. In addition, hormones are degraded by cell surface enzymes or lysosomal enzymes within the cells, or are conjugated with glucuronic acid and sulfate for excretion in the urine or bile. (From Roth 1976)

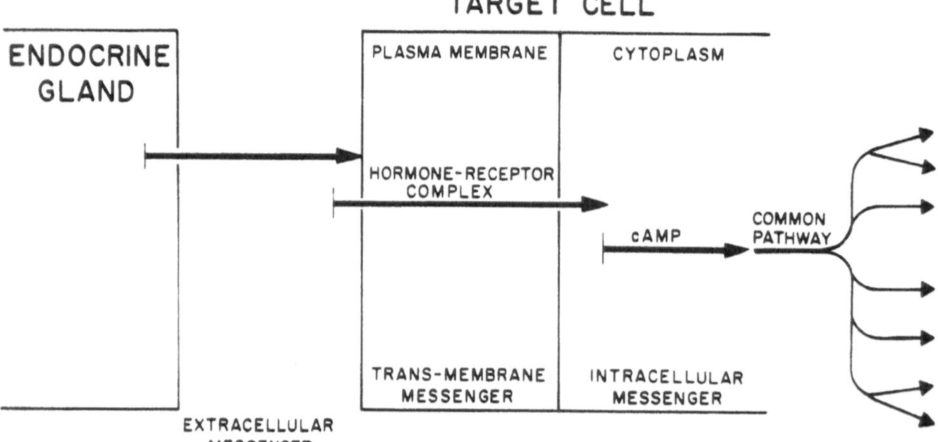

Fig. 2. Mechanism of action of polypeptide hormones on target cells. Many polypeptide hormones act on target cells by binding to specific receptors on the cell surface and activating the membrane-limited enzyme, adenylate cyclase, resulting in the intracellular formation of cyclic adenosine monophosphate (cAMP). This second messenger conveys the hormonal information within the target cell and by either common pathways (e.g., activation of protein kinases), or branch pathways which are unique for a particular hormone, elicits the biologic response of the hormone. (From Roth 1979)

assembly of hormone and a prominent Golgi apparatus for packaging of hormone into granules for intracellular storage and transport (Fig. 3). Secretory granules are unique to polypeptide hormone-secreting endocrine cells and provide a mechanism for intracellular storage of substantial amounts of preformed hormone. These membrane-limited granules represent macromolecular aggregations of active hormone, often in association with specific binding proteins. Upon receipt of an appropriate signal for hormone secretion, secretory granules are directed to the periphery of the endocrine cell, probably by the contraction of microfilaments, where the limiting membrane of the granule fuses with the plasma membrane of the cell. The hormone-containing granule core is extruded into the extracellular perivascular space either by the process of emiocytosis or exocytosis. Subsequently, the granule core is fragmented and molecules of active hormone are transported rapidly through capillary fenestrae into the circulation. Hormone synthesized in excess of the body's requirement is degraded by fusion of the hormone-containing secretory granules with lysosomes, a process termed crinophagy (Fig. 3). Endocrine glands, such as the pituitary, are concerned exclusively with endocrine function. They are small in relation to other body organs, widely distributed in the body, and connected with one another only by the bloodstream. They are richly supplied with blood and there is a close anatomic relationship between endocrine cells and the capillary network. The peripheral cytoplasmic extensions of capillary endothelial cells have fenestrae covered by a single membrane in order to facilitate rapid transport of raw materials and secretory products between the bloodstream and endocrine cells.

Structure and Function of the Adenohypophysis

The pituitary gland in an adult animal is completely separated from the oral cavity. It is situated in the sella turcica, a concavity of the sphenoid bone, and enveloped by an extension of dura mater. The pituitary gland (hypophysis) is subdivided anatomically into the adenohypophysis (anterior lobe) and neurohypophysis (posterior lobe).

Embryologic Development of the Pituitary Gland

Embryologically, the pituitary gland develops from a dorsal evagination of oropharyngeal ectoderm (Rathke's pouch) and a ventral downgrowth of diencephalic neuroectoderm (Fig. 4). The point of fusion of the two primordia develops into the pars intermedia. The pars

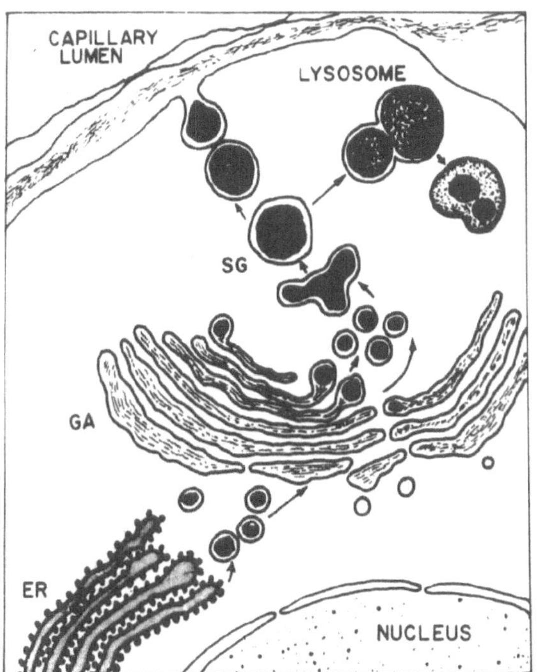

Fig. 3. Synthesis of polypeptide hormones in endocrine cells, such as the adenohypophysis, begins on ribosomes attached to membranes of the rough endoplasmic reticulum (*ER*). Precursor hormone molecules accumulate within the cisternae of the ER and are transported to the Golgi apparatus (*GA*), where they are concentrated and packaged into membrane-limited secretory granules (*SG*). Secretory granules are macromolecular aggregations of preformed active hormone that are moved to the periphery of the cell by contraction of microfilaments and released into the perivascular spaces either by exocytosis or emiocytosis Hormone synthesized in excess of the body's requirement is degraded by fusion of secretory granules with lysosomes, a process termed "crinophagy"

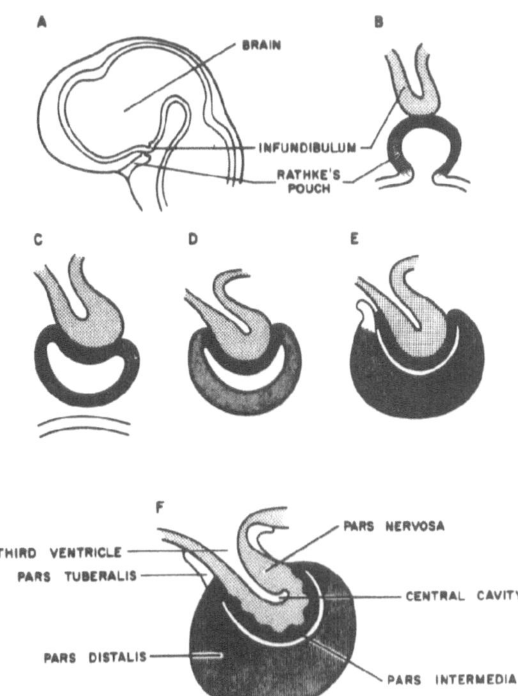

Fig. 4. Embryologic development of the adenohypophysis from a dorsal evagination of oropharyngeal ectoderm (Rathke's pouch) and the neurohypophysis from a ventral downgrowth of diencephalic neuroectoderm. (From Turner and Bagnara 1971)

distalis undergoes extensive proliferation to form the major part of the adenohypophysis and is responsible for the secretion of the tropic hormones.

The pituitary gland has two preformed cavities, the residual lumen of Rathke's pouch and the infundibular reccss of thc third vcntriclc (ccntral cavity). Separation of the developing adenohypophysis from the oropharynx is completed by formation of the sphenoid bone.

Structure of the Adenohypophysis

The adenohypophysis consists of three portions, the pars distalis, pars tuberalis, and pars intermedia. In many species the adenohypophysis completely surrounds the pars nervosa of the neurohypophyseal system (Fig. 5). The pars distalis is the largest of the three parts of the adenohypophysis and contains the multiple populations of endocrine cells that secrete the pituitary tropic hormones. The secretory cells are supplied with abundant capillaries that have fenestrae in the cytoplasm and are supported by the cytoplasmic processes of stellate follicular (sustentacular) cells (Figs. 6, 7).

The pars tuberalis consists of dorsal projections of cells along the infundibular stalk. It functions primarily as a scaffold for the capillary network of the hypophyseal portal system during its course from the median eminence to the pars distalis. The pars intermedia forms the junction between the pars distalis and pars nervosa (Howe 1973). It lines the residual lumen of Rathke's pouch and contains two populations of cells. In the dog, one of these cell types synthesizes and secretes adrenocorticotropic hormone (ACTH), similar to corticotrophs in the pars distalis (El Etreby and Dubois 1980; Halmi et al. 1981).

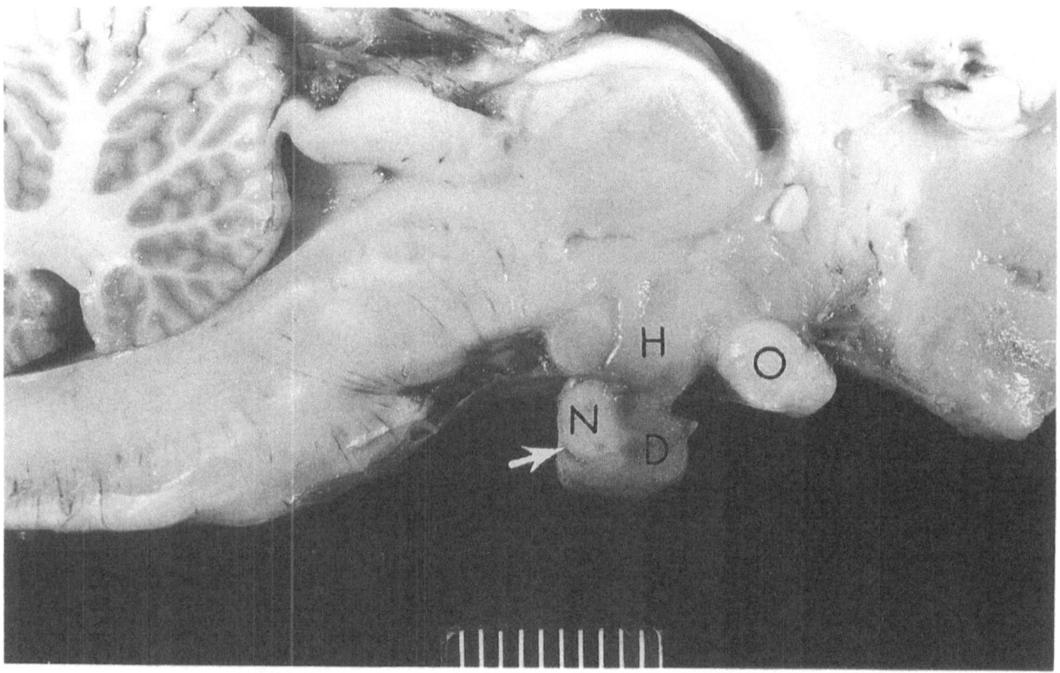

Fig. 5. The pituitary region of an adult dog, illustrating the close relationship to the optic chiasm (O), hypothalamus (H), and overlying brain. The pars distalis (D) forms a major part of the adenohypophysis and completely surrounds the pars nervosa (N). The residual lumen of Rathke's pouch (*white arrows*) separates the pars distalis and pars nervosa, and is lined by the pars intermedia. The scale at the bottom represents 1 cm

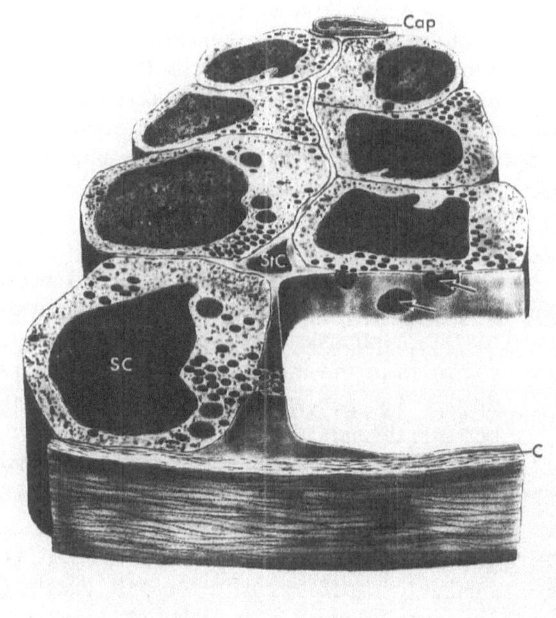

Fig. 6. Structural arrangement of secretory cells (*SC*) in the adenohypophysis. Small groups of tropic hormone-secreting cells are supported by cytoplasmic processes of sustentacular (*StC*) or follicular cells. Capillaries (*Cap*) are numerous and have fenestrae (*arrows*) within their cytoplasm (*C*)

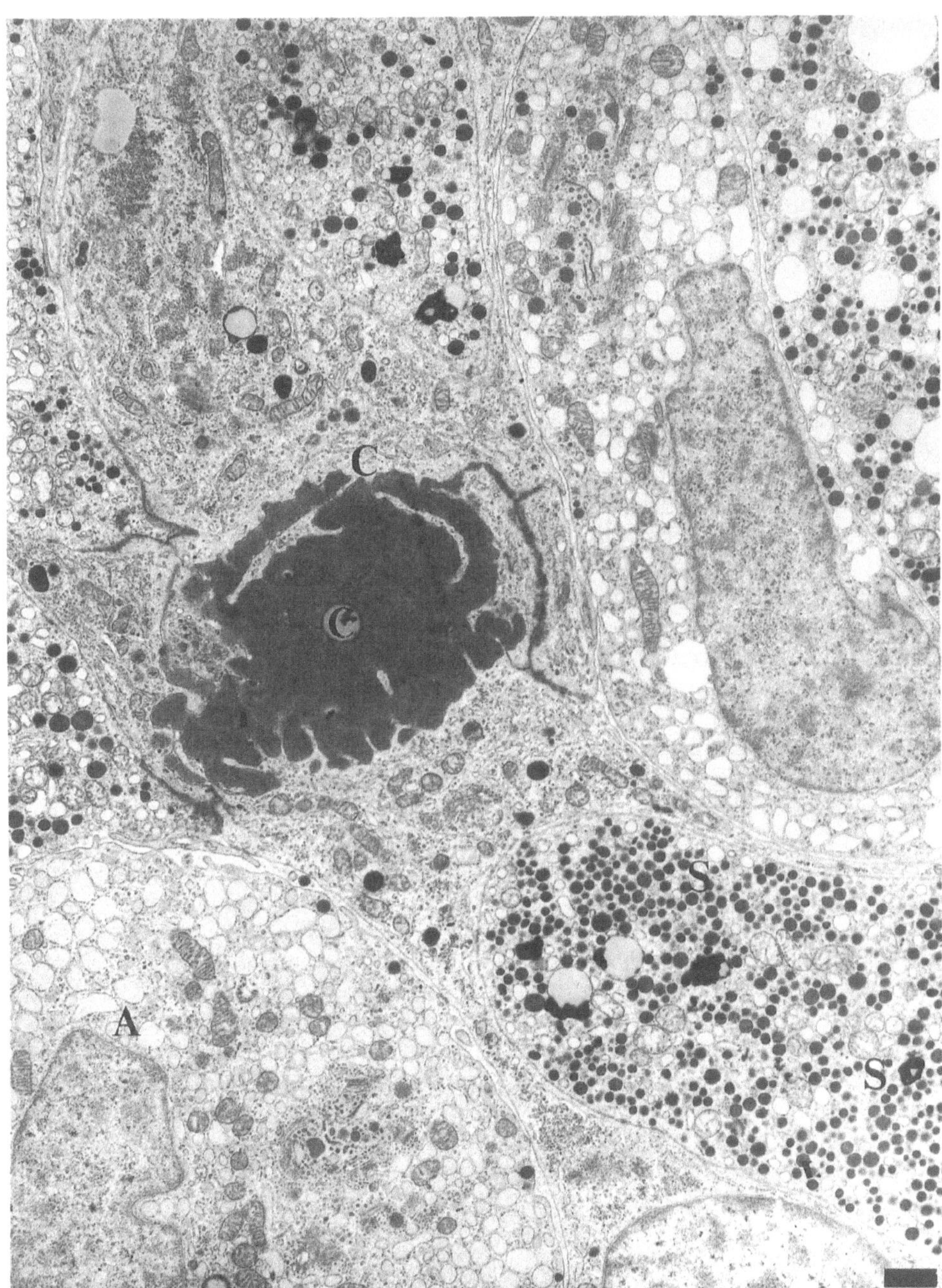

Fig. 7. Pars distalis from a dog. Acidophils in the storage (*S*) phase of the secretory cycle have numerous secretory granules and acidophils in the actively synthesizing (*A*) phase have an expanded cytoplasmic area with distended cisternae of endoplasmic reticulum (*E*) and a prominent Golgi apparatus (*A*). The acidophils are supported by the cytoplasmic processes (*arrows*) of follicular cells that surround the extracellular accumulations of colloid (*C*). *Bar*, 1 µm. (From Capen and Koestner (1967))

Functional Cytology of Adenohypophysis

A specific population of endocrine cells are present in the pars distalis (and in the pars intermedia for ACTH in the dog) that synthesize and secrete each of the pituitary tropic hormones (Ricci and Russolo 1973). Secretory cells in the adenohypophysis have been subdivided into acidophils, basophils, and chromophobes based on interaction of their secretory granules with pH-dependent histochemical stains; however, immunocytochemical staining has largely replaced histochemistry in the evaluation of changes in secretory cells of the adenohypophysis.

Acidophils are further subdivided functionally into somatotrophs and luteotrophs that secrete growth hormone (GH, somatotropin; Wilhelmi 1968) and luteotropic hormone (LTH, prolactin; Papkoff 1976), respectively. Their granules are simple proteins that stain with orange G, azocarmine or erythrosin. Basophils include both gonadotrophs that secrete luteinizing hormone (LH) and follicle stimulating hormone (FSH; El Etreby and Fath El Bab 1978b) and thyrotrophs that secrete thyrotropic hormone (TSH; El Etreby and Fath El Bab 1978c). Secretory granules of basophils are glycoproteins that react with the periodic acid-Schiff's reagent. Chromophobes are pituitary cells that do not have obvious cytoplasmic secretory granules seen with light microscopy. They include the endocrine cells concerned with the synthesis of ACTH and melanocyte-stimulating hormone (MSH), nonsecretory follicular (stellate) cells, degranulated chromophils in the actively synthesizing phase of the secretory cycle (Fig. 8), and undifferentiated stem cells of the adenohypophysis.

Immunocytochemical staining of the adenohypophysis has demonstrated that ACTH- and MSH-staining cells (antisera to porcine ACTH, synthetic $ACTH^{\beta(1-24)}$ and $ACTH^{\beta(17-39)}$, and bovine MSH^{β}) are polyhedral to round, sparsely granulated, and most numerous in the ventrocentral and cranial portions of the pars distalis, where they occur in large groups in dogs (El Etreby and Dubois 1980). They are less frequent in the dorsal and caudal regions of the pars distalis and throughout the pars tuberalis. In the pars intermedia of dogs most cells demonstrate immunoreactivity to either porcine ACTH, MSH^{α} or MSH^{β}. Thyrotrophs are large polyhedral cells situated singly or in small groups ventrocentrally in the paramedian plane of the pars distalis (El Etreby and Fath El Bab 1978c). Gonadotrophs (cells reacting with antisera to human FSH^{β} and/or bovine LHβ) are oval to polyhedral and distributed singly in the pars distalis, particularly in the dorsocranial region and in caudal extensions along the pars intermedia (El Etreby and Fath El Bab 1978b).

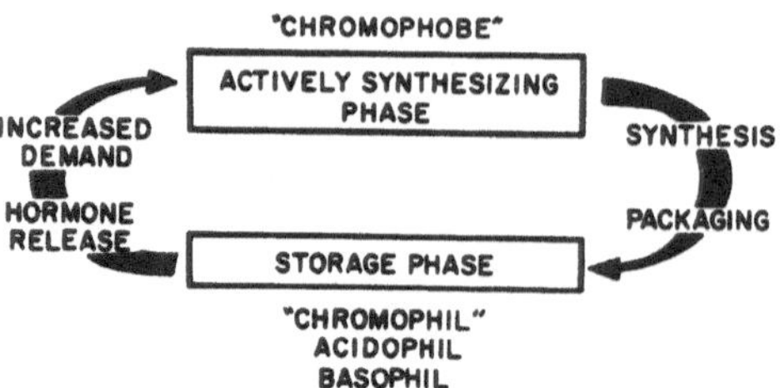

Fig. 8. Secretory cycle of endocrine cells in the adenohypophyisis. During the actively synthesizing phase all pituitary cells are "chromophobic," since their cytoplasm contains abundant endoplasmic reticulum and Golgi apparatus, but few secretory granules. When the cell enters the storage phase, the accumulation of hormone-containing secretory granules permits the cells to be subdivided into acidophils, basophils, or "chromophobes," based upon their reaction with specific pH-dependent stains

Immunoreactive prolactin cells occur in small groups of large polygonal cells with prominent granules in the ventrocentral and cranial portions of the canine pars distalis (El Etreby and Fath El Bab 1977). A diffuse increase in this population of cells occurs in females near parturition (El Etreby et al. 1980). GH-secreting cells are present singly along capillaries in the dorsal region of the pars distalis near the pars intermedia (El Etreby and Fath El Bab 1977). They are small, round to oval, and have fine cytoplasmic granules. Somatotrophs frequently undergo diffuse hyperplasia and hypertrophy in old dogs, especially females with mammary dysplasia or neoplasia (El Etreby et al. 1980).

Hypothalamic Control of the Adenohypophysis

Each population of endocrine cells in the adenohypophysis is under the control of a corresponding releasing hormone ("factor") from the hypothalamus (Fig. 9). These releasing hormones are small peptides synthesized via neurosecretion by neurons in the hypothalamus (Schally 1978). They are transported by axonal processes to the median eminence where they are released into capillaries and conveyed by the hypophyseal

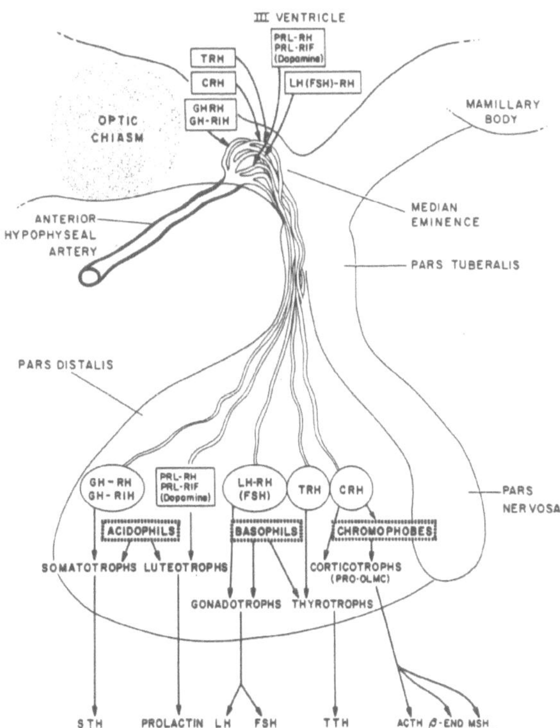

Fig. 9. Control of tropic hormone secretion from the adenohypophysis by hypothalamic releasing hormones (*RH*) and release-in-hibiting hormones (*RIH*). The releasing and release-inhibiting hormones are synthesized by neurons in the hypothalamus, transported by axonal processes, and released into a capillary plexus in the median eminence. They are transported to the adenohypophysis by the hypothalamic-hypophyseal portal system where they interact with specific populations of tropic hormone-secreting cells to govern the rate of of release of preformed hormones, such as somatotropin (*GH*, *STH*), Prolactin (*LTH*), luteinizing hormone (*LH*), follicle-stimulating hormone (*FSH*), thyrotropin (*TTH*), adrenocorticotropin (*ACTH*), and melanocyte-stimulating hormone (*MSH*). *P-RH*, Prolactin-releasing hormone; *T-RH*, Thyrotropin-releasing hormone; *C-RH*, Corticotrophic-releasing hormone. Negative feedback control is effected by the blood concentration of the secretory product of the target endocrine organ (thyroid, adrenal cortex, gonads) acting on the hypothalamus. A release-inhibiting hormone also is produced for the homeostatic control of those pituitary hormones (MSH, prolactin, and growth hormone) that do not act on a target endocrine organ

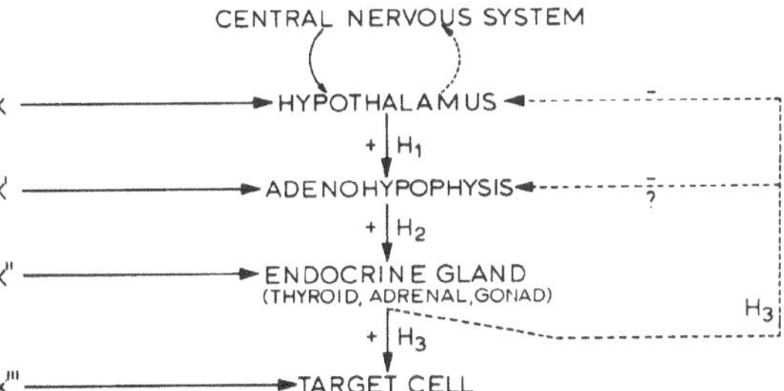

Fig. 10. Highest order of endocrine control involving interrelationship with the central nervous system. Receptors in the brain detect changes in the internal or external environment and convey this information through neural impulses to neurosecretory neurons in the hypothalamus. Releasing hormones (H_1) produced in response to the neural input stimulate the rapid release of corresponding tropic hormone (H_2) from the adenohypophysis. Tropic hormones influence the rates of existing reactions in the corresponding endocrine gland (thyroid, adrenal cortex, gonads) and increase the secretion of their hormone (H_3), which is carried by the blood stream to specific target cells to elicit a biologic response. Negative feedback control is effected by the blood concentration of the final endocrine product (H_3), primarily on cells in the hypothalamus. Local autoregulatory mechanisms (X) influence the functional activity of each component of the endocrine control system

portal system to specific endocrine cells in the adenohypophysis, where each stimulates the rapid release of a specific preformed tropic hormone. There appear to be seven different hypothalamic releasing hormones that regulate the rate of secretion of each tropic hormone secreted by the adenohypophysis. For most pituitary tropic hormones, negative feedback control is accomplished by the blood concentration of the hormone produced by the target endocrine gland, e.g., thyroid gland, adrenal cortex, ovary, or testis (Fig. 10). The hormone produced by the endocrine glands exerts negative feedback control primarily on the neurosecretory neurons in the hypothalamus that synthesize the corresponding releasing hormone. However, GH, LTH, and MSH do not act on target endocrine organs to stimulate secretion of a hormone. Negative feedback control of these three pituitary hormones is effected by production of a corresponding release-inhibiting hormone ("factor") by neurons in the hypothalamus. The relative local concentrations of the specific releasing hormone and release-inhibiting hormone appear to govern the rate of release of GH, prolactin (dopamine) and MSH from the adenohypophysis.

Structure and Function of the Neurohypophysis

The neurohypophysis has three anatomic subdivisions. The pars nervosa (posterior lobe) represents the distal component of the neurohypophyseal system. It is composed of numerous capillaries that are supported by modified glial cells (pituicytes). The capillaries in the pars nervosa are termination sites for the nonmyelinated axonal processes of neurosecretory neurons in the hypothalamus. Secretion granules that contain the neurohypophyseal hormones, i.e., oxytocin and antidiuretic hormone, are synthesized in hypothalamic neurons but are released into the bloodstream in the pars nervosa. The infundibular stalk joins the pars nervosa to the overlying hypothalamus and is composed of axonal processes from neurosecretory neurons.

Neurosecretory neurons in the hypothalamus receive neural input from higher centers and translate this into endocrine output in the form of hormonal secretion. In addition to the usual structural features of neurons, they contain prominent lamellar arrays of rough endoplasmic reticulum, large Golgi apparatuses, and numerous membrane-limited neurosecretory granules in the cell body and axonal process (Fig. 11).

The neurosecretory neurons concerned with hormone synthesis are segregated into anatomically defined regions, termed nuclei, in the hypothalamus. The supraoptic nucleus is concerned primarily with the synthesis of antidiuretic hormone, whereas oxytocin is produced predominantly by neurons in the paraventricular nucleus.

Hormones of Neurohypophysis

Antidiuretic hormone (ADH; vasopressin) and oxytocin are nonapeptides synthesized by neurons situated either in the supraoptic or paraventricular nuclei of the hypothalamus. ADH and its corresponding neurophysin appear to be synthesized as part of a common larger biosynthetic precursor molecule, termed pro-pressophysin. The hormones are packaged into membrane-limited neurosecretory granules with a corresponding binding protein (i.e., neurophysin) and transported to the para nervosa by axonal processes of the neurosecretory neurons (Fig. 11). These axons terminate on fenestrated capillaries in the pars nervosa and release ADH or oxytocin into the circulation.

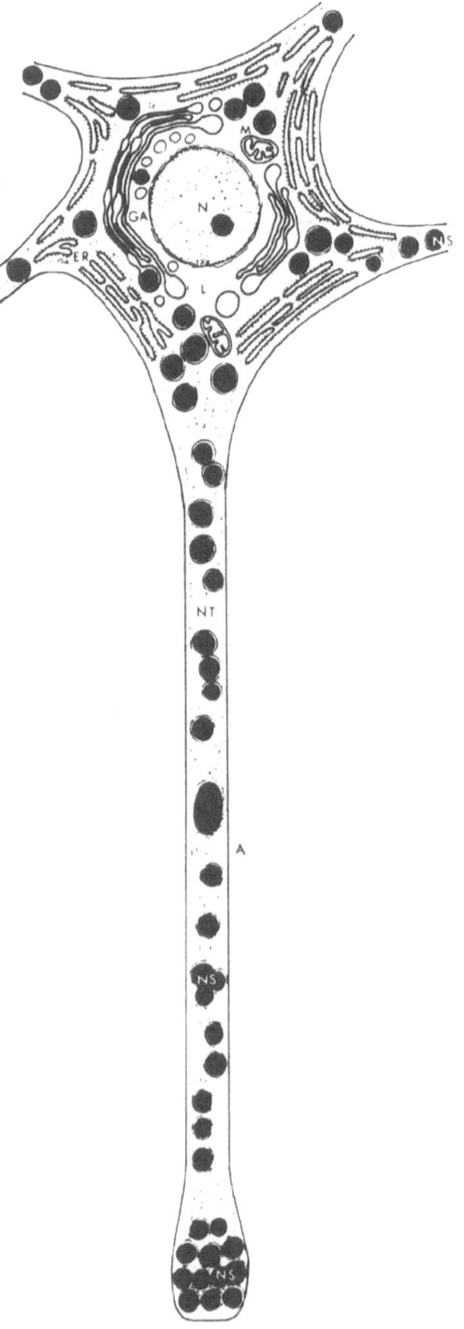

Fig. 11. Structural characteristics of a neurosecretory neuron in the hypothalamus. The nerve cell body (*N*, nucleus) has dendritic and axonal (*A*) processes with arrays of rough endoplasmic reticulum (*ER*), a prominent Golgi apparatus (*GA*), and large mitochondria (*M*). Hormone-containing, membranelimited neurosecretory granules (*NS*) are formed in the Golgi apparatus and transported along the axon to the site of release at the axon's termination on capillaries. Neurosecretory neurons synthesize the releasing and release-inhibiting hormones of the adenohypophysis and the hormones of the neurohypophysis (oxytocin, antidiuretic hormone). *NT*, Neurotubules

Blood Supply to Pituitary Gland

The neurohypophysis in most animals is supplied directly by the posterior (inferior) hypophyseal arteries that branch from the internal carotid arteries (Fig. 12). Branches of the anterior (superior) hypophyseal arteries originate from the internal carotid arteries and from the posterior communicating arteries of the cricle of Willis. Arteriolar branches penetrate the pars tuberalis, lose their muscular coat, and form a capillary plexus near the median eminence. These vessels subsequently drain into hypophyseal portal veins that supply the pars distalis. A small artery that arises from the posterior hypophyseal artery may provide a minor blood supply to the adenohypophysis (Fig. 12).

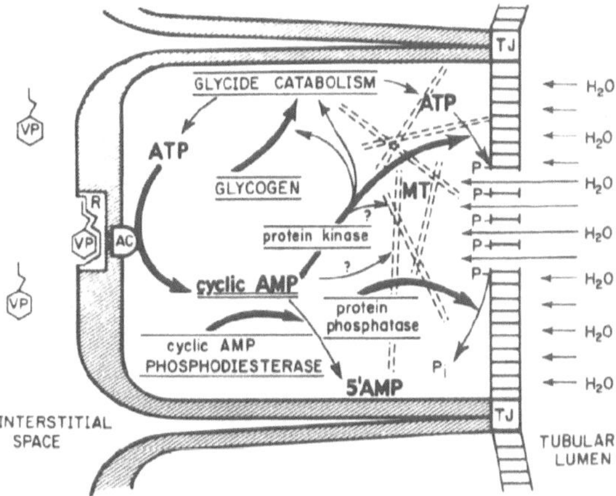

Fig. 13. Subcellular mechanism of action of antidiuretic hormone (vasopressin) in the kidney. The hormone (*VP*) binds to isoreceptors on target cells of collecting ducts and activates adenylate cyclase (*AC*) in the plasma membrane on the basilar aspect of the cell. The intracellular accumulation of cyclic adenosine monophosphate (*AMP*) activates protein kinases which phosphorylate proteins in the luminal plasma membrane that increases the permeability of the tubular cell to water. *TJ*, tight junction; *P*, proteins; *MT*, microtubules; *R*, receptor. (From Dousa 1974)

Mechanism of Action of Antidiuretic Hormone

ADH is transported by the bloodstream to its site of action in the kidney, where it binds to specific receptors on epithelial cells in the distal part of the nephron and collecting ducts. The overall effect of ADH on the kidney is to increase the active renal tubular reabsorption of water from the glomerular filtrate. The hormone (ADH)-receptor complex activates the membrane-bound enzyme, adenylate cyclase, resulting in the intracellular formation of cAMP from ATP (Dousa 1974; Fig. 13). The intracellular accumulation of cAMP appears to activate protein kinases involved in the phosphorylation of proteins in the luminal membrane of distal tubular cells that increase their permeability to water.

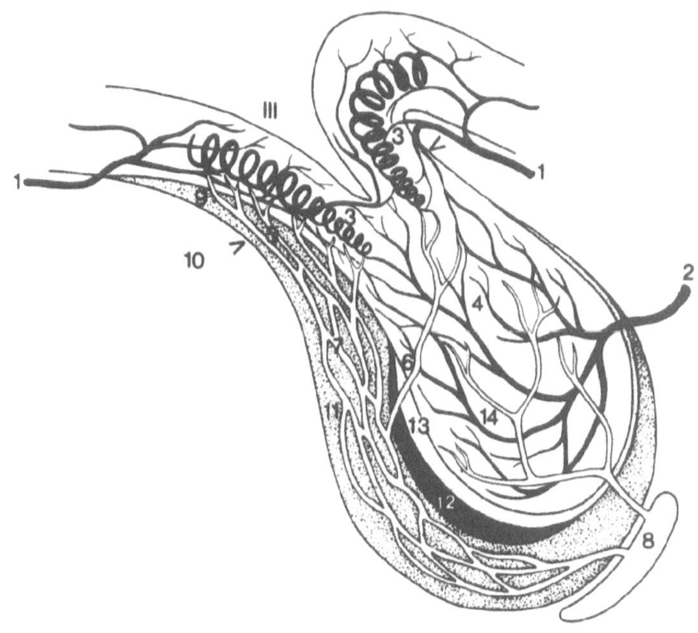

Fig. 12. Diagramatic representation of the pituitary gland and its vascular supply. *1*, superior hypophyseal artery; *2*, inferior hypophyseal artery, *3*, primary plexus of the infundibular stem; *4*, primary plexus of the infundibular process; *5*, long portal vessels; *6*, short portal vessels; *7*, secondary plexus in the adenohypophysis; *8*, collecting vein; *9*, pars tuberalis (infundibularis) of the adenohypophysis; *10*, pituitary stalk; *11*, pars distalis; *12*, residual hypophyseal lumen (intraglandular cleft); *13*, pars intermedia; *14*, infundibular process of the neurohypophysis; *III*, infundibular recess of the third ventricle. (From Meijer 1980)

Comparative Pathology of the Adenohypophysis

Introduction

The histopathological differentiation between nodular hyperplasia, adenoma, and carcinoma is often more difficult in endocrine glands such as the pituitary than in most other organs of the body. However, criteria for their differentiation should be established and applied in a uniform manner in the evaluation of proliferative lesions in endocrine glands. For many endocrine glands (especially specific trophic hormone-secreting cells of the adenohypophysis) there appears to be a continuous spectrum of proliferative lesions between diffuse or focal hyperplasia and adenomas derived from a specific population of secretory cells.

It appears to be a common feature of endocrine glands that prolonged stimulation of a population of secretory cells predisposes to the subsequent development of a higher than expected incidence of tumors. Long-term stimulation may lead to the development of clones of cells within the hyperplastic endocrine glands that grow more rapidly than the rest and are more susceptible to neoplastic transformation when exposed to the right combination of promoting carcinogens.

Focal ("nodular") hyperplasia usually appears as multiple small areas in one or both (for paired) endocrine gland(s) that are well-demarcated but not encapsulated from adjacent normal cells. Cells making up an area of focal hyperplasia closely resemble the cells of origin; however, the cytoplasmic area may be slightly enlarged and the nucleus more hyperchromatic than in the normal endocrine cell.

Adenomas are usually solitary nodules in one endocrine gland (or occasionally in both for paired endocrine glands) that are larger than the multiple areas of focal hyperplasia. They are sharply demarcated from the adjacent normal glandular parenchyma, and there is often a thin, partial to complete, fibrous capsule. The adjacent parenchyma is compressed to varying degrees depending on the size of the adenoma. Cells composing an adenoma may closely resemble the cells of origin morphologically and in their architectural pattern of arrangement; however, there often are histological differences such as multiple layers of cells lining follicles and vascular trabeculae or solid clusters of secretory cells subdivided into packets by a fine fibrovascular stroma. Carcinomas are usually larger than adenomas of an endocrine gland, such as the pituitary, and result in a macroscopically detectable enlargement. The differentiation between adenoma and carcinoma of an endocrine gland is often more difficult than in other tissues of the body using only morphological criteria. Histopathological features that are suggestive of malignancy include intraglandular invasion, invasion into and through the capsule of the gland with establishment of secondary foci of growth in the periglandular fibrous and adipose connective tissues, formation of tumor cell thrombi within vessels (especially muscular walled), and particularly the establishment of metastases at distant sites. The spread of neoplastic endocrine cells subendothelially in highly vascular benign tumors should not be mistaken for vascular invasion. Malignant endocrine cells are often more pleomorphic (including oval or spindle shaped) than normal, but nuclear pleomorphism is not a consistent criterion to distinguish adenoma from carcinoma. Mitotic figures may be frequent in malignant cells, but the significance of this criterion can vary considerably with the degree of background stimulation of the endocrine gland.

Many neoplasms derived from endocrine glands such as the pituitary are functionally active, secrete an excessive amount of hormone either continuously or episodically, and result in dramatic clinical syndromes of hormone excess. Quantitation of hormone levels in serum of plasma in the basal or stimulated state and/or the measurement of hormonal metabolites in the urine over a 24-h period of excretion is essential to confirm that an endocrine tumor is functional and releasing hormone at an abnormally elevated rate. Morphologically, an endocrine tumor can often be interpreted as endocrinologically active if the rim of normal tissue around the tumor undergoes trophic atrophy due to negative feedback inhibition by the elevated hormone levels or an altered blood constituent. In response to the autonomous secretion of hormone by the tumor these nonneoplastic secretory cells, especially the cytoplasmic area, become smaller than normal, and eventually the number of cells is decreased. Functional pituitary neoplasms secreting an excess of a particular trophic hormone (e.g., ACTH) are associated with striking hypertrophy and hyperplasia of target cells in the adrenal cortex (e.g., zonae fasciculata and reticularis) or follicular cells in the thyroid glands.

Hypophyseal Changes Associated with Alterations in Target Organs

In response to surgical removal or disease processes in a target endocrine organ of the pituitary, e.g., thyroid gland, adrenal cortex, or gonads, there is a progressive decline in the circulating concentration of hormone produced by the target organ. This reduction in circulating hormone level is detected by the hypothalamic-adenohypophyseal axis and results in structural changes in the specific tropic-hormone-secreting cell population in the pars distalis.

The initial reaction is a rapid release of storage granules containing preformed tropic hormone from one population of endocrine cells in the pars distalis. For example, only thyrotropic basophils degranulate following thyroidectomy or thyroid disease, corticotropic chromophobes degranulate after adrenalectomy, and gonadotropic basophils release their secretory granules in response to gonadectomy. After an interval of several days following surgical ablation or extensive destruction of a target endocrine organ, the corresponding degranulated tropic-hormone-secreting cell in the pars distalis undergoes hypertrophy with expansion of the cytoplasm in response to the sustained increased demand for the particular tropic hormone. The abundant cytoplasm contains extensive organelles concerned with hormonal synthesis (rough endoplasmic reticulum) and packaging into secretory granules (Golgi apparatus) plus large mitochondria.

If the demand for tropic hormone secretion is sustained for days or weeks, one specific population of endocrine cells in the pars distalis undergoes hyperplasia. Small groups of hyperplastic tropic hormone-secreting cells are present, scattered throughout an otherwise normal pars distalis. In response to long-term (weeks to months) stimulation, the hypertrophied cytoplasm of the cells becomes vacuolated due to the extensive distention of profiles of rough endoplasmic reticulum with a finely granular, moderately electron-dense material. Subsequently, the multiple small cytoplasmic vacuoles coalesce to form a large vacuole that may displace the nucleus eccentrically, characteristic of cells in the pituitary gland which degranulate following thyroidectomy, adrenalectomy, or gonadectomy.

Endocrinologically Inactive Chromophobe Adenoma Arising in the Pars Distalis

Nonfunctional pituitary tumors occur frequently in laboratory rodents, dogs, cats, and horses but are uncommon in other species (Capen 1978). Although chromphobe adenomas appear to be endocrinologically inactive, they may result in significant functional disturbances and clinical signs by virtue of compression atrophy of adjacent portions of the pituitary gland and dorsal extension into the overlying brain.

Nonfunctional pituitary adenomas often result in clinical disturbances related to lack of secretion of pituitary tropic hormones and diminished target organ function, or dysfunction of the central nervous system (Capen 1978; Gilbert and Willey 1969; Farrow 1969). Affected animals often are depressed, have incoordination and other disturbances of balance, are weak, and may collapse with exercise. In long-standing cases there may be evidence of blindness with dilated and fixed pupils due to compression and disruption of optic nerves by dorsal extension of the pituitary tumor (Fig. 14). Affected animals may undergo progressive loss of weight ("pituitary cachexia") with muscle atrophy due to a lack of the protein anabolic effects of growth hormone. Compression of the cells that secrete gonadotropic hormones or the corresponding releasing hormones results in atrophy of the gonads. The affected animals appear dehydrated, as evidenced by a lusterless, dry coat, and they consume increased amounts of water.

Clinical signs associated with nonfunctional pituitary adenomas and hypopituitarism are not highly specific and could be confused with other disorders of the central nervous system such as brain tumors and encephalitis, or with chronic renal disease. Hypopituitarism caused by pituitary tumors should be included in the differential diagnosis of diseases characterized by incoordination, depression, polyuria, blindness, and a sudden change in personality in adult or old animals. Because the blindness is central in origin, ophthalmoscopic examination usually fails to reveal significant lesions. There is no effect on body stature associated with compression of the pars distalis and

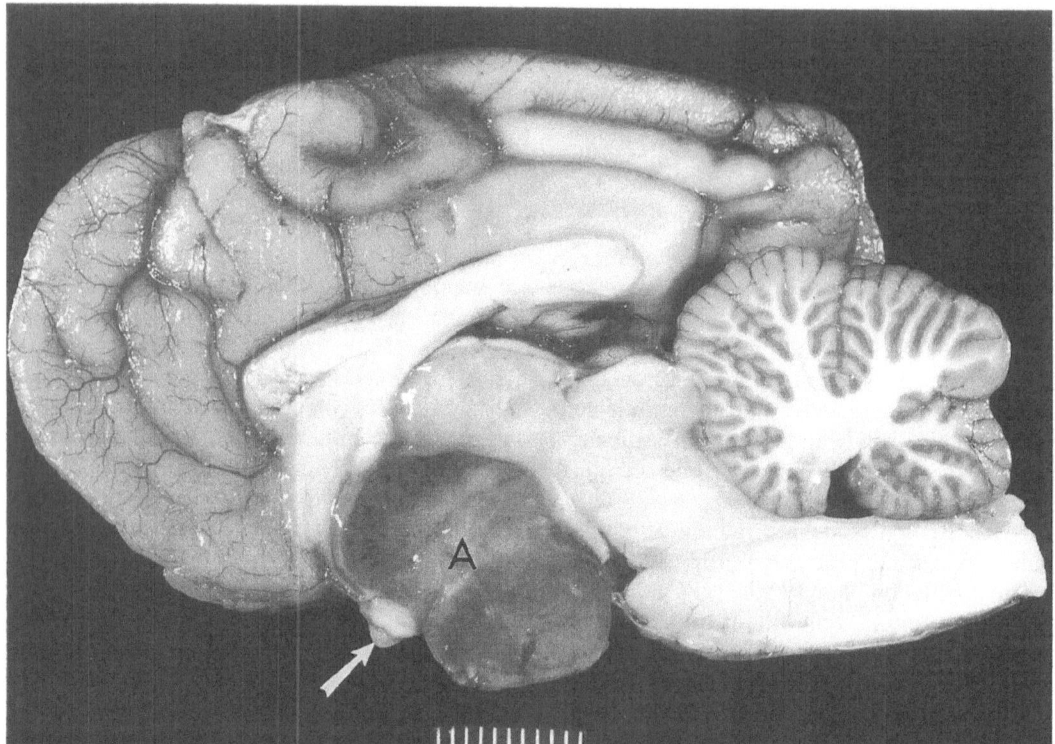

Fig. 14. Large pituitary adenoma (*A*) in a dog, extending dorsally out of the sella turcica into the overlying brain. The optic chiasm (*white arrow*) is severely compressed by the large adenoma. The adenohypophysis, neurohypophysis, and hypothalamus are incorporated and destroyed by the neoplasm, resulting in clinical disturbances of panhypopituitarism and diabetes insipidus. The scale at the bottom represents 1 cm

interference with growth hormone secretion, because these neoplasm usually arise in adult animals that have already completed their growth. However, the atrophy of the skin and loss of muscle mass may be related to a lack of the protein anabolic effects of growth hormone. Interference in the secretion of pituitary tropic hormones often leads to gonadal atrophy, resulting in either decreased libido or anestrus, reduced basal metabolic rate due to diminished thyrotropin secretion, and hypoglycemia from tropic atrophy of the adrenal cortex.

Endocrinologically inactive pituitary adenomas often attain considerable size before they cause obvious signs or kill the animal (Fig. 14). The proliferating tumor cells incorporate the remaining structures of the adenohypophysis and infundibular stalk. The neoplasms attach firmly to the base of the sella turcica, but cause no erosion of the sphenoid bone. The incomplete diaphragma sella permits dorsal growth of the adenoma along lines of least resistance. The entire hypothalamus may become compressed and replaced by the tumor.

The adrenal glands in animals with large nonfunctional pituitary adenomas are small and consist primarily of medullary tissue surrounded by a narrow zone of cortex (Fig. 15). The adrenal cortex appears as a thin yellow-brown rim composed of a moderately thickened capsule and secretory cells of the outer zona glomerulosa, which are not predominantly under the control of ACTH. The zonae fasciculata and reticularis are severely atrophied compared with these zones in normal adrenal glands. Thyroid glands in animals with large pituitary adenomas are often smaller than normal, though atrophied to a much lesser degree than the adrenal cortex (Fig. 15). The majority of the atrophic thyroid follicles are large, lined by a flattened cuboidal epithelium, and have few endocytotic vacuoles near the interface between the colloid and luminal aspect of the follicular cells. The thyroid lesion is due to lack of TSH-induced endocytosis of colloid. Seminiferous

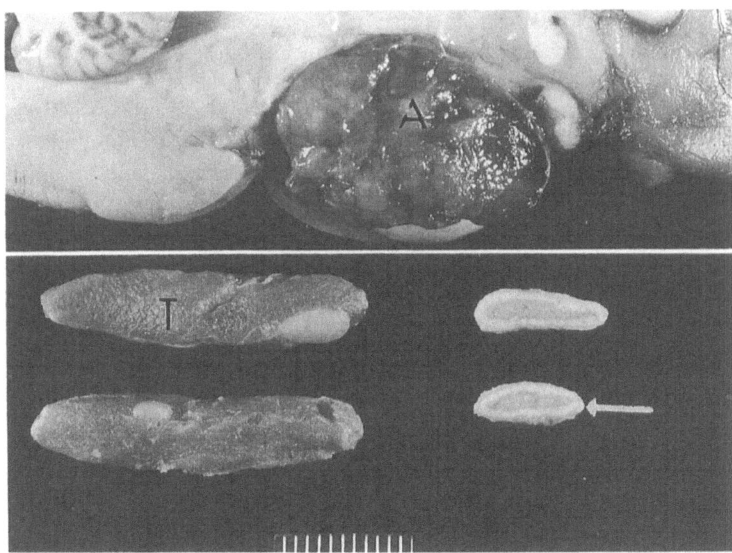

Fig. 15. Large, endocrinologically inactive, chromophobe adenoma (*A*) from a dog with extension into the hypothalamus. There is severe tropic atrophy and reduction in size of the adrenal glands (*white arrow*) due to loss of cells in the zonae fasciculata and reticularis from the subnormal secretion of ACTH. The thyroid glands (*T*) are approximately normal in size due to the distension of follicles with colloid in the absence of thyrotropin secretion. The scale at the bottom represents 1 cm

tubules of the testes are small and show little evidence of active spermatogenesis; this is due to interference with gonadotropin (GTH) secretion. The cells comprising nonfunctional pituitary adenomas are cuboidal to polyhedral and either arranged in diffuse sheets or subdivided into small packets by fine connective tissue septa. Special histochemical techniques for pituitary cytology fail to demonstrate specific secretory granules within the cytoplasm of tumor cells. The histogenesis of nonfunctional chromphobe adenomas is often difficult to define precisely, but they appear to be derived from pituitary cells that are unable to either store or secrete an excess of a specific hypophyseal tropic hormone.

Endocrinologically Active Corticotroph (ACTH-Secreting) Adenoma of the Adenohypophysis Associated with Hypercortisolism (Cushing-like Disease)

Functional tumors arising in the pituitary gland may derive from corticotroph (ACTH-secreting) cells in either the pars distalis or the pars intermedia. They cause a clinical syndrome of cortisol excess (similar to Cushing's disease). These neoplasms are encountered most frequently in dogs and infrequently in other animal species. They develop in adult to aged dogs and have been reported in a number of breeds (Capen et al. 1967; Clarkson et al. 1959; Coffin and Munson 1953; Hare 1935; Rijnberk et al. 1967, 1969; White 1938; Meijer 1980); boxers, Boston terriers, and dachshunds appear to have a higher incidence of functional (ACTH-secreting) pituitary tumors than other breeds. The spectrum of dramatic clinical manifestations and lesions that develop is primarily the result of long-term overproduction of cortisol by hyperplastic adrenal cortices (Capen and Martin 1975; Capen et al. 1967; Lubberink et al. 1971; Siegel et al. 1970). These changes are the result of the combined gluconeogenic, lipolytic, protein catabolic, and anti-inflammatory actions of glucocorticoid hormones on many organ systems of the body.

Peterson et al. (1982) reported that 84% of dogs with pituitary-dependent hyperadrenocorticism had adenomas derived from cells either of the pars distalis or pars intermedia. Immunocytochemical staining of the tumor cells gave a positive reaction for ACTH, β-lipotrophin, and β-endorphin (β-END). Low doses of dexamethasone (15 μg/kg) suppressed ACTH production and subsequently plasma cortisol levels in normal dogs but did not suppress dogs with pituitary-dependent hyperadrenocorticism or adrenal cortical neoplasms. High doses of dexamethasone (1.0 mg/kg) usually suppressed plasma cortisol levels in dogs with pituitary-dependent hyperadrenocorticism but not significantly in dogs with adrenal cortical neoplasms (Peterson and Drucker 1981).

Radioimmunoassays for plasma ACTH in the dog have demonstrated a mean concentration of 46 pg/ml (range 17–98 pg/ml; Feldman et al. 1977). Assays for plasma ACTH are useful in differentiating pituitary-dependent from other causes of adrenal cortical hyperplasia and the syndrome of cortisol excess. Dogs with functional adrenal cortical neoplasms have plasma ACTH concentrations two standard deviations or more below (<20 pg/ml) the mean value for normal dogs, whereas dogs with pituitary-dependent hyperadrenocorticism have plasma ACTH values higher than 40 pg/ml (Feldman 1981, 1983). The differentiation between pituitary- and adrenal-dependent hyperadrenocorticism by laboratory methods has been reviewed by Peterson (1984b).

The pituitary gland is consistently enlarged in animals with corticotroph adenomas (Fig. 16). Neither the occurrence nor the severity of functional disturbances appears to be directly related to the size of the neoplasm. Small adenomas are as likely to be endocrinologically active as are larger neoplasms. The larger adenomas are often firmly attached to the base of the sella turcica without evidence of erosion of the sphenoid bone. In the animal species most likely to develop pituitary neoplasms the diaphragma sella is incomplete. Therefore, the line of least resistance favors dorsal expansion of the gradually enlarging pituitary mass and invagination into the infundibular cavity, dilation of the infundibular recess and the third ventricle, with eventual compression and replacement of the hypothalamus, and extension of the tumor into the thalamus.

Dorsal expansion of larger corticotroph adenomas results in either a broadbased indentation and compression of the overlying hypothalamus (Fig. 16) or extension into and replacement of the parenchyma of the hypothalamus and occasionally the thalamus. In the larger neoplasms there are often focal areas of hemorrhage, necrosis, mineralization, and liquefaction. In addition, growth of the pituitary tumor along the basilar aspects of the brain may result in incorporation of the second, third, and fourth cranial nerves, leading to functional disturbances from a disruption of their function.

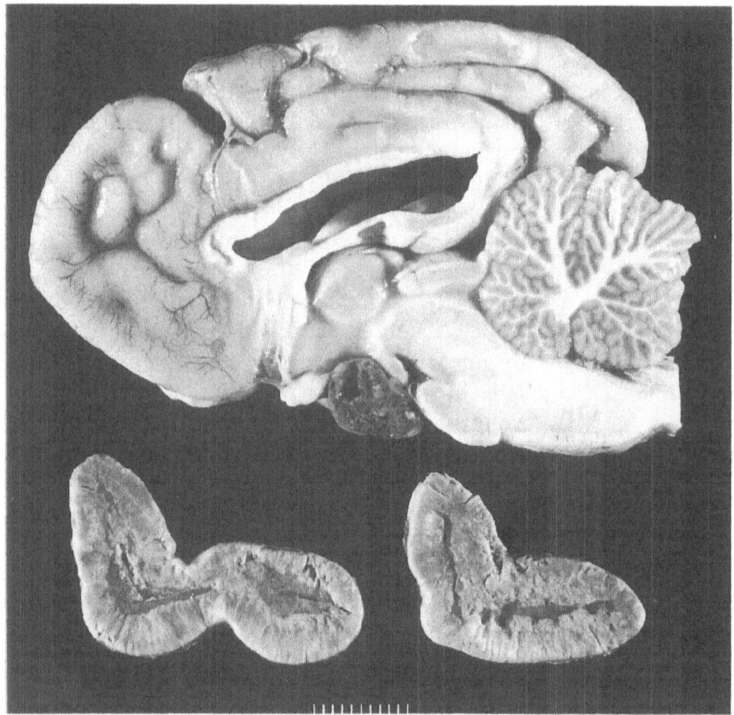

Fig. 16. Corticotropic hormone (ACTH)-secreting (chromophobe) adenoma in the pituitary gland of a dog, with bilateral enlargement of the adrenal glands. The long-term secretion of ACTH resulted in hypertrophy and hyperplasia of secretory cells of the zonae fasciculata and reticularis in the adrenal cortex and in an excessive secretion of cortisol. The scale at the bottom represents 1 cm

Bilateral enlargement of the adrenal glands occurs in dogs with functional corticotroph adenomas (Fig. 16). This enlargement is often striking and is due entirely to increased cortical parenchyma, primarily in the zonae fasciculata and reticularis. Nodules of yellow-orange cortical tissue are often found outside the capsule in the periadrenal fat, as well as extending down into the adrenal medulla. The corticomedullary junction is irregular and the medulla is compressed.

Pituitary corticotroph adenomas are composed of well-differentiated, large or small chromophobic cells supported by fine connective tissue septa. They can be subclassified into sinusoidal and diffuse types on the basis of the predominant pattern of cellular architecture. The cytoplasm of the tumor cells is devoid of secretory granules detectable by specific histochemical procedures used for pituitary cytology. However, pituitary corticotroph adenomas arising in both the pars distalis and the pars intermedia associated with the syndrome of cortisol excess are composed of polyhedral cells that immunocytochemically stain selectively for ACTH and MSH (El Etreby et al. 1980). Nodules of focal hyperplasia and microadenomas, composed of similar ACTH/MSH cells, are also present in both lobes of the adenohypophysis.

Although remnants of the pars distalis can be identified near the periphery of the adenomas, the demarcation between the neoplasm and pars distalis is not distinct. The pars distalis is either partly replaced by the neoplasm or severely compressed. The pars nervosa and infundibular stalk are either infiltrated and disrupted by tumor cells or completely incorporated within the larger neoplasms.

Cells comprising functional corticotroph adenomas have definite ultrastructural evidence of secretory activity (Capen and Koestner 1967). Organelles concerned with protein synthesis (endoplasmic reticulum) and packaging of secretory products (Golgi apparatus) are well developed in tumor cells. Hormone-containing secretory granules can be demonstrated by electron microscopy in cells comprising functional corticotroph adenomas (Fig. 17). This is in contrast to the absence of demonstrable secretory granules within neoplastic cells observed with light microscopy following application of special histochemical procedures. The granules vary in number from cell to cell, are roughly spherical, and are surrounded by a delicate limiting membrane. They are small (mean diameter, 170 µm), electrondense, and have a prominent submembranous space.

Adenoma of the Pars Intermedia

Adenomas derived from cells of the pars intermedia are the most common type of pituitary tumor in horses, the second most common type in dogs, infrequent in certain strains of laboratory rats and nonhuman primates (Chalifoux et al. 1983), and rare in other species. They develop in older horses, with females affected more frequently than males (Gribble 1972). Nonbrachycephalic breeds of dogs develop adenomas in the pars intermedia more often than brachycephalic breeds (Capen et al. 1967).

Two cell populations have been identified in the pars intermedia of normal dogs by immunocytochemistry (Halmi et al. 1981). The predominant cell type (A-cell) stains strongly for α-MSH as in the pars intermedia of other species. A second cell type (B-cell) in the canine pars intermedia stains intensely for ACTH but not for α-MSH. This second cell population may account for the high bioactive ACTH concentration found in the pars intermedia of dogs (Halmi et al. 1981) and may give rise to corticotroph adenomas of the pars intermedia in dogs having the syndrome of cortisol excess (Capen et al. 1967).

Adenomas of the pars indermedia are either (a) endocrinologically inactive and accompanied by varying degrees of hypopituitarism and diabetes insipidus or (b) associated with the secretion of excessive ACTH leading to bilateral adrenocortical hyperplasia and the syndrome of cortisol excess in dogs (Capen et al. 1967). The clinical signs with functional corticotroph adenomas arising in the pars intermedia are similar to those arising in the pars distalis in dogs, and the neoplastic cells stain immunocytochemically for ACTH and MSH (El Etreby et al. 1980).

Adenomas of the pars intermedia produce only a moderate enlargement of the pituitary gland. The pars distalis can often be identified and is sharply demarcated from the anterior margin of the neoplasm (Fig. 18). The tumor may extend across the residual hypophyseal lumen and cause compression atrophy, but it does not usually invade the parenchyma of the pars distalis. Though the posterior lobe is incorporated within the tumor, the infundibular stalk is intact. Degenerative changes within the neoplasm are minimal.

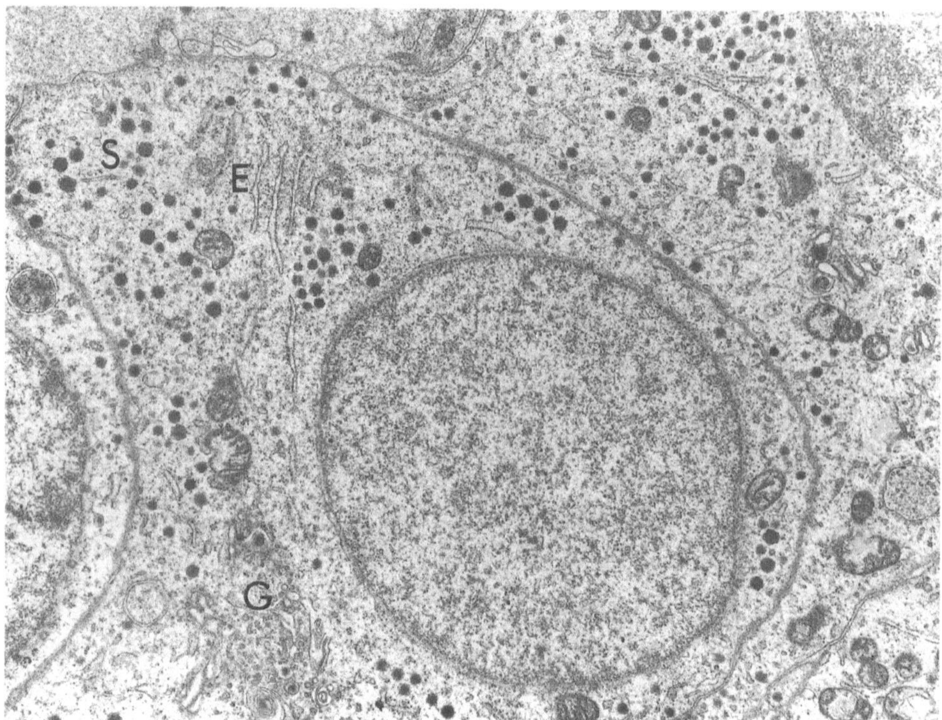

Fig. 17. Electron micrograph illustrating neoplastic cells in a functional corticotroph adenoma in the pituitary gland from a dog with cortisol excess similar to Cushing's disease. Organelles concerned with hormonal synthesis (*E*, endoplasmic reticulum) and packaging (*G*, Golgi apparatus) are well developed. Numerous small (approximately 170 µm) hormonestorage granules (*S*) are present in the cytoplasm, ×10400

Adenomas of the pars intermedia appear to arise from the epithelial lining of the residual hypophyseal lumen covering the infundibular process in dogs. They are relatively small, more strictly localized than chromophobe adenomas arising in the pars distalis, and extend across the residual hypophyseal lumen to compress the pars distalis (Fig. 19). They are sharply demarcated from the pars distalis, usually by in incomplete layer of condensed reticulum; however, they are not encapsulated. The histopathologic appearance of adenomas of the pars intermedia is unique, and strikingly different from adenomas arising in the pars distalis. They are composed of numerous large, colloid-filled follicles interspersed between nests of chromophobic cells of varying size with an eosinophilic cytoplasm. The neoplastic cells compress and frequently invade the pars nervosa and infundibular stalk resulting in disturbances of water metabolism early in the course of development of the tumor (Capen and Koestner 1967).

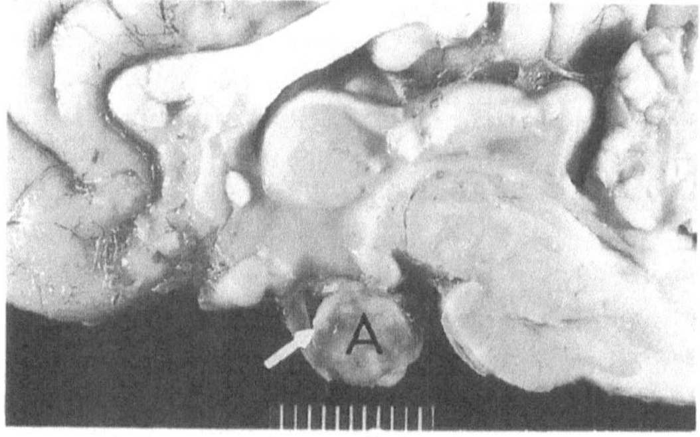

Fig. 18. Adenoma (*A*) derived from corticotrophs in the pars intermedia in a dog with a syndrome of cortisol excess. The tumor is relatively small, sharply demarcated from the compressed pars distalis (*white arrow*), and has only slightly compressed the overlying hypothalamus. The neurohypophysis was incorporated by the adenoma and the dog had evidence of disturbances in water metabolism

Adenomas originating in the pars intermedia are often associated with a unique clinical syndrome in certain species of animals due to extensive hypothalamic involvement. The syndrome associ-

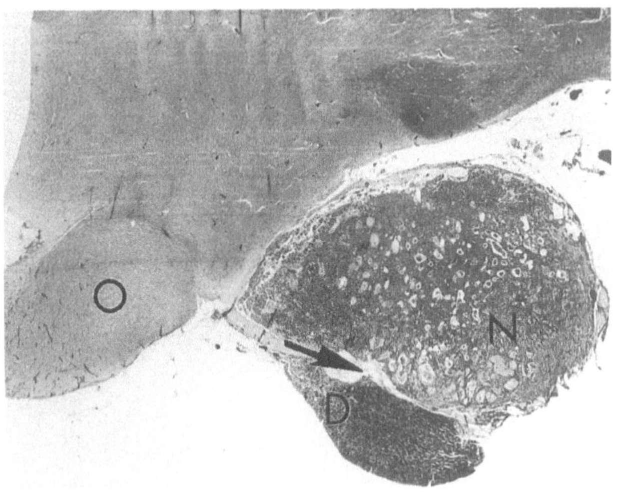

Fig. 19. Adenoma arising in the pars intermedia of the pituitary of a dog. The neoplasm (*N*) is sharply demarcated from the compressed pars distalis (*D*). The *arrow* indicates the residual hypophyseal lumen. There are numerous colloid-filled follicles in terspersed between the large nests of chromophobic cells within the adenoma. O, optic nerve

ated with tumors of the pars intermedia in horses is characterized by polyuria, polydipsia, ravenous appetite, muscle weakness, somnolence, intermittent hyperpyrexia, and generalized hyperhidrosis. Affected horses also develop a striking "hirsutism" because of a failure of the seasonal shedding of hair from disruption of hypothalamic autonomic function (Bäckström 1963; Eriksson et al. 1956; Loeb et al. 1966; Gribble 1972). The hair over most of the trunk and extremities is long (up to 4–5 in.), abnormally thick and wavy, and often matted.

Larger adenomas of the pars intermedia result in the development of persistent hyperglycemia (insulin-resistant) and glycosuria in horses (Loeb et al. 1966). This appears to be the result of disruption of the "satiety center" in the ventromedial aspects of the hypothalamus by the dorsally expanding adenoma (Fig. 20), increased (often ravenous) appetite and intake of food, elevation of the blood glucose concentration, stimulation of insulin secretion, and down-regulation of numbers of insulin receptors on target cells resulting in progressive insulin resistance.

Polyuria, polydipsia, and low urine specific gravity are the result of incorporation of the pars nervosa by the pars intermedia-derived tumor, which thereby interferes with ADH secretion. Larger adenomas extend into the hypothalamus and destroy the supraoptic nucleus, resulting in disruption of ADH synthesis by neurosecretory neurons. The intermittent hyperpyrexia and generalized hyperhidrosis appear to be the result

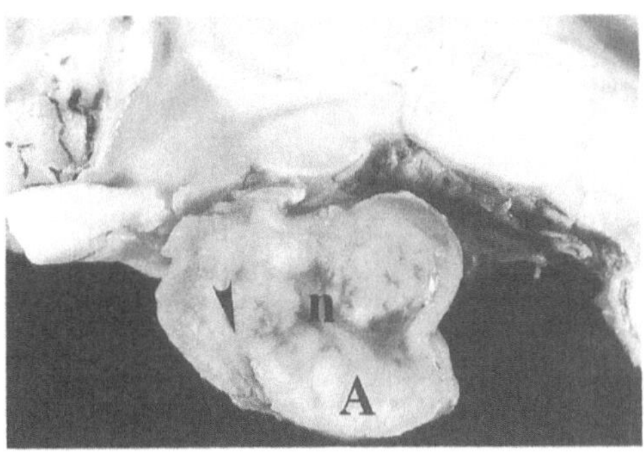

Fig. 20. Adenoma of pars intermedia from a horse. The adenoma (*A*) is sharply demarcated (*arrowhead*) from the compressed pars distalis (*left*) and incorporates the pars nervosa (*n*)

of disruption of homeostatic centers for body temperature regulation in the hypothalamus by the pituitary adenoma.

Electron microscopy of adenomas of the pars intermedia in horses reveals numerous membrane-limited secretory granules in the cytoplasm of tumor cells (Fig. 21). Their mean diameter is approximately 300 nm, and they are surrounded by a closely applied limiting membrane. The rough endoplasmic reticulum and Golgi apparatus are particularly well developed in cells constituting adenomas of the pars intermedia in horses, suggesting that they are synthesizing and packaging considerable amounts of protein (e.g., pro-OLMC) for secretion (Fig. 21). Mitotic figures are uncommon. The compressed remnant of pars distalis is atrophic but contains granulated

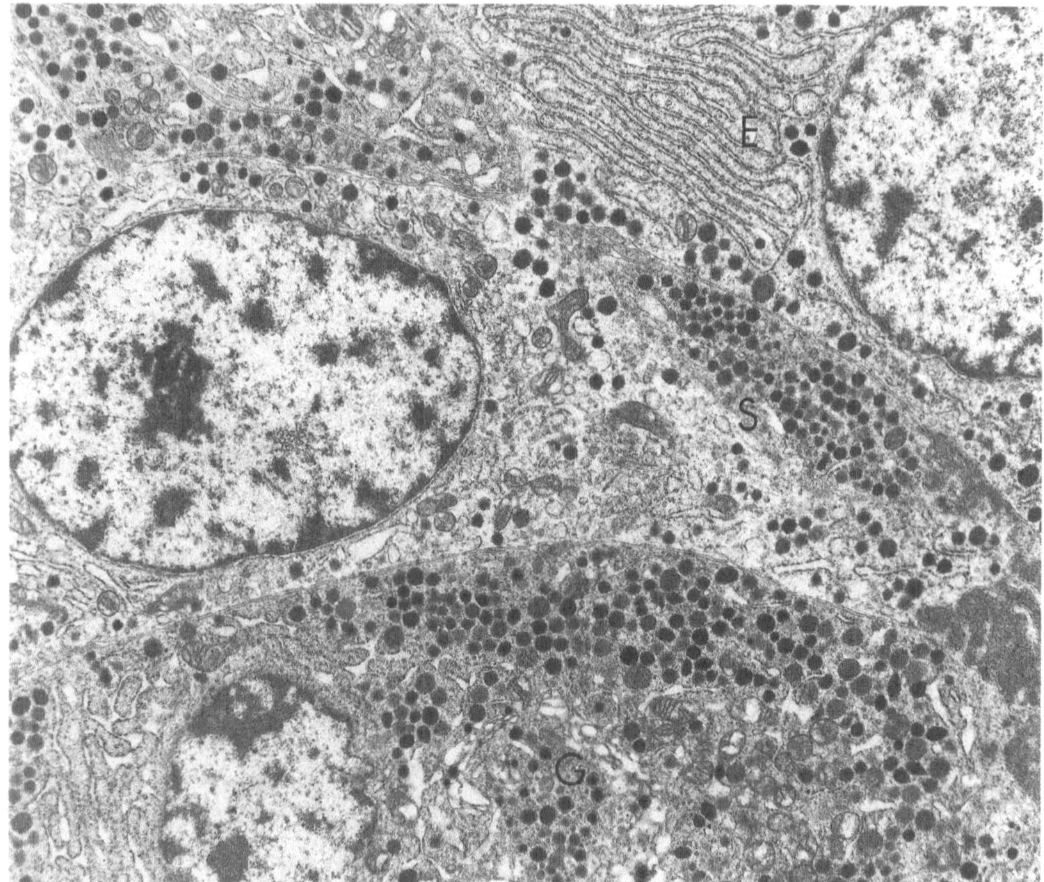

Fig. 21. Adenoma in the pars intermedia of the horse. Neoplastic cells with large lamellar arrays of rough endoplasmic reticulum (*E*), prominent Golgi apparatuses (*G*), and numerous electron-dense secretory granules (*S*), approximately 300 nm in diameter with a closely applied limiting membrane

acidophils and basophils. The neurohypophysis is often infiltrated at the periphery by neoplastic cells, compressed, and replaced by fibrous astrocytes and hemosiderin-laden macrophages. The hypothalamus is also often compressed and has increased glial cells and a loss of nerve cell bodies. In addition to the space-occupying effects, adenomas of the pars intermedia may be endocrinologically active. Plasma cortisol and immunoreactive adrenocorticotropin (iACTH; molecular weight 4500) levels may be modestly elevated in horses with pars intermedia adenomas (Orth et al. 1982). The cortisol levels often lack the normal diurnal rhythm and are not suppressed by either high or low doses of dexamethasone.

The modest elevations in plasma immunoreactive ACTH appear to be due to the different processing of pro-OLMC in tumors derived from cells of the pars intermedia. This may explain the normal or slightly elevated blood cortisol levels and normal or mildly hyperplastic adrenal cortices often observed in horses with adenomas of the pars intermedia. Wilson et al. (1982) reported that the tumor concentration of ACTH was six times that of the normal pars intermedia and approached the levels found in the pars distalis of normal horses. The plasma and tumor levels of pars intermedia-derived peptides (corticotropinlike intermediate lobe peptide, α-MSH, β-MSH, and β-END) were disproportionately elevated (40 times or more) compared to those of ACTH, apparently as the result of selective posttranslational processing of pro-OLMC in a similar manner as the normal pars intermedia.

Horses with pituitary adenomas derived from pars intermedia develop a clinical syndrome associated with the autonomous production of excess proopiomelanocortin (POMC) derived petides. Immunocytochemical evaluation of adenomas of the pars intermedia revealed a diffuse moderate to strong staining for POMC, α-MSH, and β-END (Heinrichs et al. 1990). Although many of the functional disturbances in horses with pituitary adenomas (e.g., diabetes insipidus, polyphagia, hyperpyrexia, hyperhidrosis, and hirsutism) appear to be the result of hypothalamic or neurohypophyseal dysfunction, other signs (e.g., docility and diminished responsiveness to painful stimuli) may be related to the elevated plasma and cerebrospinal levels of β-END. Although ACTH is demonstrable in adenomas of the pars intermedia, the staining intensity is patchy and considerably weaker than that of POMC, α-MSH, and β-END. These findings are in accord with biochemical studies that report markedly elevated concentrations of immunoreactive POMC and POMC-derived peptides including α- and β-MSH, corticotropinlike intermediate lobe peptide, and β-END in adenomas and plasma of affected horses relative to ACTH. The overall processing of peptides in adenomas in the pars intermedia appears to be similar to that in the normal equine pars intermedia (Heinrichs et al. 1990).

Corticotrophs in the pars distalis of horses have strong immunostaining for ACTH, whereas only a few cells stain for α-MSH. These immunocytochemical findings illustrate the differences between adenomas of the pars intermedia in horses and corticotroph adenomas of the pars distalis (also pars intermedia in dogs) that result in the classic Cushing's disease in humans and dogs. Corticotroph adenomas associated with Cushing's disease are characterized by strong immunostaining for ACTH and weak to moderate immunostaining for α-MSH.

Craniopharyngioma Associated with Hypopituitarism

Craniopharyngioma is a benign tumor which derives from epithelial remnants of the oropharyngeal ectoderm of the craniopharyngeal duct (Rathke's pouch). It occurs in animals younger than those with other types of pituitary neoplasms and is present in either a suprasellar or infrasellar location. It is one cause of panhypopituitarism and dwarfism in young dogs due to a subnormal secretion of somatotropin and other tropic hormones beginning at an early age, prior to closure of the growth plates. (Eigenmann et al. 1983).

Craniopharyngiomas have alternating solid and cystic areas (White 1938). The solid areas are composed of nests of epithelial cells (cuboidal, columnar, or squamous) with focal areas of mineralization. The cystic spaces are lined by either columnar or squamous cells and contain keratin debris and colloid.

Craniopharyngiomas are often large, and grow along the ventral aspect of the brain where they can incorporate several cranial nerves. In addition, they extend dorsally into the hypothalamus and thalamus (Fig. 22). The clinical signs resulting from this type of pituitary tumor are often a combination of (a) lack of secretion of pituitary tropic hormones resulting in tropic atrophy and subnormal function of the adrenal cortex and thyroid (Fig. 22), gonadal atrophy, and failure to attain somatic maturation due to a lack of growth hormone; (b) disturbances in water metabolism (polyuria, polydipsia, low urine specific gravity and osmolality) from interference in the release and synthesis of antidiuretic hormone by the large tumor (Saunders and Rickard 1952); (c) deficits in cranial nerve function; and (d) central nervous system dysfunction due to extension into the overlying brain.

Acidophil Adenoma of Pars Distalis

Neoplasms derived from granulated acidophils are uncommon in all domestic animal species but are common in old animals of many strains of rats. Acidophil adenomas and adenocarcinomas have been reported in the cat, dog, and sheep.

Acidophil adenomas enlarge the pituitary gland and indent the overlying hypothalamus or extend into the overlying brain to varying degrees. The enlarged hypophysis is composed of irregular columns of acidophils interspersed between numerous large blood-filled sinusoids. The fibrous stroma is sparse. Although the degree of cytoplasmic granulation of acidophils varies from cell to cell, the predominating type of neoplastic acidophil usually contains many secretory granules. The nuclei of the densely granulated acidophils are small, oval, and hyperchromatic. Sparsely granulated (chromophobic) cells are interspersed between the densely granulated

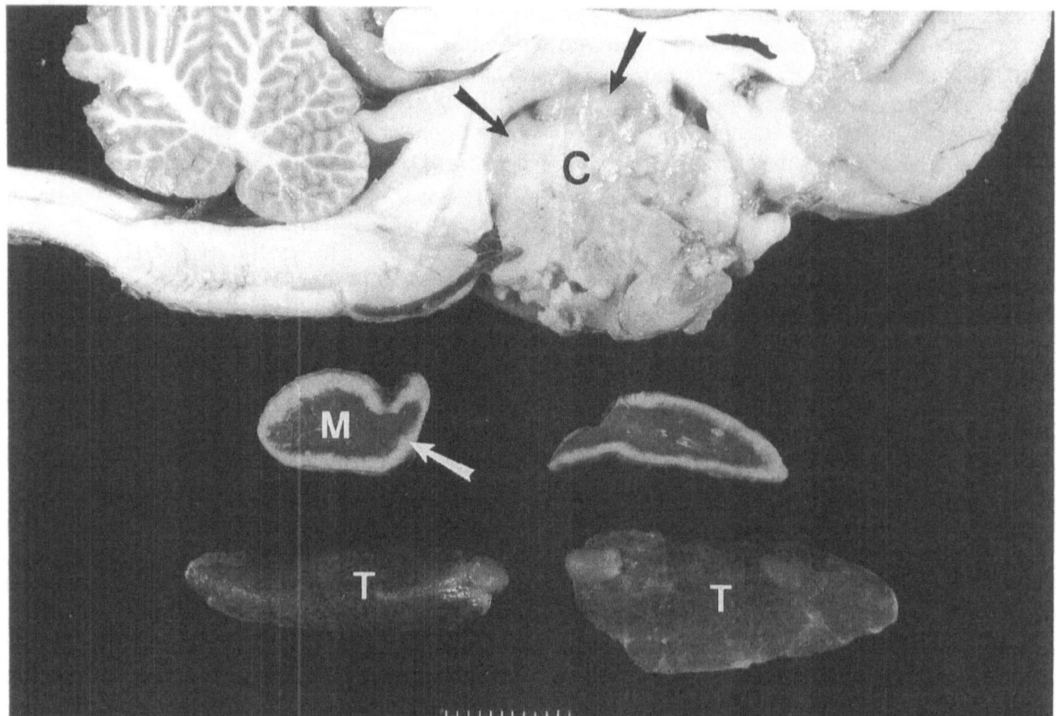

Fig. 22. Craniopharyngioma (*C*) with dorsal extension and compression of the hypothalamus and thalamus (*black arrows*). The large neoplasm has incorporated the adenohypophysis and neurohypophysis, and resulted in severe tropic atrophy of the adrenal cortex (*white arrow*). The adrenal glands consist predominantly of medulla (*M*) surrounded by a thin rim of cortex (capsule plus zona glomerulosa). Although thyroid follicular cells were flattened and atropic, the overall gland (*T*) size was within normal limits, due to distension of follicles with colloid. The scale at the bottom represents 1 cm

acidophils. Their cytoplasm is more abundant and lightly eosinophilic but contains only an occasional secretory granule. Secretory granules of the acidophils are bright red when stained with acid fuchsin-aniline blue and with Crossman's modification of Mallory's trichrome. Orange-G stains the granules an intense yellowish orange, but they are periodic acid-Schiff negative.

Electron-microscopic evaluation reveals that two types of acidophils occur within pituitary acidophil adenomas (Fig. 23). The predominating type of acidophil is smaller and contains many secretory granules. The granules are spherical to oval, uniformly electron dense, finely granular, and surrounded by a delicate limiting membrane. The submembranous space of the granule is narrow. The mean diameter of mature secretory granules in the neoplastic acidophils is 420 nm (range, 320–600 nm; Fig. 23). The less common type of neoplastic acidophil has a greater cytoplasmic and nuclear area but contains numerous organelles and few mature secretory granules. The rough endoplasmic reticulum is extensive and consists of aggregates of lamellar arrays of granular membranes. The Golgi apparatus is prominent and associated with numerous small prosecretory granules. Mitochondria are observed more often in the cytoplasm of this type of acidophil. These hypertrophied acidophils are considered to be secretorily active cells. Cells with varying amounts of organellar development and numbers of mature secretory granules are present between the extremes of storage and actively synthesizing acidophils.

Acidophil adenomas in cats have been associated with clinical signs of diabetes mellitus with degranulation of the pancreatic islets and vacuolar changes in beta cells. The persistent elevation in serum somatotropin in cats is also associated with proliferation of joint cartilage, leading to degenerative arthropathy, and with kidney disease due to periglomerular fibrosis and mesangial proliferation. Acidophil adenomas in sheep may attain considerable size (Fig. 24) and remain

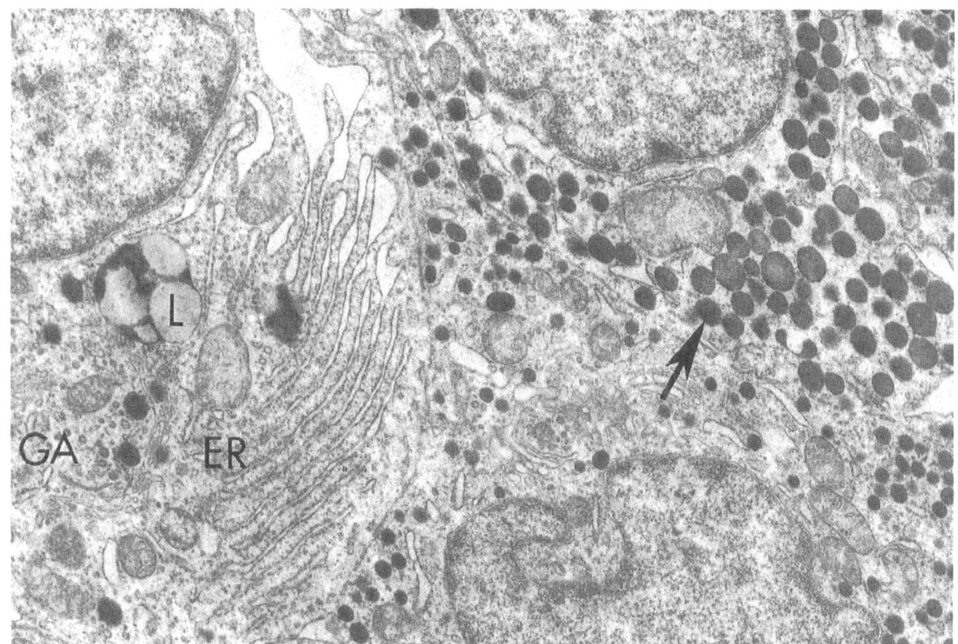

Fig. 23. Acidophil adenoma of the dog. Acidophils in the storage phase that have many large secretion granules (*arrow*). Actively synthesizing acidophils have well-developed rough endoplasmic reticulum (*ER*) and Golgi apparatus (*GA*) but few secretory granules and appear chromophobic by light microscopy. Lipofuscin granule (*L*) in tumor cell

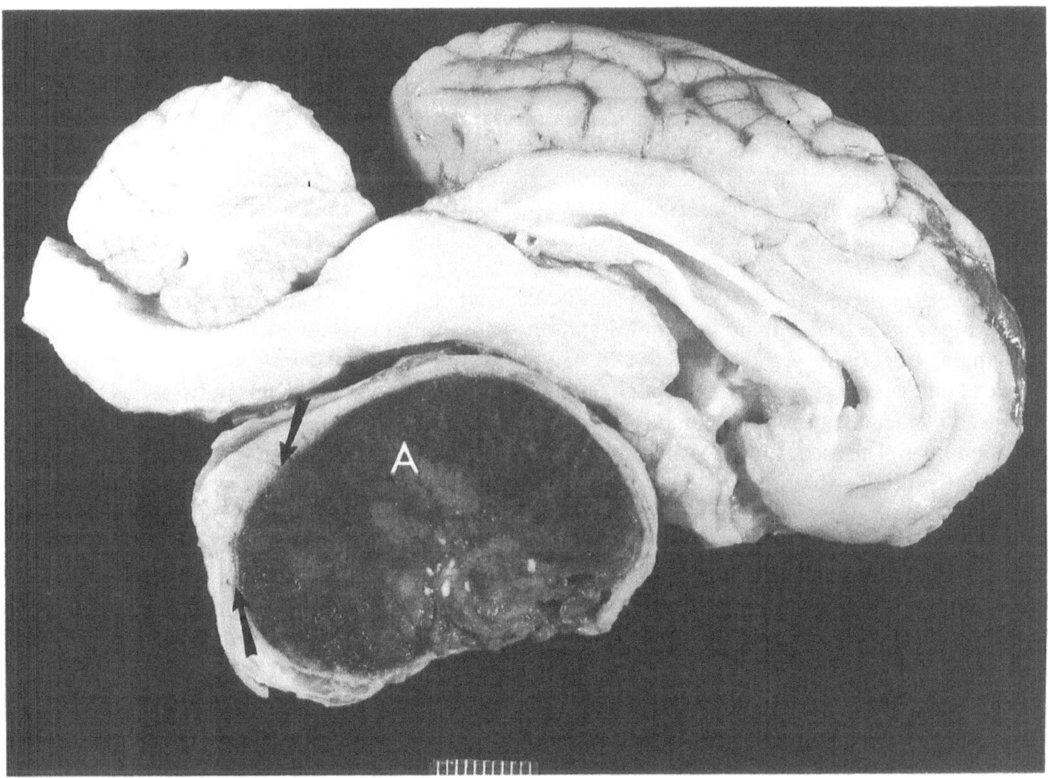

Fig. 24. Acidophil adenoma (*A*) of a ewe with severe compression of the pars distalis (*arrows*) and overlying brain

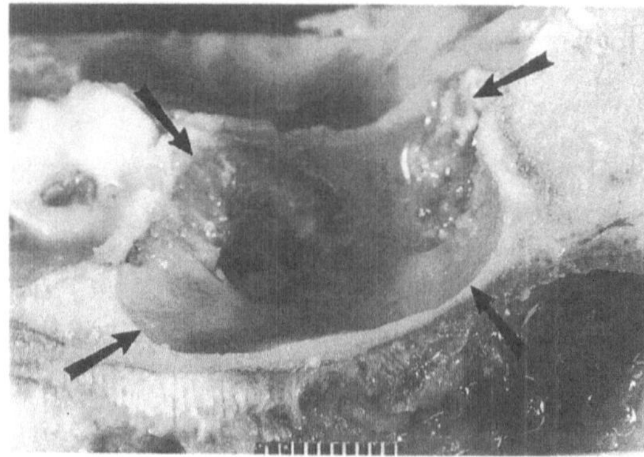

Fig. 25. Erosion of sella turcica with a large acidophil adenoma. (Same animal as in Fig. 24). The adenoma remained confined to the sella turcica due to the complete diaphragma sellae resulting in enlargement and deepening of sella turcica (*arrows*)

confined to the sella turcica because sheep have a complete diaphragma sellae separating the pituitary fossa from the brain. The remaining adeno- and neurohypophysis are compressed severely, and the sella turcica is enlarged and deepened because of pressure-induced osteolysis (Fig. 25).

Glycoprotein Hormone α-Subunit Producing Pituitary Adenomas

The pituitary gland of rats has a high incidence of spontaneous pituitary tumors (McComb et al. 1984; Sandusky et al. 1988). The incidence of pituitary tumors can be increased by treatment with certain hormones such as estrogens (DeNicola et al. 1978) or by irradiation (Condliffe et al. 1969; Furth et al. 1973). Jameson et al. (1992) reported recently that the administration of salmon calcitonin for 1 year to Sprague-Dawley and Fisher 344 rats was associated with an increased incidence of pituitary gland hyperplasia and adenomas. The association of calcitonin treatment and pituitary tumors was dose-dependent and was more pronounced with salmon calcitonin than with porcine calcitonin.

Using both immunohistochemical analysis and measurements of serum hormone levels, Jameson et al. (1992) provided evidence that prolonged administration of calcitonin resulted in pituitary tumors that produced the common α-subunit of the glycoprotein hormones LH, FSH, and TSH, a type of tumor that has been shown to comprise a significant fraction of pituitary tumors in humans (Black et al. 1987; Jameson et al. 1987). Immunohistochemistry and in situ hybridization analysis demonstrated that most pituitary tumors associated with calcitonin administration expressed a glycoprotein hormone α-subunit, whereas expression of the α-subunit was identified infrequently in hyperplastic lesions of control rats.

Serum levels of each of the major pituitary hormones were measured in both sexes of Sprague-Dawley and Fischer rats. There were no signifcant alterations in the levels of growth hormone, prolactin, or ACTH and the tumors were negative by immunohistochemical and in situ hybridization assessment for these hormones (Jameson et al. 1992). Serum LH and FSH levels were unaffected by the treatment with calcitonin; however, TSH levels were elevated 2.1-fold after calcitonin treatment in Sprague-Dawley but not Fischer rats of either sex (Fig. 26). Interestingly, thyroid weights were decreased by 43% in calcitonin-treated male rats and there was atrophy of thyroid follicular cells in some treated rats, suggesting that the immunoreactivity detected by the TSH assay was not biologically active. After treatment with calcitonin, serum α-subunit levels were increased by at least 20-fold in Sprague-Dawley males and fourfold in male Fischer rats (Figs. 26, 27). There was a good correlation between histopathologic evidence of α-subunit producing pituitary tumors and elevated serum levels. In each of the calcitonin-treated rats that had adenomas, the tumors were positive for α-subunit by immunohistochemistry and in situ hybridization for expression of α-subunit mRNA. Serum levels of α-subunit were elevated in male Sprague-Dawley rats after 2, 5, 8, 16, 24, 40, and 52 weeks to determine the time course for hormone elevation. Elevated levels of α-subunit were detected as early as 24 weeks in rats treated with calcitonin and the majority of animals had increased α-subunit levels by 40 weeks of treatment (Fig. 28), suggesting that pituitary tumors developed only after several months of exposure to calcitonin. Levels of α-subunit in vehicle-treated rats were below the detection limits of the assay at each time point.

The studies reported by Jameson et al. (1992) did not determine whether the effects of calcitonin were direct or indirect. Calcitonin is known to be produced in large amounts in the posterior hypothalamus and median eminence where it may normally exert an effect on the hypothalamus-

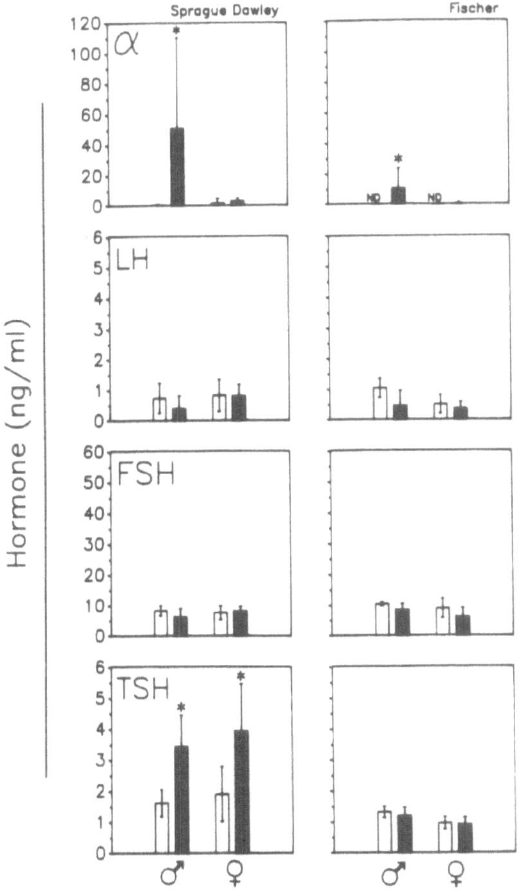

Fig. 26. Serum glycoprotein hormone levels in rats treated chronically with salmon calcitonin. Sprague-Dawley (*left panels*) or Fischer rats (*right panels*) were treated for 52 weeks with vehicle (*open bars*) or calcitonin (80 IU/kg per day; *black bars*). Results are the mean ± SD; f91p < 0.05. □, control; ■, treated. (From Jameson et al. 1992)

Fig. 27. Serum α-subunit levels in individual male rats treated chronically with calcitonin. The serum levels for individual animals are denoted: ○, vehicle; ●, calcitonin-treated. (From Jameson et al. 1992)

Fig. 28. Time course for the increase in serum α-subunit levels in male Sprague-Dawley rats. Symbols in the undetectable range represent values for more than one animal. The number of animals in each group is shown in parentheses. ○, control; ●, calcitonin-treated. (From Jameson et al. 1992)

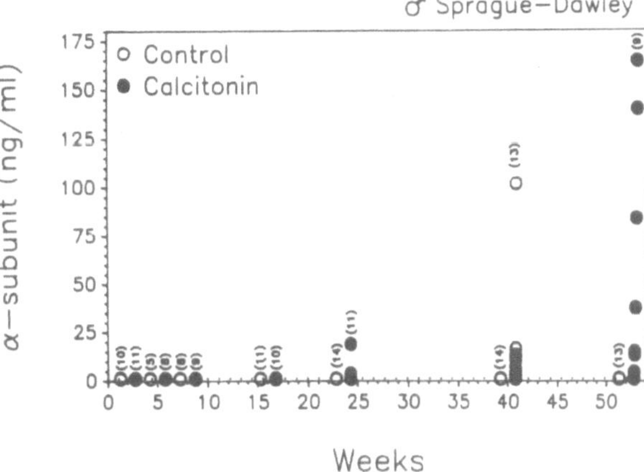

pituitary axis (Watkins et al. 1980; Fischer et al. 1981). Calcitonin receptors have been identified in the hypothalamus and lower numbers of receptors are found in the pituitary gland (Fischer et al. 1981).

A striking feature of the calcitonin-induced pituitary tumors and elevated serum α-subunit levels was the predilection for male over female rats. The basis for the sex- and species-specific effects of calcitonin was not determined (Jameson et al. 1992). The relevance of the effects of calcitonin in the rat pituitary gland to human pathophysiology is uncertain at present. Neither the treatment of patients with calcitonin nor patients with the multiple endocrine neoplasia syndrome II with medullary thyroid cancer and elevated calcitonin levels have resulted in the development of pituitary tumors. The doses of calcitonin used in the study reported by Jameson et al. (1992) were from 25- to 50-fold greater on a per-weight basis than doses administered to patients. In addition, rats of several strains are known to be highly predisposed to develop pituitary tumors compared to humans.

There are several other examples of physiologic manipulations that result in the formation of specific pituitary proliferative lesions in rodents: (a) caffeine and nonfunctional adenomas of undetermined cell types (Yamagami et al. 1983); (b) estrogen treatment and lactotroph hyperplasia and adenomas (DiNicola et al. 1978); (c) hypothyroidism and castration predisposing to the development of thyrotroph and gonadotroph hyperplasia and neoplasia; and (d) transgenic mice that overexpress GH-releasing hormone resulting in the development of somatotroph hyperplasia (Mayo et al. 1988).

Pituitary Chromophobe Carcinoma

Pituitary carcinomas are much less common than adenomas. They are usually endocrinologically inactive, but may cause significant functional disturbances by destroying the pars distalis and neurohypophyseal system, leading to panhypopituitarism and diabetes insipidus.

Pituitary carcinomas become large and invade the brain and the sphenoid bone of the sella turcica. Metastases may occur to distant sites such as the spleen or liver. Malignant tumors of pituitary chromophobes are highly cellular and often have large areas of hemorrhage and necrosis. Giant cells, nuclear pleomorphism, and mitotic figures are encountered more frequently than in adenomas.

Cysts of the Craniopharyngeal Duct

Cysts may develop from remnants of the distal craniopharyngeal duct, which normally disappears by birth in most animal species. The cysts are lined by ciliated, cuboidal to columnar epithelium and contain mucin (Rao and Bhat 1971). In dogs, especially of the brachycephalic breeds, cysts from these remnants are frequently found at the periphery of the pars tuberalis and pars distalis. Cystic remnants of the craniopharyngeal duct in one survey were found in 53% of dogs of several breeds (Schiefer and Hänichen 1967).

Craniopharyngeal duct cysts occasionally become large enough to exert pressure on the infundibular stalk and hypophyseal portal system, median eminence, or pars distalis. Structures adjacent to the cysts atrophy to varying degrees owing to compression and interference with the blood supply. Disruption of a large cyst with escape of the proteinic contents into adjacent tissues may incite an intense, local inflammation with subsequent fibrosis that interferes with pituitary function. Clinical signs may include visual difficulties due to pressure on the optic chiasm, diabetes insipidus, obesity, and hypofunction of the adenohypophysis (gonadal atrophy, decreased basal metabolic rate, and hypoglycemia).

Cysts Derived from the Pharyngeal Hypophysis

The proximal portion of the adenohypophyseal anlage may persist in the dorsal aspect of the oral cavity in adults as undifferentiated remnants of cells along the craniopharyngeal canal, or as differentiated cells similar to those of the definitive adenohypophysis. These remnants, called the pharyngeal hypophysis, have been described in dogs, cats, other animal species, and human beings (McGrath 1974; Cohrs and Nieberle 1967). The pharyngeal hypophysis is physically separated from the sellar adenohypophysis in dogs, but in cats these structures may be continuous due to persistance of the craniopharyngeal canal.

The pharyngeal hypophysis is seen most frequently in brachycephalic breeds of dogs. It is a tubular structure lined by ciliated columnar epithelium, located on the midline of the nasopharynx, and is frequently continuous with a multilocular cyst that is lined by squamous, ciliated cuboidal or columnar epithelium. The cyst contains a colloid material and cellular debris. A mass of differentiated acidophilic, basophilic, and chromophobic cells similar to those of the sellar adenohypophysis usually extends from the cyst wall.

Cysts (up to several centimeters in diameter) may be derived from the oropharyngeal end of the craniopharyngeal duct and project as a space-occupying mass into the nasopharynx in dogs. The predominant clinical sign may be related to respiratory distress due to ventral displacement of the soft palate and occlusion of the posterior nares (Slatter et al. 1976). The cyst wall may be hard on palpation, from the presence of partially mineralized woven bone. The contents of the cyst are often yellow-gray and caseous due to the accumulation of keratin and desquamated epithelial cells from the cyst lining. The squamous epithelial lining of the cyst appears to be derived from metaplasia of the remnants of the primitive oropharyngeal epithelium.

Pituitary Cyst Resulting from a Failure of Differentiation of Oropharyngeal Ectoderm of Rathke's Pouch Associated with Panhypopituitary Dwarfism

Pituitary dwarfism in German shepherd dogs usually is associated with a failure of the oropharyngeal ectoderm of Rathke's pouch to differentiate into tropic-hormone-secreting cells of the pars distalis. This results in a progressively enlarging, multiloculated cyst in the sella turcica and an absence of the adenohypophysis (Fig. 29). The cyst is lined by pseudostratified, often ciliated, columnar epithelium with interspersed mucin-secreting goblet cells (Fig. 30). The mucin-filled cysts eventually occupy the entire pituitary area in the sella turcica and severely compress the pars nervosa and infundibular stalk (Fig. 29). Few differentiated, tropic-hormone-secreting chromophils are present in the pituitary region that

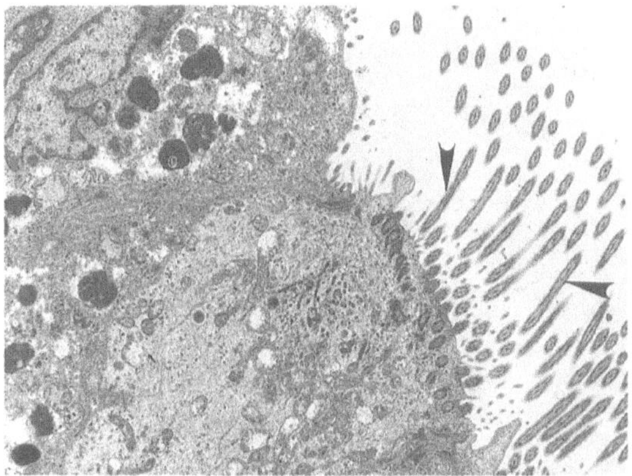

Fig. 30. Pituitary cyst associated with dwarfism in a dog. The primitive oro-pharyngeal epithelium failed to differentiate into trophic hormone-producing cells of the pituitary and have numerous cilia (*arrowheads*) projecting into the cyst

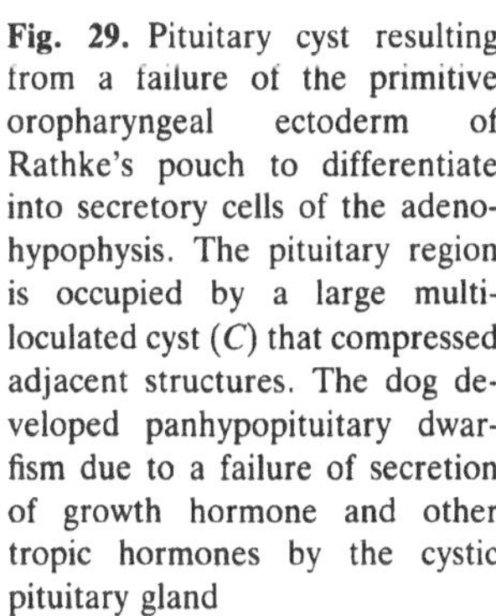

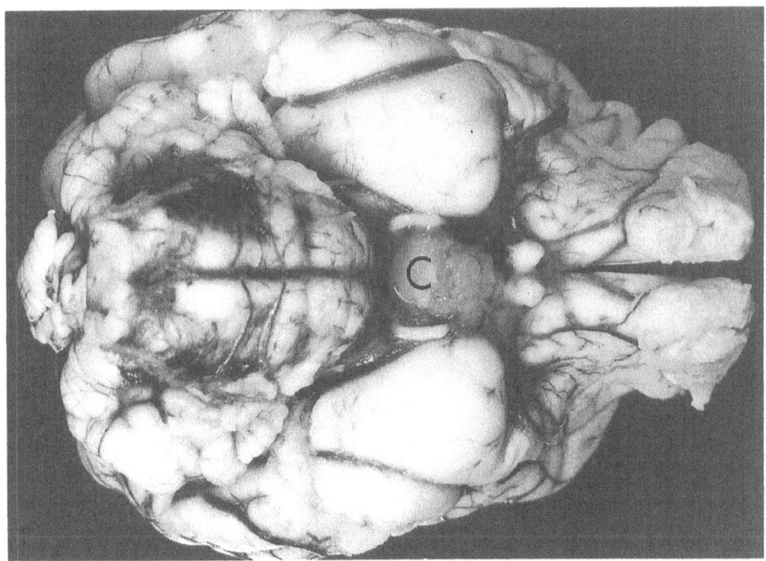

Fig. 29. Pituitary cyst resulting from a failure of the primitive oropharyngeal ectoderm of Rathke's pouch to differentiate into secretory cells of the adenohypophysis. The pituitary region is occupied by a large multiloculated cyst (*C*) that compressed adjacent structures. The dog developed panhypopituitary dwarfism due to a failure of secretion of growth hormone and other tropic hormones by the cystic pituitary gland

immunocytochemically stain for the specific tropic hormones. An occasional small nest or rosette of poorly differentiated epithelial cells are interspersed between the multiloculated cysts, but their cytoplasm is usually devoid of hormone-containing secretory granules.

Panhypopituitary dwarfism occurs most frequently in German shepherd dogs, but has been reported also in other breeds such as the spitz, toy pinscher, and Carelian bear dogs from Denmark. The dwarf pups appear normal or are indistinguishable from littermates at birth and until about 2 months of age. Subsequently the slower growth rate than the littermates, retention of puppy hair and lack of primary guard hairs gradually become evident in dwarf pups (Fig. 31). German shepherd dogs with pituitary dwarfism appear coyote- or fox-like due to their diminutive

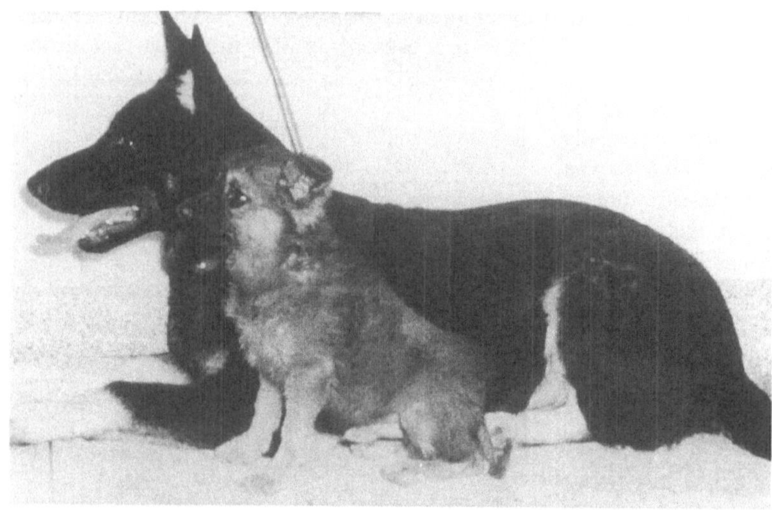

Fig. 31. Panhypopituitarism ("pituitary dwarfism") in a 5-month-old German shepherd dog. An unaffected littermate weighted 60 pounds and the dwarf 8.8 pounds. Note the retention of the puppy-hair coat on the dwarf. (Courtesy of Dr. J. Alexander and the Canadian Veterinary Journal 1962)

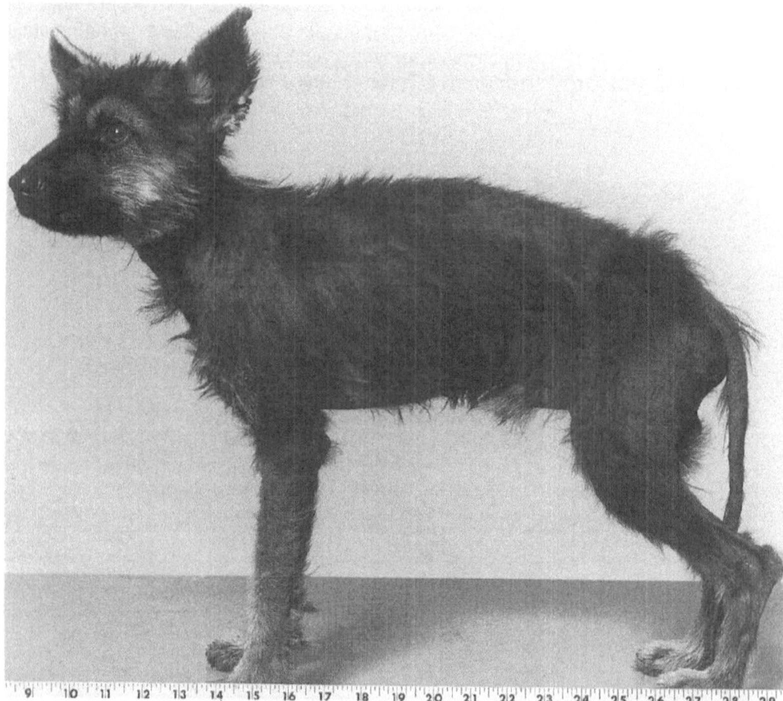

Fig. 32. Panhypopituitarism (pituitary dwarfism), German shepherd, 1 year of age

size and soft woolly coat (Fig. 32) (Muller and Jones 1973; Muller 1979). A bilaterally symmetrical alopecia develops gradually and often progresses to complete alopecia except for the head and tufts of hair on the legs. There is progressive hyperpigmentation of the skin until it is uniformly brown-black over most of the body. Adult German shepherd dogs with panhypopituitarism vary in size from as tiny as 4 lb up to nearly half normal size, apparently depending upon whether the failure of formation of the adenohypophysis is nearly complete or only partial.

Panhypopituitarism in German shepherd dogs often occurs in littermates and related litters, suggesting a simple autosomal recessive mode of inheritance (Andresen and Willeberg 1976; Andresen et al. 1974; Lund-Larsen and Grøndalen 1976; Willeberg et al. 1975; Nicholas 1978). The activity of somatomedin (a cartilage-growth-promoting peptide whose production in the liver and plasma activity are controlled by somatotropin) is low in dwarf dogs (Lund-Larsen and Grøndalen 1976). Intermediate somatomedin activity is present in the phenotypically normal ancestors suspected to be heterozygous carriers. Assays for somatomedin (a non-species-specific, somatotropin-dependent peptide) provide an indirect measurement of circulating growth-hormone activity in dogs with suspected pituitary dwarfism (Willeberg et al. 1975; Van Wyk et al. 1974).

Basal levels of circulating canine growth hormone are detectable but low (normal range, 1.75 ± 0.17 ng/ml) in pituitary dwarfs and fail to increase following a provocative test for GH secretion provided by clonidine injection as in normal dogs. Insulin hypersensitivity has been demonstrated in pituitary dwarf dogs, probably due to a change in insulin receptor numbers or affinity of binding in response to the low serum GH levels. Dwarf dogs develop more profound hypoglycemia following an insulin injection than do normal dogs, but their response is similar to that of experimentally hypophysectomized dogs.

Comparative Pathology of Neurohypophysis

Diabetes insipidus is a disorder in which inadequate ADH is produced or target cells in the kidney lack the biochemical machinery necessary to respond to the secretion of normal or elevated circulating levels of hormone. The hypophyseal form of diabetes insipidus develops as a result of compression and destruction of the pars nervosa, infundibular stalk, or supraoptic nucleus in the hypothalamus.

The lesions responsible for the disruption of ADH synthesis or secretion in hypophyseal

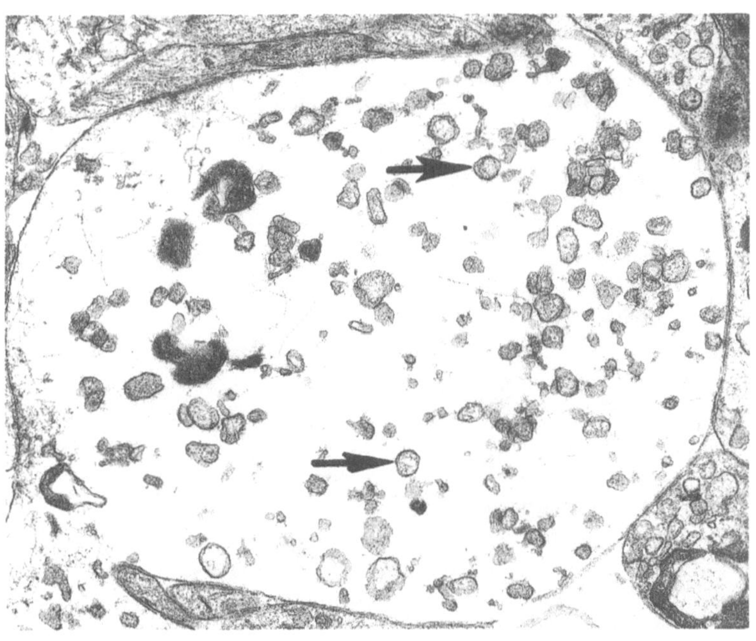

Fig. 33. Electron micrograph illustrating a cross section of an axonal process in the pars nervosa of a dog with hypophyseal diabetes insipidus associated with a large pituitary adenoma. The axonal swelling contains few neurosecretory granules with dense cores but occasional irregularly shaped. Empty vesicles. (*arrows*), ×19 800

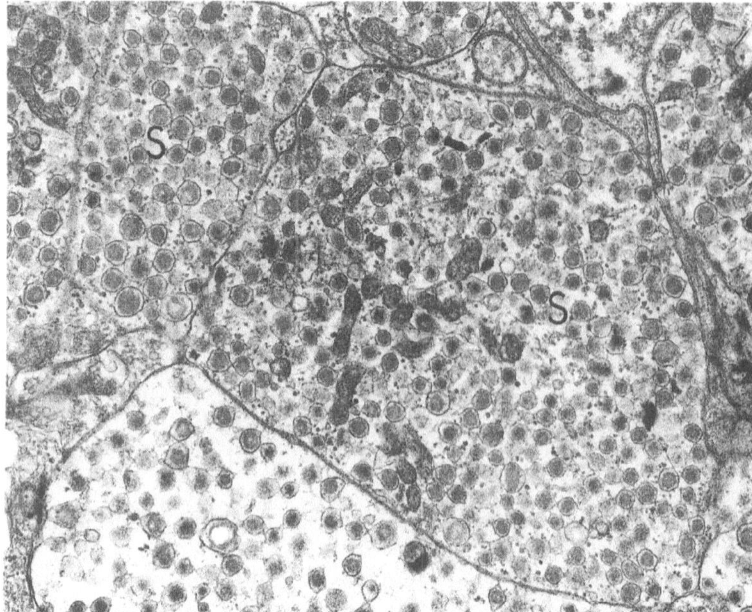

Fig. 34. Electron micrograph illustrating a cross section of an axonal process in the pars nervosa of a normal dog, showing numerous membrane-bound, ADH-containing neurosecretory granules (*S*), ×17000. (From Koestner and Capan 1967)

diabetes insipidus include large pituitary neoplasms (Koestner and Capen 1967), a dorsally expanding cyst or inflammatory granuloma, and traumatic injury to the skull with hemorrhage and glial proliferation in the neurohypophyseal system (Rogers et al. 1977). The posterior lobe, infundibular stalk, and hypothalamus are compressed or disrupted by neoplastic cells. This interrupts the nonmyelinated axons that transport ADH from its site of production, primarily in the supraoptic nucleus of the hypothalamus, to the site of release in the capillary plexus of the pars nervosa. Compression of neurosecretory neurons in the supraoptic nucleus of the hypothalamus by the dorsally expanding neoplasm may also result in decreased ADH synthesis. Axons in the compressed pars nervosa with hypophyseal diabetes insipidus associated with pituitary neoplasms are depleted of ADH-containing, dense neurosecretory granules (Fig. 33), unlike those in normal animals (Fig. 34).

Sporadic cases of hypophyseal diabetes insipidus may be the result of an inherited biochemical defect in the synthesis of ADH and its corresponding neurophysin I, as has been well characterized in the Brattleboro strain of rats (Sokol and Valtin 1965; Kalimo and Rinne 1972). In the nephrogenic form of diabetes insipidus blood levels of ADH are normal or elevated, but target cells in the distal nephron and collecting ducts are unable to respond due to a lack of adenylate cyclase in the plasma membrane (Fig. 30).

Animals with diabetes insipidus excrete large volumes of hypotonic urine, which in turn obliges them to take in equally large amounts of water to prevent hyperosmolality of body fluids and dehydration (Koestner and Capen 1967; Green and Farrow 1974). Urine osmolality is decreased below normal plasma osmolality (approximately 300 mOsM/kg) in both hypophyseal and nephrogenic forms of diabetes insipidus (Figs. 35, 36). In

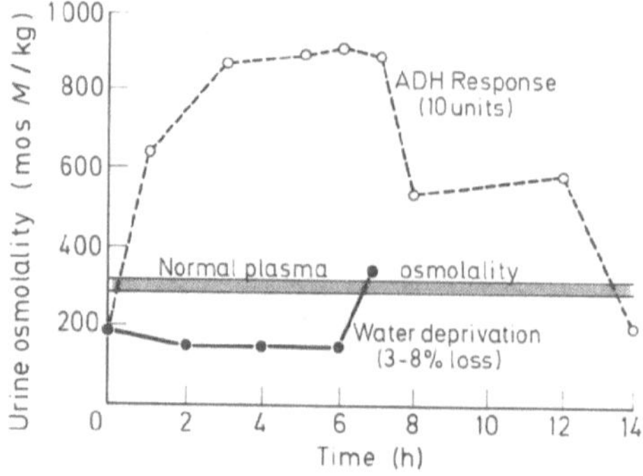

Fig. 35. Hypophyseal diabetes insipidus in a Great Dane (male, 2.5 years) illustrating the decrease in urine osmolality below that of plasma, and rapid increase of urine osmolality above normal plasma osmolality in response to exogenous ADH. (Redrawn from Richards 1970)

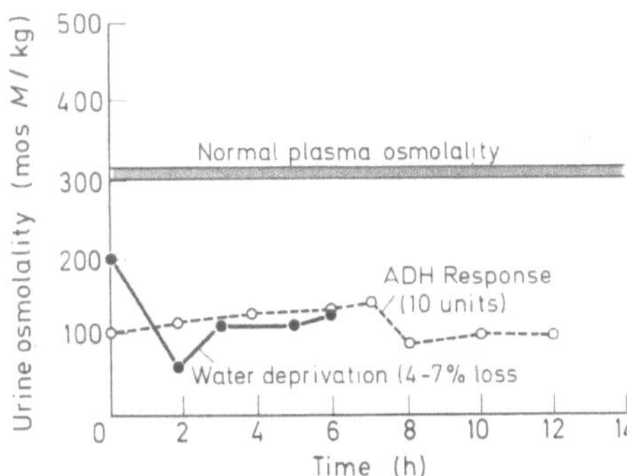

Fig. 36. Nephrogenic diabetes in a poodle (male, 4 years) illustrating the decrease in urine osmolality below plasma and lack of response both to hyperosmotic stimuli provided by water deprivation and to the administration of exogenous ADH. (Redrawn from Richards 1970)

response to water deprivation, urine osmolality remains below that of plasma in both forms of diabetes insipidus in contrast to what is observed in normal animals. The elevation of urine osmolality above that of plasma in response to exogenous ADH in the hypophyseal form (Fig. 35) but not in nephrogenic diabetes insipidus (Fig. 36) is useful in the clinical separation of these two forms of the disease (Richards 1970; Lage 1973).

References

Alexander JE (1962) Anomaly of craniopharyngeal duct and hypophysis. Can Vet J 3:83

Andresen E, Willeberg P (1976) Pituitary dwarfism in German shepherd dogs: additional evidence of simple, autosomal recessive inheritance. Nord Vet Med 28:481–486

Andresen E, Willeberg P, Rasmussen PG (1974) Pituitary dwarfism in German Shepherd dogs. Nord Vet Med 26: 692–701

Bäckström G (1963) Nägot on hirsutism i samband med hypofystumörer hos häst. Nord Vet Med 15:778–786

Black PM, Hsu DW, Klibanski A, Kliman B, Jameson L, Ridgway EC, Hedley-White ET, Zervas NT (1987) Hormone production in clinically nonfunctioning pituitary adenomas. J Neurosurg 66:244–250

Capen CC (1978) Tumors of the endocrine glands. In: Tumors in domestic animals, 2nd edn. Moulton JE (ed) University of California Press, Berkeley Los Angeles

Capen CC, Koestner A (1967) A Functional chromophobe adenomas of the canine adenohypophysis. An ultrastructural evaluation of a neoplasm of pituitary corticotrophs. Vet Pathol 4:326–347

Capen CC, Martin SL (1975) Animal model: hyperadrenocorticism (Cushing's-like syndrome and disease in dogs). Am J Pathol 81:459–462

Capen CC, Martin SL, Koestner A (1967) Neoplasms in the adenohypophysis of dogs. A clinical and pathologic study. Vet Pathol 4:301–325

Chalifoux LV, MacKey JJ, King NW (1983) A sparsely granulated, nonsecreting adenoma of the pars intermedia associated with galactorrhea in a male Rhesus monkey (*Macaca mulatta*). Vet Pathol 20:541–547

Clarkson TB, Netsky MG, de la Torre E (1959) Chromophobe adenoma in a dog: angiographic and anatomic study. J Neuropathol Exp Neurol 18:559–562

Coffin DL, Munson TO (1953) Endocrine diseases of the dog associated with hair loss. J Am Vet Med Assoc 123:402–408

Cohrs P, Nieberle K (1967) Textbook of special pathological anatomy of domestic animals. Pergamon, New York

Condliffe PG, Mochizuki M, Fontaine YA, Bates RW (1969) Purification and properties of thyrotropin from functional pituitary tumors in mice. Endocrinology 85:453–464

DeNicola AF, von Lawzewitsch I, Kaplan SE, Libertun C (1978) Biochemical and ultrastructural studies on estrogen-induced pituitary tumors in F344 rats. J Natl Cancer Inst 61:753–763

Dousa TP (1974) Cellular action of antidiuretic hormone in nephrogenic diabetes insipidus. Mayo Clin Proc 49:188–199

Eigenmann JF, Lubberink AAME, Koemann JP (1983) Panhypopituitarism caused by a suprasellar tumor in a dog. J Amer Anim Hosp Assoc 19:377–382

El Etreby MF, Dubois MP (1980) The utility of antisera to different synthetic adrenocorticotrophins (ACTH) and melanotrophins (MSH) for immunocytochemical staining of the dog pituitary gland. Histochemistry 66:245–260

El Etreby MF, Fath El Bab MR (1977) The utility of antisera to canine growth hormone and canine prolactin for immunocytochemical staining of the dog pituitary gland. Histochemisty 53:1–15

El Etreby MF, Fath El Bab MR (1978b) Effect of cyproterone acetate, d-norgestrel and progesterone on cells of the pars distalis of the adenohypophysis in the Beagle bitch. Cell Tissue Res 191:205–218

El Etreby MF, Fath El Bab MR (1978a) Effect of 17β-estradiol on cells stained for FSH^{β} and/or LH^{β} in the dog pituitary gland. Cell Tissue Res 193:211–218

El Etreby MF, Fath El Bab MR (1978c) Localization of thyrotropin (TSH) in the dog pituitary gland. A study using immunoenzyme histochemistry and chemical staining, Cell Tissue Res 186:399–412

El Etreby MF, Müller-Peddinghaus R, Bhargava AS, Trautwein G (1980) Functional morphology of spontaneous hyperplastic and neoplastic lesions in the canine pituitary gland. Vet Pathol 17:109–122

Eriksson K, Dyrendahl S, Grimfelt DA (1956) Case of hirsutism in connection with hypophyseal tumor in a horse. Nord Vet Med 8:807

Farrow BRH (1969) Chromophobe adenoma of the pituitary in a dog. Vet Rec 84:609–610

Feldman EC (1981) Effect of functional adrenocortical tumors on plasma cortisol and corticotropin concentrations in dogs. J Am Vet Med Assoc 178:823–826

Feldman EC (1983) Distinguishing dogs with functioning adrenocortical tumors from dogs with pituitary-dependent hyperadrenocorticism. J Am Vet Med Assoc 183:195–200

Feldman EC, Bohannon NV, Tyrrell JB (1977) Plasma adrenocorticotropin levels in normal dogs. Am J Vet Res 38:1643–1645

Fischer JA, Tobler PH, Kaufmann M, Born W, Henke H, Cooper PS, Sagar SM, Martin JB (1981) Calcitonin: regional distribution of the hormone and its binding sites in the human brain and pituitary. Proc Natl Acad Sci USA 78: 7801–7805

Furth J, Ueda G, Clifton KH (1973) The pathophysiology of pituitaries and their tumors. Methods Cancer Res 10: 1011–1015

Gilbert GJ, Willey EN (1969) Pituitary chromophobe adenoma in the bulldog. J Am Vet Med Assoc 154:1071–1074

Green RA, Farrow CS (1974) Diabetes insipidus in a cat. J Am Vet Med Assoc 164:524–526

Gribble DH (1972) The endocrine system. In: Catcott EJ, Smithcors JR (eds) Equine medicine and surgery, 2nd ed. American Veterinary Publications, Wheaton, Illinois, pp 433–457

Halmi NS, Peterson ME, Colurso GJ, Liotta AS, Krieger DT (1981) Pituitary intermediate lobe in dog: two cell types and high bioactive adrenocorticotropin content. Science 211: 72–74

Hare T (1935) Chromophobe cell adenoma of the pituitary gland associated with dystrophia adiposogenitalis in a maiden bitch. Proc R Soc Med 25:1492–1495

Heinrichs M, Baumgärtner W, Capen CC (1990) Immunocytochemical demonstration of proopiomelanocortin-derived peptides in pituitary adenomas of the pars intermedia in horses. Vet Pathol 27:419–425

Howe A (1973) The mammalian pars intermedia: a review of its structure and function. J Endocrinol 59:385–409

Jameson JL, Klibanski A, Black PM, Zervas NT, Lindell CM, Hsu DW, Ridgway EC, Habener JF (1987) Glycoprotein hormone genes are expressed in clinically nonfunctioning pituitary adenomas. J Clin Invest 80:1472–1478

Jameson JL, Weiss J, Polak JM, Childs GV, Bloom SR, Steel JH, Capen CC, Prentice DE, Fetter AW, Langloss JM (1992) Glycoprotein hormone alpha-subunit-producing pituitary adenomas in rats treated for one year with calcitonin. Am J Pathol 140:75–84

Kalimo H, Rinne UK (1972) Ultrastructural studies on the hypothalamic neurosecretory neurons of the rat. II. The hypothalamo-neurohypophysial system in rats with hereditary hypothalamic diabetes insipidus. Z Zellforsch Mikrosk Anat 134:205–225

Koestner A, Capen CC (1976) Ultrastructural evaluation of the canine hypothalamic-neurohypophysial system in diabetes insipidus associated with pituitary neoplasma. Vet Pathol 4:513–536

Lage AL (1973) Nephrogenic diabetes insipidus in a dog. J Am Vet Med Assoc 163:251–253

Loeb WF, Capen CC, Johnson LE (1966) Adenomas of the pars intermedia associated with hyperglycemia and glycosuria in two horses. Cornell Vet 56:623–639

Lubberink AAME, Rijnberk A, der Kinderen PJ, Thijssen JHH (1971) Hyperfunction of the adrenal cortex: a review. Aust Vet J 47:504–509

Lund-Larsen TR, Grøndalen J (1976) Ateliotic dwarfism in the German shepherd dog: low somatomedin activity associated with apparently normal pituitary function (2 cases) and with panadenopituitary dysfunction (1 case). Acta Vet Scand 17:293–306

Mayo KE, Hammer RE, Swanson LW, Brinster RL, Rosenfeld MG, Evans RM (1988) Dramatic pituitary hyperplasia in transgenic mice expressing a human growth hormone-releasing factor gene. Mol Endocrinol 2:606–612

McComb DJ, Kovacs K, Beri J, Zak F (1984) Pituitary adenomas in old Sprague-Dawley rats: a histologic, ultrastructural, and immunocytochemical study. J Natl Cancer Inst 73:1143–1166

McGrath P (1974) The pharyngeal hypophysis in some laboratory animals. J Anat 117:95–115

Meijer JC (1980) An investigation of the pathogenesis of pituitary-dependent hyperadrenocorticism in the dog. Thesis, University of Utrecht, The Netherlands

Muller GH (1979) Pituitary dwarfism: cutaneous manifestations of an endocrine disorder. Vet Clin North Am 9:41

Muller GH, Jones SR (1973) Pituitary dwarfism and alopecia in a German shepherd with cystic Rathke's cleft. J Am Anim Hosp Assoc 9:567–572

Nicholas F (1978) Pituitary dwarfism in German shepherd dogs: a genetic analysis of some Australian data. J Small Anim Pract 19:167–174

Orth DN, Holscher MA, Wilson MG, Nicholson WE, Plue RD, Mount CD (1982) Equine Cushing's disease: plasma immunoreactive proopiolipomelanocortin peptide and cortisol levels basally and in response to diagnostic tests. Endocrinology 110:1430–1441

Papkoff H (1976) Canine pituitary prolactin: isolation and partial characterization. Proc Soc Exp Biol Med 153:498–500

Peterson ME (1984a) Feline hyperthyroidism. Vet Clin North Am 14:809–826

Peterson ME (1984b) Hyperadrenocorticism. Vet Clin North Am 14:731–749

Peterson ME, Drucker WD (1981) Advances in the diagnosis and management of canine Cushing's syndrome. In: Proceedings of the 31st Gaines Veterinary Symposium, pp 17–24

Peterson ME, Kreiger DT, Drucker WD, Halmi NS (1982) Immunocytochemical study of the hypophysis in 25 dogs with pituitary-dependent hyperadrenocorticism. Acta Endocrinol 101:15–24

Rao RR, Bhat NG (1971) Incidence of cysts in pars distalis of mongrel dogs. Indian Vet J 48:128–133

Ricci V, Russolo M (1973) Immunocytological observations on the localization of ACTH in the hypophysis of the dog. Acta Anat (Basel) 84:10–18

Rijnberk A, der Kinderen PJ, Thijssen JHH (1967) "Cushing's syndrome" (spontaneous hyperadrenocorticism) in the dog. J Endocrinol 37:1–43

Rijnberk A, der Kinderen PJ, Thijssen JHH (1969) Canine Cushing's syndrome. Zentralbl Veterinaermed (A) 16: 13–28

Richards MA (1970) Polydipsia in the dog – Symposium 1, 2, and 3. The differential diagnosis of polyuric syndromes in the dog. J Small Anim Pract 10:651–667

Rogers WA, Valdez H, Anderson BC, Comella C (1977) Partial deficiency of antidiuretic hormone in a cat. J Am Vet Med Assoc 170:545–547

Roth J (1976) Introduction to session. In: Beers RF Jr, Bassett EG (eds) Cell membrane receptors for viruses, antigens and antibodies, polypeptide hormones, and small molecules. Raven Press, New York

Roth J (1979) Receptors for peptide hormones. In: De Groot LJ (ed) Endocrinology vol III. Grune and Stratton, New York

Sandusky GE, Van Pelt CS, Todd GC, Wightman K (1988) An immunocytochemical study of pituitary adenomas and focal hyperplasia in old Sprague-Dawley and Fischer 344 rats. Toxicol Pathol 16:376–380

Saunders LZ, Rickard CG (1952) Craniopharyngioma in a dog with apparent adiposogenital syndrome and diabetes insipidus. Cornell Vet 42:490–495
Schally AV (1978) Aspects of hypothalamic regulation of the pituitary gland. Its implications for the control of reproductive processes. Science 202:18–28
Schiefer B, Hänichen T (1967) Zur Kenntnis und möglichen Bedeutung von Hypophysencysten beim Hund. Acta Neuropathol (Berl) 7:232–241
Siegel ET, Kelly DF, Berg P (1970) Cushing's syndrome in the dog. J Am Vet Med Assoc 157:2081–2089
Slatter DH, Schirmer RG, Krehbiel JD (1976) Surgical correction of cystic Rathke's cleft in a dog. J Am Anim Hosp Assoc 12:641
Sokol HW, Valtin H (1965) Morphology of the neurosecretory system in rats homozygous and heterozygous for hypothalamic diabetes insipidus (Brattleboro strain). Endocrinology 77:692–700
Turner CD, Bagnara JT (1971) General endocrinology, 5th edn. Saunders, Philadelphia
Van Wyk JJ, Underwood LE, Hintz RL, Clemmons DR, Voina SJ, Weaver RP (1974) The somatomedins: a family of insulin-like hormones under growth hormone control. Recent Prog Horm Res 30:259–318
Watkins WB, Moore RY, Burton D, Bone HG, Catherwood BD, Deftos LJ (1980) Distribution of immunoreactive calcitonin in the rat pituitary gland. Endocrinology 106: 1966–1970
White EG (1938) A suprasellar tumor in a dog. J Pathol Bacteriol 47:323–326
Wilhelmi AE (1968) Canine growth hormone. Yale J Biol Med 41:199–207
Willeberg P, Kastrup KW, Andresen E (1975) Pituitary dwarfism in German shepherd dogs: studies on somatomedin activity. Nord Vet Med 27:448–454
Wilson MG, Nicholson WE, Holscher MA, Sherrell BJ, Mount CD, Orth DN (1982) Proopiolipomelanocortin peptides in normal pituitary, pituitary tumor, and plasma of normal and Cushing's horses. Endocrinology 110:941–954
Yamagami T, Handa H, Takeuchi J, Munemitsu H, Aoki M, Kato Y (1983) Rat pituitary adenoma and hyperplasia induced by caffeine administration. Surg Neurol 20:323–331

Histology, Ultrastructure, and Immunochemistry, Pituitary Gland, Rat

R. Yoshiyuki Osamura

The pituitary gland of the rat is located in the midline at the base of the brain on the sella turcica, which is rather flat in this animal. Superiorly, it is connected with the hypothalamus by the stalk. The pituitary gland of the rat is divided into three major anatomical parts: the pars distalis, the pars intermedia, and the pars nervosa. The pars tuberalis, composed of cells resembling those of the pars distalis, is present around the stalk up to the hypothalamus.

The hormones produced or secreted by the pituitary are listed in Table 1.

The glycoprotein hormones are composed of two subunits, α and β; they share comman α subunits and posses a specific β subunit that controls their specific structure and function.

The morphological approach has been focused mainly on the identification of specific hormone-producing cells, especially in the pars distalis. Historically, this identification has been accomplished by using various dyes, such as periodic acid-Schiff (PAS) and orange G. Ultrastructural observations and immunohistochemical staining has, in more recent times, made it possible to identify these hormone-secreting cells.

Histology

With H and E staining of formalin-fixed and paraffin-embedded tissue, a lower-power view of horizontal sections of the pituitary gland reveals the anterior pars distalis, pars intermedia, and pars nervosa (Fig. 37). In a higher-power view of the pars distalis, polygonal or polyhedral cells separated by sinusoidal structures may be seen (Fig. 38). These anterior pituitary cells may be recognized as basophilic, acidophilic or chromophobic cells, based on the tinctorial features of their cytoplasm.

When PAS and orange G stain are applied to formalin-fixed paraffin sections it is possible to distinguish basophilic cells (PAS-positive) from acidophilic cells (orange G-positive). By applying PAS-orange G stains in conjunction with aldehyde fuchsin or aldehyde thionine stains, the pituitary cells may be divided into the following subgroups: basophilic cells into adrenocorticotropic hormone (ACTH), follicle-stimulating hormone (FSH), luteinizing hormone (LH), and thyroid-stimulating hormone (TSH); acidophilic cells into growth hormone (GH) and luteotropic

Table 1. Hormones secreted by the pituitary

Pars distalis	
Peptide hormones	*Glycoprotein hormones*
Adrenocorticotropic hormone (ACTH)	Follicle-stimulating hormone (FSH)
Growth hormone (GH) (Somatotropin, STH)	Luteinizing hormone (LH)
Prolactin (PRL) (Luteotropin, LTH)	Thyroid-stimulating hormone (TSH) (Thyrotropin, TTH)
Pars nervosa	
Vasopressin	
Oxytocin	
Pars intermedia	
Adrenocorticotropic hormone (ACTH)(some species)	
Melanocyte-stimulating hormone (MSH)(some species)	

hormone (LTH) cells. However, this separation is not specific and further identification in this field has been aided by electron microscopic observations.

Ultrastructure

Ultrastructurally, further identification of cell types, especially GH and LTH cells, has become possible to some extent. As seen under the electron microscope, GH cells are round to oval and contain many round, dense-cored secretion granules with a diameter of about 300–350 nm (Rodin 1974), distributed throughout the cytoplasm (Fig. 39). Some rough endoplasmic reticulum is present near the nucleus. LTH cells are characterized by the presence of many large ovoid or polymorphic secretory granules of about 600–900 nm in diameter clustered near the nucleus, and lamellated rough endoplasmic reticulum at the periphery of the cytoplasm. A well-developed

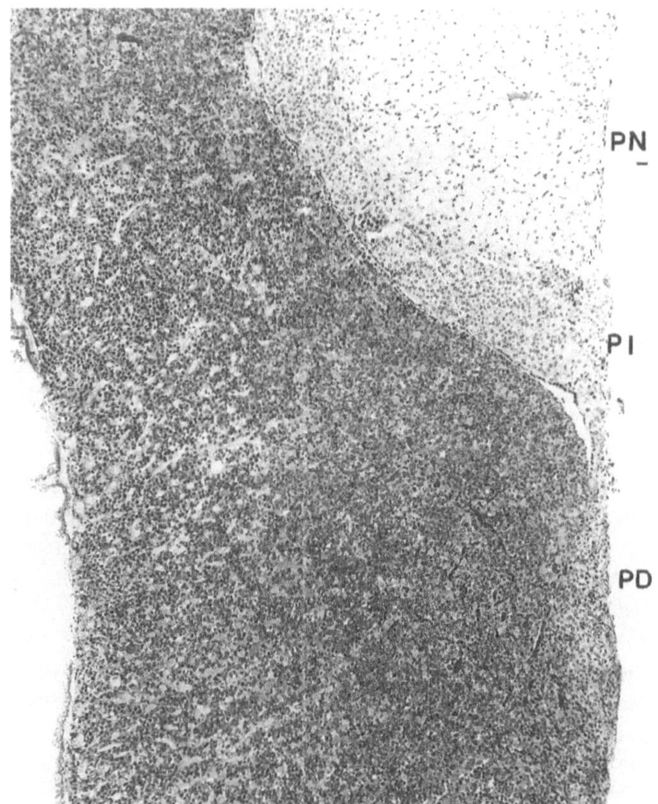

Fig. 37. Low magnification of normal adult pituitary gland, divided into pars distalis (*PD*) pars intermedia (*PI*), and pars nervosa (*PN*). H&E, ×75

Fig. 38. Higher magnification of pars distalis which is composed of many large round cells (probably gonadotrophs) and many smaller compact cells. H&E, ×300

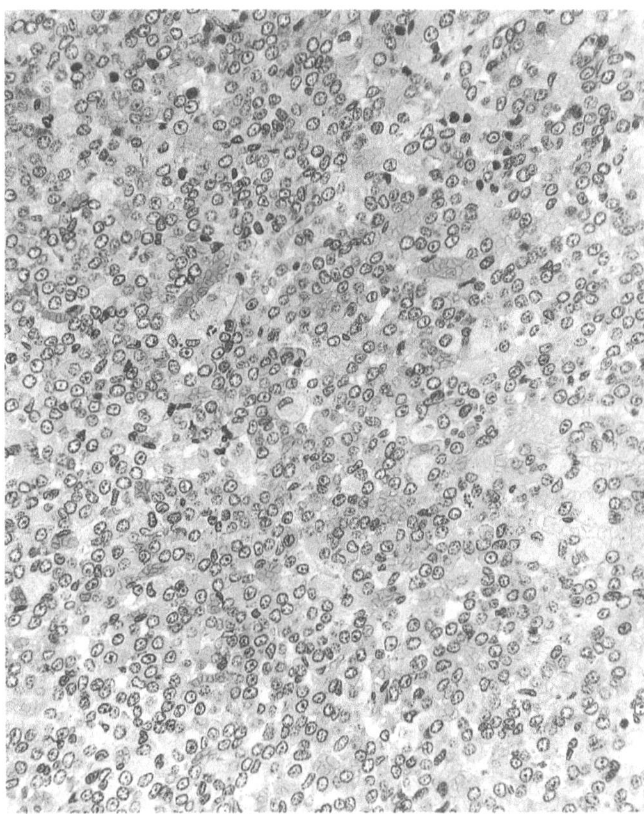

Golgi apparatus is present in close relationship with the secretory granules, and mitochondria are sparse. The gonadotropic (LH and FSH) cells are recognized by the presence of ample cytoplasm containing abundant dilated, rough endoplasmic reticulum, and scattered round secretory granules, 100–300 nm in diameter (Fig. 40).

The identification of the other types of hormone-secreting cells, especially ACTH and TSH cells, relies upon immunohistochemical staining. However, ultrastructurally, these ACTH cells contain relatively small dense-cored secretory granules averaging 200 nm in diameter, located in the periphery of the cytoplasm (Fig. 39). The perinuclear area contains rough endoplasmic reticulum (RER) and Golgi apparatus. These characteristics do not permit precise identification of cells which secrete ACTH (Kawarai 1981; Moriarty 1973; Osamura et al. 1980, 1981).

The cells of the pars intermedia are round to ovoid and contain many electron-dense to more lucent secretory granules with an average diameter of 200 nm (Rodin 1974). RER is not prominent. Sometimes electron-dense secretory granules are adjacent to a conspicuous Golgi apparatus (Fig. 41).

The cells of the pars nervosa are characteristically clustered and surrounded by a basement membrane. Each cell contains many electron-dense cored secretory granules about 100–300 nm in diameter (Rodin 1974), and many smaller vesicles. Frequent parallel arrangement of tubules is also seen. Large osmiophilic lipid globules (Fig. 42) are prominent.

Immunocytochemistry

In our studies for light microscopic localization of hormones and identification of cell types we have utilized Nakane's peroxidase-labeled antibody method applied to formalin-fixed and paraffin-embedded tissue. This method is specific and enables one to accurately classify all pituitary cells (Nakane 1968, 1970, 1975) according to their function.

Many ACTH cells are widely distributed in the pars distalis, and the pars intermedia is composed

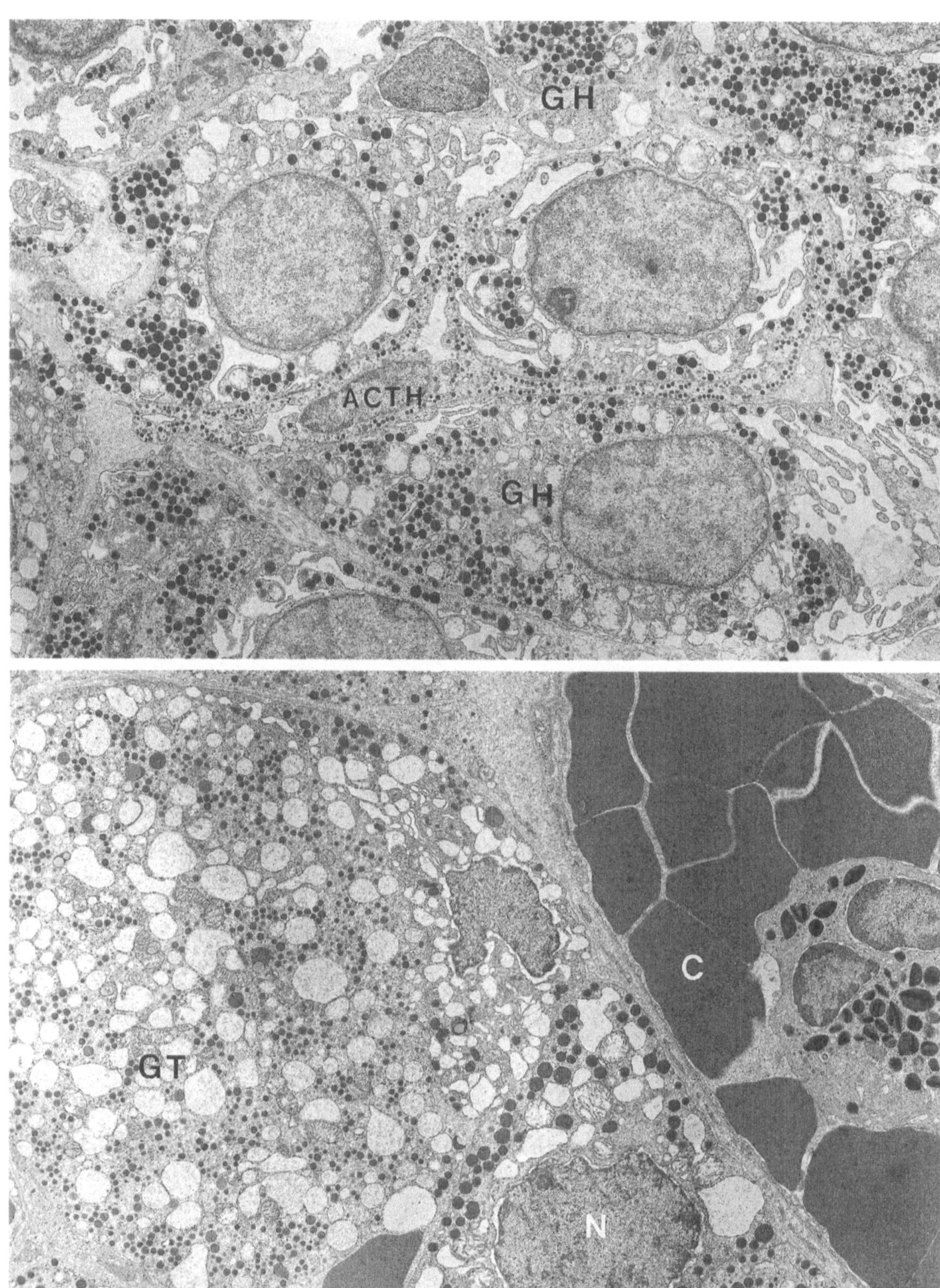

Fig. 39. (*above*) Ultrastructure of pars distalis. The growth hormone (*GH*) cells with many round, dense secretory granules are easily recognizable. The central stellate cells with slender cytoplasmic processes and peripheral small secretory granules are probably ACTH cells, ×6300

Fig. 40. (*below*) Ultrastructure of pars distalis. The gonadotrophs (*GT*) contain dilated and vesicular rough endoplasmic reticulum and scattered round, small secretory granules. The lactotroph (*LT*) contains polymorphic secretory granules in the female rat. *N*, nucleus; *C*, capillary, ×6300

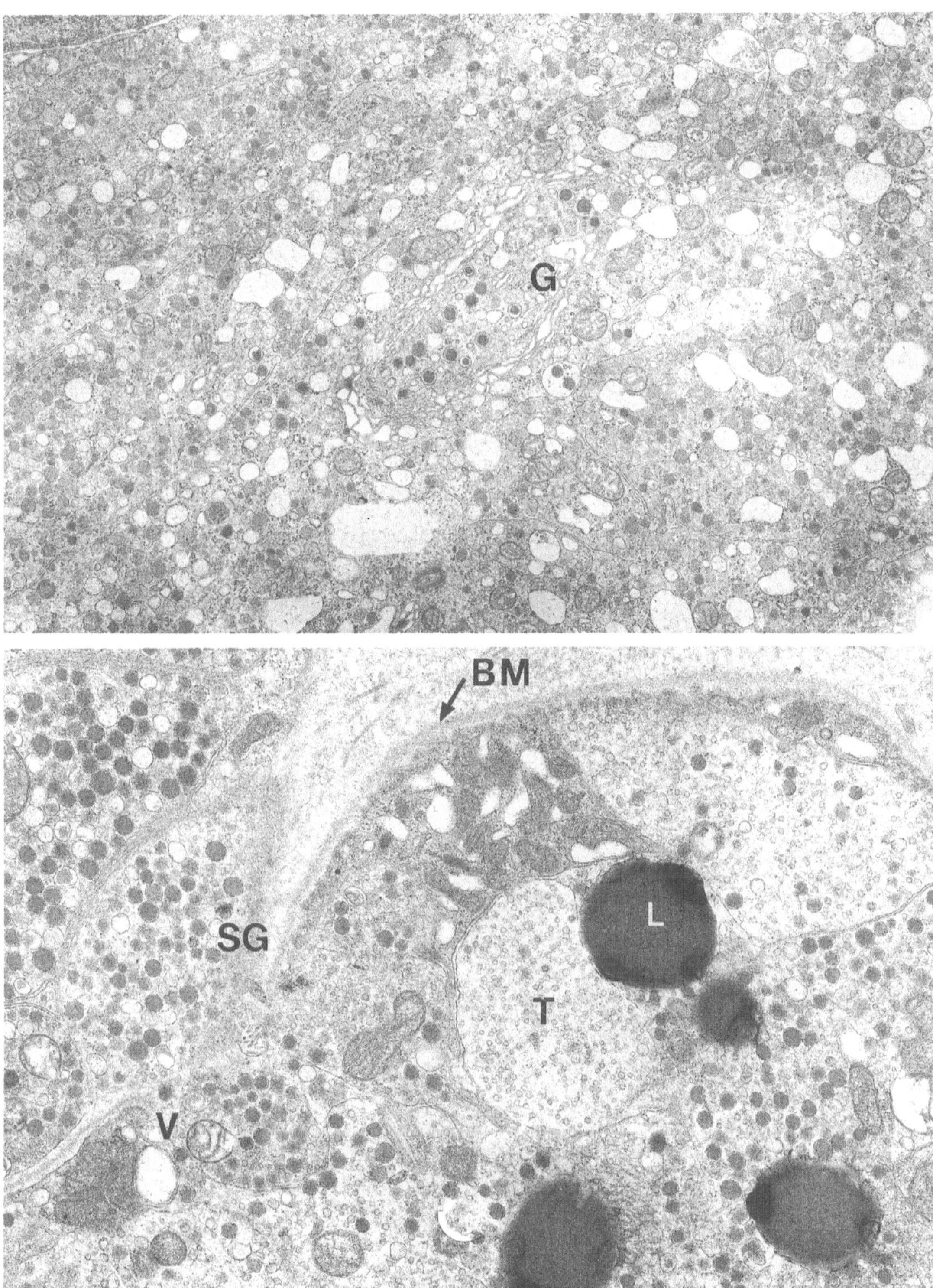

Fig. 41. (*above*) Ultrastructure of pars intermedia. The cells contain many small, dense-cored secretory granules as well as a prominent Golgi apparatus (*G*). The secretory granules near the Golgi apparatus are more eletron-dense than others in the same cell, ×6300

Fig. 42. (*below*) Ultrastructure of pars nervosa. Cells contain many nerve fibers and small secretory granules (*SG*), vesicles (*V*), tubules (*T*), and large osmiophilic lipid globules (*L*). The pars nervosa cells are in clusters surrounded by basement membrane (*BM*), ×6300

exclusively of them (Fig. 43). The ACTH cells in the pars distalis are characterized by elongated cytoplasm which is in contact with the capillaries (Fig. 44). These elongated cells are usually in close relationship with other types of hormone-secreting cells, including GH cells. The cells in the pars intermedia react mainly with antibody against ACTH, and they are round or ovoid with round nuclei.

The GH cells are distributed throughout the pars distalis; they are round to oval and contain evenly distributed immunoreactive GH in the cytoplasm. The LTH cells are present throughout the pars distalis, but they are more concentrated in the dorsocephalic area ("sex zone"). Individual LTH cells are cup-shaped and are in close relationship with gonadotrophs (Fig. 45). Prolactin is located not only in the secretory granules but also in the cisternae of RER, Golgi, and perinuclear spaces (Figs. 46–49). These localizations are in argreement with those of other investigators and support a pathway proposed by Farquhar (1971). In this concept, the hormone is produced in the RER and moves to the Golgi apparatus, where it is included in secretory granules. These granules are then extruded into extracellular spaces (secretion). In the rat, LH and FSH are present in most of the same gonadotropin-secreting cells. Some cells in the center of the pars distalis contain only FSH. In our studies on the rat using antibody against human chorionic gonadotropin, which cross reacts with rat LH, the LH cells are concentrated in the so-called sex zone. These cells are round or oval (Fig. 50). The cells that contain thyrotropin (TSH), according to Nakane, are more frequently found in clusters in the center of the gland. They are polygonal to stellate in shape. In our recent observation utilizing antibody against TSH subunit (supplied by the National Institutes of Health, Bethesda, Maryland, USA), TSH cells were localized in clusters in the center of the gland and were ovoid or angular shape, confirming Nakane's findings. Immunoreactive TSH is present throughout the cytoplasm (Fig. 51).

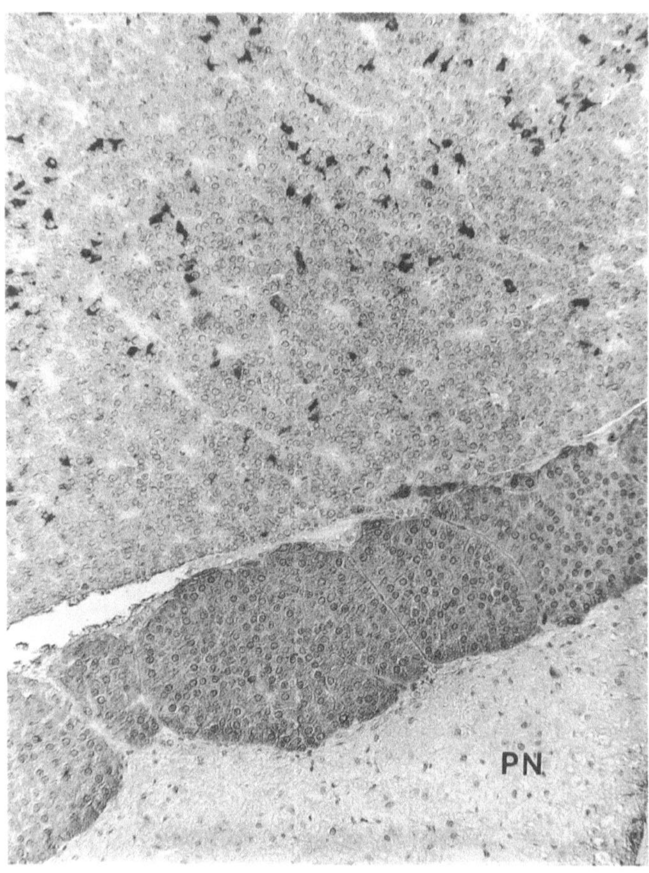

Fig. 43. Immunohistochemical staining for ACTH. The pars distalis contains scattered ACTH-positive cells and the pars intermedia is diffusely stained for ACTH. *PN*, pars nervosa. Peroxidase-labeled antibody method, ×150

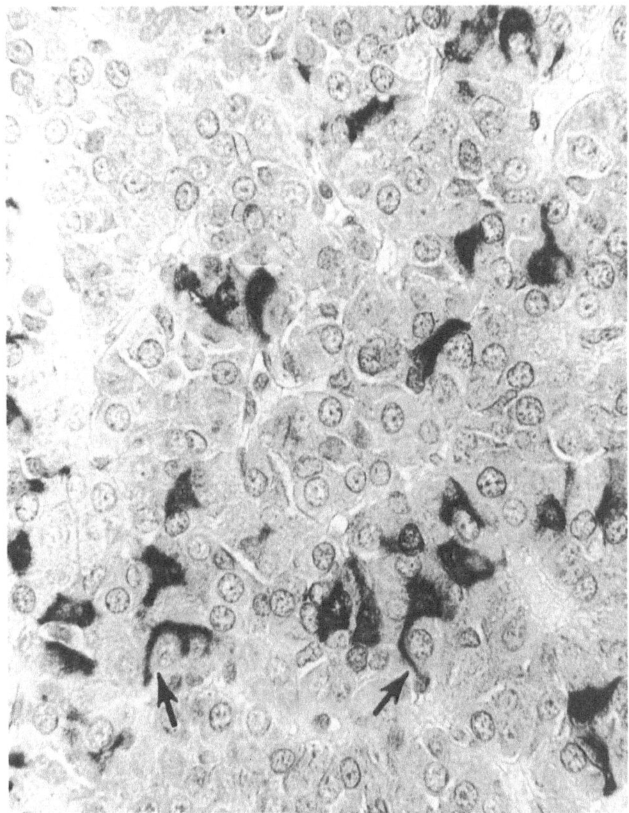

Fig. 44. The ACTH cells in pars distalis have characteristic, slender cytoplasmic processes (*arrows*) and are labeled by the peroxidase-labeled antibody method, ×600

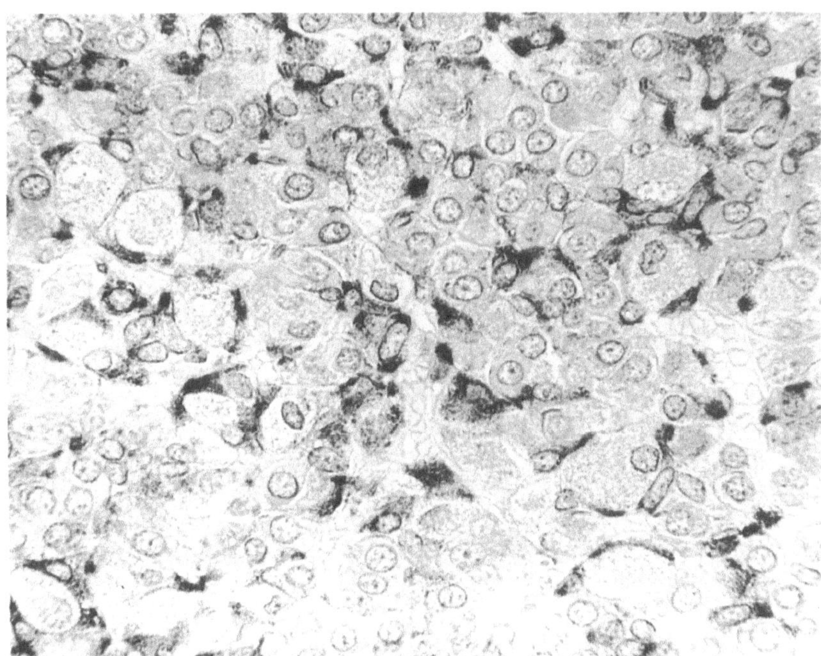

Fig. 45. The LTH-positive cells in the pars distalis are flat or cup-shaped and in close proximity to the gonadotrophs. Peroxidase-labeled antibody method, ×600

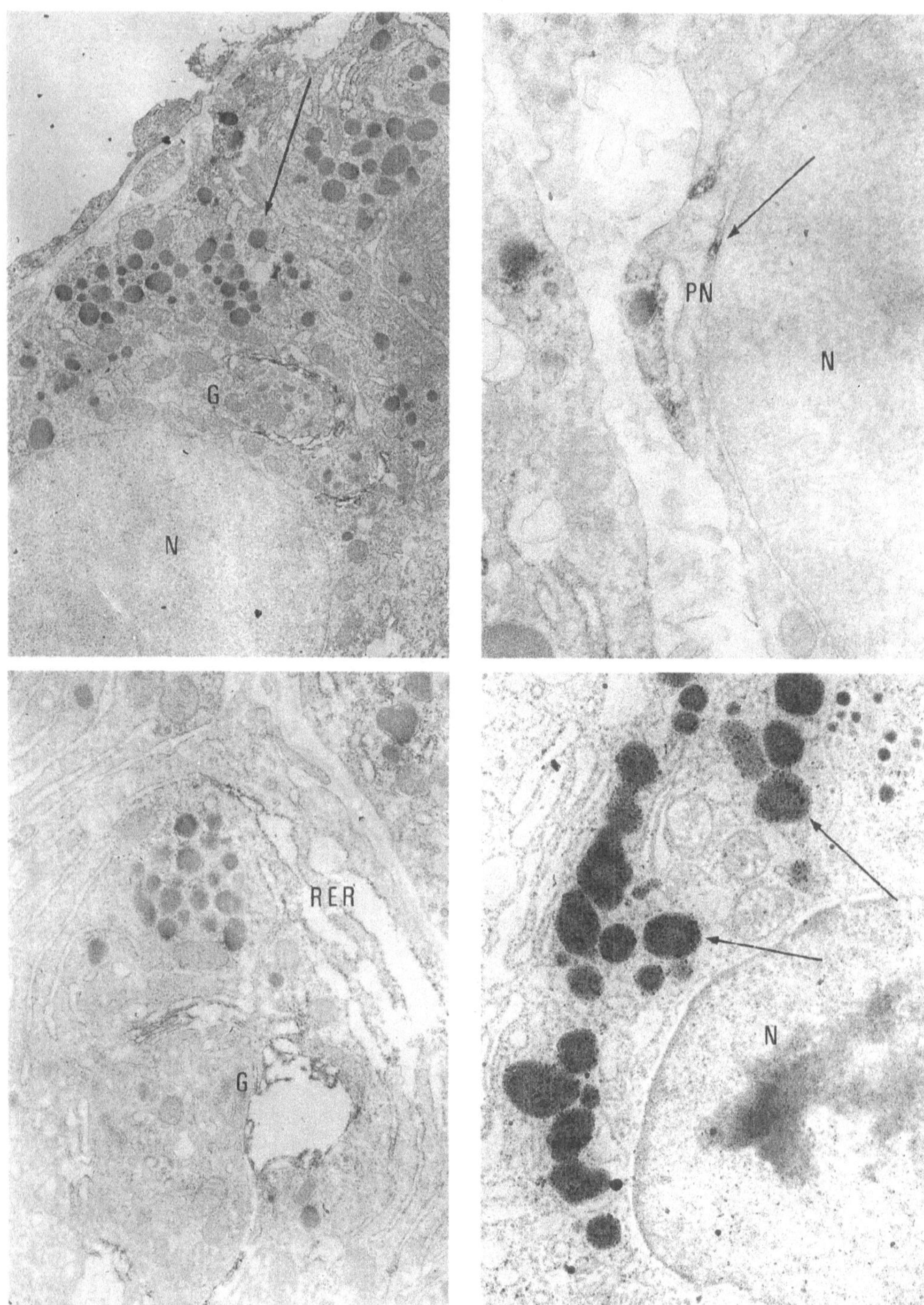

Fig. 46. (*upper left*) Immunoelectron microscopic localization of LTH in normal rats. Prolactin is localized in Golgi saccules (*G*) and secretory granules (*arrows*). *N*, nucleus. Immunoelectron microscopy pre-embedding, ×6300

Fig. 48. (*lower left*) Same as in Fig. 46, but ×16000. Localization in cisternae of rough endoplasmic reticulum (*RER*)

Fig. 47. (*upper rigght*) Same as in Fig. 46, but ×31000. Localization in perinuclear spaces (*PN*)

Fig. 49. (*lower right*) Immunoelectron microscopic localization of LTH exclusively in secretory granules (*arrows*). *N*, nucleus. Post-embedding, ×30000

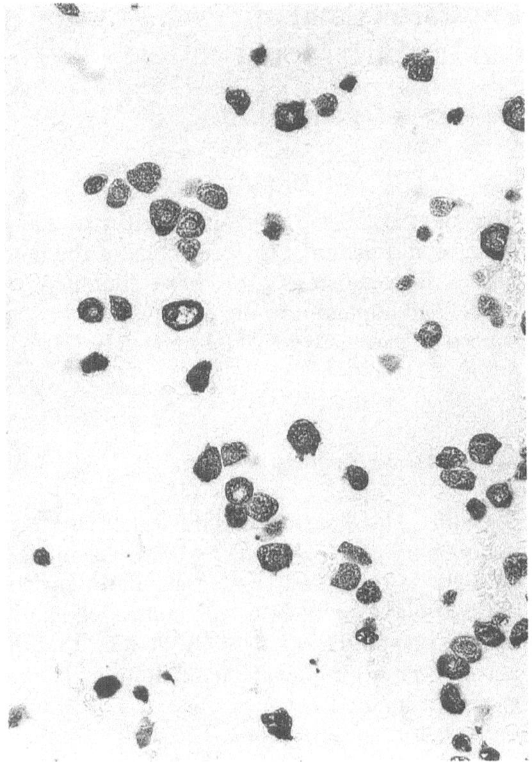

Fig. 50. The LH cells in the pars distalis are round or ovoid and contain LH evenly distributed in the cytoplasm. Peroxidase-labeled antibody method, ×300

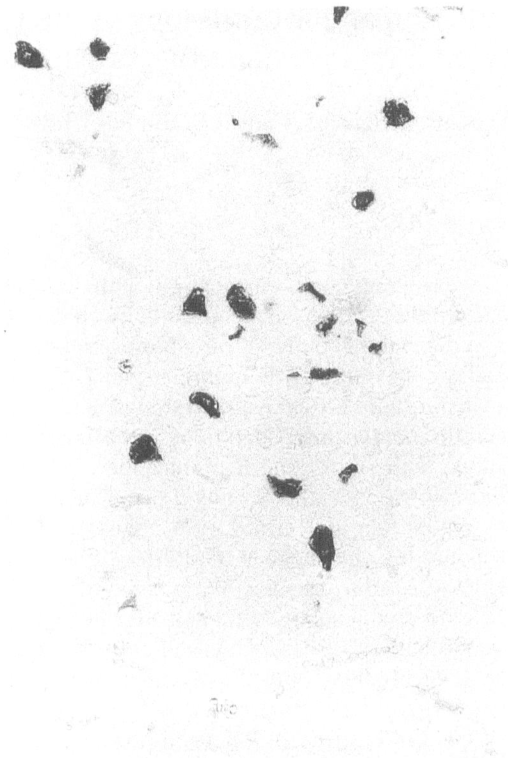

Fig. 51. The TSH cells in the pars distalis are smaller than LH cells and have an angular shape. Peroxidase-labeled antibody method, ×300

References

Farquhar M (1971) Processing of secretory products by cells of the anterior pituitary gland. In: Memoirs of the Society for Endocrinology, 19. Subcellular organization and function in endocrine tissue. Cambridge University Press, London, pp 79–124

Kawarai Y (1981) Cell identification in rat anterior pituitary with the comparative light- and electron microscopic immunohistochemical technique on adjacent thin and thick sections. Acta Histochem Cytochem 14:376–382

Moriarty GC (1973) Adenohypophysis: ultrastructural cytochemistry. A review. J Histochem Cytochem 21:855–894

Nakane PK (1968) Simultaneous localization of multiple tissue antigens using the peroxidase-labeled antibody method: a study of pituitary glands of the rat. J Histochem Cytochem 16:557–560

Nakane PK (1970) Classifications of anterior pituitary cell types with immunoenzyme histochemistry. J Histochem Cytochem 18:9–20

Nakane PK (1975) Recent progress in the peroxidase-labeled antibody method. Ann N Y Acad Sci 254:203–211

Osamura RY, Komatsu N, Nakahashi E, Watanabe K (1980) Light and electron microscopical combined staining by immunohistochemical and enzyme histochemical methods using rat prolactin-secreting pituitary tumours. Histochem J 12:371–379

Osamura RY, Komatsu N, Izumi S, Yoshimura S, Murakoshi M, Watanabe K (1981) Pre-embedding immunoelectron microscopy by peroxidase-labeled antibody method. Applications to endocrinology. Acta Histochem Cytochem 14: 383–390

Rodin JAG (1974) Histology, a text and atlas. Oxford University Press, New York, pp 427–439

Function and Morphology of the Rat Pituitary Gland, Combined Investigations by Means of an In Vitro Model

Annamaria Baiocco, Claude E. Boujon, Gilberto E. Bestetti, and Giovanni L. Rossi

Introduction

The combination of biochemical with morphological investigations can substantially contribute to reducing the number of laboratory animals used for the study of the pituitary gland. Several in vitro systems are available to study the pituitary secretion under basal conditions and after stimulation with different hypothalamic releasing factors (Arimura and Schally 1975; Mitsuma et al. 1990; Vale and Grant 1975). However, the structure of the incubated pituitary gland has seldom been investigated. Farquhar et al. (1975) reported that in hemipituitary glands "the cellular fine structure was reasonably well preserved up to 1 h of incubation," but "with longer incubation times there was progressive deterioration in the condition of the tissue, in that the center of the pieces showed increasing nuclear pyknosis, autophagy, and cell death." Perez and Hymer (1990) described a tissue slicing method for the study of the function and position of somatotrophs in the rat pituitary gland and reported that, 1 h after gyrotory incubation, by light microscopy the tissue had good cell integrity, and by ultrastructural study the characteristics of the adenohypophyseal cells were maintained. They also examined the basal growth hormone (GH) secretion from pituitary slices placed in gyrotory incubation for three consecutive 20-min periods and stated that "in preliminary experiments GHRH had no effect on GH release from tissue placed in rotary incubation."

The morphological evaluation of the in vitro treated pituitary tissue is, among other factors, essential to confirm the biochemical results, because only data obtained from well-preserved tissue are reliable. Moreover, the use of the same gland for both biochemical and morphological studies (a) allows morphofunctional correlations, (b) reduces the number of animals per experiment, and (c) avoids extrapolation of results from different groups. Finally, the use of hemipituitary glands instead of dispersed cells allows the study of different cell types in their natural anatomical environment.

Boujon et al. (1987) developed an in vitro model for morphofunctional investigations of the mediobasal hypothalamus. We have modified this model and applied it to the investigation of some aspects of various types of pituitary cells (Baiocco et al. 1994).

Materials and Methods

Animals. The study was undertaken on eight male albino rats (360 ± 32.1 g body weight). The animals were housed under standard environmental conditions at 22°C with controlled lighting (on at 0600 hours, off at 1800). Standard rat diet and tap water were available ad libitum. The rats were decapitated between 0800 and 1030 hours under halothane anesthesia. The skull was opened and the pituitary gland rapidly removed and bisected in the sagittal plane under a stereomicroscope (5×), without removing the neurohypophysis. Pilot experiments with entire or quartered pituitary glands gave unsatisfactory results.

Incubation. The in vitro system is similar to that previously described by Boujon et al. (1987), with some modifications. Briefly, a gas bottle containing 95% O_2 and 5% CO_2 connected through vinyl tubes to two massflowmeters (model 5850 TR; Brooks Instrument, Veenendaal, The Netherlands) and coupled with two massflow controllers and reading systems (model 5876; Brooks) conveyed 4 ml/min gas mixture through vinyl tubes into two humidification bottles. From each bottle a silicon capillary tube conveyed the gas to an incubation chamber. After bubbling through the medium the gas exited the incubation chambers through two needle segments mounted on the stopper. We used an incubation and a reserve chamber, each connected to the massflow controller and to the reading system. The two chambers were supported by an acrylic rack mounted in a shaker water bath at 37°C and 140 oscillations per min. Each chamber contained 0.4 ml Locke's medium. The basal medium had the following composition: 2 m*M* HEPES, 154 m*M* NaCl, 5.6 m*M* KCl, 1 m*M* $MgCl_2$, 6 m*M* $NaHCO_3$, 10 m*M* glucose, 1.25 m*M* $CaCl_2$, and 2×10^{-2} mm bacitracin (Sigma, St. Louis, MO, USA). Four pituitary glands were incubated in basal medium alone and four stimulated with 3 ng/ml thyroid-releasing hormone (TRH; Bachem, Bubendorf, Switzerland). The two pituitary halves of each rat were incubated together in the same chamber, according to the following schema: two 10-min washings and one 20-min preincubation in basal medium, and two 20-min incubations either in basal medium alone or with added TRH. At the end of each incubation period the medium was collected in tubes and frozen at −80°C. The tubes were previously washed in Tween 20 diluted 1:20 in distilled water and then rinsed several times in distilled water.

Biochemical Studies. The TSH released into the medium during the two incubation periods was quantified by double-antibody radioimmunoassay, using a commercial kit (Repromed, Hamburg, Germany). The thyrotropin (TSH) standard used was NIADDK-r-TSH-RP-2. Briefly, 200 µl medium diluted 1:2 with PBS-BSA buffer was incubated for 24 h at 4°C with rabbit antirat TSH diluted 1:8000 in PBS-BSA. Then ^{125}I-labeled rat TSH (total activity 10 000 cpm/100 µl) was added and incubated for 24 h at 4°C. Incubation for 15 min at room temperature with goat antirabbit antiserum diluted 1:50 in phosphate buffer followed. The separation of bound from free TSH was achieved by centrifugation for 15 min at 2000 *g*. All samples were assayed in duplicate. The counting time was 1 min.

Tissue Processing. At the end of the incubation the two pituitary halves were fixed in 2% glutaraldehyde/1.5% paraformaldehyde in phosphate buffer (pH 7.4). After rinsing in S-collidine buffer, a 0.3 mm frontal slice was cut from each pituitary half at the level of its maximal height (Pitton et al. 1987). Subsequently, one slice from each hemipituitary was postfixed in 2% osmium tetroxide (pH 7.4) for 2 h; the other was not postfixed and used for immunocytochemistry. All specimens were embedded in Spurr's low viscosity medium, and semithin sections were cut. The sections from postfixed slices were stained by toluidine blue. Thin sections of both kinds of specimens were then cut for electron microscopy.

Immunocytochemistry. The immunocytochemical labeling of GH, prolactin, adrenocorticotropin, TSH, follicle-stimulating hormone, and luteinizing hormone was performed on semithin sections as described by Bestetti et al. (1987). Briefly, after etching in Mayor and acetic acid (1:7) inhibition of the endogenous phosphatase, the sections were incubated with rabbit anti-human GH (Dako, Santa Barbara, CA, USA), antihuman PRL (Dako), anti-human adrenocorticotropin (Dako), anti-human TSH (Dako), anti-bovine follicle-stimulating hormone (UCB-Bioproducts, Brussels, Belgium), and anti-human luteinizing hormone (Dako) antisera, all diluted 1:200 in PBS, and goat anti-rabbit IgG labeled with alkaline phosphatase (Sigma, St. Louis, MO, USA), diluted 1:100 in acetate buffer. The sections were finally washed in PBS-Tween 20 (1:200). To assay the immunoreaction specificity we either omitted the primary antisera or preabsorbed it with specific purified rat hormones (4 pg/100 µl; UCB-Bioproducts) according to the protocol of Lloyd and Childs (1988).

Electron Microscopy. Thin sections from postfixed specimens were counterstained with uranyl acetate and lead citrate. To demonstrate TSH thin sections were cut from not postfixed specimens and stained for immunocytochemistry as described by Bestetti et al. (1987), using rabbit anti-human TSH (Dako) diluted 1:200 and goat anti-rabbit IgG conjugated to 15 nm colloidal gold particles (Jansen Life Science Products, Beerse, Belgium) diluted 1:40 in PBS-Tween 20 (1:200). No etching was performed.

Statistics. Group mean and standard error were calculated. The significance of differences between groups was tested by the Kruskall-Wallis *H* test (Sachs 1974).

Results

Biochemistry. The amounts of TSH released during the two incubation periods in basal conditions were similar (Fig. 52). The addition of 3 ng/ml TRH into the medium resulted in a markedly increased TSH release during the second incubation period (Fig. 52).

Morphology. By conventional light microscopy of semithin sections, the incubated tissue was well

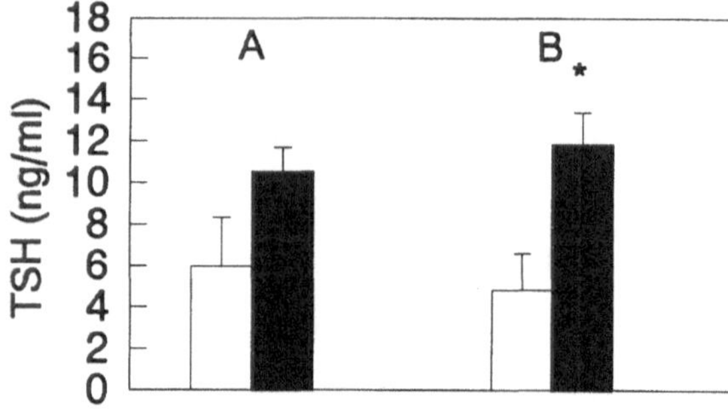

Fig. 52. TSH release during incubation 1 (*A*) and 2 (*B*) in basal medium (*empty bars*) and after stimulation with TRH at a dose of 3 ng/ml medium (*solid bars*). $^{*}p < 0.05$. (From Baiocco et al. 1994)

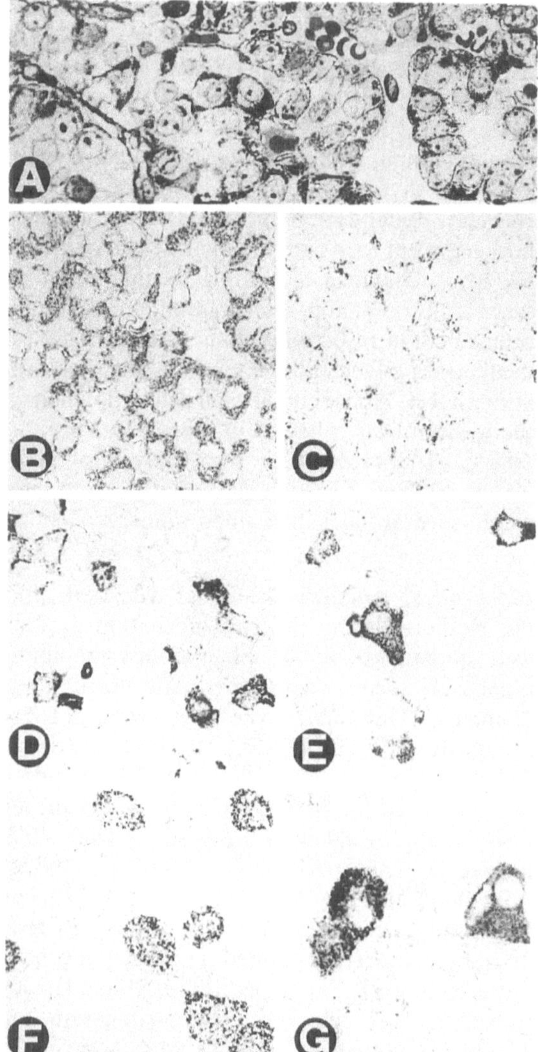

Fig. 53. Conventional (**A**) and immunocytochemical (**B–G**) light microscopy of pituitary tissue after incubation. Toluidine blue staining (**A**). Anti-GH (**B**), -PRL (**C**), -ACTH (**D**), -TSH (**E**), -FSH (**F**), and -LH (**G**) alkaline phosphatase method. ×530. (From Baiocco et al. 1994)

preserved at the periphery and in the center of the pituitary halves. (Fig. 53A). There was no sign of cell degeneration or necrosis. The nuclei were normal, the nucleoli clearly visible, and the cytoplasm was granulated. By light microscopical immunocytochemistry, somatotrophs, lactotrophs, corticotrophs, thyrotrophs, and gonadotrophs could be labeled with their corresponding anti-hormones (Fig. 53B–G). By conventional electron microscopy, the incubated tissue had a normal structure. The various pituitary cells (Fig. 54A–D) presented their typical features (Rappay 1984). The nuclear and cellular membranes as well as all intracytoplasmatic organelles were well preserved. By immunocytochemical electron microscopy the secretory granules of the thyrotrophs could be labeled for TSH (Fig. 54E).

Discussion

The functional data indicate that in our model the basal TSH secretion was stable after 40 min and remained constant during the following 40 min. The dose of 3 ng/ml TRH used for thyrotroph stimulation is within the range of the physiological TRH concentration in the pituitary portal blood (Ching and Utiger 1983; De Greef and Visser 1981; Fink et al. 1982; Guillaume et al. 1986; Sheward et al. 1983). Because of high individual variations the difference between secretion in basal condition and under TRH stimulation was not significant during the first incubation period. Our results show that the isolated pituitary gland can respond to a physiological stimulus. To ensure good tissue preservation until the end of the in vitro treatment we used pituitary halves. In fact, preliminary experiments showed that with entire pituitary glands nuclear pyknosis and cytoplasm shrinkage occurred in the central tissue portions, probably because the diffusion of medium and oxygen is confined to the gland periphery. Quartered glands were also useless because gas bubbles caused the specimens to float on the fluid surface inducing hypoxia and necrosis of the superficial cell layers. The removal of neurohypophysis before incubation was omitted to avoid the consequent mechanical damage.

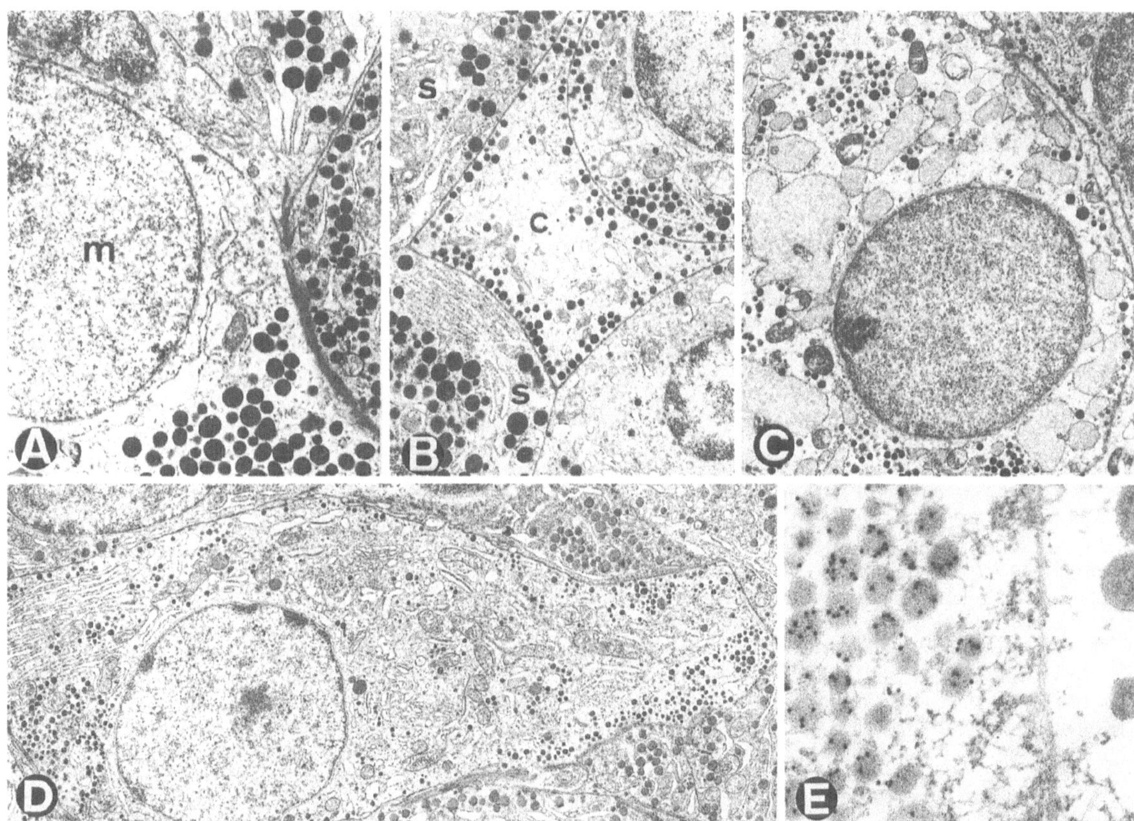

Fig. 54. Conventional (**A–D**) and immunocytochemical (**E**) electron microscopy of pituitary tissue after incubation. Mammotroph (**A**, *m* ×6600, somatotroph (**B**, *s*) and corticotroph (**B**, *c*, ×6600), gonadotroph (**C**, ×6600), and thyrotroph (**D**, ×4500). Thyrotroph with secretory granules labeled by anti-TSH (colloidal gold method, **E**, ×30000). (From Baiocco et al. 1994)

Farquhar et al. (1975) reported that pituitary dissection may cause cell death because of the discharged intracellular proteases on the surface of the cut. These proteases could again catabolize the hormones released into the medium. Therefore bacitracin, a protease inhibitor, was added to the medium.

To preserve the incubated tissue, pH must be close to neutrality (Paul 1970). Medium composition, temperature, and gas flow can influence pH. We used a HEPES-buffered Locke's medium according to Boujon et al. (1987). This medium, maintained at 37°C with a gas flow of 4 ml/min per 0.4 ml, has a pH of about 7. Our morphological results demonstrate that the present model is suitable for conventional light and electron microscopical studies on various cell types in the isolated pituitary gland. Moreover, by means of immunocytochemistry we could label immunoreactive cells and granules. Thus, the tissue could also be used for densitometrical evaluations of the hormone content in single pituitary cells. Since the results of both functional and morphological investigations were satisfactory, we propose our in vitro model to be used for combined studies which would permit reduction of the number of animals needed for an experiment, avoid the extrapolation of results from different groups, and replace an in vivo by an in vitro experiment.

Acknowledgments. This work was supported by the Swiss Federal Veterinary Office grant no. 014.89.4 to G.E:B. and in part by the Swiss National Research Foundation grant no. 3-28273.90 to G.L.R. and G.E.B. We thank Ms. U. Forster, Mr. S. Grimm, and Mr. G. DiLullo for skillful technical assistance. We thank also Prof.

Wanner for the permission to publish the figures that are copyrighted by the Schweizer Archiv for Tierheilkunde.

References

Arimura A, Schally AV (1975) Methods for estimating the biologic activity of the luteinizing hormone- and follicle stimulating hormone-releasing hormone. In: O'Malley BW, Harriman JG (eds) Methods in enzymology, vol 37. Academic, New York, pp 233–238

Baiocco A, Boujon CE, Bestetti GE, Rossi GL (1994) An "in vitro" model for combined functional and morphological investigations on the rat pituitary gland. Schweiz Arch Tierheilkd 136:242–247

Bestetti GE, Reymond MJ, Perrin IV, Kniel PC, Lemarchand-Béraud T, Rossi GL (1987) Thyroid and pituitary secretory disorders in streptozotocin-diabetic rats are associated with severe structural changes of these glands. Virchows Arch [B] 53:69–78

Boujon CE, Bestetti GE, Reymond MJ, Rossi GL (1987) A model for combined morphological and functional investigations on the isolated mediobasal rat hypothalamus. Neuroendocrinology 45:311–317

Ching MCH, Utiger RD (1983) Hypothalamic portal blood immunoreactive TRH in the rat: lack of effect of hypothyroidism and thyroid hormone treatment. J Endocrinol Invest 6:347–352

De Greef WJ, Visser TJ (1981) Evidence for the involvement of hypothalmic dopamine and thyrotrophin-releasing hormone in suckling-induced release of prolactin. J Endocrinol 91:213–223

Farquhar MG, Skutelsky EH, Hopkins CR (1975) Structure and function of the anterior pituitary and dispersed pituitary cells. In "vitro" studies. In: Tixier-Vidal A, Farquhar MG (eds) The anterior pituitary. Academic, New York, pp 106–107

Fink G, Koch Y, Ben Aroya N (1982) Release of thyrotropin releasing hormone into hypophysial portal blood is high relative to other neuropeptides and may be related to prolactin secretion. Brain Res 243:186–189

Guillaume V, Oakif LH, Dutour A, Castanas E, Oliver C (1986) Immunoreactive TRH and TRH-OH in rat hypophysial portal blood. In: Medereiros-Neto G, Gaitan E (eds) Frontiers of thyroidology. Plenum, New York, pp 295–298

Lloyd JM, Childs GV (1988) Differential storage and release of luteinizing hormone and follicle-releasing hormone from individual gonadotropes separated by centrifugal elutriation. Endocrinology 122:1282–1290

Mayor HD, Hampton JC, Rosario B (1961) A simple method for removing the resin from epoxy-embedded tissue. J Bioph Biochem Cytol 9:909–910

Mitsuma T, Hirooka Y, Kimura M, Nogimori T (1990) Failure to demonstrate the effect of various prepro TRH fragments on TSH and PRL release from rat pituitary "in vitro". Endocrinol Exp 24:333–339

Paul J (1970) The cell and its environment. In: Paul J (ed) Cell and tissue culture. Livingstone, Edinburgh, p 55

Perez FM, Hymer WC (1990) A new tissue-slicing method for the study of function and position of somatotrophs contained within the male rat pituitary gland. Endocrinology 127: 1877–1886

Pitton I, Bestetti GE, Rossi GL (1987) The changes in the hypothalamo-pituitary-gonadal axis of streptozotocin-treated male rats depend from age at diabetes onset. Andrologia 19:464–473

Rappay G (1984) Ultrastructural features of adrenocortical and hypophyseal cells in culture. In: Motta PM (ed) Ultrastructure of endocrine cells and tissue. Nijhoff, Boston, p 206

Sachs L (1974) Angewandte Statistik. Springer, Berlin Heidelberg New York

Sheward WJ, Harmar AJ, Fraser HM, Fink G (1983) Thyrotropin releasing hormone in rat pituitary stalk blood and hypothalamus: studies with high performance liquid chromatography. Endocrinology 113:1865–1869

Vale W, Grant G (1975) In "vitro" pituitary hormone secretion assay for hypophysiotropic substances. In: O'Malley BW, Harriman JG (eds) Methods in enzymology, vol 37. Academic, New York, pp 82–93

Modern Approaches to Classification of Pituitary Tumors in Human Subjects and Animals

L. Stefaneanu and K. Kovacs

Normal Pituitary

Development and Anatomy. The adenohypophysis originates in a diverticulum of stomodeal ectoderm called Rathke's pouch. A ventral evagination of diencephalon-saccus infundibuli contacts Rathke's pouch and gives rise to the neurohypophysis. The adenohypophysis has an anterior lobe, pars intermedia, and pars tuberalis. The anterior lobe (pars distalis, pars glandularis) is composed mainly of hormone-producing cells. The chronologic appearance of different cell types during intrauterine development has been established by immunocytochemistry (Setalo and Nakane 1976; Chatelain et al. 1979; Osamura and Watanabe 1985). In man and rodents the first detected are adrenocorticotropin (ACTH) immunoreactive cells and growth hormone (GH) immunoreactive cells (5–18 weeks and 16 days of gestation, respectively) followed by cells containing glycoprotein hormones such as thyrotropin (TSH), follicle-stimulating hormone (FSH), and luteinizing hormone (LH; 12 weeks and 17–18 days, respectively). The last to appear are prolactin (PRL) immunoreactive cells; their number increases markedly at term in man and postnatally in the rat.

The intermediate lobe in humans is rudimental, being represented by a few follicles. Their cavities are the vestigial lumen of Rathke's pouch. In rodents the intermediate lobe is well developed and is separated from the anterior lobe by a cleft, the residual cavity of Rathke's pouch. It is formed by cells immunoreactive for ACTH and other proopiomelanocortin (POMC) derived peptides that are detected in the rat during gestation at day 17.

The pars tuberalis is formed by clusters of glycoprotein hormone-containing cells. In the human pituitary, islets of squamous cells are present as well.

The neurohypophysis consists of the median eminence, hypophysial stalk and posterior lobe. The hypophysial stalk is composed mainly of axons and portal vessels. The axons originate in magnocellular neurons of supraoptic and paraventricular nuclei of the hypothalamus that transport vasopressin and oxytocin to the posterior lobe. The portal vessels transport the hypothalamic releasing and inhibiting hormones to the adenohypophysis.

Morphology: Adenohypophysis. On horizontal cross-section the anterior lobe of human adenohypophysis is divided in a central mucoid wedge and two lateral wings, delineated by a thin fibrous trabecula. The somatotrophs are located mainly in the lateral wings, and the corticotrophs and thyrotrophs in the mucoid wedge. The lactotrophs and gonadotrophs are scattered throughout the gland. The hormone-containing cells are dispersed in acini surrounded by a basement membrane (Kovacs and Horvath 1986).

In rodents the glandular cells have no clear-cut preference for a certain area of anterior lobe (Poole and Kornegay 1982), and no acinar structures are found. The groups of cells are separated by a rich fibrovascular network. The different cell types of the adenohypophysis are characterized based on hormone content and ultrastructural features (Fig. 55; Kurosumi 1968; Horvath and Kovacs 1988).

Somatotrophs (GH cells) are acidophilic and are the predominant cell type (40%–50%; Fig. 56). Electron microscopy reveals densely granulated cells with secretory granules ranging in diameter between 300 and 400 nm in rat and mouse and up to 500 nm in man. A minority of cells possess

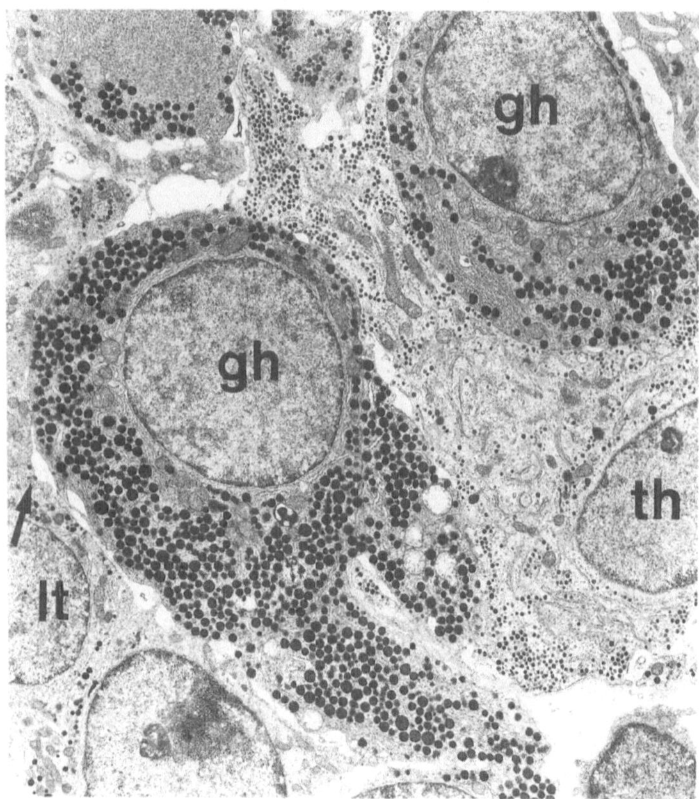

Fig. 55. Normal rat anterior lobe depicting somatotroph (*gh*), a thyrotroph (*th*), and a lactotroph (*lt*) with an extruded secretory granule (*arrow*). TEM, ×4500

small secretory granules of 150 nm. GH secretion is under the hypothalamic control. Growth hormone releasing hormone (GRH) via portal vessels stimulates GH release, while somatostatin (SRIF) has the opposite effect.

Lactotrophs (PRL cells, mammotrophs) in humans vary in number according to age, sex, parity, and hormonal status. In rodents the lactotrophs are more numerous in females (45%) than in males (24%; Fig. 57; Sasaki and Iwama 1988). During pregnancy in women a gradual, diffuse lactotroph hyperplasia occurs that is easily identified by light microscopy (Stefaneanu et al. 1992a) while in rats the diffuse increase in number of lactotrophs is mild. In most lactotrophs PRL immunostaining shows a paranuclear globular pattern corresponding to the Golgi apparatus rich in forming secretory granules. In humans the secretory granules are rather small (about 150–200 nm) while in rodents they are markedly pleomorphic, measuring up to 800 nm. The extrusion of secretory granules into the intercellular space, the hallmark of human lactotrophs, occurs in rat and mouse, not only in this cell type but in somatotrophs as well. Under sustained GRH stimulation the frequency of extruded granules increases in somatotrophs (Stefaneanu et al. 1993). In humans rare densely granulated lactotrophs with secretory granules of 250–450 nm are identified. In rodents a second type of lactotroph with small secretory granules (200 nm) is present, especially in males.

PRL secretion is inhibited by dopamine produced by the hypothalamus. As PRL-releasing factors, thyrotropin-releasing hormone (TRH), vasoactive intestinal polypeptide (VIP), angiotensin II, and neurotensin are proposed. Among peripheral hormones estrogen is a powerful stimulator of PRL production.

Mammosomatotrophs, bihormonal cells producing GH and PRL, have been identified in a small percentage by different techniques, such as reverse hemolytic plaque assay, immunocytochemistry at the light and electron microscopic level and in situ hybridization combined with immunocytochemistry (Frawley and Boockfor 1991).

Corticotrophs (ACTH cells) are basophilic cells, immunoreactive for POMC derived peptides, such as ACTH, melanocyte-stimulating hormones

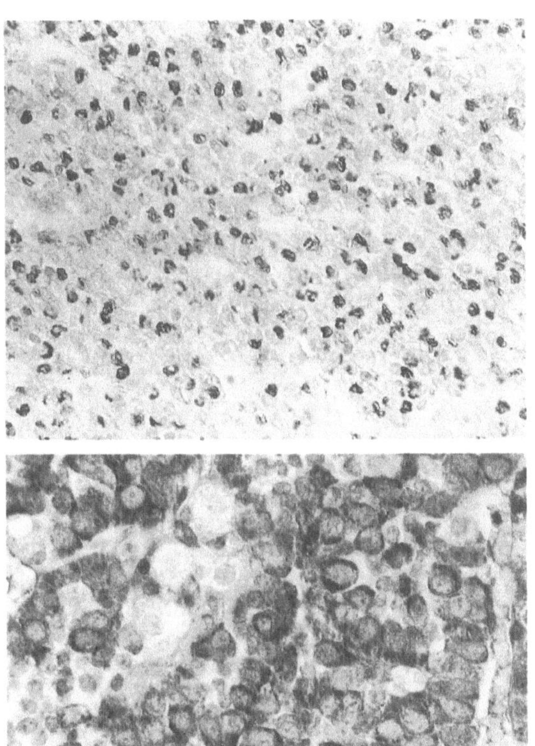

Fig. 56. (*above*) Immunostaining for GH indicates that GH cells are predominant in the pituitary of a rat. ×500

Fig. 57. (*below*) In a female rat pituitary, the PRL cells are numerous and exhibit the characteristic juxtanuclear globular immunoreactivity. ×500

(MSH), β-lipotropin, and β-endorphin. In humans the corticotrophs are ovoid or spherical, PAS positive, and contain a paranuclear vacuole that corresponds to phagolysosome at the ultrastructural level. The secretory granules are round, drop- or heart-shaped, and measure around 300 nm. The presence of bundles of type I microfilaments is characteristic for human corticotrophs. In rodents the corticotrophs have a stellate contour (Fig. 58) and small secretory granules (150–200 nm). No cytokeratin filaments are present in their cytoplasm. ACTH secretion is stimulated by hypothalamic corticotropin-releasing factor (CRF). Glucocorticoids exert an inhibitory effect. In man excessive glucocorticoids inhibit the corticotrophs that become filled with type 1 filaments known as Crooke's hyaline change. Crooke's cells do not develop in rodents in such conditions.

Thyrotrophs (TSH cells) in humans and rodents, are basophilic, markedly angular, and account for about 5% of the cells (Fig. 59). They contain spherical euchromatic nuclei and small secretory granules (150–200 nm). TSH secretion is stimulated by TRH. Thyroid hormones and glucocorticoids play an inhibitory role. Chronic hypothyroidism or thyroidectomy induces the formation of "thyroidectomy cells," the stimulated thyrotrophs.

Gonadotrophs (FSH/LH cells) are basophilic cells and are easily identified in rodents with PAS staining. Most gonadotrophs are bihormonal cells immunoreactive for FSH and LH (Fig. 60). The number of gonadotrophs varies depending on sex, age, and hormonal status. In humans the secretory granules are small (200 nm) or large (300–600 nm), the latter being predominant in women. In rodents gonadotrophs with predominant, large secretory granules of 450–700 nm prevail in males, and others with small secretory granules of 200 nm are more numerous in females (Childs 1984). Gonadotropin-releasing hormone (GnRH) is considered to stimulate both FSH and LH release. Gonadal steroids modulate the response of gonadotrophs to GnRH. Hypogonadism or gonadectomy induces the presence of so-called "gonadectomy cells," the stimulated gonadotrophs in which the rough endoplasmic reticulum (RER) enlarges and fuses to form a large cyst pushing the nucleus to the periphery (signet ring cells).

Folliculostellate cells contain no adenohypophysial hormones and are easily identified by immunocytochemistry for S-100 protein (Fig. 61). They are slender cells with long cellular processes intermingled with hormone-producing cells. It is suggested that they play a supporting, phagocytic, paracrine, and/or immunologic role (Marin et al. 1991).

Melanotrophs (intermediate lobe corticotrophs) are present in the distinct intermediate lobe of the rodent pituitary. In these cells the POMC-derived ACTH is further cleaved in α-MSH and corticotropin-like intermediate lobe peptide (CLIP). Melanotrophs are inhibited by dopamine. α-MSH secretion is stimulated by estrogen (Ellerkman et al. 1992).

In addition to the classical hormones, increasing evidence indicates that the adenohypophysial cells produce many biologically active peptides,

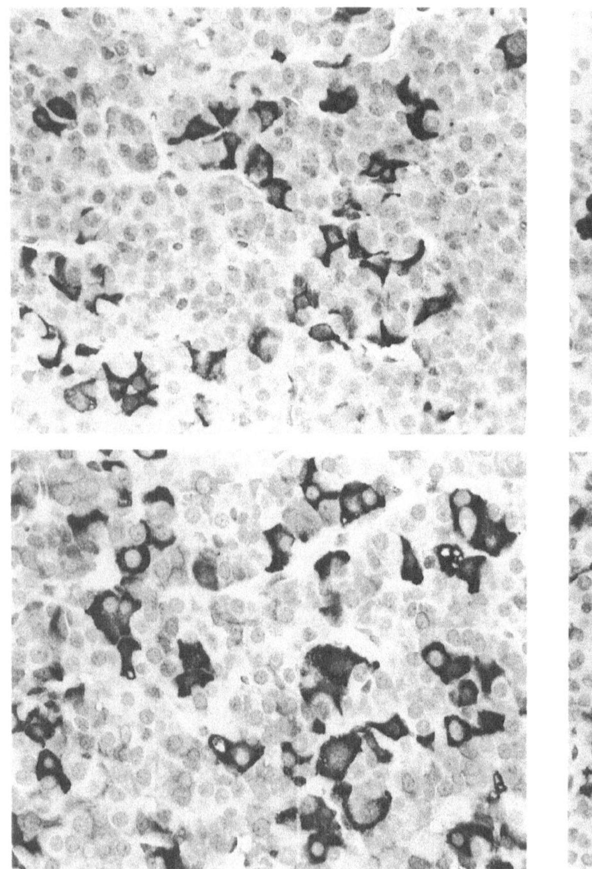

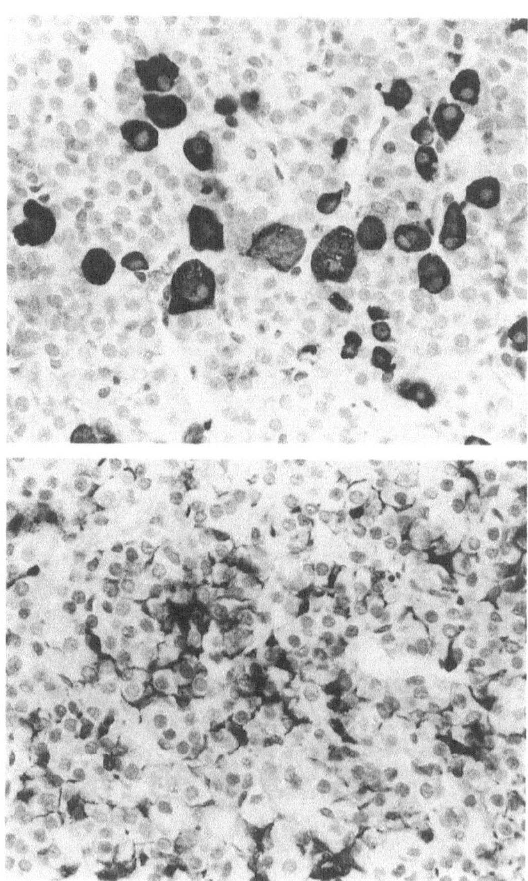

Fig. 58. (*upper left*) Rat anterior lobe contains ACTH immunoreactive cells with an angular contour. ×500

Fig. 59. (*lower left*) Thyrotrophs are immunoreative for TSH and have an angular shape in rat pituitary. ×500

Fig. 60. (*upper right*) Gonadotrophs immunoreactive for LH are large, ovoid cells in rat pituitary. ×500

Fig. 61. (*lower right*) Folliculostellate cells with long, slender cytoplasmic processes among hormone-producing cells, immunoreactive for S-100 protein. ×500

including growth factors, cytokines, and other hormones (Houben and Denef 1990; Lloyd 1993). Recent studies using mainly mRNA detection techniques also demonstrate that the pituitary produces some of its own hypothalamic releasing and inhibiting hormones, such as GRH, CRF, TRH, GnRH, VIP, and SRIF (Nagy et al. 1988; Pagesy et al. 1989, 1992; Peillon et al. 1989; Levy and Lightman 1992, 1993). There is evidence that some of these peptides have a paracrine effect; however, the precise role of most of them is obscure.

Human Pituitary Tumors

Pituitary adenomas are benign epithelial neoplasms originating in and composed of adenohypophysial cells. In the human pituitary, they occur in 6%–22% of unselected adult autopsies and represent approximately 10%–15% of intracranial tumors.

The present classification is based on histologic and ultrastructural features as well as hormone content, as assessed by immunocytochemistry and clinical correlations (Kovacs and Horvath 1986; Table 2). Molecular pathology will obviously have a major impact on this classification. Information emerging from in situ hybridization studies shows that the presently prevailing

Table 2. Frequency of human pituitary adenomas (based on unselected surgical material of 1910 cases)

Adenoma Type	Percentage
GH cell adenoma, densely granulated	7.2
GH cell adenoma, sparsely granulated	6.4
PRL cell adenoma, densely granulated	0.4
PRL cell adenoma, sparsely granulated	26.5
Mixed (GH cell - PRL cell) adenoma	3.7
Mammosomatotroph adenoma	1.3
Acidophil stem cell adenoma	1.7
Corticotroph adenoma	9.9
Silent "corticotroph" adenomas	5
Thyrotroph adenoma	1.0
Gonadotroph adenoma	9.3
Null cell adenoma	12.7
Oncocytoma	13.1
Unclassified adenoma	1.8

classification will be modified in the future (Jameson et al. 1987; Nagaya et al. 1990; McNicol et al. 1991; Uhlig et al. 1991; Li et al. 1993).

Somatotroph adenomas produce GH. In addition, they may produce PRL, α-subunit (α-SU) and/or TSH and are associated with acromegaly or gigantism. They are divided into two main types of tumors: densely granulated and sparsely granulated. The densely granulated somatotroph adenomas are acidophilic and PAS negative by light microscopy. Ultrastructural analysis reveals adenoma cells with well-developed RER and Golgi complexes and many randomly distributed secretory granules measuring 400–600 nm (Fig. 62).

Sparsely granulated somatotroph adenomas are chromophobic and PAS negative by histology. Electron microscopy is very characteristic. The RER is moderately developed, the Golgi complex is conspicuous, and several centrioles are noted. Secretory granules are sparse, irregular, randomly distributed, and measure 250 nm. A characteristic feature of this adenoma type is the so-called fibrous body consisting of aggregates of keratin positive type II microfilaments entrapping secretory granules, centrioles, mitochondria, and lysosomes (Fig. 63).

Lactotroph adenomas are associated with the galactorrhea-amenorrhea syndrome, infertility, and in men decreased libido and impotence. Currently they are rarely operated on because medical treatment with dopamine agonists such as bromocriptine not only ameliorates the clinical features and decreases blood PRL levels but also causes significant shrinkage of the tumors.

Lactotroph adenomas are divided into densely and sparsely granulated variants (Horvath and Kovacs 1988). The densely granulated tumors are very rare and are characterized by adenoma cells which contain many large, oval, spherical, or irregular secretory granules measuring 500–600 nm. The adenoma cells have well-developed RER and Golgi complexes, but the cytoplasmic organelles are overshadowed by the abundance of secretory granules. Another feature of these cells is exocytosis, the extrusion of secretory granules into the intercellular space.

Sparsely granulated lactotroph adenomas are the most frequently occurring adenoma type in the human pituitary. They are immunoreactive for PRL and contain no other hormones. Electron microscopy demonstrates very conspicuous RER, nebenkern formation, prominent Golgi areas, and irregular sparse secretory granules measuring 150–300 nm and exocytoses both on the capillary and lateral sides of the cells (Fig. 64). Lactotroph adenomas, primarily in women, are often microadenomas. However, they may reach a large size, primarily in men, invade surrounding tissues, cause local symptoms and lead to the patient's death.

Corticotroph adenomas produce ACTH and other POMC-derived peptides. These tumors are basophilic and PAS positive. In most cases they are monohormonal but rarely contain α-SU and LH. The tumors are often microadenomas, densely granulated tumors with well-developed RER, Golgi complexes, and numerous secretory granules measuring 200–450 nm. The tumor cells contain a few bundles of type I filaments (Fig. 65). There are several variants of corticotroph adenomas. One is the adenoma with Nelson's syndrome. In these tumors the microfilaments are missing. The sparsely granulated type is usually macroadenoma and has a more rapid growth rate. The Crooke's cell adenoma is full of bundles of keratin-positive microfilaments. Contrary to generally held views, Crooke's hyaline can be excessive in some adenomas. These adenomas are probably not autonomous, but the clinical correlations require further study.

Thyrotroph adenomas may be associated with hypo-, eu-, or hyperthyroidism. They are rare, chromophobic tumors possessing a few or several small cytoplasmic PAS positive globules. The presence of TSH is demonstrated by immunocytochemistry. However, some adenomas show no TSH immunoreactivity. Electron micro-

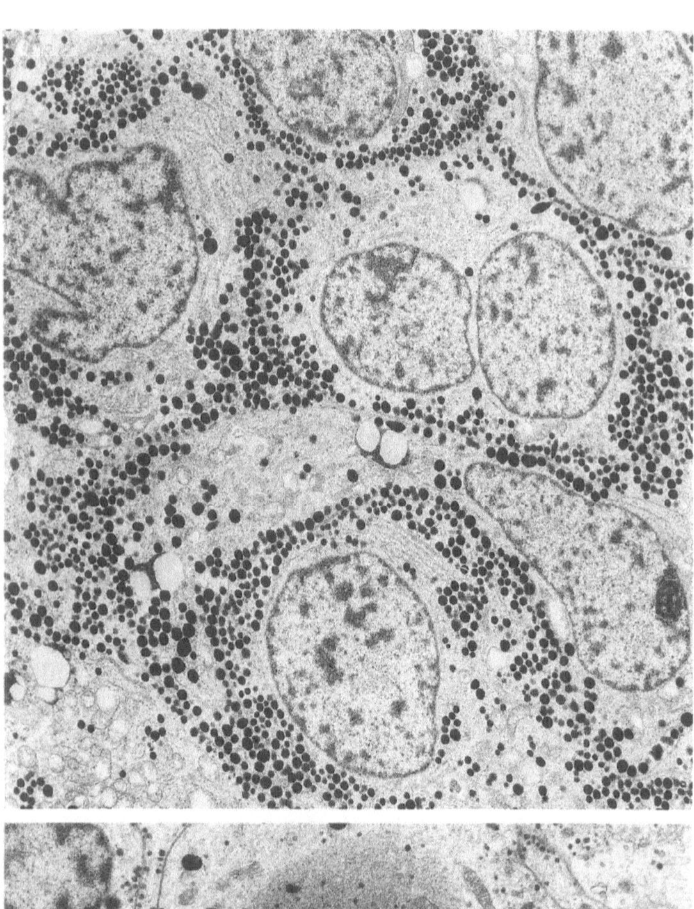

Fig. 62. Human densely granulated somatotroph adenoma is composed of cells with many secretory granules measuring about 500 nm. TEM, ×4500

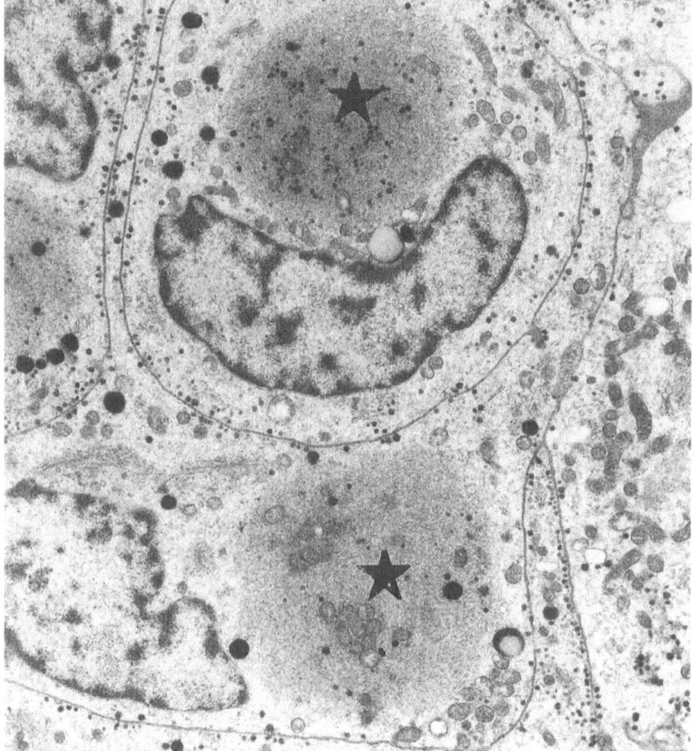

Fig. 63. Human sparsely granulated adenoma contains paranuclear fibrous bodies (*stars*) with diagnostic significance. TEM, ×7000

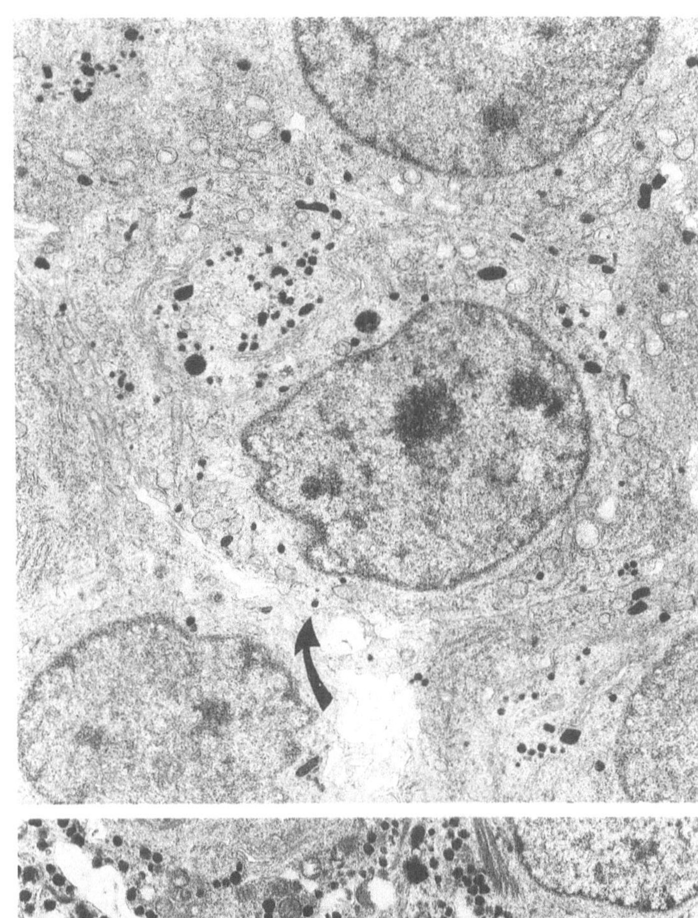

Fig. 64. Human sparsely granulated lactotroph adenoma with prominent Golgi apparatus forming secretory granules. An extruded granule (*arrow*) is depicted, as well. TEM, ×8000

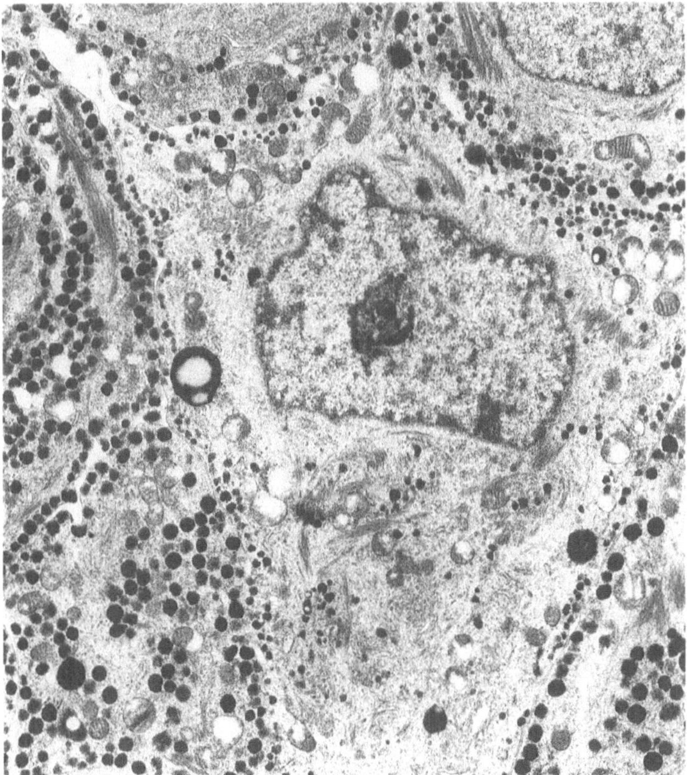

Fig. 65. Human corticotroph adenoma. The adenoma cells are rich in secretory granules and contain bundles of filaments. TEM, ×7500

scopy reveals oval, elongated tumor cells with moderately developed RER and Golgi apparatus and a few small secretory granules lining up under the cell membrane and measuring 100–200 nm.

Null cell adenomas are not associated with hormone excess. These tumors are either immunonegative for adenohypophysial hormones or contain a few to several cells exhibiting immunoreactivity, most frequently for α-SU, FSH, and LH, less frequently for TSH, GH, and PRL, and exceptionally for ACTH. Electron microscopy reveals cells in which RER and Golgi complexes are poorly represented. A few randomly distributed small secretory granules are always noticeable (Fig. 66).

Oncocytoma is a variant of null cell adenoma which contains a large number of mitochondria. They can be so numerous as to fill the entire cytoplasm and obscure other cytoplasmic constituents (Fig. 67). Neither clinically, immunocytochemically, in vitro, nor by in situ hybridization is there a difference between null cell and oncocytic adenomas. The cause of oncocytic transformation is not known. Oncocytes and oncocytic tumors occur in several other organs, such as thyroid and parathyroid.

Gonadotroph adenomas are clinically nonfunctioning; however, serum FSH and LH levels may be elevated, especially in men. They contain FSH and/or LH and α-SU immunoreactivity in more than 25% of the cells. Electron microscopy shows a sexual dichotomy (Horvath and Kovacs 1984). Male gonadotroph adenomas resemble null cell adenomas while female gonadotroph adenomas show a characteristic feature, the so-called honeycomb Golgi apparatus – this occurs in approximately 80% of cases and is of diagnostic significance. There is an overlap between null cell adenomas and gonadotroph adenomas by immunocytochemistry and electron microscopy. This suggests that perhaps almost all tumors arise in gonadotrophs and represent only one tumor type. Alternatively, we favor the view that these tumors arise in precursor cells which can undergo uni- or multidirectional differentiation and produce various hormones, most often FSH and α-SU, less frequently other hormones (Kovacs et al. 1990). The results of in situ hybridization studies are in accordance with the latter theory, showing that these tumors most frequently express the glycoprotein hormone genes but in some cases other hormones, such as TSH, PRL, and ACTH (Lloyd et al. 1991).

This description shows that all known pituitary hormones can be produced by pituitary adenomas, and every known adenohypophysial cell type can be present in adenomas. Many pituitary tumors closely resemble their nontumorous counterparts. There are tumors, however, which have no nontumorous counterparts, although null cells and oncocytes have been described in the normal human pituitary.

There are four more entities which should be discussed in addition to the cell types discussed in this chapter: plurihormonal adenomas, silent adenomas, invasive adenomas, and adenohypophysial carcinomas. Plurihormonal pituitary adenomas are intriguing neoplasms. Previously it was thought that one cell type can produce only one hormone. Immunocytochemical, ultrastructural, and biochemical investigations, however, have clearly shown that the one cell–one hormone theory is not true, and that several pituitary tumors produce more than one hormone. Immunocytochemistry reveals that the most frequent combination is the production of GH and PRL, followed by GH and α-SU, GH, PRL, α-SU, and TSH. Other combinations occur but are rare and of limited significance.

Morphologically these plurihormonal tumors may be monomorphous or polymorphous. The former are composed of one cell type, and two or more hormones can be demonstrated in the same cell by immunocytochemistry. Two or more cell types can be identified in the latter, each of which produces only one hormone. Acidophil stem cell adenomas and mammosomatotroph adenomas are monomorphous tumors. Mixed somatotroph-lactotroph adenomas are bimorphous – GH is located in one cell type and PRL in the other. However, mixed somatotroph-lactotroph adenomas may contain adenoma cells immunoreactive for both GH and PRL. In situ hybridization studies also show that the sharp separation of these various ultrastructural subtypes is not justified (Li et al. 1993). The cytogenesis of plurihormonal adenomas is unresolved. Preliminary evidence indicates that plurihormonal clones occur in the nontumorous adenohypophysis. If this is so, plurihormonal adenomas can arise from nontumorous plurihormonal cells. Alternatively, it is possible that these tumors arise in a noncommitted precursor cell, and that after neoplastic transformation or during progression the transformed cell undergoes multidirectional differentiation and begins to produce multiple

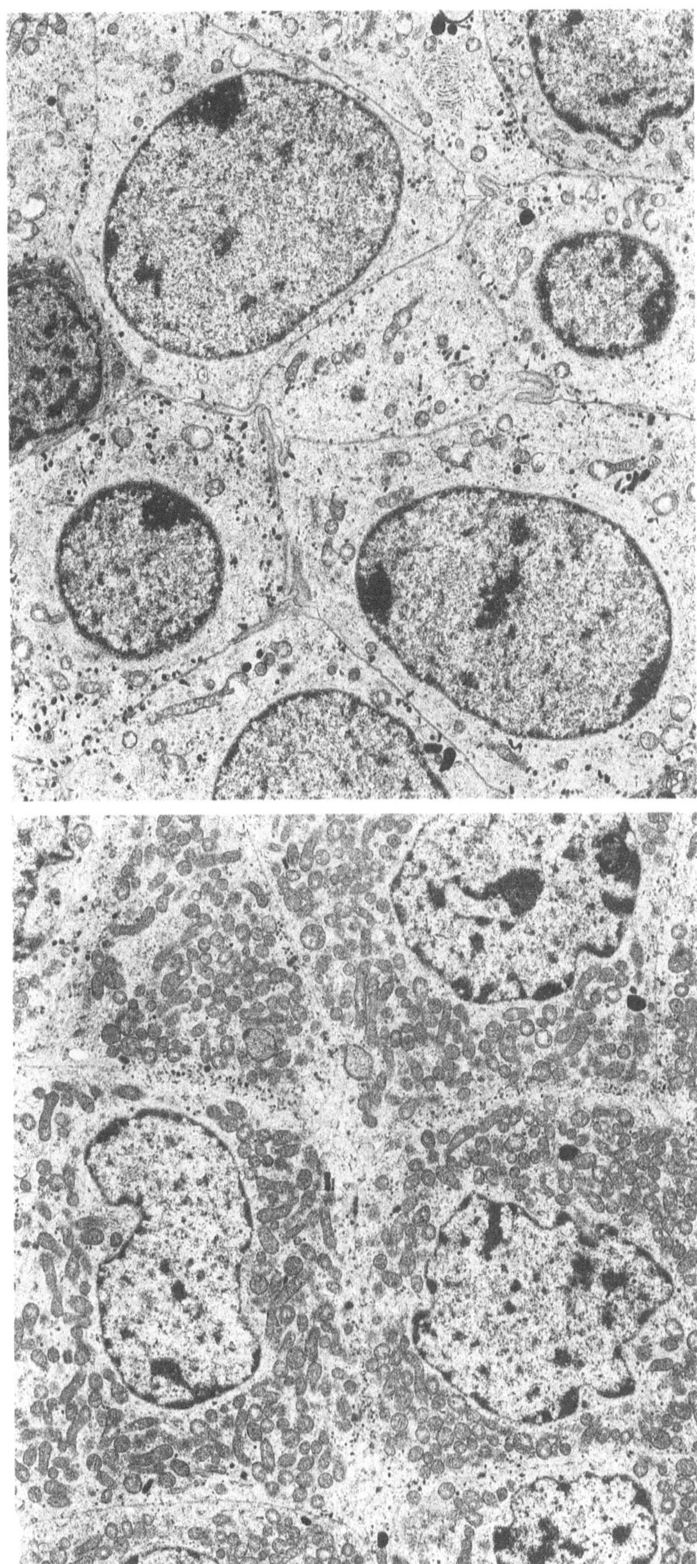

Fig. 66. Human null cell adenoma with a few small secretory granules and scarce RER. TEM, ×5000

Fig. 67. Human pituitary oncocytoma is composed of cells packed with mitochondria. TEM, ×5000

hormones (Kovacs et al. 1989). It should be noted that the factors accounting for multidirectional differentiation are completely unknown.

Silent pituitary adenomas raise questions that are as yet unresolved. The characteristic feature of these tumors is that the adenoma cells are immunoreactive for one or two or more hormones, but they are not associated with elevated blood hormone levels or with clinical symptoms indicative of hormone excess. The most frequent type is the silent corticotroph adenoma, which is morphologically identical to that which actively secretes ACTH and is associated with Cushing's disease.

Invasive adenomas infiltrate and destroy neighboring tissues and have no distinct border. These tumors have a poorer prognosis, are more difficult to operate on, and recur more frequently than tumors which have an expansive growth pattern. Gross invasion occurs in approximately 35% of pituitary adenomas, while microscopic invasion occurs in 55%–60% of pituitary tumors (Pernicone and Scheithauer 1993). Large adenomas invade more frequently than small tumors. Invasiveness in the pituitary is not regarded as a sign of malignancy.

Pituitary carcinomas are very rare. The criterion for the diagnosis of carcinoma is the documented presence of distant metastases. Pleomorphism, mitotic figures, necrosis, and invasiveness do not permit the diagnosis of carcinoma. Pituitary carcinomas may give rise to metastases in the spinal cord, bones, liver, heart, lung, lymph nodes, etc. They may produce GH, PRL, or ACTH and are clinically and biochemically associated with hormone excess and the relevant hypersecretory endocrine syndrome. In other cases, however, pituitary carcinomas produce no hormones and are associated with only local symptoms and general symptoms depending on the size and site of the primary tumor and the metastases (Pernicone and Scheithauer 1993).

Pituitary Tumors in Experimental Animals

Spontaneous pituitary tumors in various species have long been recognized (Fisher 1926; Wolfe et al. 1938). Most of these studies report pituitary adenomas in rats, less frequently in mice, and only occasionally in other species such as fish, parakeet, cow, horse, buffalo, and dog. In the rat the incidence of spontaneous tumors has been extensively documented in different strains over the past four decades, and the morphologic descriptions are based mainly on routine histologic stainings. Immunohistochemical demonstration of hormone content is less documented, and the ultrastructural studies are sporadic (Jacobs and Huseby 1967; Sass et al. 1975; Kovacs et al. 1977; Magnusson et al. 1979; Ueberberg and Lutzen 1979; Kroes et al. 1981; McComb et al. 1984, 1985).

Pituitary tumors can be induced by physical and/or chemical agents, target organ ablation, and recently by genetic manipulation. Both spontaneous and induced pituitary tumors can be maintained by serial transplantation offering the possibility to study their behavior in such conditions (Lloyd et al. 1991). Transgenic animals are valuable experimental models for studying the pathogenesis of pituitary tumors.

Spontaneous Tumors in Rats. The frequency of pituitary adenomas increases with age. The incidence and tumor types depends on the strain. Frequently the adenoma is preceded by diffuse hyperplasia and/or nodular hyperplasia. In diffuse hyperplasia the reticulin stain indicates the preservation of fibrillar network, and immunocytochemistry shows that the proliferating cell type is intermingled with other cell types. Nodular hyperplasia can be single or multiple (Fig. 68). The distinction between hyperplastic nodules and adenomas is sometimes difficult. A focal proliferation is called nodule when there is no sharp border and no compression of adjacent

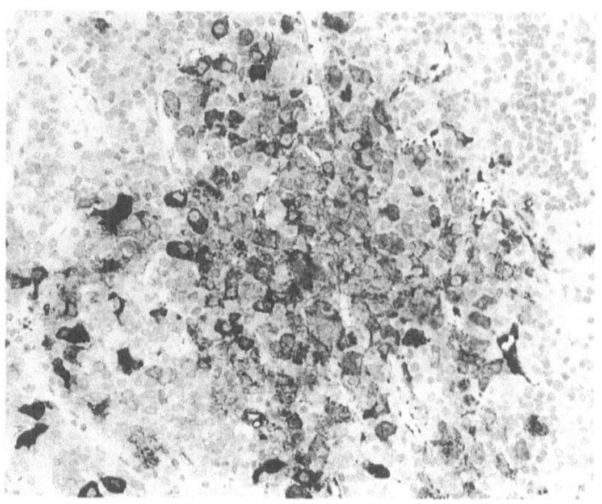

Fig. 68. Focal thyrotroph hyperplasia in an old rat. TSH immunostaining. ×250

tissue as assessed by reticulin staining (Fig. 69). Adenohypophysial tumors can be microscopic with a normal gross appearance of the pituitary, or they can be large, weighing up to 200–300 mg (normal pituitary weight is 10–15 mg) and compress the brain. In the latter case one wing or the whole gland is enlarged, and the tumor is frequently hemorrhagic (Fig. 70).

Histologic appearance varies from a solid pattern to cords of cells separated by hemorrhagic areas of different sizes and dilated capillaries filled with red blood cells. Usually the adenoma compresses the surrounding nontumorous pituitary, with the formation of a pseudocapsule. Pleomorphic nuclei and mitoses may be present. The hematoxylin-eosin stain distinguishes acidophilic, basophilic, chromophobic, and mixed tumors. The basophilic tumors are PAS positive due to the glycoprotein component of prehormones or hormones. Pituitary tumors are classified based on immunocytochemistry for adenohypophysial hormones, ultrastructural features, and recently by in situ hybridization for hormones mRNAs (Kovacs et al. 1977; Trouillas et al. 1982; McComb et al. 1984, 1985; Sandusky et al. 1988; Sano et al. 1989).

Lactotroph (PRL) adenomas, as in human patients, are chromophobic, sparsely granuled, and rarely acidophilic, densely granulated tumors. By light microscopy most lactotroph adenomas are hemorrhagic, and the large tumors contain necrotic areas with macrophages loaded with PAS-positive pigment and iron.

Sparsely granulated adenomas show typical PRL immunoreactivity as a juxtanuclear globule (Fig. 71). Ultrastructurally the abundant cytoplasm

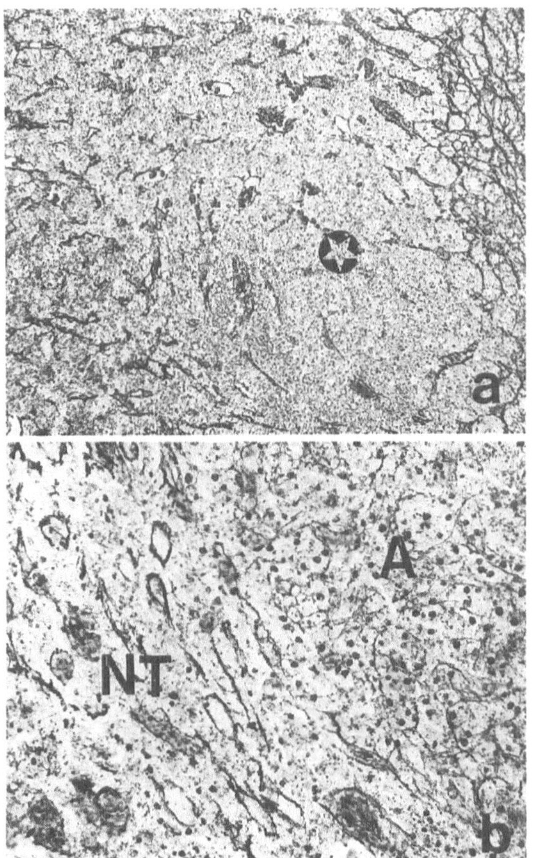

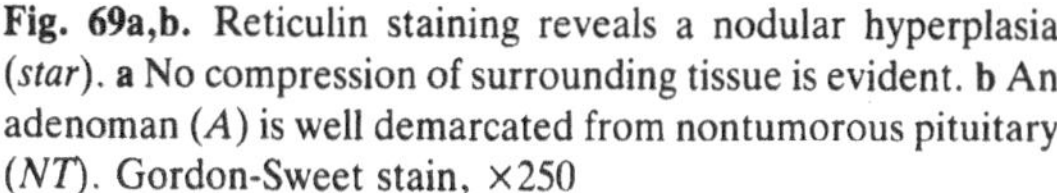

Fig. 69a,b. Reticulin staining reveals a nodular hyperplasia (*star*). **a** No compression of surrounding tissue is evident. **b** An adenoman (*A*) is well demarcated from nontumorous pituitary (*NT*). Gordon-Sweet stain, ×250

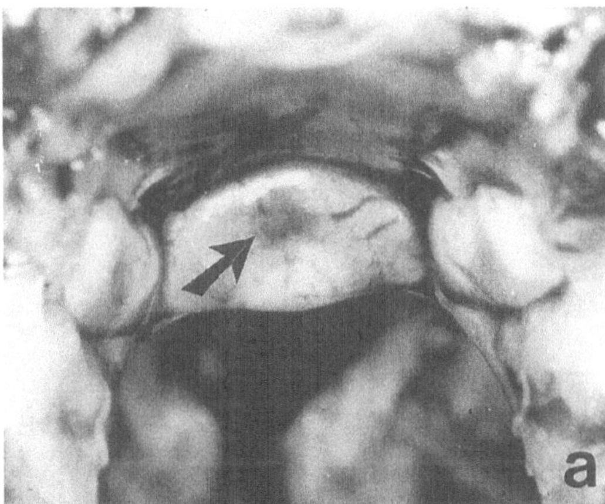

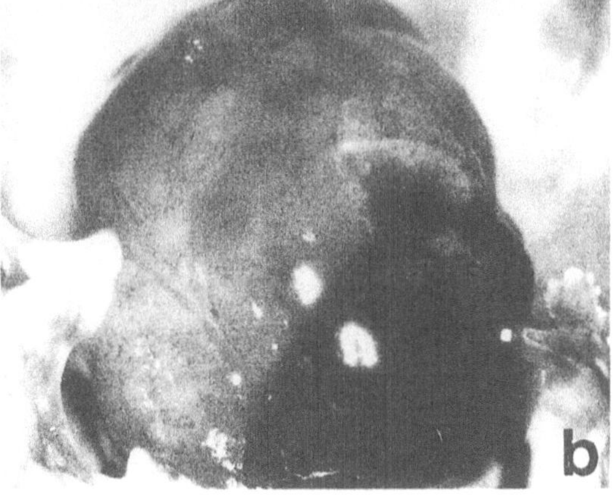

Fig. 70. **a** The gross appearance of the pituitary of an old rat is normal, except for a small hemorrhagic area (arrow). **b** A large, hemorrhagic, well demarcated tumor is evident in an old rat

contains extensively developed RER disposed in parallel arrays or fingerprint (nebenkern) patterns. Secretory granules (150–200 nm) are abundant in the large Golgi area and scattered throughout the cytoplasm. As in human adenomas, extrusion of secretory granules is frequently seen (Fig. 72).

Densely granulated adenomas have a diffuse PRL immunoreactivity over the cytoplasm. Electron microscopy shows the cytoplasm to contain numerous irregular, large secretory granules of 300–600 nm, some of which are extruded.

Somatotroph (GH cell adenomas) are rare. Only one adenohypophysial adenoma immunoreactive for GH and associated with elevated plasma GH levels has been reported so far (McComb et al. 1984). This acidophilic tumor by electron microscopy has a variable number of secretory granules (300–400 nm), single or multiple extruded secretory granules, moderate to numerous

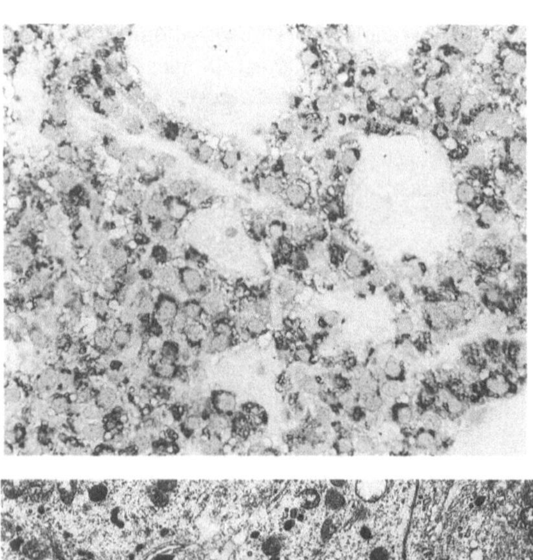

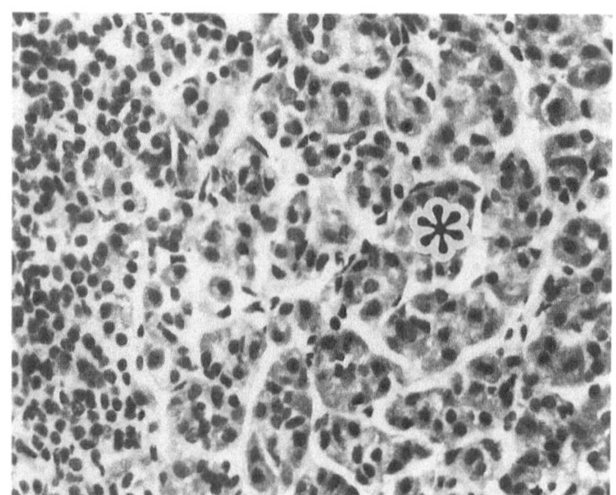

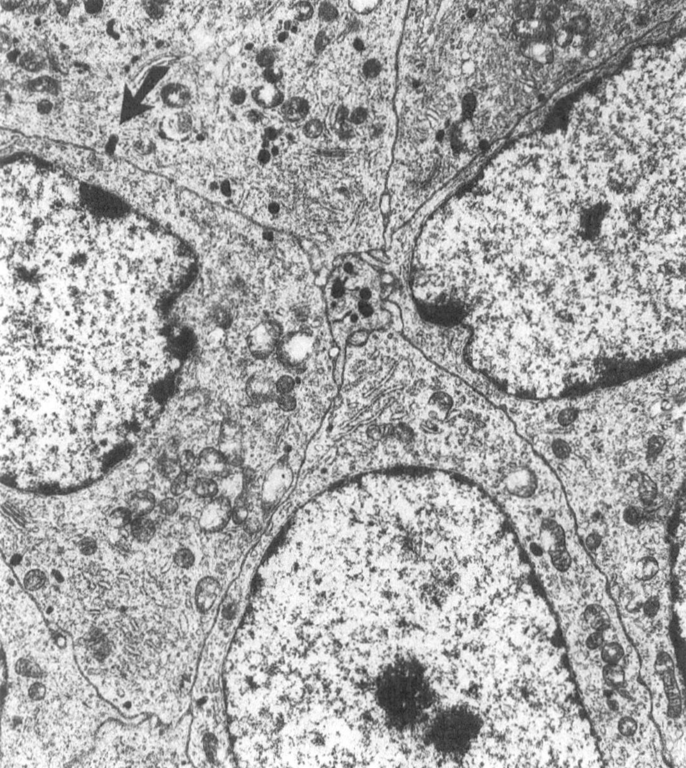

Fig. 71. (*upper left*) Old rat pituitary contains a lactotroph adenoma. PRL immunoreactivity is located adjacent to nuclei. ×500

Fig. 72. (*below*) Sparsely granulated lactotroph adenoma of a rat. Note extruded secretory granules (*arrow*) TEM, ×5500

Fig. 73. (*upper right*) Pituitary of an old Lobund-Wistar rat. A gonadotroph nodule, PAS positive (asterisk), with a trabecular pattern is seem. PAS, ×250

mitochondria, and some large filamentous perinuclear aggregates reminiscent of a fibrous body, the marker of human sparsely granulated somatotroph adenoma.

GH-PRL producing adenomas are acidophilic or chromophobic and are divided into two groups based on the pattern of GH and PRL immunoreactivity: monomorphous adenoma in which GH and PRL are colocalized in the same cell, and bimorphous adenoma in which GH and PRL are localized in different cells or in the same cell. Monomorphous GH-PRL adenoma contains a few small secretory granules (100–150 nm), some extruded, modest RER, and vesicular Golgi complex. Both serum hormone levels are elevated. Bimorphous GH-PRL adenoma is composed of sparsely granulated lactotrophs and densely granulated somatotrophs. This adenoma type resembles human mixed lactotroph-somatotroph adenoma. Serum PRL and GH or only PRL levels are elevated (McComb et al. 1984).

Thyrotroph adenoma is a rare tumor type described as an adenoma or nodule. It can be acidophilic, chromophobic, and PAS positive. Ultrastructurally the adenoma is composed of large cells which resemble stimulated thyrotrophs with dilated vesicular RER.

Gonadotroph adenoma can be acidophilic, chromophobic, or PAS positive. It has a solid or trabecular pattern. Immunocytochemistry reveals the presence of FSH and LH. The solid proliferations can be nodular or adenomatous, and there are no clear cut criteria for their distinction (Fig. 73). Only the trabecular variant has been studied by electron microscopy. Densely granulated adenomas resemble nontumorous gonadotrophs (Fig. 74). Sparsely granulated tumors are composed of cells with euchromatic nuclei, prominent Golgi complexes, and a variable number of small secretory granules.

ACTH-immunoreactive adenoma is rare in rats (Holmes and Mandle 1961; Berkvens et al. 1980; Lee et al. 1982; McComb et al. 1984). In some animals the examination of adrenal glands revealed cortical hyperplasia, indicating ACTH secretion by the pituitary tumor (Holmes and Mandle 1961; Kaspareit-Rittinghausen et al. 1990). ACTH immunoreactive adenomas are chromophobic,

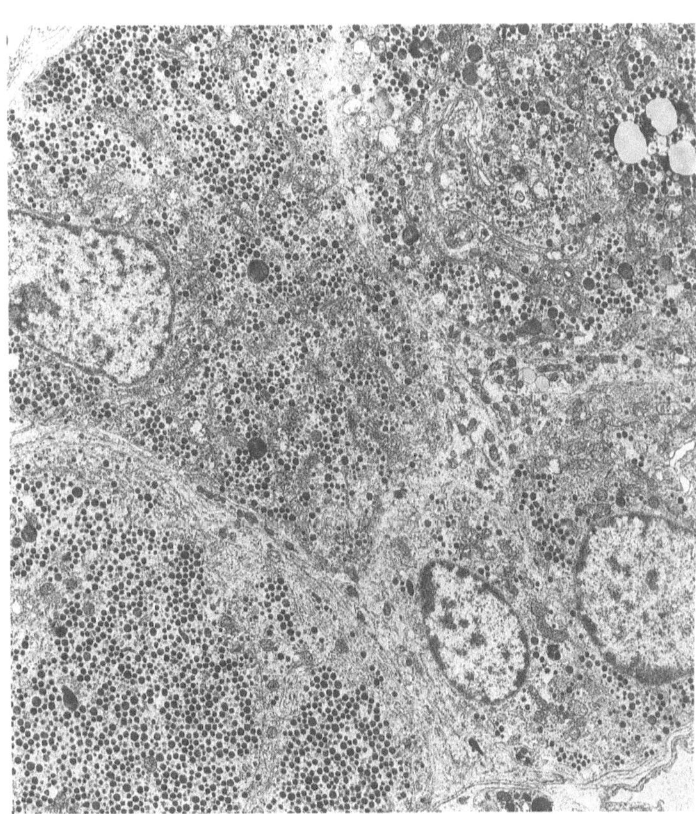

Fig. 74. Rat, pituitary, contains a densely granulated gonadotroph "nodule" composed of cells resembling the normal gonadotrophs. TEM, ×4000

with a solid pattern, and may contain spaces filled with blood. No ultrastructural description is available so far.

In the nontumorous adenohypophysis adjacent to a functioning ACTH adenoma no ACTH immunoreactive cells have been identified, suggesting the loss of hormonal content by the inhibited corticotrophs (Kaspareit-Rittinghausen et al. 1990). This finding is in contrast to that in human patients in whom the presence of Crooke's cells indicates a functioning corticotroph adenoma.

Plurihormonal adenoma most commonly contains GH and PRL immunoreactivity. Occasionally other combinations of hormones occur, such as PRL, TSH, and LH; GH and LH; PRL and ACTH; PRL and TSH; and PRL and LH.

Immunonegative adenomas contain no hormone by immunocytochemistry. It is chromophobic or PAS positive. Ultrastructurally differentiated cells are described with no resemblance to nontumorous cells.

Intermediate lobe adenoma in the rat is much rarer than that of the anterior lobe. It is chromophobic or basophilic, sometimes hemorrhagic, and often extends into the posterior lobe. Many cells are immunoreactive for ACTH and MSH. Ultrastructural examination reveals secretory granules with variable electron density of 100–300 nm, dispersed at the periphery of the cells. Intermediate lobe tumors are very frequently found in horses (Heinrichs et al. 1990) and are common in dogs (El Etreby et al. 1980).

As in human pituitary tumors, the local invasion of surrounding tissues is not considered a criterion of malignancy. The presence of distant metastases indicates malignancy. To our knowledge, no metastases have been reported in spontaneous rodent pituitary tumors.

Experimental Pituitary Tumors. Pituitary tumors can be induced by chemicals, irradiation, and homeostatic derangements (Furth and Clinton 1966; Furth et al. 1976).

Natural and synthetic estrogens have been used extensively in different doses and durations to induce a wide spectrum of lesions from diffuse lactotroph hyperplasia to nodules and adenomas (Stefaneanu and Kovacs 1991). In 1936 Cramer and Horning (1936), McEwen et al. (1936), and Zondek (1936) reported for the first time that estrogens can induce pituitary tumors. The pioneering work of Furth and colleagues (1959) on transplantable tumors opened a path which continues to yield new information on the histology of pituitary tumors. Estrogen-induced lactotroph adenomas are chromophobic or acidophilic, and most cells are immunoreactive for PRL; a minority of cells show GH immunoreactivity. By electron microscopy the adenomas resemble the spontaneous ones; however, isolated somatotrophs or those dispersed in small groups are present (Ueda et al. 1970; McComb et al. 1981).

Many transplantable tumors were induced by estrogens by Furth and colleagues (Furth 1955; Furth et al. 1976; Ueda et al. 1968). The best studied transplanted tumors are MtT/W5, MtT/WlO, MtT/Wl5, MtT/F4, and 7315a. Initially these tumors produced PRL, and during subsequent transplantation GH and sometimes ACTH production became evident (McComb et al. 1980). In MtT/W5 three cell types are seen: one producing GH, another PRL, and a small percentage immunopositive for both GH and PRL (Parsons et al. 1980). MtT/F4 tumors are composed of undifferentiated cells with scarce secretory granules. Both MtT/Wl5 and MtT/F4 are growth inhibited by chronic estrogen treatment (Morel et al. 1982; Trouillas et al. 1984; Lloyd et al. 1985). In the former the GH production and GH mRNA are increased, while PRL secretion is inhibited by estrogen (Lloyd et al. 1988). In MtT/F4 an opposite effect is seen, i.e., PRL secretion is increased while the tumor cells become more differentiated (Trouillas et al. 1984). The predominance of GH production by other transplantable tumors induced by radiation and chemicals is reported as well (MacLeod et al. 1966; Hollander and Hollander 1971). MtT/5A5 transplantable tumor established by Makino et al. (1984) predominantly produces GH.

Most transplantable tumors do not metastasize. However, the GH variant of MtT/W5 induced by radiation proved highly malignant, and MtT/Wl5 produced metastases to ovaries and bones (Hollander and Hollander 1971).

High doses of calcitonin administered for a minimum of 6 months are associated with increased incidence of pituitary tumors in rats (Ishii et al. 1991; Jameson et al. 1992). Immunocytochemistry and in situ hybridization reveals that the adenomas produce α-SU of glycoprotein hormones. Although calcitonin receptor has been demonstrated in pituitary cells, it is not known whether the proliferation of a subset of glycoprotein hormone-producing cells is a direct or indirect effect of calcitonin (Jameson et al. 1992).

Thyroidectomy, iodine deficient diets, and propylthiouracyl induce thyrotroph hyperplasia and eventually TSH-producing adenomas. Bilateral gonadectomy results in basophilic pituitary tumors, with cells resembling normal gonadotrophs (Griesbach and Purves 1960). Low doses of ^{131} I induce thyrotroph and gonadotroph adenomas (Furth et al. 1959).

Transgenic mice with foreign genes incorporated permanently into their genome offer a novel experimental model for various diseases, including tumors. A high incidence of pituitary tumors has been reported in transgenic mice carrying genes encoding hormones, oncogenes, or mutated tumor suppressor genes.

Mice transgenic for human GRH fused with metallothionein promoter develop gigantism. The increased ectopic GRH production stimulates the pituitary which becomes enlarged and shows massive somatotroph and mammosomatotroph hyperplasia (Mayo et al. 1988; Stefaneanu et al. 1989). Later, in old age, pituitary adenomas develop; these are diffusely immunoreactive for GH and contain a strong signal for GH mRNA. PRL and its mRNA are expressed focally. A few adenomas contain islets of TSH immunoreactive cells. Ultrastructurally most tumors are well differentiated, with cells resembling the hyperplastic somatotrophs (Fig. 75). Other tumors contain cells with a few small secretory granules and enlarged Golgi apparatus reminiscent of glycoprotein hormone-producing cells (Asa et al. 1992; Lloyd et al. 1992).

Somatotroph hyperplasia also develops in mice transgenic for GH promoter/cholera toxin fusion gene (Burton et al. 1991). The expression of this activator of Gs protein induces high concentrations of cAMP (the second mediator of GRH) in somatotrophs. No pituitary tumors are reported in these transgenics.

Mice transgenic for SV40 large T antigen fused with arginine-vasopressin promoter develop pituitary and endocrine pancreatic tumors at a young age (Murphy et al. 1987; Stefaneanu et al. 1992b). Most pituitary tumors are focally immunoreactive for GH and rarely for TSH. In situ hybridization shows diffuse signal for GH mRNA, indicating that the tumors are derived from somatotrophs. Ultrastructurally the tumor cells are very undifferentiated (Fig. 76). In a few mice a second tumor is found originating in the intermediate lobe. These tumors are ACTH immunoreactive and contain abundant POMC and mRNA. Both anterior and intermediate tumors are immunoreactive for large T antigen and p53 protein, suggesting their direct involvement in tumor formation. Since no somatotroph hyperplasia is evident in the surrounding nontumorous tissue, this transgenic model resembles the human somatotroph adenoma.

The insertion of SV40 oncogene fused with α-SU promoter, leads to transgenic mice that develop pituitary gonadotroph adenomas (Windle et al. 1990). In these tumors the presence of neural tissue suggests the expression of a neurotrophic factor by the adenoma cells (Schechter et al. 1992).

ACTH-secreting adenomas are reported in mice transgenic for polyoma large T antigen fused with polyoma early region promoter. The transgenic mice and nontransgenics bearing transplanted tumors have increased body weight and enlarged cortices, indicating elevated ACTH levels (Helseth et al. 1992).

Heterozygous mice in which one allele of the retinoblastoma (RB) gene was disrupted develop pituitary tumors invading the brain. This experimental model confirms the role of this tumor-suppressor gene in tumor formation (Jacks et al. 1992).

Pathogenesis

Pituitary tumorigenesis has been dominated by two theories, one supporting an intrinsic pituitary abnormality and the other emphasizing an abnormal regulatory mechanism. New data indicate that probably both mechanisms are involved in the complex, multistep process of pituitary tumor formation (Davis and Haggard 1993; Levy and Lightman 1993).

Clonality studies analyzing allelic X chromosome inactivation pattern have proven most human pituitary tumors to be monoclonal (Alexander et al. 1990; Herman et al. 1990). These results support the concept that a somatic mutation in a single cell is the initial event in adenoma formation. Abnormalities in Gs (α) protein offer an example of a somatic mutation that could be directly involved in tumor growth. However, only 40% of somatotroph adenomas contain Gs (α) mutation (Spada et al. 1990). Other candidate proteins, which when mutated can act as initiators,

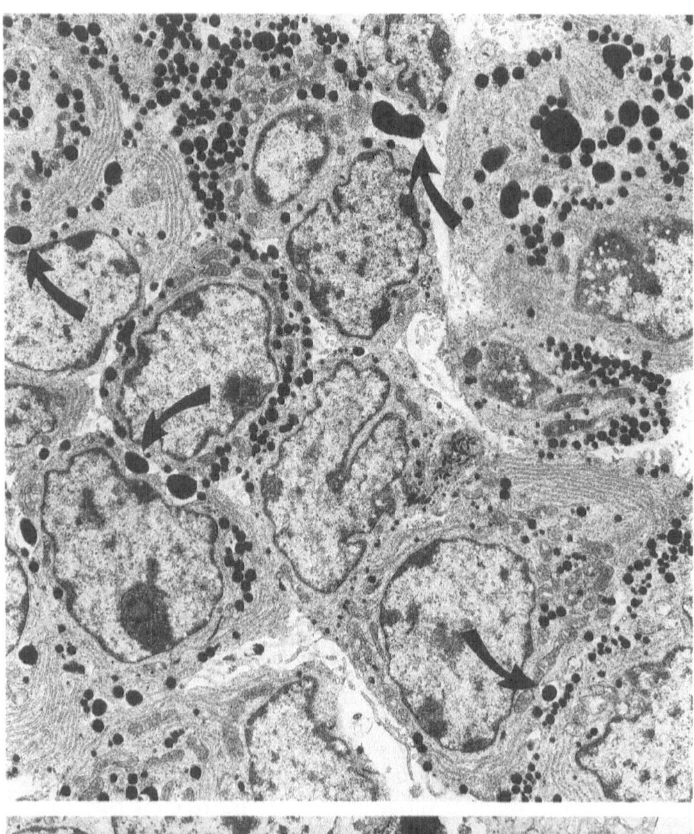

Fig. 75. Pituitary adenoma in a GRH transgenic mouse. The adenoma cells resemble the hyperplastic somatotrophs and contain large deposits of extruded secretory material (*arrows*). TEM, ×4000

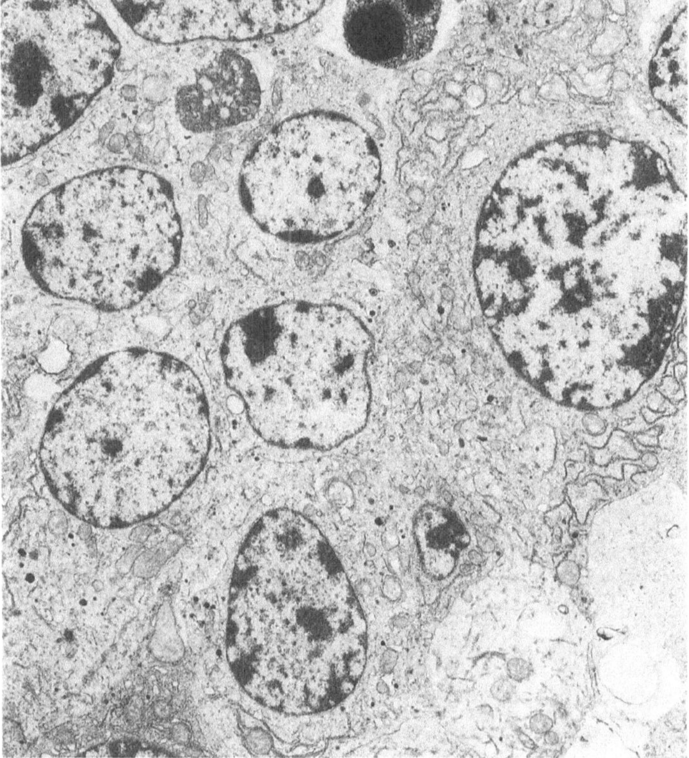

Fig. 76. Pituitary tumor of an AVP/SV40 transgenic mouse. Note undifferentiated cells with rare, tiny secretory granules. TEM, ×4000

include growth factors, receptors, and tumor suppressor genes. The fact that some adenomas are preceded by hyperplasia suggests that hypothalamic or other stimulating hormone, or the escape from hypothalamic inhibition may act as tumor promoters. The demonstration of the production of high levels of hypothalamic releasing factors by the pituitary tumors suggests their possible involvement in an autocrine or paracrine fashion to tumorigenesis.

Advances in molecular biology techniques in the near future should further expand our understanding of pituitary tumorigenesis.

Acknowledgements. This work was supported in part by grant MT-11270 from the Medical Research Council of Canada and by the generous donation of Mr. and Mrs. Jarislowsky. We are indebted to Dr. E. Horvath for providing us with the electron micrographs of human pituitary adenomas, to Ms. Elizabeth Chambers for technical assistance, and to Mrs. Wanda Wlodarski for secretarial work.

References

Alexander JM, Biller BM, Bikkal H, Zervas NT, Arnold A, Klibanski A (1990) Clinically nonfunctioning pituitary tumors are monoclonal in origin. J Clin Invest 86:336–340

Asa SL, Kovacs K, Stefaneanu L, Horvath E, Billestrup N, Gonzalez-Manchon C, Vale W (1992) Pituitary adenomas in mice transgenic for growth hormone-releasing hormone. Endocrinology 131:2083–2089

Berkvens JM, van Nesselrooy JHJ, Kroes R (1980) Spontaneous tumours in the pituitary gland of old Wistar rats. A morphological and immunocytochemical study. J Pathol 130:179–191

Burton FH, Hasel KW, Bloom FE, Sutcliffe JG (1991) Pituitary hyperplasia and gigantism in mice caused by a cholera toxin transgene. Nature 350:74–77

Chatelain A, Dupouy JP, Dubois MP (1979) Ontogenesis of cells producing polypeptide hormones (ACTH, MSH, LPH, GH, prolactin) in the fetal hypophysis of the rat: influence of hypothalamus. Cell Tissue Res 196:409–427

Childs GV (1984) Fluidity of gonadotropin storage in cycling female rats. In: McKerns KW (ed) Hormonal control of the hypothalamo-pituitary-gonadal axis. Plenum, New York, pp 181–198

Cramer W, Horning ES (1936) Experimental production by oestrin of pituitary tumors with hypopituitarism. Lancet 1:247–249

Davis JR, Haggard N (1993) Towards the pathogenesis of human pituitary tumours (commentary). J Endocrinol 136:3–6

El Etreby MF, Muller-Peddinghaus R, Bhargava AS, Trautwein G (1980) Functional morphology of spontaneous hyperplastic and neoplastic lesions in the canine pituitary gland. Vet Pathol 17:109–122

Ellerkmann E, Nagy GM, Frawley LS (1992) -Melanocyte-stimulating hormone is a mammotrophic factor released by neurointermediate lobe cells after estrogen treatment. Endocrinology 130:133–138

Fischer O (1926) Über Hypophysen Geschwulste der Weissen Ratten. Virchows Arch Pathol Anat 259:9–29

Frawley LS, Boockfor FR (1991) Mammosomatotropes: presence and functions in normal and neoplastic pituitary tissue. Endocr Rev 12:337–355

Furth J (1955) Experimental pituitary tumors. Recent Prog Horm Res 11:221–255

Furth J, Clifton KH (1966) Experimental pituitary tumors. In: Harris GW, Donovan BT (eds) The pituitary gland, vol 2. Butterworths, London, pp 460–497

Furth J, Haran-Ghera N, Curtis HJ, Buffe HRF (1959) Studies on the pathogenesis of neoplasms by ionizing radiation. I. Pituitary tumors. Cancer 19:550

Furth J, Nakane PK, Pasteels JL (1976) Tumors of the pituitary gland. In: Turusov VS (ed) Pathology of tumors in laboratory animals, vol 1, part 2. International Agency for Research on Cancer, Lyon, pp 201–237

Griesbach WE, Purves HD (1960) Basophil adenomata in the rat hypophysis after gonadectomy. Br J Cancer 14:49–59

Heinrichs M, Baumgartner W, Capen CC (1990) Immunocytochemical demonstration of proopiomelanocortin-derived peptides in pituitary adenomas of the pars intermedia in horses. Vet Pathol 27:419–425

Helseth A, Siegal GP, Haug E, Bautch VL (1992) Transgenic mice that develop pituitary tumors. A model for Cushing's disease. Am J Pathol 140:1071–1080

Herman V, Fagin J, Gonsky E, Ezrin C, Kovacs K, Melmed S (1990) Clonal origins of pituitary adenomas. J Clin Endocrinol Metab 71:1427–1433

Hollander N, Hollander VP (1971) Development of a somatotropic variant of the mammosomatotropic tumor MtT-W5. Proc Soc Exp Biol Med 137:1157–1162

Holmes RL, Mandle A (1961) A spontaneous pituitary tumor in a rat associated with adrenal hypertrophy. J Endocrinol 22:29–30

Horvath E, Kovacs K (1984) Gonadotroph adenomas of the human pituitary: sex-related fine-structural dichotomy. A histologic, immunocytochemical, and electron microscopic study of 30 tumors. Am J Pathol 117:429–440

Horvath E, Kovacs K (1986) Pathology of prolactin adenomas of the human pituitary. Semin Diagn Pathol 3:4–17

Horvath E, Kovacs K (1988) Fine structural cytology of the adenohypophysis in rat and man. J Electron Microsc Tech 8:401–432

Houben H, Denef C (1990) Regulatory peptides produced in the anterior pituitary. TEM Nov/Dec 398–403

Ishii J, Katayama S, Itabashi A, Takahama M, Kawazu S (1991) Salmon calcitonin induces pituitary tumors in rats. Endocrinol Jpn 38:705–709

Jacks T, Fazeli A, Schmitt EM, Bronson RT, Goodell MA, Weinberg RA (1992) Effects of an Rb mutation in the mouse. Nature 359:295–300

Jacobs BB, Huseby RA (1967) Neoplasms occurring in aged Fischer rats with special reference to testicular, uterine, and thyroid tumors. J Natl Cancer Inst 39:303–309

Jameson JL, Klibanski A, Black PM, Zervas NT, Lindell CM, Hsu DW, Ridgway EC, Habener JF (1987) Glycoprotein hormone genes are expressed in clinically nonfunctioning pituitary adenomas. J Clin Invest 80:1472–1478

Jameson JL, Weiss J, Polak JM, Childs GV, Bloom SR, Steel JH, Capen CC, Prentice DE, Fetter AW, Langloss JM (1992) Glycoprotein hormone alpha-subunit-producing pituitary adenomas in rats treated for one year with calcitonin. Am J Pathol 140:75-84

Kaspareit-Rittinghausen J, Hense S, Deerberg F (1990) Cushing's syndrome, and disease-like lesions in rats. Z Versuchstierkd 33:229-234

Kovacs K, Horvath E (1986) Tumors of the pituitary gland. In: Armed Forces Institute of Pathology (ed) Atlas of tumor pathology, second series, fascicle 21. Armed Forces Institute of Pathology, Washington DC

Kovacs K, Horvath E, Ilse RG, Ezrin C, Ilse D (1977) Spontaneous pituitary adenomas in aging rats: a light microscopic, immunocytological and fine structural study. Beitr Pathol 161:1-16

Kovacs K, Horvath E, Asa SL, Stefaneanu L, Sano T (1989) Pituitary cells producing more than one hormone. TEM Nov/Dec 104-107

Kovacs K, Asa SL, Horvath E, Ryan N, Singer W, Killinger DW, Smyth HS, Scheithauer BW, Ebersold MJ (1990) Null cell adenomas of the pituitary: attempts to resolve their cytogenesis. In: Lechago J, Kameya T (eds) Endocrine pathology update. Field and Wood, New York, pp 17-31

Kroes R, Garbis-Berkvens JM, DeVries T, van Nesselrooy JH (1981) Histological profile of a Wistar rat stock including a survey of the literature. J Gerontol 36:256-259

Histopathological profile of a Wistar rat stock including a survey of the literature. J Gerontol 36:259-279

Kurosumi K (1968) Functional classification of cell types of the anterior pituitary gland accomplished by electron microscopy. Arch Histol Jpn 29:329-362

Kurosumi K (1986) Cell classification of the rat anterior pituitary by means of immunoelectron microscopy. J Clin Electron Microsc 19:299-319

Lee AK, De Lellis RA, Blount M, Nunnemacher G, Wolfe H (1982) Pituitary proliferative lesions in aging male Long-Evans rats. A model of mixed multiple endocrine neoplasia syndrome. Lab Invest 47:595-602

Levy A, Lightman SL (1992) Growth hormone-releasing hormone transcripts in human pituitary adenomas. J Clin Endocrinol Metab 74:1474-1476

Levy A, Lightman SL (1993) The pathogenesis of pituitary adenomas. Review. Clin Endocrinol 38:559-570

Li J, Stefaneanu L, Kovacs K, Horvath E, Smyth HS (1993) Growth hormone (GH) and prolactin (PRL) gene expression and immunoreactivity in GHL- and PRL-producing human pituitary adenomas. Virchows Arch [A] 422:193-201

Lloyd RV (1991) Ultrastructure of spontaneous and transplanted pituitary tumors in laboratory animals. J Electron Microsc Tech 19:64-79

Lloyd RV (1993) Cytology and function of the pituitary gland. In: Lloyd RV (ed) Surgical pathology of the pituitary gland. Philadelphia, Saunders, pp 5-17 (Major problems in pathology, vol 27)

Lloyd RV, Landefeld TD, Maslar I, Frohman LA (1985) Diethylstilbestrol inhibits tumor growth and prolactin production in rat pituitary tumors. Am J Pathol 118:379-386

Lloyd RV, Cano M, Landefeld TD (1988) The effects of estrogens on tumor growth and on prolactin and growth hormone mRNA expression in rat pituitary tissues. Am J Pathol 133:397-406

Lloyd RV, Jin L, Fields K, Chandler WF, Horvath E, Stefaneanu L, Kovacs K (1991) Analysis of pituitary hormones and chromogranin A mRNAs in null cell adenomas, oncocytomas, and gonadotroph adenomas by in situ hybridization. Am J Pathol 139:553-564

Lloyd RV, Jin L, Chang A, Kulig E, Camper SA, Ross BD, Downs TR, Frohman LA (1992) Morphologic effects of hGRH gene expression on the pituitary, liver and pancreas of MT-hGRH transgenic mice. An in situ hybridization analysis. Am J Pathol 141:895-906

MacLeod RM, Smith MC, DeWitt GW (1966) Hormonal properties of transplanted pituitary tumors and their relation to the pituitary gland. Endocrinology 79:1149-1156

Magnusson G, Majeed SK, Gopinath C (1979) Infiltrating pituitary neoplasms in the rat. Lab Anim 13:111-113

Makino S, Mori H, Koizumi K, Yamashita H, Hayashi Y, Aono T, Matsumoto K (1984) Functional and morphological characteristics of transplantable rat pituitary tumors established in nude mice. Cancer Res 44:4487-4495

Marin F, Stefaneanu L, Kovacs K (1991) Folliculo-stellate cells of the pituitary (review). Endocr Pathol 2:180-192

Mayo KE, Hammer RE, Swanson LW, Brinster RL, Rosenfeld MG, Evans RM (1988) Dramatic pituitary hyperplasia in transgenic mice expressing a human growth hormone-releasing factor gene. Mol Endocrinol 2:606-612

McComb DJ, Ilse G, Ryan IN, Horvath E, Kovacs K, Nagy E, Berczi I (1980) Histologic, immunocytologic and subcellular changes in the rat adenohypophysis caused by prolactin, growth hormone and ACTH-producing transplanted pituitary tumors: a comparison with spontaneous prolactin-producing adenomas. Exp Pathol 18:213-222

McComb DJ, Ryan N, Horvath E, Kovacs K, Nagy E, Berczi J, Domokos J, Laszlo FA (1981) Five different adenomas derived from the rat adenohypophysis: immunocytochemical and ultrastructural study. J Natl Cancer Inst 66: 1103-1111

McComb DJ, Kovacs K, Beri J, Zak F (1984) Pituitary adenomas in old Sprague Dawley rats: a histologic, ultrastructural and immunocytochemical study. J Natl Cancer Inst 73:1143-1166

McComb DJ, Kovacs K, Beri J, Zak F, Milligan JV, Shin SH (1985) Pituitary gonadotroph adenomas in old Sprague-Dawley rats. J Submicrosc Cytol 17:517-530

McEwen CS, Selye H, Colip JB (1936) Some effects of prolonged administration of oestrin in rats. Lancet 1: 775-776

McNicol AM, Walker E, Farquharson MA, Teasdale GM (1991) Pituitary macroadenomas associated with hyperprolactinaemia: immunocytochemical and in situ hybridization studies. Clin Endocrinol (Oxf) 35:239-244

Morel Y, Albaladejo V, Bouvier J, Andre J (1982) Inhibition by 17 beta-estradiol of the growth of the rat pituitary transplantable tumor MtF4. Cancer Res 42:1492-1497

Murphy D, Bishop A, Rindi G, Murphy MN, Stamp GW, Hanson J, Polak JM, Hogan B (1987) Mice transgenic for a vasopressin-SV40 hybrid oncogene develop tumors of the endocrine pancreas and the anterior pituitary. A possible model for human multiple endocrine neoplasia type I. Am J Pathol 129:552-566

Nagaya T, Seo H, Kuwayama A, Sakurai T, Tsukamoto N, Sugita K, Matsui N (1990) Prolactin gene expression in human growth hormone-secreting pituitary adenomas. J Neurosurg 72:879-882

Nagy G, Mulchahey JJ, Neil JD (1988) Autocrine control of prolactin secretion by vasoactive intestinal peptide. Endocrinology 122:364-366

Osamura RY, Watanabe K (1985) Histogenesis of the cells of the anterior and intermediate lobes of human pituitary glands: immunohistochemical studies. Int Rev Cytol 95: 103–129

Pagesy P, Li JY, Rentier-Delrue F, LeBouc Y, Martial JA, Peillon F (1989) Evidence of pre-prosomatostatin MRNA in human normal and tumoral anterior pituitary gland. Mol Endocrinol 3:1289–1294

Pagesy P, Li JY, Berthet M, Peillon F (1992) Evidence of gonadotropin-releasing hormone mRNA in the rat anterior pituitary. Mol Endocrinol 6:523–528

Parsons JA, Baskin DG, Erlandsen SI (1980) Heterogeneity of the MtTWI5 mammosomatotropic tumor. II. Characterization of parenchimal cells by superimposition immunocytochemistry and electron microscopy. Anat Rec 196:301–311

Peillon F, LeDafniet M, Garnier P, Feinstein MC, Donnadieu M, Barret A, Gautron JP, Brandi AM, Benlot C, Lagoguey A (1989) Neurohormones coming from the normal and tumoral human anterior pituitary. Secretion and regulation in vitro. Pathol Biol (Paris) 37:840–845

Pernicone PJ, Scheithauer BW (1993) Invasive pituitary adenomas and pituitary carcinomas. In: Lloyd RV (ed) Surgical pathology of the pituitary gland. Philadelphia, Saunders, pp 121–136 (Major problems in pathology, vol 27)

Poole MC, Kornegay WD III (1982) Cellular distribution within the rat adenohypophysis: a morphometric study. Anat Rec 204:45–53

Sandusky GE, van Pelt CS, Todd GC, Wightman K (1988) An immunohistochemical study of pituitary adenomas and focal hyperplasia in old Sprague-Dawley and Fischer 344 rats. Tox Pathol 16:376–380

Sano T, Kovacs K, Stefaneanu L, Asa SL, Snyder L (1989) Spontaneous pituitary gonadotroph nodules in aging male Lobund-Wistar rats. Lab Invest 61:343–349

Sasaki F, Ivema Y (1988) Sex differences in prolactin and growth hormone cells in mouse adenohypophysis: stereological, morphometric and immunohistochemical studies by light and electron microscopy. Endocrinology 123:905–912

Sass B, Rabstein LS, Madison R, Nims RM, Peters RL, Kelloff GJ (1975) Incidence of spontaneous neoplasms in F344 rats throughout the natural life span. J Natl Cancer Inst 54:1449–1456

Schechter J, Windle JJ, Stauber C, Mellon PL (1992) Neural tissue within anterior pituitary tumors generated by oncogene expression in transgenic mice. Neuroendocrinology 56: 300–311

Setalo G, Nakane P (1976) Functional differentiation of the fetal anterior pituitary cells in the rat. Endocr Exp 10: 155–166

Spada A, Arosio M, Bochicchio D, Bazzoni V, Vallar L, Bassetti M, Faglia G (1990) Clinical, biochemical and morphological correlates in patients bearing growth hormone-secreting pituitary tumors with or without constitutively active adenylyl cyclase. J Clin Endocrinol Metab 71:1421–1426

Stefaneanu L, Kovacs K (1991) Effects of drugs on pituitary fine structure in laboratory animals. J Electron Microsc Tech 19:80–89

Stefaneanu L, Kovacs K, Horvath E, Asa SL, Losinski NE, Billestrup N, Price J, Vale W (1989) Adenohypophysial changes in mice transgenic for human growth hormone-releasing hormone: a histological, immunocytochemical and electron microscopic investigation. Endocrinology 125: 2710–2718

Stefaneanu L, Kovacs K, Lloyd RV, Scheithauer BW, Young WFJR, Sano T, Jin L (1992a) Pituitary lactotrophs and somatotrophs in pregnancy: a correlative in situ hybridization and immunocytochemical study. Virchows Arch [B] 62: 291–296

Stefaneanu L, Rindi G, Horvath E, Murphy D, Polak JM, Kovacs K (1992b) Morphology of adenohypophysial tumors in mice transgenic for vasopressin-SV40 hybrid oncogene. Endocrinology 130:1789–1795

Stefaneanu L, Kovacs K, Horvath E, Clark RG, Cronin MJ (1993) Effect of intravenous infusion of growth hormone-releasing hormone (GRH) on the morphology of rat pituitary somatotrophs. Endocr Pathol 4:131–139

Takizawa S, Moy P, Marolla J, Furth J (1968) Characterization of four transplantable mammotropic pituitary tumor variants in the rat. Cancer Res 28:1963–1975

Trouillas J, Girod C, Claustrat B, Cure M, Dubois MP (1982) Spontaneous pituitary tumors in the Wistar/Furth/Ico rat strain. An animal model of human prolactin adenoma. Am J Pathol 109:57–70

Trouillas J, Morel Y, Pharaboz MO, Cordier G, Girod C, Andre J (1984) Morpho-functional modifications associated with the inhibition by estradiol of MtTF4 rat pituitary tumor growth. Cancer Res 44:4046–4052

Ueberberg H, Lutzen L (1979) The spontaneous rate of tumours in the laboratory rat: strain C4bb: Thom (SPF) Arzneimittelforschung 29:1876–1879

Ueda G, Tanizawa O, Hamanaka N, Nishiura H (1970) Changes of growth hormone-containing cells during tumorigenesis and subpassages of estrogen-induced pituitary tumors in rat. Endocrinol Jpn 17:447–452

Uhlig H, Saeger W, Fehr S, Ludecke DK (1991) Detection of growth hormone, prolactin and human β-chorionic gonadotropin messenger RNA in growth-hormone-secreting pituitary adenomas by in situ hybridization. Virchows Arch [A] 418:539–546

Windle JJ, Weiner RI, Mellon PL (1990) Cell lines of the pituitary gonadotrope lineage derived by targeted oncogenesis in transgenic mice. Mol Endocrinol 4:597–603

Wolfe JM, Bryan WR, Wright AW (1938) Histologic observations on the anterior pituitaries of old rat with particular reference to the spontaneous appearance of pituitary adenomata. Am J Cancer 34:352–372

Zondek B (1936) Tumors of the pituitary induced with follicular hormone. Lancet 1:776–778

Histochemical Identification of Hormones in Pituitary Tumors, Rat

R. Yoshiyuki Osamura and Shozo Takayama

The most reliable means of identifying the hormone-secreting cells in the pituitary gland is immunohistochemical staining. This method has been used by various investigators to classify human and animal pituitary tumors. For many years, the classification of pituitary tumors into three types – acidophilic, basophilic, and chromophobic – was based on their staining by dyes, such as hematoxylin and eosin (H and E), periodic acid Schiff (PAS), orange G, aldehyde fuchsin, and erythrosin. It was believed that the chromophobic tumors did not produce hormone. However, immunohistochemical methods have clearly shown that many chromophobic adenomas do produce hormones; for example, almost all prolactin-secreting tumors are chromophobic (Osamura and Watanabe 1976; Osamura et al. 1978, 1980).

The current concensus is that the identification and classification of pituitary tumors based upon immunohistochemical identification of the hormones that the tumors produce provides a useful approach which includes understanding of the functional effects of the tumors.

In laboratory animals, pituitary tumors may be induced by radiation, estrogen, or thyroidectomy, or they may occur spontaneously. Most of these tumors are chromophobic by ordinary staining methods.

In order to specifically identify pituitary hormones in cells, we have utilized Nakane's peroxidase-labeled antibody method applied to formalin-fixed paraffin sections, to 6-μm frozen sections (pre-embedding method) for light microscopy, or to ultrathin plastic sections (postembedding method) for examination with the electron microscope (Nakane 1975; Osamura and Watanabe 1976).

Spontaneous Pituitary Tumors

Spontaneous pituitary tumors have been reported frequent in Wistar, Yale, Amsterdam, Columbia-Sherman, and Charles River rats (Furth and Clifton 1966; Furth et al. 1976). In a series studied by Takayama (personal observations) pituitary tumors were found in 34% of male and 40% of female Wistar rats more than 2 years of age. In one report, the frequency of tumors was higher in males than in females (Ito et al. 1972), however, later reports indicate that the tumors may be more frequent in females (Berkvens et al. 1980; Furth et al. 1976).

Spontaneous pituitary tumors in female and male rats are similar in histologic appearance. The tumors are usually well encapsulated and solid or markedly congested. Some congested tumors are commonly labeled as "hemorrhagic adenomas". These tumors are composed of a mixture of neoplastic anterior pituitary cells and networks of vascular spaces. In the hemorrhagic areas, the pools of blood are frequently lined by tumor cells. When stained with H and E the tumor cells are chromophobic, and vary in appearance from rather uniform round epithelial cells with large hyperchromatic nuclei and amphophilic cytoplasm (Fig. 77) to focally anaplastic areas with many giant cells and mitoses (Fig. 78). The exact biologic nature of these atypical cells has not been determined, although focal carcinomatous transformation has been suggested (Furth et al. 1976). The function of these spontaneous tumors is indicated by immunohistochemical staining of prolactin in the uniform as well as in the anaplastic cells (Figs. 79, 80). Although Ito et al. (1972) claim that spontaneous chromophobic pituitary tumors in male rats are mammotropic (secrete Luteotropic hormanes LTH), in our experience, spontaneous pituitary tumors containing LTH are found exclusively in female rats. Spontaneous mammary tumors were seen in Takayama's series only in female, not in male rats (Takayama personal observations 1981). We have demonstrated in female rats both LTH-positive pituitary tumors and mammary tumors with lactating ducts. This suggests a relationship between these two tumors. Cystic mammary hyperplasia is also commonly seen in association with pituitary tumors made up of LTH cells.

Other immunohistochemically identified types of natural pituitary tumors that secrete LTH alone, LTH and growth hormone (GH), LTH and thyroid stimulating hormone (TSH) or adrenocorticotropic hormone (ACTH) have been reported in

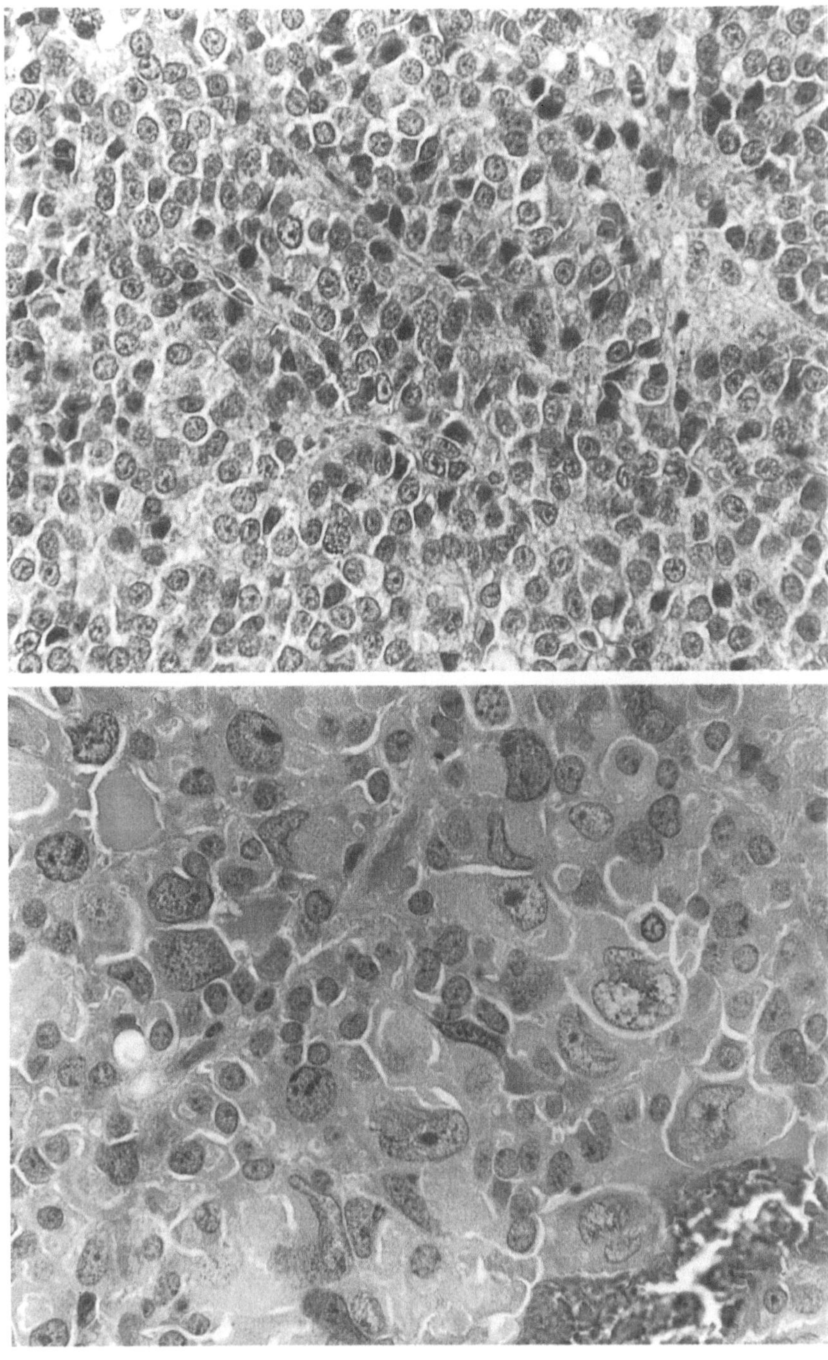

Fig. 77. (*above*) Spontaneous pituitary tumor in a rat. The tumor is chromophobic and has many uniform cells with round to ovoid nuclei and close relationship to capillaries. H&E, ×300

Fig. 78. (*below*) Another part of the same tumor shown in Fig. 77, with many large anaplastic cells with bizarre nuclei. H&E, ×600

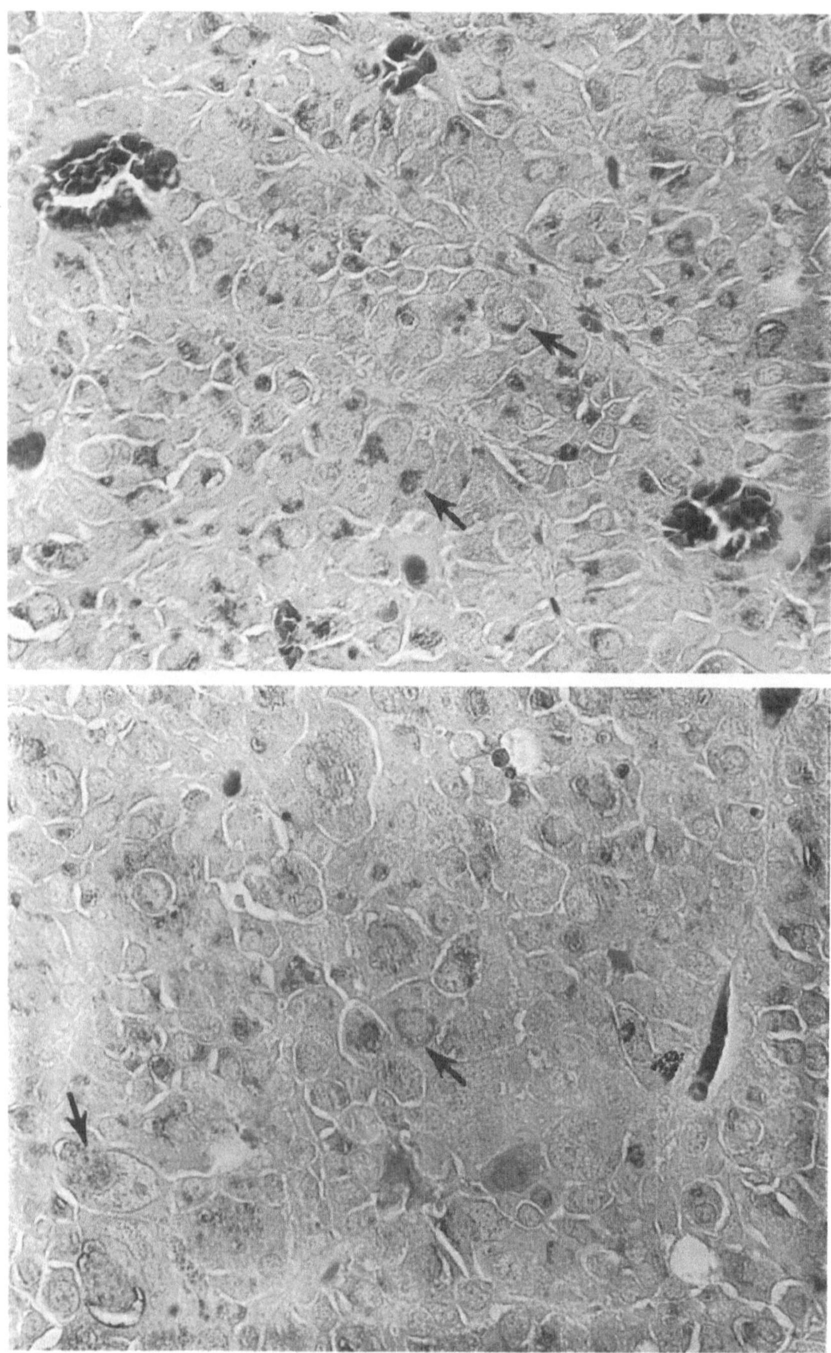

Fig. 79. Prolactin (*top*) in cells of spontaneous pituitary tumor. Area shown similar to that in Fig. 77. Stained by peroxidase-labeled antibody method, ×300

Fig. 80. Prolactin (*bottom*) in large cells with bizarre nuclei seen in Fig. 78. Stained by peroxidase-labeled antibody method, ×600

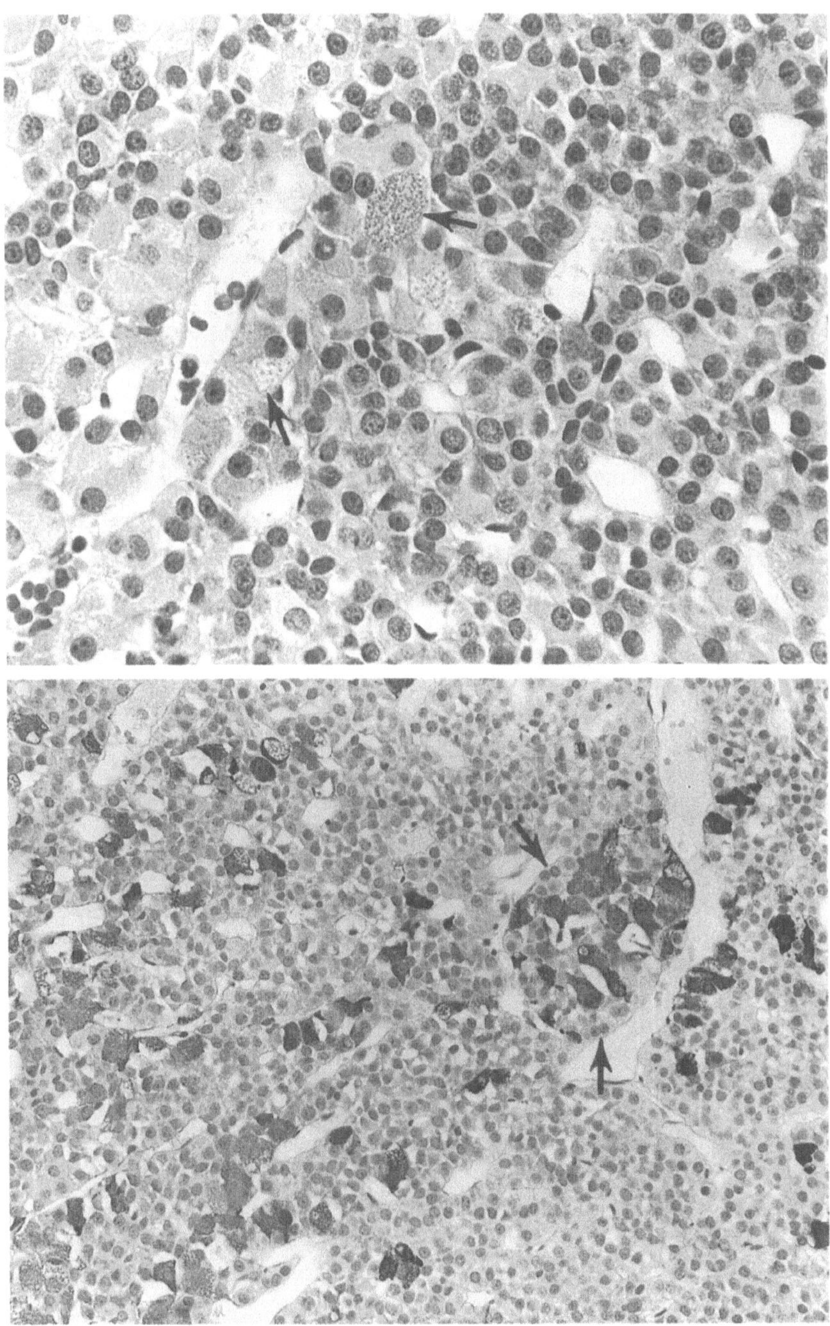

Fig. 81. (*above*) The pars distalis in a rat, 16 weeks after thyroidectomy. The large cells, some containing granular cytoplasm (*arrows*), have been called "thyroidectomy cells." H&E, ×300

Fig. 82. (*below*) Nodular hyperplasia (*arrows*) and TSH cells (*darkly stained*) in the same pituitary as in Fig. 81, following thyroidectomy. Peroxidase-labeled antibody method, ×300

rats (Berkvens et al. 1980; Kovacs et al. 1980). Pituitary tumors made up of LTH cells are much more frequent than those containing GH, TSH or ACTH.

Pituitary Tumors Induced by Thyroidectomy

In rats and mice, thyroid hormone deficiency (as a result of radiation, diet, chemicals, or surgical thyroidectomy) may result in hyperplasia of TSH cells and adenoma formation (Furth et al. 1973). Axelrad and Leblond (1955) reported the sequential formation of adenomas from large swollen "thyoidectomy cells." Large cells forming multicentric nodules considered to be basophilic occupied most of the gland (Furth and Clifton 1966; Furth et al. 1973, 1976).

Sixteen weeks after surgical thyroidectomy in rats, many swollen anterior pituitary glands develop rather chromophobic "thyroidectomy cells" some of which have granules in their cytoplasm (Fig. 81). Immunohistochemical staining for TSH reveals that the hyperplastic nodules consist of cells containing TSH (Fig. 82). These hyperplastic nodules are considered likely to give rise to TSH-secreting adenomas. With the electron microscope, these cells may be seen to contain many vesicular spaces outlined by RER, a few small secretory granules, and an occasional Golgi apparatus. Ultrastructural changes in the "thyroidectomy cells" have been also reported by Farquhar (1971).

Pituitary Tumors Induced by Estrogen

It is well known that estrogen treatment of rats and mice results in LTH-secreting pituitary tumors (Farquhar 1971; Furth and Clifton 1966; Furth et al. 1976). The tumors are usually chromophobic and composed exclusively of LTH-positive cells. The details of these tumors are discussed separately on p. 90.

References

Axelrad AA, Leblond CP (1955) Induction of thyroid tumors in rats by a low iodine diet. Cancer 8:339–367

Berkvens JM, van Nesselrooy JHJ, Kroes R (1980) Spontaneous tumours in the pituitary gland of old Wistar rats. A morphological and immunocytochemical study. J Pathol 130:179–191

Farquhar M (1971) Processing of secretory products by cells of the anterior pituitary gland. In: Memoris of the Society for Endocrinology, No. 19 Subcellular organization and function in endocrine tissue. Cambridge University Press, London, pp 79–124

Furth J, Clifton K (1966) Experimental pituitary tumors. In: Harris GW, Donovon BT (eds) The pituitary gland, vol 2. Butterworths, London, pp 460–497

Furth J, Moy P, Hershman JM, Ueda G (1973) Thyrotropic tumor syndrome. A multiglandular disease induced by sustained deficiency of thyroid hormone. Arch Pathol Lab Med 96:217–226

Furth J, Nakane P, Pasteels JL (1976) Tumours of the piuitary gland. In: Turusov VS (ed) Pathology of tumours in laboratory animals, vol I: tumours of the rat. IARC scientific publ no 6, Lyon, part 2, pp 201–237

Ito A, Moy P, Kaunitz H, Kortwright K, Clarke S, Furth J, Meites J (1972) Incidence and character of the spontaneous pituitary tumors in strain CR and W/Fu male rats. JNCI 49:701–711

Kovacs K, Ilse G, Ryan N, McComb DJ, Horvath E, Chen HJ, Waifish PG (1980) Pituitary prolactin cell hyperplasia. Hormone Res 12:87–95

Nakane PK (1975) Recent progress in peroxidase-labeled antibody method. Ann N Y Acad Sci 254:203–211

Osamura RY, Watanabe K (1976) Peroxidase-labeled antibody method: principle and applications to endocrinology (in Japanese). Clin Endocrinol 24:1074–1087

Osamura RY, Watanabe K, Teramoto A, Hirakawa K, Kawano N, Morii S (1978) Male prolactin secreting pituitary adenomas in humans studied by peroxidase-labeled antibody method. Acta Endocrinol 88:643–652

Osamura RY, Komatsu N, Nakahashi E, Watanabe K (1980) Light and electron microscopical combined staining by immunohistochemical and enzyme histochemical methods using rat prolactin-secreting pituitary tumours. Histochem J 12:371–379

Adenoma and Carcinoma, Pars Distalis, Anterior Pituitary Gland, Rat

William W. Carlton and Christian L. Gries

Synonyms. Chromophobe, basophil, and acidophil adenoma and carcinoma,[1] adenocarcinoma, pars distalis, rat.

Gross Appearance

Pituitary neoplasms vary greatly in size, from single or multiple microscopic foci to large masses that replace the whole gland, markedly enlarging it up to a diameter of 20 mm and a weight of 350 mg or more (Kovacs et al. 1977b; Fig. 83). The neoplasms are generally well defined, spherical, circumscribed, soft, friable, and smooth, but they may have an irregular nodular surface, and they are not encapsulated. Either they are solid, or they contain cavernous vessels with hemorrhages and congestion (Andersson 1969). The neoplasms are separated from the brain, but a few invade the adjacent brain and meninges. Large neoplasms protrude from the sella and produce compression atrophy of the adjacent brain parenchyma (Wolfe et al. 1938; Ross et al. 1970; Kovacs et al. 1977b). The cut surface is light brown to dark red depending on the vascularity of the neoplasm.

Microscopic Features

Pituitary neoplasms vary in size, vascularity, and cytologic features (Wolf et al. 1938; Wolfe and Wright 1947; Thompson et al. 1961; Ross et al. 1970; Berkvens et al. 1980). Large neoplasms replace much of the gland (Fig. 84), and both small and large neoplasms often contain blood-filled spaces (Fig. 85) and foci of hemorrhage (sometimes called hemorrhagic or cavernous angiomatous adenoma). The neoplasms produce compression of the surrounding nonneoplastic parenchyma but are not encapsulated (Fig. 86). Usually the circumscribed neoplasms are of a diffuse pattern and composed of cells in sheets, clusters, or anastomosing cords of variable thickness separated by compressed capillaries and fragile connective tissue (Fig. 87). In the hemorrhagic adenoma the cell cords are separated by wide spaces filled with blood. These blood-filled spaces may be either vascular (lined by endothelium) or nonvascular (lined by pituitary gland cells; Fig. 88). Macrophages filled with hemosiderin are commonly located adjacent to congested or hemorrhagic areas in angiomatous adenomas. Pigment granules, yellow-brown and iron negative, occur in some adenoma cells (Fig. 89; Kovacs et al. 1977b).

The cells of the neoplasms vary in size and shape from small round, oval, or polyhedral cells to enormously large, bizarre forms (Fig. 90). Generally the nuclei of neoplastic cells are larger than those of normal cells. In sections stained with H&E the slight to moderately abundant cytoplasm is pale to darkly basophilic and contains moderate to large, pale, round to oval nuclei, usually centrally located and vesicular with a distinct nuclear membrane and nucleoli (Fig. 91). The nucleoli may be basophilic and multiple. Mitotic figures are generally few but may be common in some neoplasms. Focally a few to many cells have slightly to extensively vacuolated cytoplasm (Fig. 92). Cytologic atypia include nuclear pleomorphism (Fig. 93), hyperchromasia and polyploidy.

The cells of most pituitary neoplasms do not contain granules in routine H&E stained sections. Differential staining techniques are not especially useful for identifying the cells in pituitary adenomas of rats. The cytoplasm of neoplastic cells does not usually stain either with PAS, aldehyde fuchsin, or aldehyde thionin, but certain neoplasms have cells that give a positive reaction to prolactin by Herlant's erythrosin or Brookes'

[1] Benign or malignant neoplasia and hyperplasia of the pars distalis are best distinguished by means of tissue and cellular stains, such as H&E. In this section the authors propose that tumors of the pars distalis of the rat be classified as adenomas or carcinomas, and that the descriptive terms chromophobe, basophil, and acidophil not be used. This is proposed because tintorial staining features do not indicate cellular function, i.e., the type of or presence of hormone production. The identity of the hormones secreted by the cells involved in these lesions must be determined by use of other techniques, such as immunoperoxidase methods, described elsewhere in this volume (p. 33). After the secretory products of the affected cells have been determined, descriptive terms may be added to further distinguish the neoplasm.

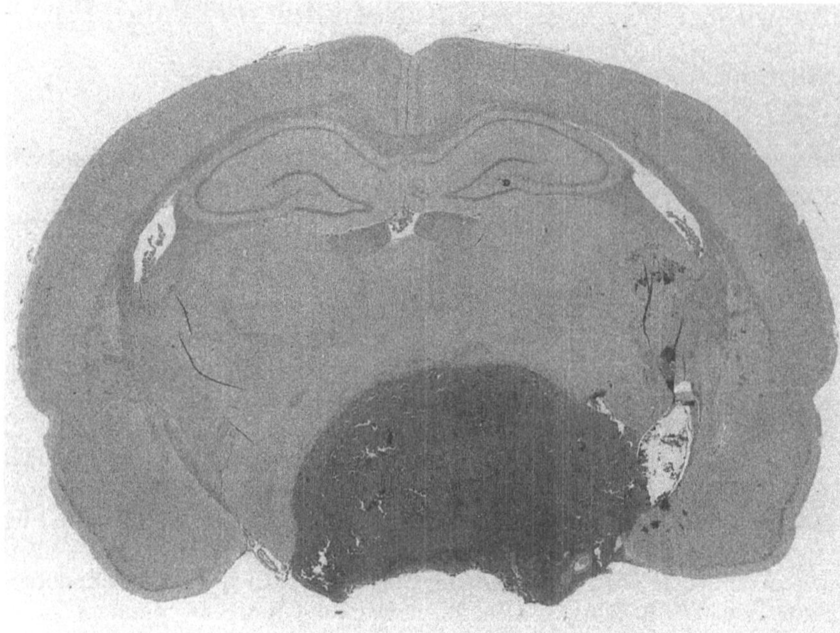

Fig. 83. Pituitary adenoma, rat. Expanisive growth has replaced gland and caused compression atrophy of overlying brain. H&E, ×6

carmoisin methods (Kovacs et al. 1977b; Berkvens et al. 1980).

Ultrastructure

The ultrastructural features of spontaneous pituitary gland "chromophobe adenomas" observed in Sprague-Dawley rats have been reported by Majeed et al. (1980). In their series the ultrastructural appearance was uniform, and one cell type was dominant. The neoplastic cells were generally without desmosomes and had irregularly shaped nuclei with dense marginal chromatin and large nucleoli. The cytoplasmic granules varied greatly in number among different neoplasms and between areas of the same neoplasm, as well as in size and shape. The rough endoplasmic reticulum was well developed and sometimes arranged in concentric whorls. The Golgi complexes were prominent in the neoplastic cells. The mitochondria had well-developed cristae and varied in number and size. The ultrastructural features were suggestive of active mammotropic cells.

The ultrastructure of prolactin-secreting cells in adenomas of the pituitary gland of female Long-Evans rats was studied by Kovacs et al. (1977b) and Lee et al. (1982). These neoplasms were composed of oval to polyhedral cells with large oval to irregular nuclei, rich in chromatin and with a prominent nucleolus. The cytoplasm contained parallel cisternae or concentric whorls of rough-surfaced endoplasmic reticulum. A modest number of rod-shaped, moderately dense mitochondria were present. The Golgi system was usually extensively developed. Spherical and/or pleomorphic secretory granules occurred in the neoplastic cells but varied greatly in number from neoplasm to neoplasm and from cell to cell within the same neoplasm. Most neoplasms were composed of sparsely granulated cells, with most secretory granules measuring 250–300 nm in diameter. Misplaced exocytosis was a feature of many neoplastic cells. Multiple centrioles, rudimentary cilia, and pigment granules were fairly common in cells of some adenomas. (See also Schelin and Lundin 1971.)

Differential Diagnosis

Pituitary adenomas must be differentiated from focal and diffuse hyperplasias, and the adenoma differentiated from carcinoma. Focal hyperplasias

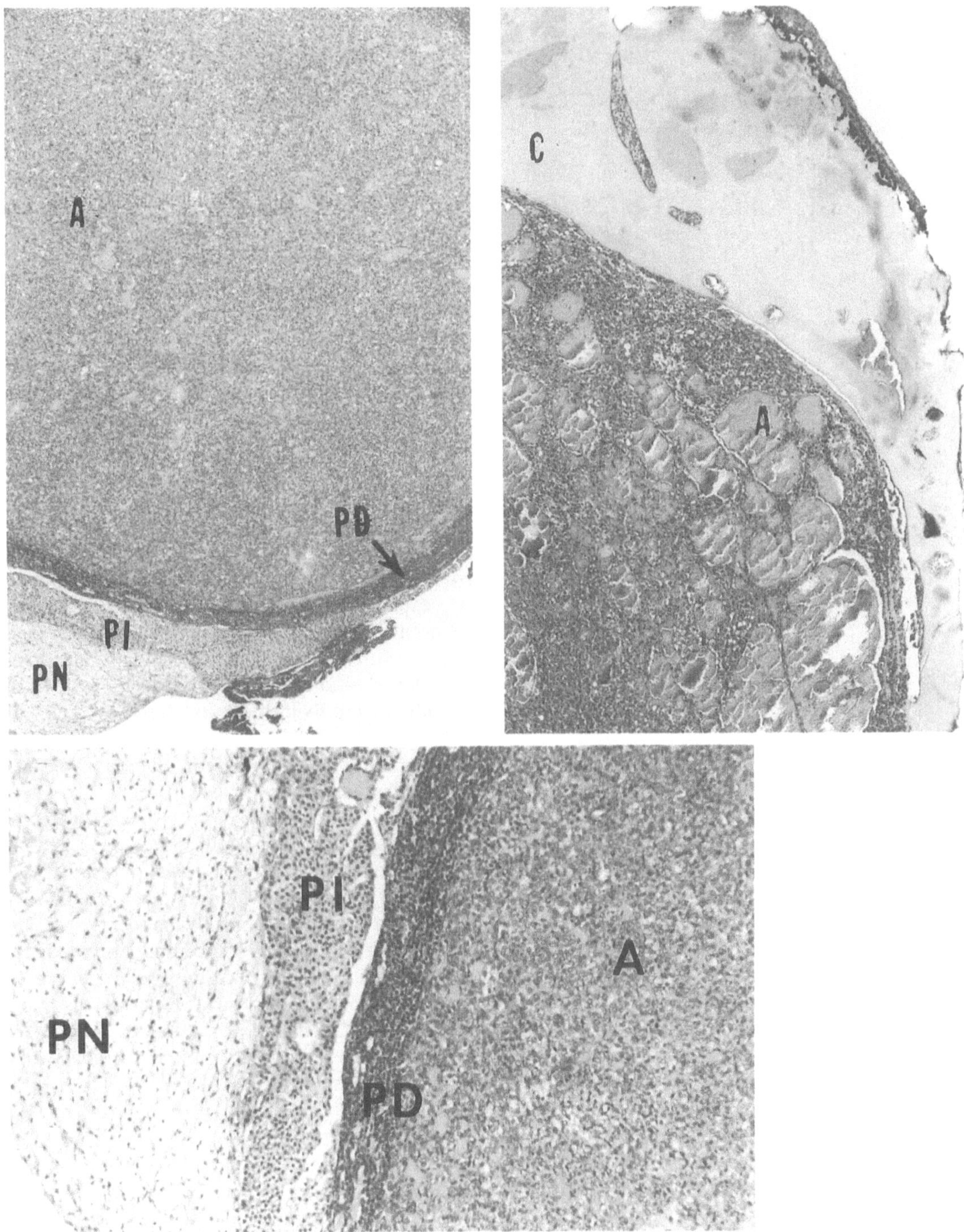

Fig. 84. (*upper left*) Pituitary adenoma (*A*), rat. Central round mass stains with less intensity than the compressed rim of non-neoplastic pars distalis (*PD*). Pars nervosa (*PN*) and adjacent pars intermedia (*PI*) are also shown. H&E, ×35

Fig. 85. (*upper right*) "Angiomatous" pituitary adenoma (*A*) rat. Numberous spaces of variable size, filled with blood, lie adjacent to colloid-filled cyst (*C*). H&E, ×35

Fig. 86. (*below*) Pituitary adenoma (*A*), rat. Closely packed cells have compressed adjacent non-neoplastic pars distalis. Pars intermedia (*PI*) lies between compressed pars distalis (*PD*) and pars nervosa (*PN*). H&E, ×56

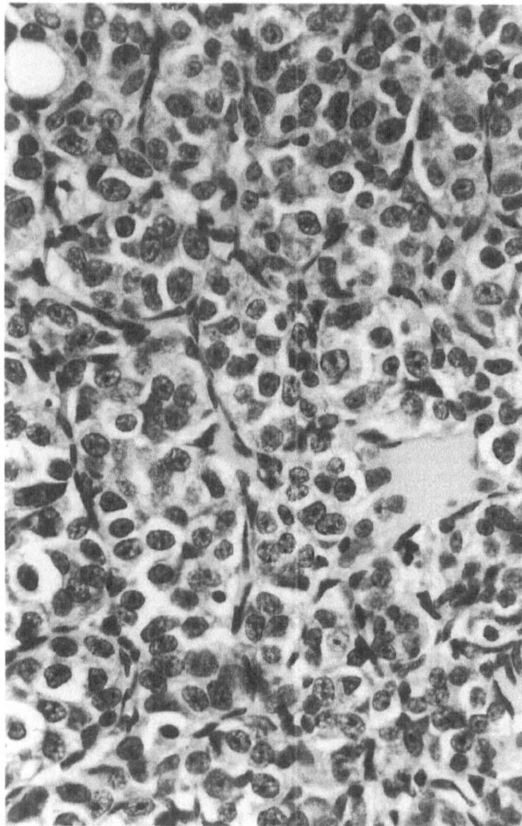

Fig. 87. Pituitary adenoma, rat. A delicate stroma divides variably sized collections of closely packed, fairly uniform epithelial cells. H&E, ×350

of the pituitary gland are common and occur in association with micro- or gross adenomas. The adenoma is distinguished by increased vascularity with a few to numerous dilated vascular spaces, by compression of the adjacent nonneoplastic parenchyma, and by changes in cellular and/or nuclear size. Generally the nuclei of neoplastic cells are larger than those of nonneoplastic cells. Cytoplasmic volume of neoplastic cells may be reduced or increased, and neoplastic cells often appear palely basophilic in H&E stained sections. The most useful criterion for designating a pituitary neoplasm as a carcinoma is its infiltration of the adjacent brain and meninges. The presence of giant cells, normal or abnormal mitotic figures, abnormal nuclei, and focal necrosis indicates malignancy. However, neoplasms with such histologic features may be found without evidence of local invasion, and other neoplasms that invade the brain are histologically indistinguishable from noninvasive pituitary gland adenomas (MacKenzie and Garner 1973).

[Editors note: The equivalent term for the malignant variety used in the WHO international classification is "adenocarcinoma, pars distalis (M)" (Mohr et al. 1994).]

Without the information obtainable using the techniques of transmission electron microscopy and immunohistochemical staining, the common pituitary neoplasms as seen with routine H&E stained sections are probably best designated as adenoma or carcinoma of the pars distalis. The designation chromophobe adenoma adds no specificity to the diagnosis and is considered obsolete. A definitive diagnosis is based on the demonstration of specific cell types in the neoplasms.

Biologic Features

Most pituitary gland neoplasms are benign, grow by expansion, and do not usually infiltrate adjacent brain and meninges. Metastasis beyond the cranium appears to be exceedingly rare. Rats with large pituitary gland neoplasms with focal atrophy of the hypothalamus often have signs of lethargy and anorexia. These rats undergo a period of progressive weight loss prior to death (Boorman and Hollander 1973).

Most pituitary gland adenomas of aged rats are either mammotropic (Berkvens et al. 1980) or mammosomatotropic neoplasms (Furth et al. 1976). In a study of 26 spontaneous pituitary neoplasms in female Long-Evans rats, Kovacs et al. (1977b) reported that the immunoperoxidase technique established the presence of immunoreactive prolactin in the cytoplasm of many adenoma cells. Rats with these mammotropic neoplasms have elevated serum prolactin activity. Prolactin-positive adenomas are the most frequent. Other adenomas may be positive for luteinizing hormone, thyroid-stimulating hormone, or growth hormone, but these usually account for only a few adenomas (McComb et al. 1984). Few pituitary gland neoplasms of rats contain adrenocorticotropin (ACTH) reacting cells identified by immunocytochemical techniques, and only one or two such neoplasms have been found among populations of Fischer 344, Sprague-Dawley, Wistar, and Long-Evans rats (Sandusky et al. 1988; Berkvens et al. 1980; Lee et al. 1982; McComb et al. 1984). None of the affected rats

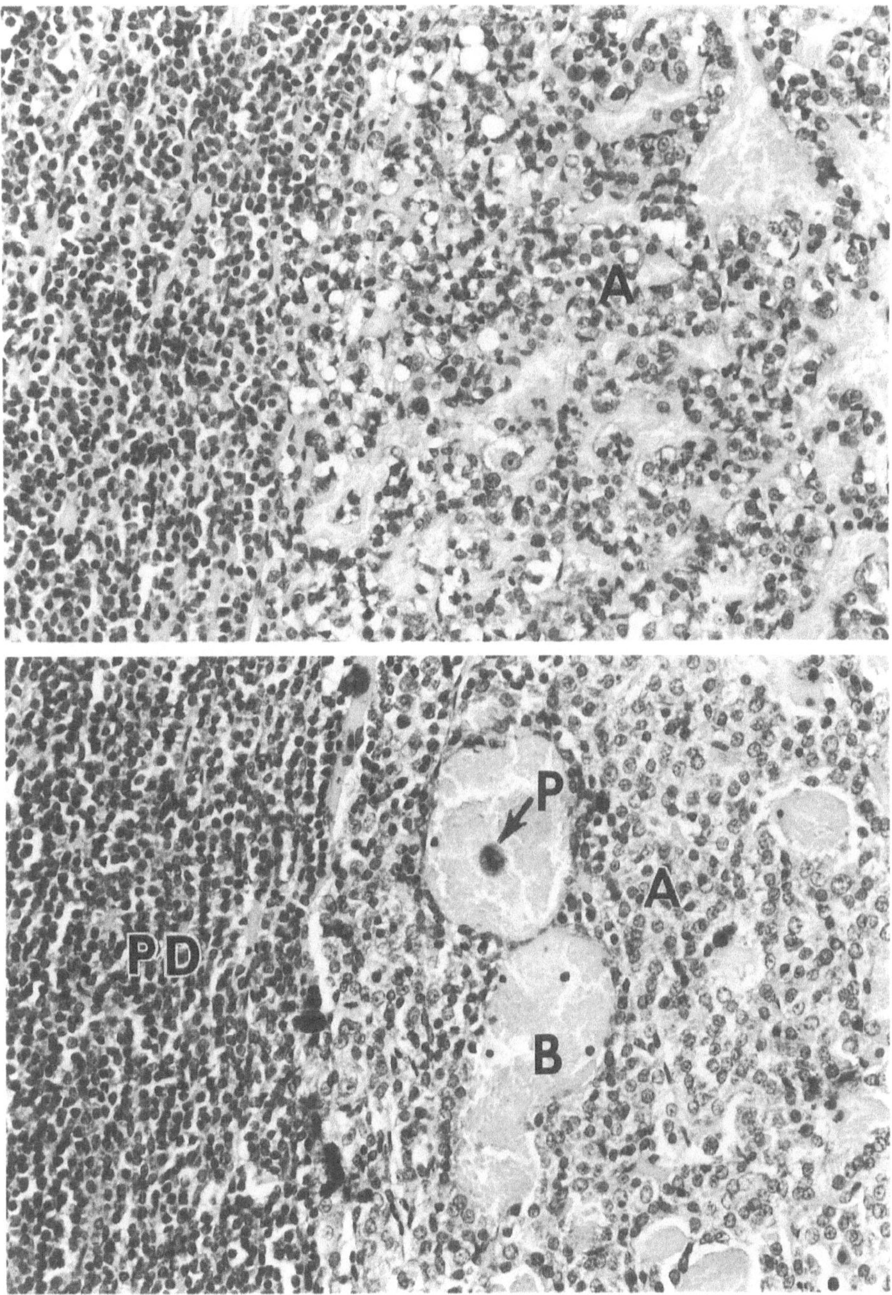

Fig. 88. (*above*) Pituitary adenoma (*A*), rat. Sinusoidal pattern with interconnecting cords of tumor cells separated by blood-filled spaces. H&E, ×224

Fig. 89. (*below*) Pituitary adenoma, rat. Composed of closely packed epithelial cells (*A*) with larger, more vesicluar nuclei than those found in adjacent compressed non-neoplastic parenchyma (*PD*). Spaces are filled with blood (*B*) and pigment clumps (*P*). H&E, ×224

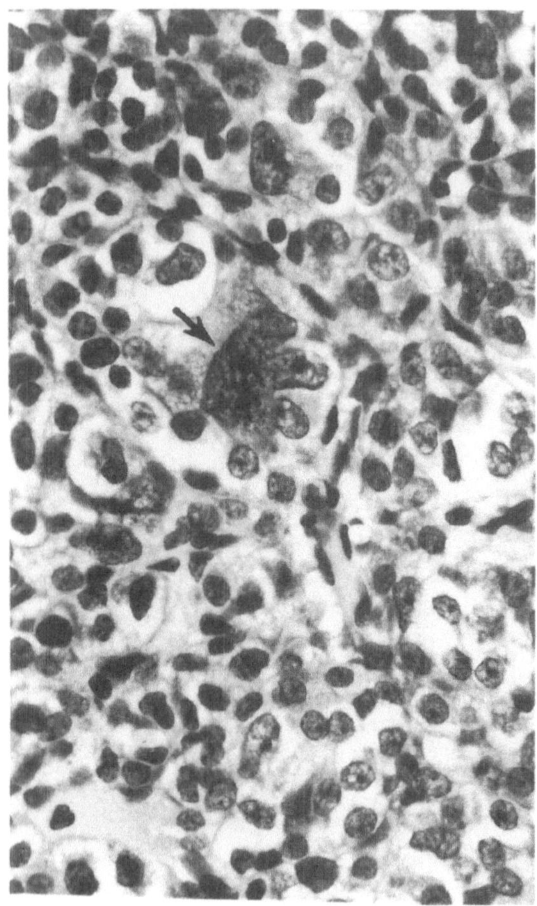

Fig. 90. Pituitary adenoma, rat. Diffuse pattern is composed of closely packed epithelial cells with variably sized nuclei and pale-staining or vacuolated cytoplasm. A giant, bizarre nucleus (*arrow*) is present. H&E, ×560

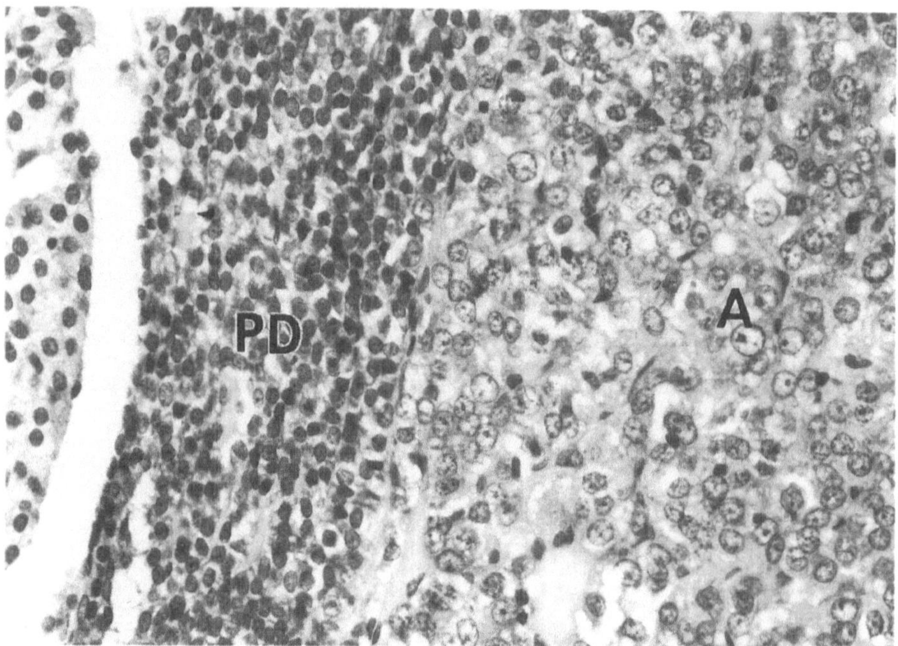

Fig. 91. Pituitary adenoma (*A*) of diffuse pattern, sharply delimited from compressed non-neoplastic parenchyma (*PD*) and composed of closely packed, large epithelial cells with indistinct borders and large, vesicular, variably sized nuclei. H&E, ×350

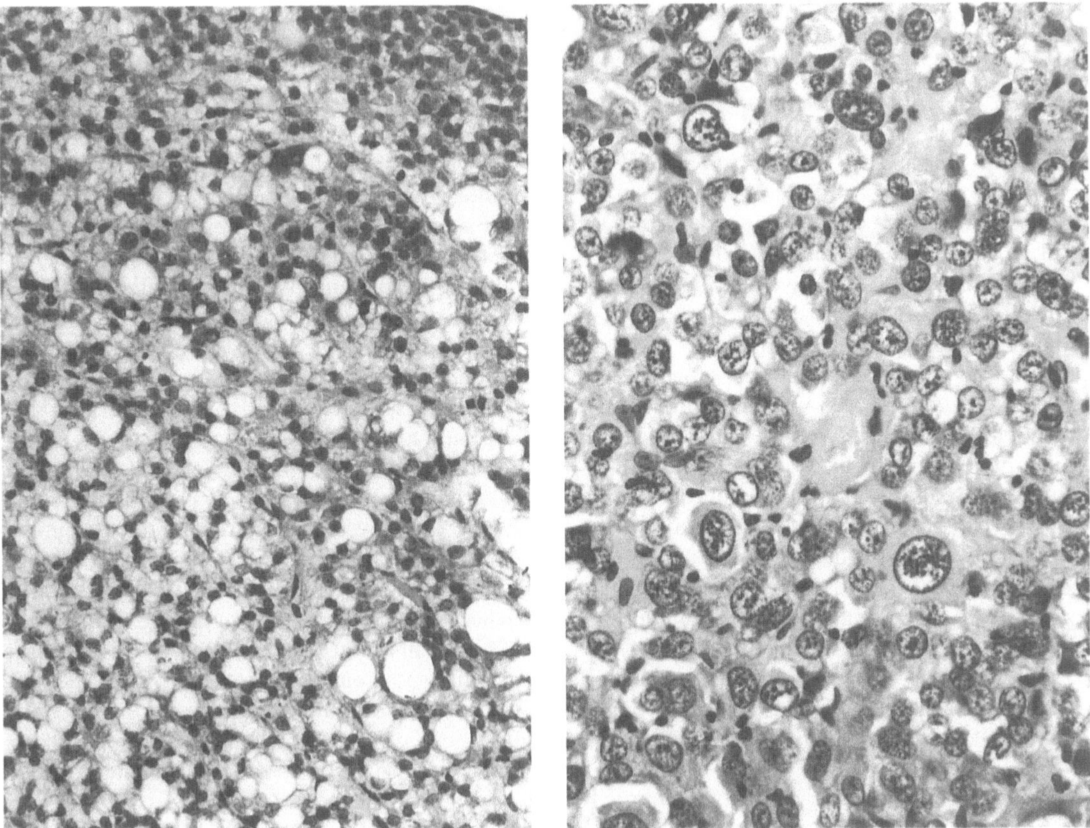

Fig. 92. (*left*) Pituitary adenoma with extensive cytoplasmic vacuolation. H&E, ×224

Fig. 93. (*right*) Pituitary adenoma, rat. Diffuse pattern, composed of closely packed epithelial cells with nuclei of many sizes and shapes, and varying chromatin content and arrangement. H&E, ×350

had clinical signs associated with ACTH hormone secretion. Cushing's disease (syndrome) has been observed in two Lew/Han rats with pituitary neoplasms containing ACTH-positive cells. The affected rats had an enlarged pendulous abdomen, were obese, and had lesions of bilateral adrenal cortical hyperplasia as well as fatty degeneration of the liver (Kaspareit-Rittinghausen et al. 1990). Proliferative lesions of gonadotroph cells are rarely reported in rats (Griesbach 1967; Lee et al. 1982; McComb et al. 1985), but a rather high incidence (27/130 rats) was observed in aging male Lobund-Wistar rats (Sano et al. 1989). The development of the lesions was delayed by feed restriction and germ-free status.

Pathogenesis. Pituitary gland neoplasms arise from cells that have suffered some derangement of the normal feedback mechanism between the pituitary cell and its target tissue (Furth et al. 1973). The operation of an extrinsic agent (viral, chemical, or physical) is not necessary for pituitary gland tumorigenesis. In contrast to the normal pituitary gland cell which produces a single hormone per cell type (exception is the gonadotroph), the cells of the pituitary gland adenoma, while of a single cell type, have the potential of secreting more than one hormone (adenomas are monomorphous but multihormonal). Immunoperoxidase staining has localized both prolactin and growth hormone in the cytoplasm of the same pituitary adenoma cells (Ito et al. 1971, 1972b). Rats bearing primary pituitary gland adenomas have, in some studies, slight to moderate stimulation of the mammary glands (Bielschowsky 1954). Microscopically both acini and ductal structures are increased in number and are distended with amorphous acidophilic material (Kim et al. 1960; Ito et al. 1972a).

Etiology. Anterior pituitary neoplasms have been induced in rats by three major procedures: (a) prolonged specific hormone imbalance, (b) exposure to ionizing radiation, and (c) combined hormone imbalance and ionizing radiation (Furth et al. 1973; Russfield 1966). Estrogens (estrone, diethylstilbestrol) are effective agents for inducing pituitary neoplasms in the rat, and the neoplasms induced are estrogen dependent when first transplanted; however, autonomy is achieved after several generations of transplantation. Most of the estrogen-induced pituitary gland neoplasms are mammosomatotropic.

Chronic thyroid deficiency, subtotal thyroidectomy, or subtotal thyroidectomy and administration of ^{131}I has produced thyrotropic pituitary gland adenomas (Furth et al. 1973). Pituitary gland neoplasms have also been induced in rats by exposure of the head and neck to 8 Gy X-irradiation. These neoplasms were transplantable and stimulated somatic growth as well as growth and activity of the mammary glands (Russfield 1966).

The incidence of pituitary gland adenoma has been modified by dietary manipulation. The prevalence of this neoplasm was markedly reduced by caloric restriction (Saxton et al. 1948; Berg and Simms 1961; Ross et al. 1970). The proportion of protein in the diet also modified the incidence of pituitary gland adenoma. In studies by Ross et al. (1970) restriction in protein intake reduced the number of pituitary gland neoplasms, but the greatest reduction occurred in groups restricted in both caloric and protein intakes.

Frequency. Spontaneous primary pituitary gland neoplasms of the chromophobe type are common in certain strains of the laboratory rat (Table 3). Prevalence of the neoplasm has varied among groups of rats of the same strain obtained from different commercial sources (MacKenzie and Garner 1973), as well as among strains. Sex may also have an effect on the incidence. In most reports giving the sex of the rats the number of pituitary gland neoplasms was greater in the female (Kociba et al. 1979; Magnusson et al. 1979), but in a few early reports with the Osborne-Mendel strain the number of pituitary gland neoplasms was greater in males (Saxton et al. 1948; Saxton and Graham 1944). These neoplasms are found in older rats; few are found in rats younger than 15–18 months (Crain 1958; Gilbert and Gillman 1958; Boorman and Hollander 1973; Kociba et al. 1979).

Acidophil adenomas appear to be rare pituitary gland neoplasms, as few have been reported (Wolfe and Wright 1947; Fitzgerald et al. 1971). Two acidophil adenomas were found in 2-year-old female Holtzman rats. The lesions were circumscribed, nonencapsulated nodules composed of hypertrophied cells containing large rounded nuclei with prominent nucleoli. The abundant granular cytoplasm contained PAS-positive granules in some cells.

Basophil adenomas are also infrequent in the pituitary gland of the rat (Griesbach 1967). One found in a series of neoplasms from Sprague-Dawley rats consisted of a small nodule composed of cells containing PAS-positive cytoplasmic granules (Schardein et al. 1968). Basophil adenomas were found in aged rats chronically deficient in iodine (Bielschowsky 1953). Three basophil adenomas were described in the Holtzman rat strain (Fitzgerald et al. 1971), all in males; two of them were found in rats killed at 1 year of age. The circumscribed, nonencapsulated nodules of the anterior lobe were composed of uniform, hypertrophied cells with PAS-positive cytoplasmic granules.

Pituitary gland carcinomas, differentiated from adenomas by their infiltration of the adjacent brain or meninges, are not common; 11 cases were found among 1038 pituitary gland neoplasms from 2609 approximately 2-year-old Sprague-Dawley rats of both sexes (Magnusson et al. 1979). These infiltrating neoplasms were vascular solid masses composed of predominantly uniform, relatively small cells with few mitotic figures. Extracranial metastases were not found. In a study of 492 Sprague-Dawley rats Kociba et al. (1979) recorded 44 pituitary gland carcinomas, with extension to the brain in 13.

Comparison with Other Species

Neoplasms of the pars distalis in domestic animals include functional (corticotroph) and nonfunctional chromophobe adenomas, basophil and acidophil adenomas, and chromophobe carcinomas. The latter three pituitary neoplasms are considered rare (Capen 1990). Functional (corticotroph) adenomas occur most frequently in the

Table 3. Spontaneous neoplasms of the anterior pituitary (pars distalis), rat

Strain	Age (months)	Pituitary (Male/Female)	Tumors/no. rats examined (%)	Reference
Vanderbilt	17–30	2/17 male	12	Wolfe et al. 1938
		11/38 female	29	
Wistar	Old	26/38	68	Wolfe et al. 1938
Yale (OM)	13–30	16/30 male	53	Saxton 1941
		1/13 female	8	
Yale (OM)	8–30	70/158 male	44	Saxton and Graham 1944
		22/125 female	18	
Osborne-Mendel	7–37	45/99 male	45	Saxton et al. 1948
		24/99 female	24	
Rochester (Wistar)	18–24	11/786	1	Crain 1958
Wistar	10–38	52/612 male	8	Gilbert and Gillman 1958
		75/609 female	12	
Sprague-Dawley	17–42	251/1211	21	Simms and Berg 1957
W/FU (Wistar)	17–33	20/73	27[a]	Kim et al. 1960
Sprague-Dawley	12–30	8/50	16[a]	Thompson and Hunt 1963
Fisher	22–24	9/92 male	10	Jacobs and Huseby 1967
		3/102 female	3	
SD (Holtzman)	6–18	9/806 male	1	Schardein et al. 1968
		23/618 female	4	
SD (Charles River)	–	512/1242	42	Ito et al. 1972a
WAG/Rij (Wistar)	12–43	199/290	69	Boorman and Hollander 1973
Sprague-Dawley	24	10/258	4[a]	MacKenzie and Garner 1973
Sprague-Dawley (Holtzman)	24	14/268	5[a]	
Sprague-Dawley (Diablo)	24	14/2176[a]	–	
Sprague-Dawley (Charles River)	24	48/5358[a]	–	
Osborne-Mendel	24	20/131	15[a]	
Oregon	24	11/673	5[a]	
Sprague-Dawley	13–24	68/236 male	19	
		135/236 female	57	Kociba et al. 1979
Sprague-Dawley	24	442/1371 male	32	Magnusson et al. 1979
		596/1238 female	48	
Wistar (Chbb: Thom SPF)	21–30	30/400 male	7.5	Ueberberg and Lutzen 1979
		65/400 female	16	

[a] Sex not recorded.

dog but are also described in other species, including the cat and the horse. These ACTH-secreting neoplasms produce the syndrome of hyperadrenocorticism (see p. 15). Spontaneous ACTH-secreting neoplasms are rare in the rat and have not been induced experimentally, but adrenotropic cell lines have been developed from a variant of a mammosomatotropic neoplasm (Ito 1976; Furth et al. 1976). Sandusky et al. (1988) found only two ACTH-positive adenomas in 62 Fischer 344 rats with pituitary neoplasms. Only two single ACTH-positive neoplasms were found in studies on Wistar (Berkvens et al. 1980), Long-Evans (Lee et al. 1982) and Sprague-Dawley rats (McComb et al. 1984). In the rat most pituitary adenomas are mammotropic or mammosomatotropic in respect to hormone production.

Nonfunctional chromophobe adenomas occur in the dog, cat (Zaki and Liu 1973), and horse and, while endocrinologically inactive, produce clinical disease due to damage to the overlying brain or nearby structures such as the optic nerves. Histologically the polyhedral cells arranged in a diffuse pattern have no histochemically demonstrable secretory granules.

Few adenomas of the pituitary gland have been described in nonhuman primates, and those described include an adenoma of the anterior pituitary gland in a rhesus monkey (*Macaca mulatta*; Kent and Pickering 1958), a chromophobe adenoma in a *M. arctoides* (Seibold and Wolf 1973), and a thyrotropic cell adenoma in a *M. fasicularis* (Tsuchitani and Narama 1984).

Acidophil adenomas are rare in domestic animals but are most often described in the dog. Hypersecretion of neither somatotropin nor prolactin has been demonstrated in this species. A few acidophilic pituitary gland adenomas have been described in the cat and have been associated with diabetes mellitus and production of growth hormone (Heinrichs et al. 1989; Lichtensteiger et al. 1986). In the cat the neoplasms are multinodular, nonencapsulated, sharply defined, and composed of large polygonal cells with abundant finely granular acidophilic cytoplasm in H&E and trichrome-stained sections. The nuclei are relatively large and round with a prominent nucleolus.

Pituitary gland carcinomas are uncommon in domestic animals; the majority have been seen in aged dogs. These neoplasms may extensively invade the brain, and metastasis may occur rarely to distant sites (Powers and Winkler 1977).

Neoplasms of the pituitary gland of humans include adenomas of the adenohypophysis classified previously as acidophil, basophil and chromophobe adenomas, and carcinomas (Russell and Rubinstein 1972). Most of the adenomas arise from the pars distalis. The chromophobe adenoma accounts for about 79% of the pituitary gland adenomas, the acidophil adenoma for 15%, and the basophil adenoma for 6%. Histologically the chromophobe adenoma occurs in two principal architectural forms: sinusoidal and diffuse. In the sinusoidal type elongated, tapering cells are orientated toward the supporting blood vessels, producing an appearance of papillary growth. The diffuse type consists of variably sized groups of polygonal cells without any specific orientation to the blood vessels. The cytoplasm of cells of certain of these adenomas is vacuolated, and in biopsy specimens resembles oligodendroglioma. The solid rat pituitary gland adenoma most nearly resembles the diffuse pattern described for the human pituitary gland chromophobe adenoma.

The acidophil adenoma is composed of compact collections of polygonal cells in a diffuse pattern containing fine to coarse acid-fuchsin positive cytoplasmic granules, and in human patients it is often associated with gigantism and acromegaly. The basophilic adenoma, which occurs most often in young people, is associated with Cushing's syndrome. Histologically these neoplasms consist of polygonal cells in a diffuse pattern and the cells contain PAS-positive granules. Ultrastructural and immunohistochemical studies in combination with clinical and pathologic evaluation of pituitary gland syndromes have established that not all chromophobe adenomas are inactive, and hormone secretion by a number of these neoplasms has been demonstrated. Histologically pure chromophobe adenomas have been associated with acromegaly, Cushing's syndrome, and Forbes-Albright syndrome. Nonfunctioning adenomas may include chromophobe, eosinophil and basophil adenomas. Endocrine-active adenomas also include all histologic types (Blaylock and Kempe 1977).

Classification of human pituitary neoplasms has been modified in recent years to include groups based on the histochemical and ultrastructural features. These groups include (Kovacs et al. 1977a):

- Prolactin cell adenomas
  - Densely granulated
  - Sparsely granulated
- Growth hormone cell adenomas
  - Densely granulated
  - Sparsely granulated
- Mixed prolactin growth hormone cell adenoma
- Acidophil stem cell adenoma
- Corticotropic cell adenoma
  - Functioning
  - Silent
- Gonadotroph cell adenoma
- Thyrotroph cell adenoma
- Undifferentiated (null cell) adenoma
  - Nononcocytic
  - Oncocytic

The prolactin-producing cell adenomas are the most common and most of these are sparsely granulated. The null cell adenomas are the second most common of the adenomas.

Carcinomas of the human pituitary gland are uncommon, and most have been associated with Cushing's syndrome. Carcinomas with extracranial metastasis are rare (D'Abrera et al. 1973); in the reported cases metastases have been found in the liver, spinal cord, cauda equina, and upper cervical lymph nodes.

References

Andersson P (1969) High incidence of chromophobe pituitary adenoma-like lesions in an inbred Sprague-Dawley breeding rat colony. Acta Vet Scand 10:111–117

Berg BN, Simms HS (1961) Nutrition and longevity in the rat. J Nutr 74:23–32

Berkvens JM, van Nesselrooy JHJ, Kroes R (1980) Spontaneous tumours in the pituitary of old Wistar rats. A morphological and immunocytochemical study. J Pathol 130:179–191

Bielschowsky F (1953) Chronic iodine deficiency as a cause of neoplasia in thyroid and pituitary of aged rats. Br J Cancer 7:203–213

Bielschowsky F (1954) Functional acidophilic tumors of the pituitary of the rat. Br J Cancer 8:154–160

Blaylock RL, Kempe LG (1977) Pituitary adenomas – a reappraisal of their pathology and treatment. Neurochirugia (Stuttg) 10:63–78

Boorman GA, Hollander CF (1973) Spontaneous lesions in the female WAG/Rij (Wistar) rat. J Gerontol 28:152–159

Capen CC (1990) Tumors of the endocrine glands. In: Moulton JE (ed) Tumors in domestic animals, 2nd edn. University of California Berkeley Press, Berkeley

Crain RC (1958) Spontaneous tumors in the Rochester strain of the Wistar rat. Am J Pathol 34:311–343

D'Abrera VS, Burke WJ, Bleasel KF, Bader L (1973) Carcinoma of the pituitary gland. J Pathol 109:335–343

Fitzgerald JE, Schardein JL, Kaump DH (1971) Several uncommon pituitary tumors in the rat. Lab Anim Sci 21: 581–584

Furth J, Ueda G, Clifton KH (1973) The pathophysiology of pituitaries and their tumors: Methodological advances. In: Busch H (ed) Methods in cancer research, vol 10. Academic, New York, pp 201–277

Furth J, Nakane P, Pasteels JL (1976) Tumours of the pituitary gland. In: Turusov VS (ed) Pathology of tumours in laboratory animals, vol I, part 2. IARC, Lyon, pp 201–237 (IARC scientific publication no 6)

Gilbert C, Gillman J (1958) Spontaneous neoplasms in albino rats. S Afr J Med Sci 23:257–272

Griesbach WE (1967) Basophil adenomata in the pituitary glands of 2-year-old male Long-Evans rats. Cancer res 27:1813–1818

Heinrichs M, Baumgartner W, Krug-Manntz S (1989) Immunocytochemical demonstration of growth hormone in an acidophilic adenoma of the adenohypophysis in a cat. Vet Pathol 26:179–180

Ito A (1976) Animal model of human disease: pituitary tumors. Am J Pathol 83:423–426

Ito A, Martin JM, Grindeland RE, Takizawa S, Furth J (1971) Mammotropic and somatotropic hormones in sera of normal rats and in rats bearing primary and grafted pituitary tumors. Int J Cancer 7:416–429

Ito A, Moy P, Kaunitz H, Kortwright K, Clarke S, Furth J, Meites J (1972a) Incidence and character of the spontaneous pituitary tumors in strain CR and W/Fu male rats. JNCI 49:701–711

Ito A, Furth J, Moy P (1972b) Growth hormone-secreting variants of a mammotropic tumor. Cancer Res 32:48–56

Jacobs BB, Huseby RA (1967) Neoplasms occurring in aged Fischer rats, with special reference to testicular, uterine and thyroid tumors. JNCI 39:303–309

Kaspareit-Rittinghausen J, Hense S, Deerberg F (1990) Cushing's syndrome and disease-like lesions in rats. Z Versuchstierkd 33:229–234

Kent SP, Pickering JE (1958) Neoplasms in monkeys (Macaca mulatta); spontaneous and irradiation induced. Cancer 11: 138–147

Kim U, Clifton KH, Furth J (1960) A highly inbred line of Wistar rats yielding spontaneous mammo-somatotropic pituitary and other tumors. JNCI 24:1031–1055

Kociba RJ, Keyes DG, Lisowe RW, Kalnins RP, Dittenber DD, Wade CE, Gorzinski SJ, Mahle NH, Schwetz BA (1979) Results of a two-year chronic toxicity and oncogenic study of rats ingesting diets containing 2,4,5-trichlorophenoxyacetic acid (2,4,5-T). Food Cosmet Toxicol 17:205–221

Kovacs K, Horvath E, Egrin C (1977a) Pituitary adenomas. Pathol Annu 12(II):341–382

Kovacs K, Horvath E, Ilse RG, Ezrin C, Ilse D (1977b) Spontaneous pituitary adenomas in aging rats. A light microscopic, immunocytological and fine structural study. Beitr Pathol 161:1–16

Lee AK, DeLellis RA, Blount M, Nunnemacher G, Wolfe HJ (1982) Pituitary proliferative lesions in aging male Long-Evans rats. Lab Invest 47:595–602

Lichtensteiger CA, Wortman JA, Eigenmann JE (1986) Functional pituitary acidophil adenoma in a cat with diabetes mellitus and acromegalic features. Vet Pathol 23:518–521

McComb DJ, Kovacs K, Beri J, Zak F (1984) Pituitary adenomas in old Sprague-Dawley rats: a histologic, ultrastructural, and immunocytochemical study. J Natl Cancer Inst 73:1143–1166

McComb DJ, Kovacs K, Beri J, Zak F, Milligan JV, Shin SH (1985) Pituitary gonadotroph adenomas in old Sprague-Dawely rats. J Submicrosc Cytol 17:517–530

MacKenzie WF, Garner FM (1973) Comparison of neoplasms in six sources of rats. J Natl Cancer Inst 50:1243–1257

Magnusson G, Majeed SK, Gopinath C (1979) Infiltrating pituitary neoplasms in the rat. Lab Anim 13:111–113

Majeed SK, Gopinath C, Magnusson G (1980) Ultrastructure of spontaneous pituitary neoplasms in the rat. J Comp Pathol 90:239–246

Mohr U, et al. (1994) International classification of rodent tumors, part I: the rat 6. Endocrine system. International Agency for Research on Cancer (WHO), Lyon

Powers RD, Winkler JK (1977) Pituitary carcinoma with extracranial metastasis in a cow. Vet Pathol 14:524–526

Ross MH, Bras G, Ragbeer MS (1970) Influence of protein and caloric intake upon spontaneous tumor incidence of the anterior pituitary gland of the rat. J Nutr 100:177–189

Russell DS, Rubinstein LG (1972) Pathology of tumors of the nervous system, 3rd edn. Williams and Wilkins, Baltimore

Russfield AB (1966) Tumors of endocrine glands and secondary sex organs. US Government Printing Office, Washington DC (USHEW PHS publication no 1332)

Sandusky GE, van Pelt CS, Todd GC, Wightman K (1988) An immunocytochemical study of pituitary adenomas and focal hyperplasia in old Sprague-Dawley and Fischer 344 rats. Toxicol Pathol 16:376–380

Sano T, Kovacs K, Stefaneanu L, Asa SL, Snyder DL (1989) Spontaneous pituitary gonadotroph nodules in aging male Lobund-Wistar rats. Lab Invest 61:343–349

Saxton JA Jr (1941) The relation of age to the occurrence of adenoma-like lesions in the rat hypophysis and to their growth after transplantation. Cancer Res 1:277–282

Saxton JA Jr, Graham JB (1944) Chromophobe adenoma-like lesions of the rat hypophysis: frequency of spontaneous lesions and characteristics of growth of homologous intraocular transplants. Cancer Res 4:168–175

Saxton JA Jr, Sperling GA, Barnes LL, McCay CM (1948) The influence of nutrition upon the incidence of spontaneous tumors of the albino rat. Acta Unio Int Contra Cancrum 6:423–431

Schardein JL, Fitzgerald JE, Kaump DH (1968) Spontaneous tumors in Holtzman-source rats of various ages. Vet Pathol 5:238–252

Schelin U, Lundin PM (1971) An electron microscopic study of normal and neoplastic acidophil cells of the rat pituitary. Acta Endocrinol (Copenh) 678:29–39

Seibold HR, Wolf RH (1973) Neoplasms and proliferative lesions in 1065 nonhuman primates necropsies. Lab Anim Sci 23:533–539

Simms HS, Berg BN (1957) Longevity and onset of lesions in male rats. J Gerontol 12:244–252

Thompson SW, Hunt RD (1963) Spontaneous tumors in the SpragueDawley rat: incidence rates of some types of neoplasms as determined by serial section versus single section technics. Ann NY Acad Sci 108:832–845

Thompson SW, Huseby RA, Fox MA, Davis CL, Hunt RD (1961) Spontaneous tumors in the Sprague-Dawley rat. J Natl Cancer Inst 27:1037–1057

Tsuchitani M, Narama I (1984) Pituitary thyrotroph cell adenoma in a cynomolgus monkey (Macaca fascicularis). Vet Pathol 21:444–447

Ueberberg H, Latzen L (1979) The spontaneous rate of tumors in the laboratory rat: strain chbb: Thom (SPF). Drug Res 29:1876–1879

Wolfe JM, Wright AW (1947) Cytology of spontaneous adenomas in the pituitary gland of the rat. Cancer Res 7:759–773

Wolfe JM, Bryan WR, Wright AW (1938) Histologic observations on the anterior pituitaries of old rats with particular reference to the spontaneous appearance of pituitary adenomata. Am J Cancer 34:352–372

Zaki FA, Liu SK (1973) Pituitary chromophobe adenoma in a cat. Vet Pathol 10:232–237

Adenoma, Pars Intermedia, Anterior Pituitary, Rat

William W. Carlton and Christian L. Gries

Gross Appearance

Adenomas of the pars intermedia of the pituitary gland (as defined by the WHO*/IARC international classification of rodent tumors) vary in size and may cause enlargement of the gland. The gross appearance is similar to the solid chromophobe adenoma of the pars distalis.

Microscopic Features

Adenomas of the pars intermedia vary in size and occur as circumscribed, nonencapsulated, nodular masses that cause compression of the adjacent nonneoplastic tissue (Fig. 94). The neoplasms are composed of closely packed, enlarged, agranular epithelial cells with round to oval nuclei and moderately abundant, palely basophilic cytoplasm (MacKenzie and Boorman 1990; Fig. 95). In small neoplasms the neoplastic cells are only larger and less basophilic than the nonneoplastic cell (Fig. 96; McEwen et al. 1939; Wolfe and Wright 1947). In pigmented rats some neoplastic cells contain melanin granules such as are usually found in normal intermediate lobe cells. Large neoplasms of the intermediate lobe occupy most of the pituitary gland and are composed of large, round to polygonal, pleomorphic cells with relatively small nuclei and few mitotic figures and are arranged about sinusoids and in cords (Berkvens et al. 1980). The neoplastic cells of larger neoplasms may infiltrate the pars nervosa (Lee et al. 1982). Many cells have clear, slightly eosinophilic cytoplasm with a clear zone at the periphery of the cell (Fig. 97). The cells of these intermediate lobe neoplasms are chromophobic by several conventional stains and no hormones are detected by the immunoperoxidase reaction (Berkvens et al. 1980).

Ultrastructure

A published description of the ultrastructural morphology of adenomas of the intermediate lobe of the rat pituitary gland has not been found. However, Ward (unpublished observations) has noted large cytoplasmic granules similar to those seen in normal cells of the pars intermedia in one such neoplasm.

* World Health Organization, International Classification of Rodent Tumors (Mohr 1994).

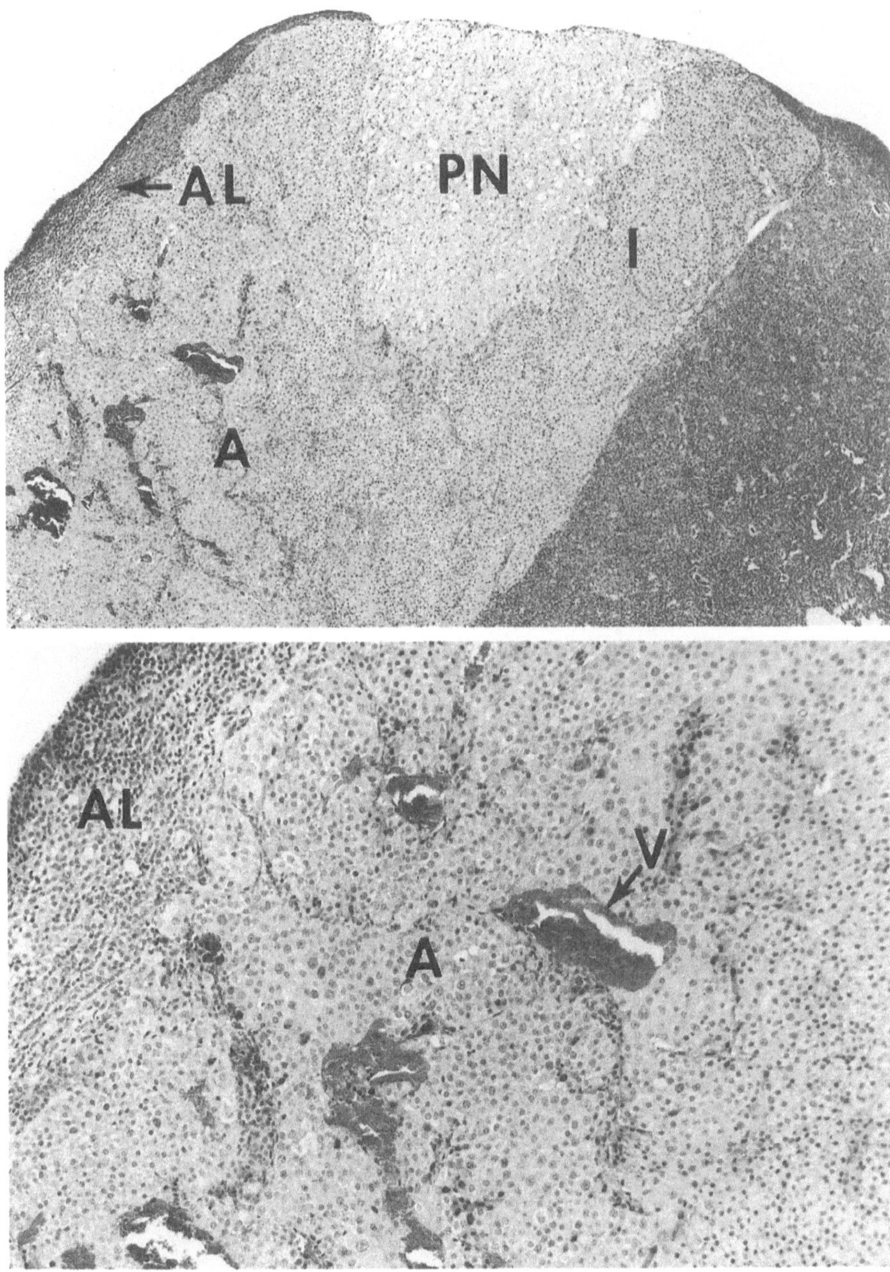

Fig. 94. (*above*) Adenoma (*A*) pars intermedia, rat pituitary. Compression of the surrounding anterior lobe (*AL*). *PN*, Pars nervosa; *I*, intermediate lobe. (Courtesy of Dr. R. Kociba, Dow Chemical USA) H&E, ×35

Fig. 95. (*below*) Adenoma (*A*) pars intermedia, rat pituitary. Blood-filled vascular spaces (*V*) and compression of adjacent anterior lobe (*AL*). (Courtesy of Dr. R. Kociba, Dow Chemical USA) H&E, ×88

Differential Diagnoses

The cells of the intermediate lobe neoplasms are agranular under light microscopy and can be separated from adenomas of the pars distalis by morphologic features that are elucidated by transmission electron microscopy. Berkvens et al. (1980) described a peripheral clear zone in neo-

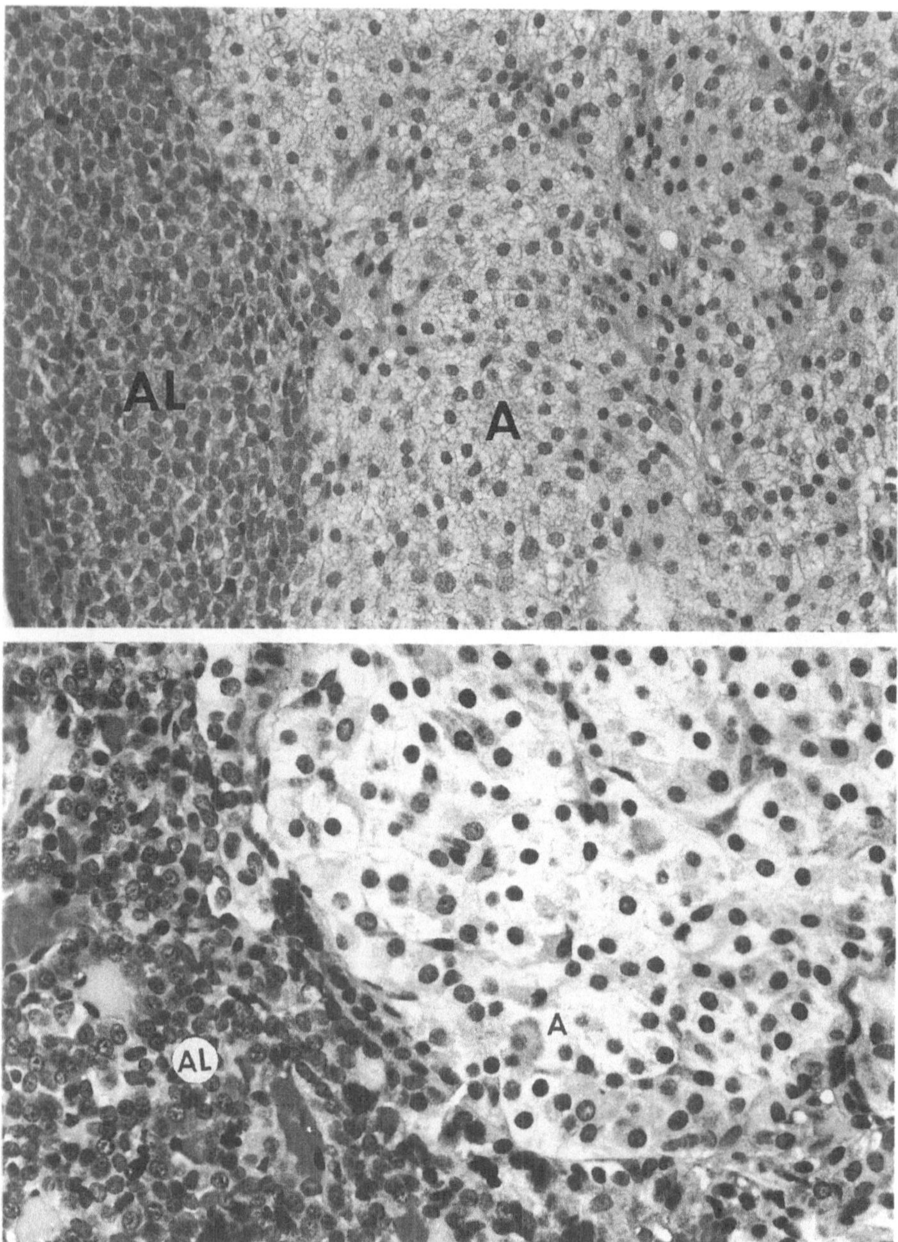

Fig. 96. (*above*) Adenoma (*A*), pars intermedia, rat pituitary. Compressed and sharply delineated anterior lobe (*AL*). (Courtesy of Dr. R. Kociba, Dow Chemical USA) H&E, ×224

Fig. 97. (*below*) Adenoma (*A*), pars intermedia, rat pituitary. *AL*, Anterior lobe. (Courtesy of Dr. R. Kociba, Dow Chemical USA) H&E, ×350

plastic cells lying next to sinusoids in four pars intermedia adenomas and considered this a characteristic feature of these neoplasms.

Adenoma must be separated from focal or diffuse hyperplastic changes in the pars intermedia. In diffuse hyperplasia irregular thickening occurs along the entire length of the pars intermedia, and the general architecture and cellular morphology of the pars intermedia remains normal. Infiltration of other portions of the pituitary gland

and compression of adjacent nonneoplastic tissues does not occur with hyperplasias but does occur with adenoma (Berkvens et al. 1980).

Biologic Features

Spontaneous adenomas of the pars intermedia of the rat hypophysis are rare and few cases have been reported (Russfield 1966). An intermediate lobe adenoma was found in an aged, dwarfed female rat (Fischer 1926), two in aged rats of the Vanderbilt strain (Wolfe and Wright 1947), one in one of 36 aged Long-Evans rat (Lee et al. 1982), one among 55 adenomas from 66 aged Sprague-Dawley rats (McComb et al. 1984), and one in 472 aged Sprague-Dawley rats (Kociba et al. 1979). Four intermediate lobe neoplasms were found among 69 pituitary neoplasms in 114 aged Wistar rats (Berkvens et al. 1980).

Intermediate lobe neoplasms have not been produced experimentally in the rat, but an intermediate lobe neoplasm was observed in an albino rat treated with estrone for 331 days (McEwen et al. 1936) and in a hooded rat given estrogens for 860 days (McEwen et al. 1939). No evidence indicates that the estrogenic stimulation in these two rats was etiologically significant in the development of the intermediate lobe adenomas. The usual response of the pituitary gland of rats exposed to estrogens is the development of adenomas of the pars distalis (Russfield 1966). This is in contrast to the situation in the Syrian hamster, in which the expected response to estrogen stimulation is the development of hyperplasias and adenomas of the intermediate lobe (Koneff et al. 1946; Vasquez-Lopez 1944).

Carcinomas of the intermediate lobe have not been described. Metastasis of intermediate lobe neoplasms is not recorded, and studies of transplantability of these neoplasms apparently have not been carried out.

Adenomas of the intermediate lobe appear to be endocrinologically inactive. The cells are chromophobic with conventional stains and prolactin, growth hormone, or thyroid-stimulating hormone and adrenocorticotropin were not detected by the immunoperoxidase reaction (Berkvens et al. 1980).

Comparison with Other Species

The pars intermedia is poorly developed in the adenohypophysis of the human pituitary gland. Neoplasms of the pars intermedia have not been described in human patients (Russell and Rubinstein 1972). A sparsely granulated, nonsecreting adenoma of the pars intermedia was found in a male rhesus monkey with galactorrhea (Chalifoux et al. 1983). The neoplastic cells were negative for prolactin and other pituitary gland hormones by immunohistochemical methods.

Adenomas of the pars intermedia are the most common neoplasms of the pituitary gland in the horse and the second most common in the dog (Capen 1990); they are rare in other species. Most of the intermediate lobe adenomas in the dog and the horse are endocrinologically inactive, and the clinical syndromes are due to disturbed hypothalamic function. However, a few neoplasms secrete excessive adrenocorticotropin, which results in adrenal cortical hyperplasia. In the dog intermediate lobe adenomas are associated with hypopituitarism and diabetes insipidus. Horses with adenomas of the intermediate lobe have a clinical syndrome characterized by polyuria, polydipsia, ravenous appetite, muscular weakness, hyperhidrosis, and hirsutism (Horvath et al. 1988).

Grossly, adenomas of the pars intermedia in horses cause enlargement of the pituitary gland. These neoplasms extend out of the sella turcica and compress the overlying hypothalamus to displace and compress the optic nerves.

Histologically the intermediate lobe adenomas in the horse may be seen to replace the pars nervosa and cause compression atrophy of the pars distalis. Fine connective tissue subdivides the neoplasms into variably sized aggregates of polyhedral to cylindrical cells with eosinophilic granular cytoplasm arranged in cords and nests. Histologic patterns vary, and follicular structures filled with colloid and sarcomatous areas of spindle-shaped cells are occasionally found. In the dog the intermediate lobe adenoma is composed of nests and cords of chromophobic cells interspersed among colloid-containing follicles lined by cuboidal, partly ciliated cells.

References

Berkvens JM, van Nesselrooy JHJ, Kroes R (1980) Spontaneous tumors in the pituitary gland of old Wistar rats. A morphological and immunocytochemical study. J Pathol 130:179–191

Capen CC (1990) Tumors of the endocrine glands. In: Moulton JE (ed) Tumors in domestic animals, 3rd edn. University of California Press, Berkeley, chap 13

Chalifoux LV, MacKey JJ, King NW Jr (1983) A sparsely granulated, nonsecreting adenoma of the pars intermedia associated with galactorrhea in a male rhesus monkey (*macaca mulatta*). Vet Pathol 20:541–547

Fischer O (1926) Über Hypophysengeschwülste der weissen Ratten. Virchows Arch Pathol Anat 259:9–29

Horvath CJ, Ames TR, Metz AL, Larson VL (1988) Adenocorticotropin-containing neoplastic cells in a pars intermedia adenoma in a horse. J Am Vet Med Assoc 192:367–371

Kociba RJ, Keyes DG, Lisowe RW, Kalnins RP, Dittenber DD, Wade CE, Gorzinsk SJ, Mahle NH, Schwetz BA (1979) Results of a two-year chronic toxicity and oncogenic study of rats ingesting diets containing 2,4,5-trichlorophenoxyacetic acid (2,4,5-T). Food Cosmet Toxicol 17:205–221

Koneff AA, Simpson ME, Evans HM (1946) Effects of chronic administration of diethylstilbestrol on the pituitary and other endocrine organs of hamsters. Anat Rec 94:169–195

Lee AK, DeLellis RA, Blount M, Nunnemacher G, Wolfe HJ (1982) Pituitary proliferative lesions in aging male Long-Evans rats. Lab Invest 47:595–602

MacKenzie WF, Boorman GA (1990) Pituitary gland, chapter 30. In: Boorman GA, Eustis SL, Elwell MR, Montgomery CA Jr, MacKenzie WF (eds) Pathology of the Fischer rat. Academic, San Diego, pp 493–494

Mohr U (1994) International classification of rodent tumours, part 1. World Health Organization, IARC Science Publication no 122

McComb DJ, Kovacs K, Beri J, Zak F (1984) Pituitary adenomas in old Sprague Dawley rats: a histologic, ultrastructural, and immunocytochemical study. J Natl Cancer Inst 73:1143–1156

McEwen CS, Selye H, Collip JB (1936) Some effects of prolonged administration of oestrin in rats. Lancet 1:775–776

McEwen CS, Selye H, Collip JB (1939) A pigmented adenoma of the intermediate lobe in a rat chronically treated with oestrin. Proc Soc Exp Biol Med 40:241–246

Russell DS, Rubinstein LJ (1972) Pathology of tumors of the nervous system, 3rd edn. Williams and Wilkins, Baltimore

Russfield AB (1966) Tumors of endocrine glands and secondary sex organs. US Government Printing Office, Washington DC (USDHEW PHS publication no 1332)

Vasquez-Lopez E (1944) The reaction of the pituitary gland and related hypothalamic centers in the hamster to prolonged treatment with estrogens. J Pathol 56:1–14

Wolfe JM, Wright AW (1947) Cytology of spontaneous adenomas in the pituitary gland of the rat. Cancer Res 7:759–773

Craniopharyngioma, Pituitary Gland, Rat

William W. Carlton and Christian L. Gries

Synonyms. Craniopharyngioma, benign; craniopharyngioma, malignant (WHO).*

Gross Appearance

This neoplasm either arises within or invades the anterior lobe of the pituitary gland and causes enlargement of the gland and compression atrophy of the overlying hypothalamus. The neoplasm can have both solid and cystic areas.

Microscopic Features

Histologically the craniopharyngioma is composed of papillary formations, cords, columns, and nests of keratinizing squamous epithelium and variably sized cystic spaces filled with keratin and cellular debris (Fig. 98). The well-differentiated squamous epithelium of the papillary formations and the lining of the cysts (Fig. 99) has marked hyper-

* World Health Organization, International Classification of Rodent Tumors (Mohr 1994).

▶

Fig. 98. (*upper left*) Craniopharyngioma, pituitary, rat. Papillary formations arising from the squamous epithelium line cystic spaces filled with keratin and cellular debris. (Courtesy of Dr. R. Marler, Dow Chemical USA) H&E, ×35

Fig. 99. (*upper right*) Craniopharyngioma, pituitary, rat. Squamous lining of a cyst with associated rim of anterior lobe cells. (Courtesy of Dr. R. Marler, Dow Chemical USA) H&E, ×350

Fig. 100. (*lower left*) Craniopharyngioma, pituitary, rat. Anastomosing cords of keratinizing squamous epithelium with hyperkeratosis and parakeratosis. (Courtesy of Dr. R. Marler, Dow Chemical USA) H&E, ×88

Fig. 101. (*lower right*) Craniopharyngioma, pituitary, rat. Nests and cords of keratinizing squamous epithelium. (Courtesy of Dr. R. Marler, Dow Chemical USA) H&E, ×88

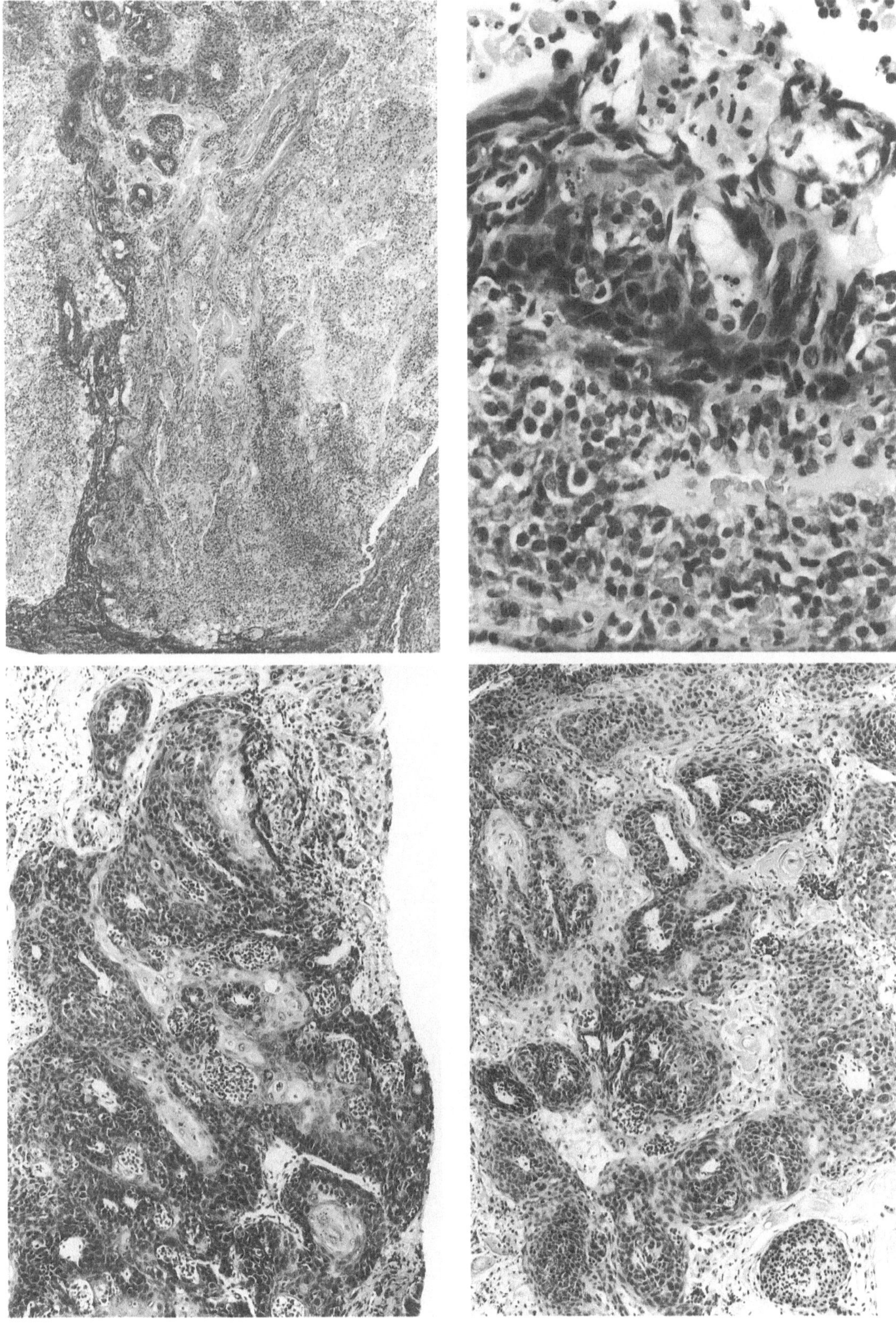

keratosis and prominent parakeratosis (Figs. 100, 101). The neoplasm may invade the adjacent brain and anterior pituitary by cords and nests of keratinizing squamous epithelium (Fig. 102; Fitzgerald et al. 1971). In other places the cords of squamous epithelium are separated by a zone of anterior pituitary gland cells (Fig. 103).

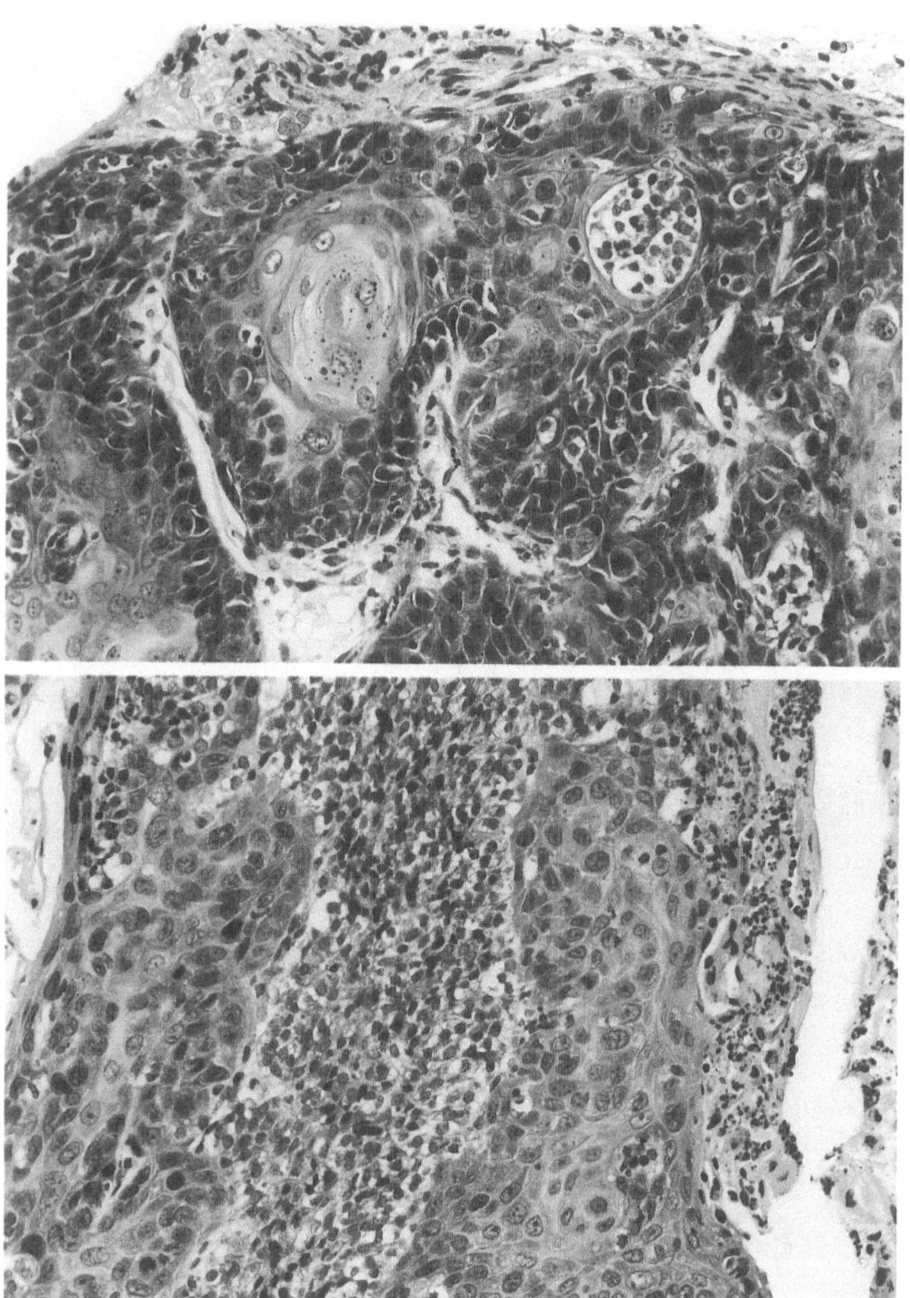

Fig. 102. (*above*) Craniopharyngioma, pituitary, rat. Well-differentiated keratinizing squamous epithelium. (Courtesy of Dr. R. Marler, Dow Chemical USA) H&E, ×224

Fig. 103. (*below*) Craniopharyngioma, pituitary, rat. Two tongues of keratinizing squamous epithelium are separated by a zone of anterior lobe cells. (Courtesy of Dr. R. Marler, Dow Chemical USA) H&E, ×224

Ultrastructure

Ultrastructural studies of craniopharyngiomas in the rat have not been reported. Typical craniopharyngiomas from human patients have areas with ultrastructural features of stratified squamous epithelium including ovoid euchromatic nuclei, infolded nuclear membranes, intercellular bridges, tonofibrils, desmosomes, keratohyaline granules, and interfacial clefs (Liszczak et al. 1978). In certain areas of the neoplasms the cells are polyhedral, and in others the compressed cells are arranged in onion-skin layerings.

Differential Diagnosis

The craniopharyngioma must be differentiated from nonneoplastic epidermoid cysts in the region of the pituitary gland. The epidermoid cysts are entirely benign and have a lining of simple stratified squamous epithelium. In the craniopharyngioma cords of squamous epithelium extend into and destroy portions of the anterior pituitary gland.

Craniopharyngiomas from human patients may be differentiated from squamous epithelium and from epidermoid, dental, and dentigerous cysts by a positive histochemical staining for alkaline phosphatase in the intermediate reticulate zone. The epithelia of the other structures are negative for the enzyme (Timperley et al. 1971). The epithelial portions of craniopharyngiomas have a positive reaction for keratin by the immunoperoxidase technique (Asa et al. 1981). Adenohypophyseal cells, neurohypophysis, and pituitary adenomas are negative for keratin.

Biologic Features

Craniopharyngioma is a rare neoplasm in the rat and few cases are described (Fitzgerald et al. 1971). These lesions are considered to originate from squamous cell remnants of Rathke's pouch, an evagination of the primitive stomodeum. After losing contact with the oral ectoderm this pouch develops into the adenohypophysis (Rhodin 1974). These neoplasms are locally invasive, but extracranial metastases are not described.

Comparison with Other Species

These neoplasms are rare in rodents, but a case has been described in a laboratory mouse (Helder 1986). The neoplasm compressed and displaced the pituitary gland and was composed of cords of squamous epithelium with cysts lined by cuboidal or stratified squamous epithelium and filled with necrotic cells or proteinaceous material. The neoplasm extended into the hypothalamus and peduncular region of the mesencephalon and the periocular region.

Pituitary lesions in domestic animals comparable to the human craniopharyngioma appear to be rare and have been reported only in the dog (White 1938; Saunders and Rickard 1952; Hawkins et al. 1985). The lesions described in dogs have been large and have caused compression and destruction of the pituitary gland and the overlying hypothalamus. Clinically the signs were those of the adiposogenital syndrome and diabetes insipidus (Neer and Reavis 1983).

Histologically the lesions have varied, but all were cystic and had formations of epithelial cells including squamous epithelium (White 1938; Saunders and Rickard 1952; Hawkins et al. 1985). The "ameloblastoma" type of craniopharyngioma described in human patients has not been reported in the pituitary gland of domestic animals. Histologically the canine lesions resembled those seen in the rat and the squamous cell portions of the cases from humans.

Craniopharyngiomas in human patients represent about 3% of all intracranial tumors (Russell and Rubinstein 1972). These slowly growing lesions are usually composed of solid and cystic portions and vary greatly in size; and the larger neoplasms compress the optic chiasm, the pituitary gland, and the cavity of the third ventricle. Histologically the cystic portions of these neoplasms are lined by stratified keratinizing squamous epithelium supported by fibrous connective tissue and have solid nests of squamous cells with "pearl" formations. The solid areas are composed of interconnecting cords and trabeculae of squamous and basal cells supported by loose, poorly cellular, vascular connective tissue. The ameloblastoma type of craniopharyngioma has areas in which stellate cells are surrounded by a layer of single or pseudostratified columnar cells resting upon a basement membrane. Degenerative changes occur in the inner epithelial cells causing loosening of the more central stellate cells and development of microcystic cavitation (Petito et al. 1976).

References

Asa SL, Kovacs K, Bilbao JM, Penz G (1981) Immunohistochemical localization of keratin in craniopharyngiomas and squamous cell nests of the human pituitary. Acta Neuropathol (Berl) 54:257–260

Fitzgerald JE, Schardein JL, Kaump DH (1971) Several uncommon pituitary tumors in the rat. Lab Anim Sci 21: 581–584

Hawkins KL, Diters RW, McGrath JT (1985) Craniopharyngioma in a dog. J Comp Pathol 95:469–474

Heider K (1986) Spontaneous craniopharyngioma in a mouse. Vet Pathol 23:522–523

Liszczak T, Richardson EP, Phillips JP, Jacobsen S, Kornblith PL (1978) Morphological, biochemical, ultrastructural, tissue culture and clinical observations of typical and aggressive craniopharyngiomas. Acta Neuropathol (Berl) 43:191–203

Mohr U (1994) International classification of rodent tumours, part 1. World Health Organization, IARC Science Publication no 122

Neer TM, Reavis DU (1983) Craniopharyngioma and associated central diabetes insipidus and hypothyroidism in a dog. J Am Vet Med Assoc 182:519–520

Petito CK, DeGirolami U, Earle KM (1976) Craniopharyngiomas: a clinical and pathological review. Cancer 37: 1944–1952

Rhodin JG (1974) Histology: a text and atlas. Oxford University Press, New York

Russell DS, Rubinstein LJ (1972) Pathology of tumors of the nervous system, 3rd edn. Williams and Wilkins, Baltimore

Saunders LZ, Rickard CG (1952) Craniopharyngioma in a dog with apparent adiposogenital syndrome and diabetes insipidus. Cornell Vet 42:490–495

Timperley WR, Turner P, Davies S (1971) Alkaline phosphatase in craniopharyngiomas. J Pathol 103:257–262

White EG (1938) Suprasellar tumor in a dog. J Pathol 47:323–326

Pituitary Tumors Induced by Estrogen, Rat

R. Yoshiyuki Osamura

Gross Appearance

As early as 1 month after intramuscular administration of estrogen (Teikokuzoki) at the rate of 5 mg/rat/month, the pituitary gland becomes hyperplastic. At this stage, the pituitary gland is enlarged two to three times its normal size and is usually white to tan. Six months after the start of the estrogen injections the gland is tumorous, markedly congested, and enlarged up to tenfold. The tumor mass is well encapsulated and does not invade the adjacent tissue. The intermediate lobe is difficult to distinguish at this stage.

Microscopic Features

The pituitary gland, 6 months after the first administration of estrogen, is composed of many rather uniform chromophobic cells with a few scattered acidophilic cells (Figs. 104, 105). The sinusoids are markedly dilated and sometimes form pools of red blood cells bordered by tumor cells. Immunohistochemical staining (Nakane 1975) reveals the tumor to be composed of many round or oval cells containing prolactin (LTH cell). The hormone is usually present in the Golgi areas adjacent to and partially surrounding the nucleus (Fig. 106). The tumor also has spherical cells containing growth hormone (GH). ACTH cells are not usually a component of the tumor. Cells containing luteinizing hormone (LH) are markedly decreased in number.

Ultrastructure

The tumor cells are seen under the electron microscope to contain well-developed rough endoplasmic reticulum (RER) in the enlarged cytoplasm; the RER is lamellated or whorled in configuration (Fig. 107). The Golgi apparatus is occasionally conspicuous. The secretory granules are scattered among the prominent RER and are smaller than those in normal LTH cells, but still retain their characteristic polymorphism.

The postembedding method (p. 34) and electron microscopy reveal the LTH to be localized in the secretory granules. The preembedding method demonstrates LTH present in Golgi saccules and RER as well as in secretory granules (Fig. 108).

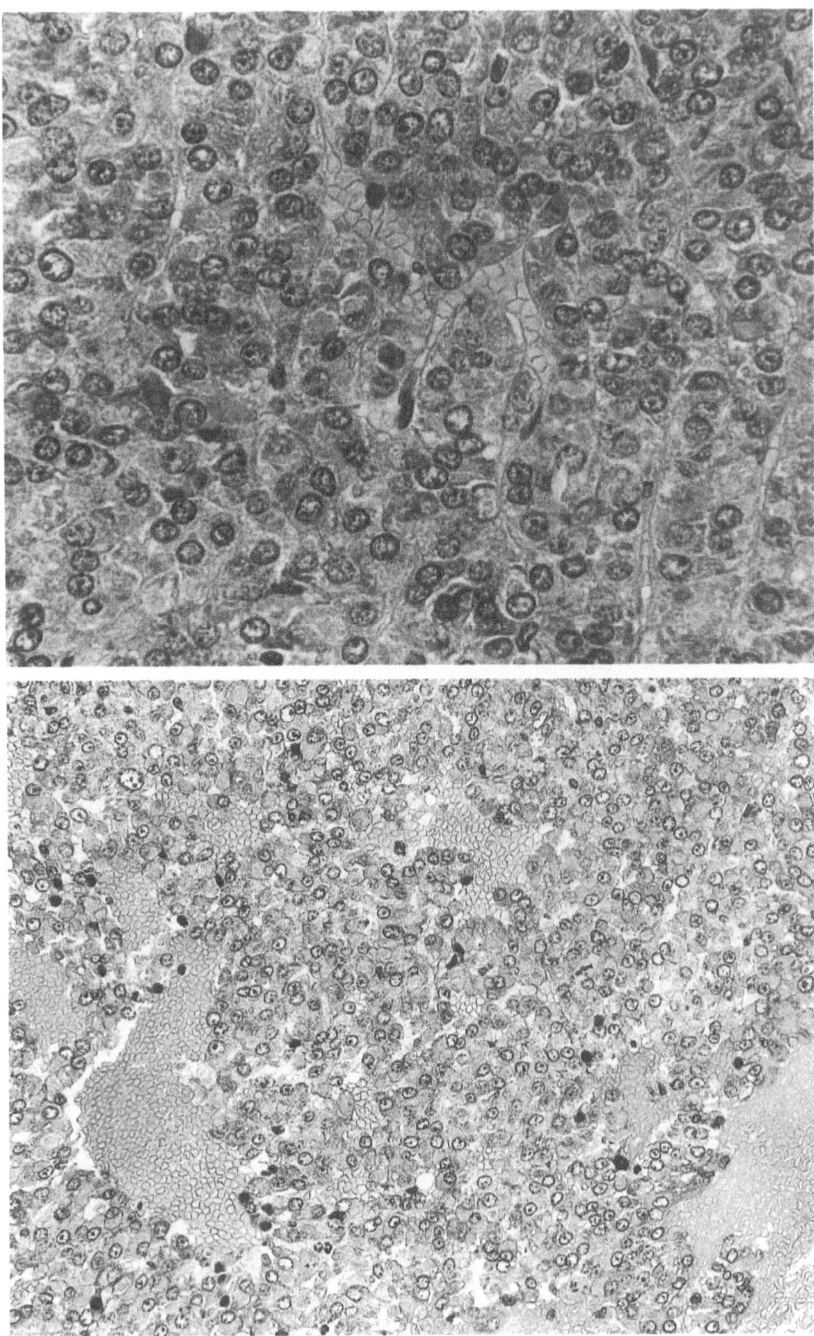

Fig. 104. (*above*) Estrogen-induced rat pituitary tumor. H&E, ×300

Fig. 105. (*below*) Tumor in anterior pituitary of a rat following prolonged administration of estrogen. Uniform, spherical cells in proximity to many capillaries. H&E, ×600

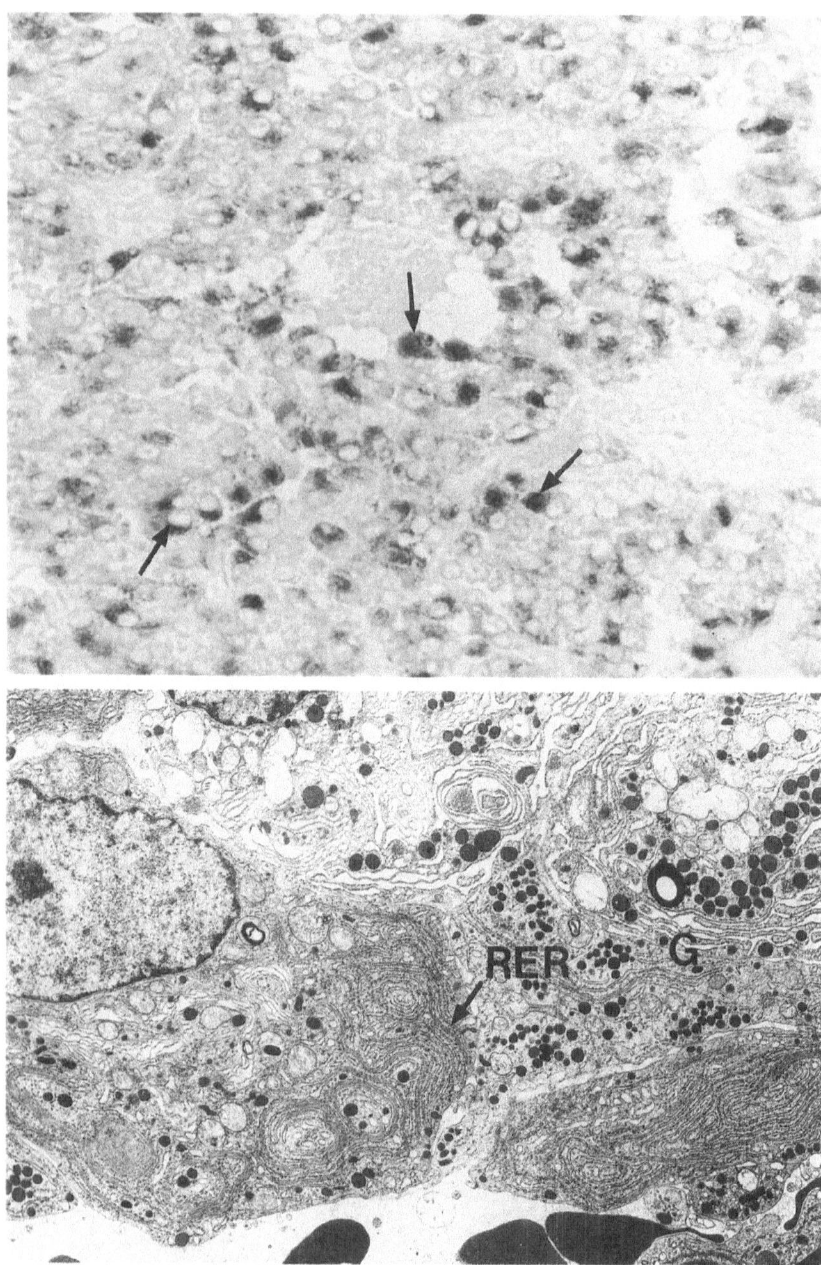

Fig. 106. (*above*) Immunohistochemical localization of LTH in estrogen-induced rat pituitary tumor (Fig. 105). Cells containing LTH (*arrows*). Peroxidase-labeled antibody method, ×500

Fig. 107. (*below*) Estrogen-induced rat pituitary tumor cell. Whorled rough endoplasmic reticulum (*RER*) and many Golgi apparatuses (*G*), ×6200

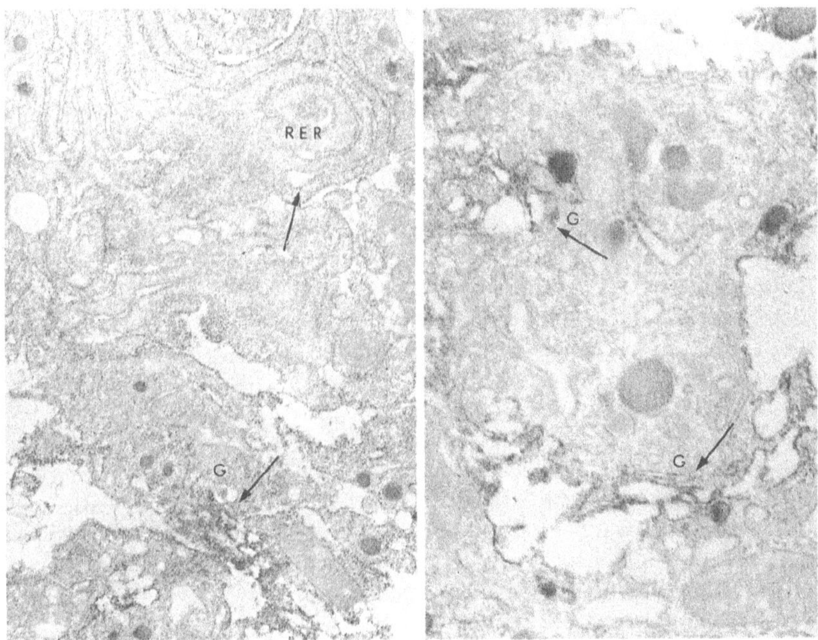

Fig. 108. Prolactin in extrogen-induced rat pituitary tumors. Golgi apparatus (*G*) and cisternae of rough endoplasmic reticulum (*RER*) contain LTH (*arrows*). Peroxidase-labeled antibody method, ×23000

(Nakane 1975; Osamura and Watanabe 1976; Osamura et al. 1980, 1981).

Differential Diagnosis

These tumors are distinguished from one another by the specific immunoperoxidase identification of the hormone which their cells produce.

Biologic Features

The estrogen-induced pituitary tumors in both female and male rats are known to be composed of cells that produce LTH. It appears that serum LTH levels might increase as the tumors become larger.

At the outset, this tumor can be transplanted only to estrogen-treated hosts, but after repeated passages it can be transplanted to nontreated hosts and it acquires the ability to grow autonomously. As autonomy is gained the tumor usually loses the capacity to produce hormone (Furth and Clifton 1966; Furth et al. 1976). Finally, the transplanted tumor acquires the potential to metastasize. After the tumor is transplanted it may develop the ability to produce GH or ACTH.

Pathogenesis

Whether estrogen acts on the pituitary gland directly or by way of the hypothalamic or some other pathway has been discussed. From our experiments with estrogen-induced tumorigenesis in splenic autografts of the pituitary, it seems that estrogen can act directly on the pituitary glands.

Bromocriptine Treatment

Recently, human pituitary prolactinomas have been treated successfully with the dopa agonist bromocriptine (BRM). In most cases of the pituitary prolactinomas, treatment with the BRM lowers serum PRL levels and decreases the size of the tumors when they are macroadenoma. In rat pituitary tumors induced by estrogen administration, BRM treatment apparently lowers serum PRL levels and decreases the weights of the pituitary glands. This can be considered as a good experimental model for human adenomas. In

BRM-treated rat pituitary PRL secreting tumor induced by estrogen the tumor cells are atrophic and contain increased small secretory granules in the cytoplasm. This suggests secretory inhibition at exocytosis levels.

Comparison with Similar Lesion in Man

In human beings, LTH-secreting pituitary adenomas are relatively common, and are probably the most frequently occurring type among pituitary adenomas. As in the rat estrogen-induced tumor, the cells of human tumors secrete prolactin (prolactinomas) and are sometimes mixed with GH cells. The tumor cells have similar ultrastructural features, including well-developed lamellated RER, Golgi apparatus, and scattered secretory granules. Immunohistochemically, the human tumor cells do contain LTH in the perinuclear Golgi areas adjacent to the nucleus, which is similar to that of rat pituitary tumors. Immunocytochemical methods on the tumor cells demonstrate the presence of LTH in the Golgi saccules as well as in the adjacent RER (Horvath et al. 1977; Osamura et al. 1978).

References

Furth J, Clifton K (1966) Experimental pituitary tumors. In: Harris GW, Donovan BT (eds) The pituitary gland, vol 2. Butterworths, London, pp 460–497

Furth J, Nakane P, Pasteels JL (1976) Tumours of the pituitary gland. In: Turusov VS (ed) Pathology of tumours in laboratory animals, vol I: tumours of the rat. IARC scientific publ no 6, Lyon, part 2, pp 201–237

Horvath E, Kovacs K, Singer W, Ezrin C, Kerenyi NA (1977) Acidophil stem cell adenoma of the human pituitary. Arch Pathol Lab Med 101:594–599

Nakane PK (1975) Recent progress in the peroxidase-labeled antibody method. Ann N Y Acad Sci 254:203–211

Osamura RY, Watanabe K (1976) Peroxidase-labeled antibody method: its principle and applications to endocrinology. Clin Endocrinol 24:1074–1087

Osamura RY, Watanabe K, Teramoto A, Hirakawa K, Kawano N, Morii S (1978) Male prolactin secreting pituitary adenomas in humans studied by peroxidase-labeled antibody method. Acta Endocrinol 88:643–652

Osamura RY, Komatsu N, Nakahashi E, Watanabe K (1980) Light and electron microscopical combined staining by immunohistochemical and enzyme histochemical methods using rat prolactin-secreting pituitary tumours. Histochem J 12:371–379

Osamura RY, Komatsu N, Izumi S, Yoshimura S, Murakoshi M, Watanabe K (1981) Pre-embedding immunoelectron microscopy by peroxidase-labeled antibody method. Applications to endocrinology. Acta Histochem Cytochem 14: 383–390

Osamura RY, Teramoto A, Watanabe K (1986) Ultrastructural localization of prolactin in the human pituitary prolactinomas and its changes by bromocriptine treatment. Acta Pathol Jpn 36(8):1123–1130

Osamura RY, Watanabe K (1986) Ultrastructural localization of prolactin in estrogen induced prolactinoma of the rat pituitary; experimental models for the human prolactinomas and the effects of bromocriptine. Acta Pathol Jpn 36(8): 1131–1137

Pituicytoma, Neurohypophysis, Rat

William W. Carlton and Christian L. Gries

Synonyms. Astrocytic glioma, neurohypophyseal astrocytoma.

Gross Appearance

This neoplasm of the pars nervosa is solid, relatively firm, and causes enlargement of the pituitary gland and compression atrophy of the overlying hypothalamus. Its size may vary from microscopic dimensions to several millimeters in diameter.

Microscopic Features

Histologically the pituicytoma is a circumscribed, nonencapsulated mass that causes compression atrophy of the anterior lobe of the pituitary gland. The neoplasm is composed of closely packed, small spindle cells arranged in indistinct cords and interlacing bundles (Fig. 109). The neoplastic cells have small, round to ovoid, darkly basophilic nuclei and a slight amount of indistinct cytoplasm (Fig. 110). Multiple foci of mineralization are present in some neoplasms. Some nuclear pleomorphism is present in certain areas of the neoplasm (Figs. 111–113).

Differential Diagnosis

The pituicytoma of the neurohypophysis must be differentiated from other neoplasms that occur in the vicinity of the pituitary gland, especially neoplasms of glial cells of the hypothalamus. Differentiation of these neoplasms is especially difficult when a neoplasm is massive and topographical relationships are lost so that origin in the neurohypophysis cannot be established. Both the hypothalamic glioma and the pituicytoma are phosphotungstic acid–hematoxylin (PTAH) positive. The pituicytes include forms designated bipolar, astrocytic, triangular, and glomerular (Liss 1956). Neoplasms may be derived from one or several of these histologic types. Thus an astrocytic form of pituicytoma indistinguishable from the brain astrocytoma is possible in the neurohypophysis. The pituicytoma could be confused with a meningioma occurring near the pituitary gland. The whorled or organoid patterns of the meningioma are not described in the pituicytoma, and the meningioma should be PTAH negative.

Biologic Features

Neoplasms of the neurohypophysis are rare in rodents, domestic animals, and human patients. Present evidence indicates that the glial pituicyte may be the cell of origin of a primary neoplasm of the neurohypophysis, the pituicytoma. The neoplasm can grow to large proportions, resulting in destruction of hypothalamic structures and other portions of the pituitary gland.

Intracranial or extracranial metastases have not been described.

The frequency of this lesion in rats has not been documented. Since this is a lesion apparently of very rare occurrence, some question may arise about its precise identity. We have included

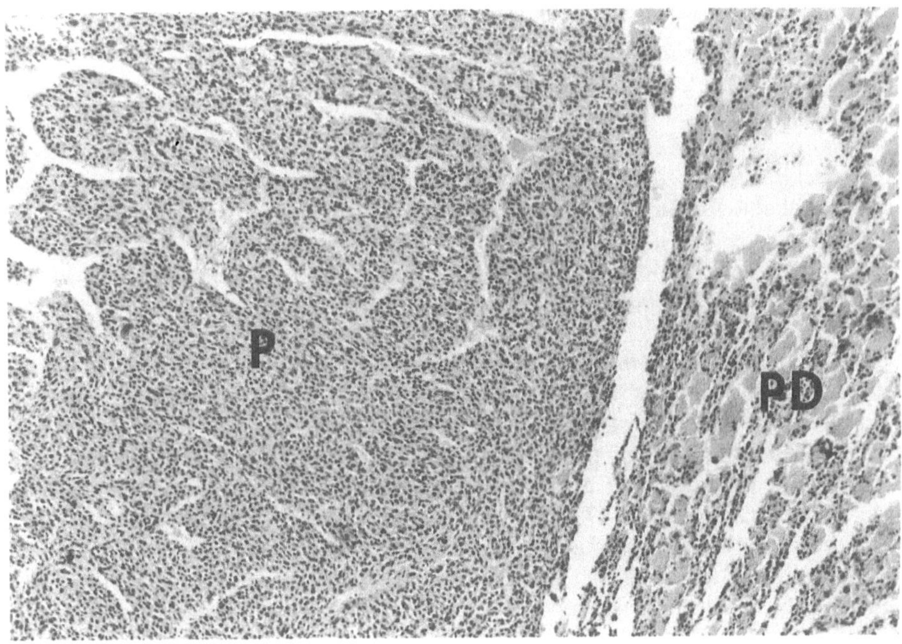

Fig. 109. Pituicytoma (*P*), neurohypophysis, rat (case 1). Highly cellular, it has caused compression atrophy of adjacent congested pars distalis (*PD*). H&E, ×88

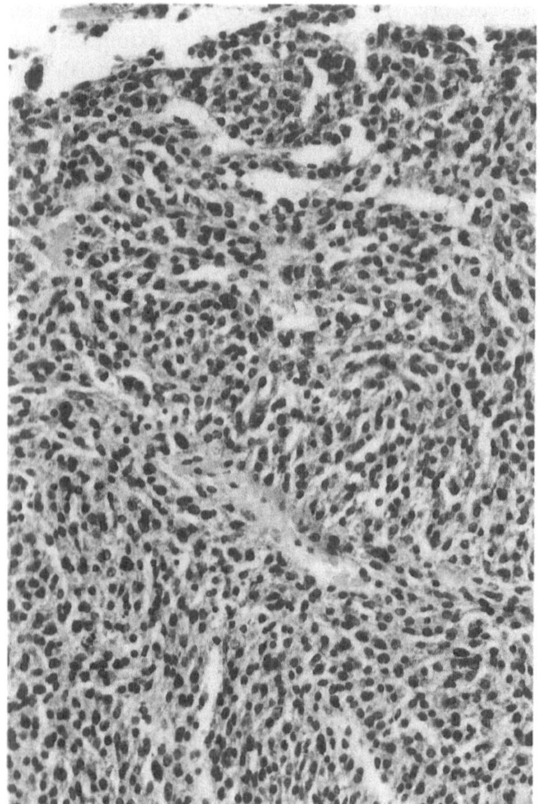

Fig. 110. Pituicytoma (*P*), neurohypophysis, rat (case 1). Composed of closely packed spindle cells with small, dark, basophilic nuclei and a slight amount of indistinct cytoplasm. H&E, ×224

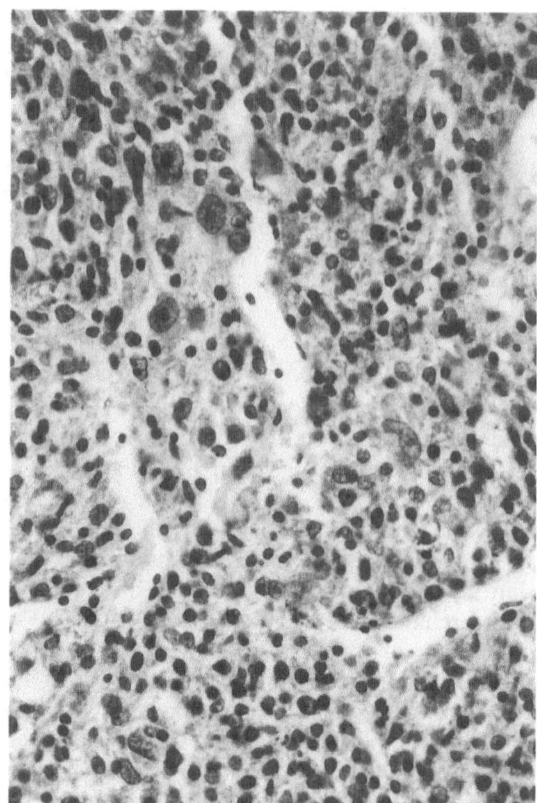

Fig. 111. Pituicytoma, neurohypophysis, rat. Large, round to ovoid to irregular vesicular nuclei with large basophilic nucleoli, scattered among smaller cells. H&E, ×350

illustrations from three similar cases in rats with the expectation that more cases may be identified and be available for further study.

Comparison with Other Species

These neoplasms are as rare in other species as they are in the rat and few cases have been described. A pituicytoma of the neurohypophysis in a Siamese cat enlarged the pituitary gland, expanded the posterior lobe, and compressed the anterior lobe (Zaki et al. 1975). The nonencapsulated vascular mass was composed of bipolar or polyhedral cells arranged in loose interlacing bundles. The neoplastic cells stained positive with PTAH and had either spindle, oval, or round nuclei. A neoplasm involving the hypothalamus, infundibulum, and neurohypophysis was observed in a dog with diabetes insipidus and adiposogenital syndrome. The lesion was considered a glial tumor with features of an infundibuloma (Saunders et al. 1951). A neurohypophyseal astrocytoma (pituicytoma) was described in a 21-year-old female rhesus monkey (HogenEsch et al. 1992). Microscopically the circumscribed white nodule with 4-mm diameter was a well-demarcated, nonencapsulated compressive lesion composed of interwoven bundles and nests of elongate to plump oval cells with indistinct cytoplasmic margins and a variable amount of pale eosinophilic cytoplasm. The neoplastic cells often radiated about blood vessels and had elongate to oval to round nuclei with inconspicuous nucleoli. The cells stained positively for glial fibrillary acidic protein, vimentin, and S-100 protein. Primary neoplasms of the human neurohypophysis are infrequently encountered and

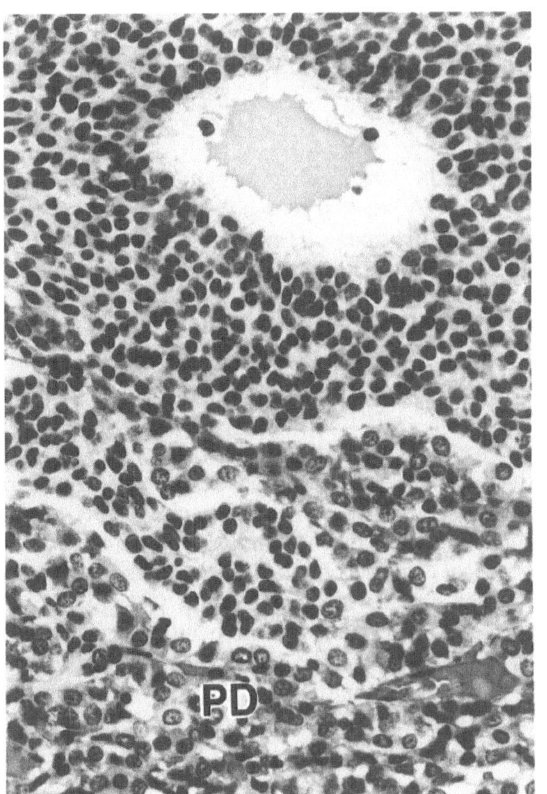

Fig. 112. Pituicytoma (case 2) from aged Sprague-Dawley rat lies adjacent to pars distalis (*PD*). Note a "cyst" surrounded by sheet of small cells with round to ovoid hyperchromatic nuclei and ill defined scant cytoplasm. H&E, ×350. (Provided by Dr. T.W. Slone)

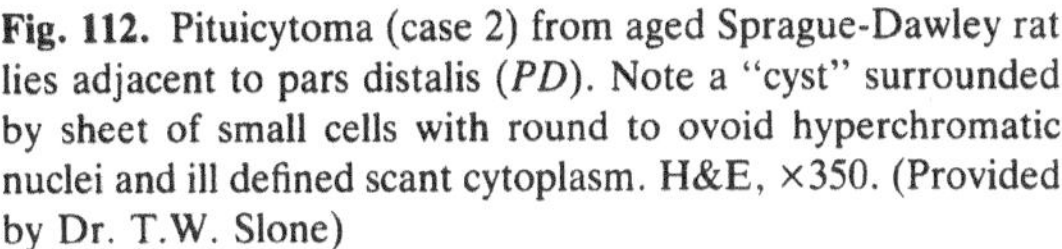

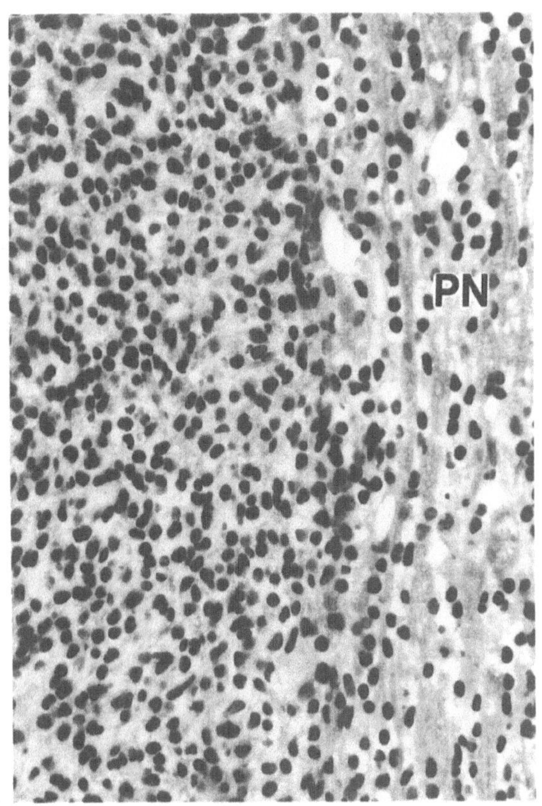

Fig. 113. Pituicytoma (case 3) from aged Sprague-Dawley rat lies adjacent to pars nervosa (*PN*) and is composed of a sheet of small cells with hyperchromatic nuclei and scant, ill-defined cytoplasm. Note nuclei and cytoplasmic features and adjacent nonneoplastic pars nervosa. H&E, ×350. (Provided by Dr. T.W. Slone)

have been described as glioma, infundibuloma, and pituicytoma (Liss and Kahn 1958; Rossi et al. 1987; Scothorne 1955).

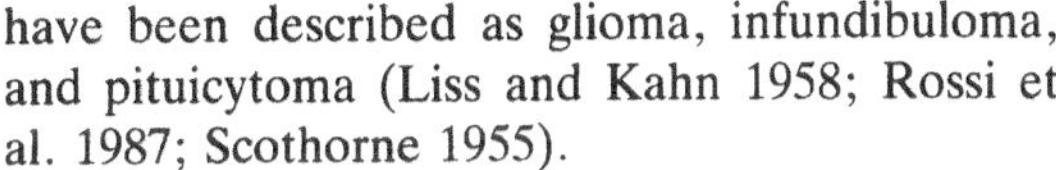

References

HogenEsch H, Broerse JJ, Zurcher C (1992) Neurohypophyseal astrocytoma (pituicytoma) in a rhesus monkey (*Macaca mulatta*). Vet Pathol 29:359–361

Liss L (1956) The cellular elements of the human neurohypophysis; a study with silver carbonate. J Comp Neurol 106:507–525

Liss L, Kahn E (1958) Pituicytoma, tumor of the sella turcica; a clinicopathological study. J Neurosurg 15:481–488

Rossi ML, Bevan JS, Esiri MM, Hughes JT, Adams CB (1987) Pituicytoma (pilocytic astrocytoma). Case report. J Neurosurg 67:768–772

Saunders LZ, Stephenson HC, McEntee K (1951) Diabetes insipidus and adiposogenital syndrome in a dog due to an infundibuloma. Cornell Vet 41:445–458

Scothorne C (1955) A glioma of the posterior lobe of the pituitary gland. J Pathol Bacteriol 69:109–112

Zaki F, Harris J, Budzilovich G (1975) Cystic pituicytoma of the neurohypophysis in a Siamese cat. J Comp Pathol 85:467–471

Gangliocytoma, Pituitary Gland, Rat

James E. Heath

Synonyms. Ganglioneuroma, ganglion cell tumor, ganglioglioma.

Gross Appearance

Pituitary gland gangliocytomas may not be grossly visible. Larger tumors may appear as flesh colored or brown nodules up to 3 mm in diameter. The tumors are not known to infiltrate adjacent structures.

Microscopic Appearance

Gangliocytomas arising in the pituitary gland of rats are composed of large polygonal cells with vesicular nuclei, prominent nucleoli, and variably abundant cytoplasm which may show Nissl substance. These large ganglionic cells usually occur in clusters and are often intermingled with smaller satellite cells having more deeply staining nuclei and scanty cytoplasm (Figs. 114, 115). Both cell types are frequently interspersed with varying density within an eosinophilic fibrillary matrix which typically blends imperceptibly with the cytoplasm of the large vesicular cells. These cells may undergo considerable pleomorphism, with variably sized and occasionally multiple nuclei (Figs. 116, 117).

Ultrastructure

Ultrastructural studies of pituitary gland gangliocytomas in the rat have not been reported.

Differential Diagnosis

Pituitary gangliocytomas must be differentiated from other neoplasms originating in the pituitary gland. Pituitary adenomas of the pars distalis are commonly observed neoplasms in rats and are usually composed of relatively small, monomorphic cells that bear little resemblance to the large vesicular cells of gangliocytoma. Carcinomas of the pars distalis are more likely than adenomas to contain large, pleomorphic cells that may superficially resemble pleomorphic nerve cells of gangliocytoma. However, the eosinophilic fibrillary matrix commonly seen in gangliocytoma is not a feature of pituitary gland carcinoma. Craniopharyngioma arises from remnants of Rathke's pouch and is distinguished by anastomosing cords of keratinizing squamous epithelial cells and cystic spaces lined with squamous epithelium. Pituicytoma (see p. 94, this volume) is also an extremely rare tumor in rats that consists of sheets of closely arranged, small spindle cells which originate in the pars nervosa, but which may encroach on the pars intermedia and/or pars distalis. Ganglioma or hamartoma arising from the oculomotor or other cranial nerve could result in a ganglion cell mass in the vicinity of the pituitary gland and might mimic pituitary gland gangliocytoma.

Biologic Features

Natural History and Pathogenesis. Gangliocytomas are considered to be rare central nervous system tumors characterized by the presence of ganglion cells, unmyelinated nerve fibers, and a glial matrix (Fischer et al. 1983). Ganglioneuroma, the peripheral counterpart of gangliocytoma, differs histologically from gangliocytoma only in having a fibrous rather than a glial matrix. Gangliocytomas of the pituitary gland are believed to arise from residual nerve cells in the neurohypophysis, as ganglionic cells have been shown to occur in the fetal posterior lobe (Jakumeit et al. 1974). Well-differentiated or "mature" tumors, whether arising in the brain, peripheral nerves, or even more rarely in such sites as the pituitary or adrenal gland, usually consist of widely scattered, well-differentiated ganglion cells within a fibrillar matrix. In other instances the ganglion cells are surrounded by variable numbers of smaller satellite cells. Such tumors are considered slow growing, indolent lesions with little or no propensity for aggressive behavior and have even been regarded by some workers as hamartomas (Serebrin and Robertson 1984). However, postsurgical follow-up studies

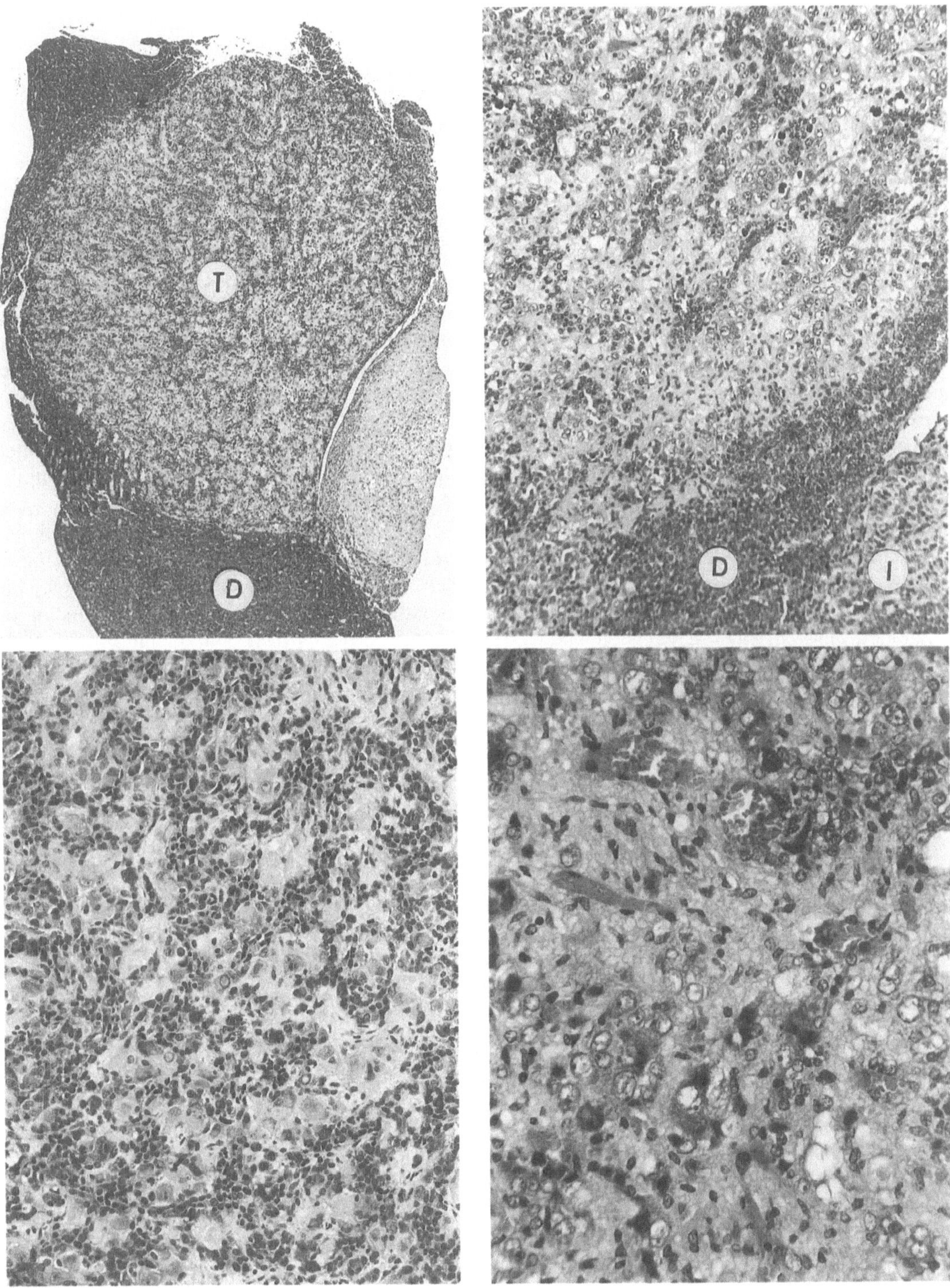

Fig. 114. (*upper left*) Pituitary gland, gangliocytoma, rat. Well-circumscribed tumor (*T*) is encroaching on the pars distalis (*D*). H&E, ×40

Fig. 115. (*lower left*) Higher magnification of Fig. 114. Note well-differentiated, large ganglion cells interspersed with smaller, deeply staining satellite cells. H&E, ×200

Fig. 116. (*upper right*) Gangliocytoma, pituitary gland, rat. Pleomorphic cell type adjacent to pars distalis (*D*) and pars intermedia (*I*). H&E, ×100

Fig. 117. (*lower right*) Higher magnification of Fig. 116. Note large, vesicular ganglionic cells and smaller satellite cells interspersed within glial matrix. H&E, ×250

in human beings indicate that these lesions are progressive and should be regarded as neoplasms. Less well-differentiated tumors composed of anaplastic or "immature" ganglion cells are reported in humans (Harkin and Reed 1969; Willis 1967; Burchiel et al. 1983). These tumors are characteristically more highly cellular than the mature variant. The individual cells, while usually retaining the large vesicular nuclei characteristic of ganglion cells, show varying degrees of pleomorphism, and multinucleated forms and mitotic figures may occur. These neoplasms, which some regard as a transitional variant toward neuroblastoma, typically grow more rapidly and are more aggressive than the more mature ganglion cell tumors.

Gangliocytomas and ganglioneuromas are considered to derive from the diffuse endocrine system. The central division of this system contains neuroendocrine and endocrine cells of the hypothalamic-pituitary axis which produce hormonally active amines and peptide hormones (Voorhess 1980; Pearse and Takor 1979). Some ganglioneuromas in man have been shown to secrete polypeptide hormones, including catecholamines and vasoactive intestinal peptides (Swift et al. 1975; Greenberg and Gardiner 1959). These tumors have been associated with a variety of clinical abnormalities including watery diarrhea, opsoclonus, myoclonus, and cerebellar ataxia. Similar syndromes in the rat resulting from ganglion cell neoplasms have not been reported.

Pituitary gangliocytomas in man have been reported as occurring simultaneously with adenomas (Kamel et al. 1989; Burchiel et al. 1983). It has been proposed that the neuronal cells of gangliocytomas may secrete a growth hormone-releasing factor which subsequently promotes the development of a growth hormone cell adenoma (Asa et al. 1980). This hypothesis suggests a functional relationship between the gangliocytoma and adenoma similar to that which occurs in the normal hypothalamic-pituitary axis.

Etiology. Pituitary gland gangliocytomas appear to be spontaneous lesions. No causative or contributory factors have been identified for these tumors in human beings or animals.

Frequency. Pituitary gangliocytomas in rats are extremely rare, and no data on incidence are available. The author has recognized this tumor in only one F344 rat (a 26-month-old male) in the evaluation of approximately 5500 (2750 male, 2750 female) Fischer 344 control and treated rats from 11 chronic toxicity studies at Southern Research Institute.

Comparison with Other Species

There are no reports in the literature on pituitary gland gangliocytoma in laboratory or domestic animals. In human beings gangliocytoma (or ganglioneuroma) occurring in the pituitary gland or the region of the sella turcica has been reported rarely (Jakumeit et al. 1974; Serebrin and Robertson 1984). A review of 21 cases revealed a mean age of 37 years, a 2:1 female to male sex predilection, and an average of 5.8 years from beginning of symptoms to tumor diagnosis (Fischer et al. 1983). Twelve of these patients had clinical evidence of pituitary hormonal hypersecretion, including acromegaly, Cushing's syndrome, and amenorrhea-galactorrhea. Mixed tumors of the pituitary fossa, which contain intermingled elements of gangliocytoma and pituitary adenoma, have been reported rarely in human beings (Kamel et al. 1989; Li et al. 1989).

References

Asa SL, Bilbao JM, Kovacs K, Linfoot JA (1980) Hypothalamic neuronal hamartoma associated with pituitary growth hormone cell adenoma and acromegaly. Acta Neuropathol (Berl) 52:231–234

Burchiel KJ, Shaw CM, Kelly WA (1983) A mixed functional microadenoma and ganglioneuroma of the pituitary fossa. Case report. J Neurosurg 58:416–420

Fischer EG, Morris JH, Kettyle WM (1983) Intrasellar gangliocytoma and syndromes of pituitary hypersecretion. Case report. J Neurosurg 59:1071–1075

Greenberg RE, Gardener LI (1959) New diagnostic test for neural tumors of infancy: increased urinary excretion of 3-methoxy-4-hydroxymandelic acid and norepinephrine in ganglioneuroma with chronic diarrhea. Pediatrics 24: 683–684 (letter)

Harkin JC, Reed RJ (1969) Atlas of tumor pathology – tumors of the peripheral nervous system. Armed Forces Institute of Pathology, Washington DC, pp 145–149

Jakumeit HD, Zimmerman V, Guiot G (1974) Intrasellar gangliocytomas. Report of four cases. J Neurosurg 40: 626–630

Kamel OW, Horoupian DS, Silverberg GD (1989) Mixed gangliocytoma-adenoma: a distinct neuroendocrine tumor of the pituitary fossa. Hum Pathol 20(12):1198–1203

Li JY, Racadot O, Kujas M, Kouadri M, et al. (1989) Immunocytochemistry of four mixed pituitary adenomas

and intrasellar gangliocytomas associated with different clinical syndromes: acromegaly, amenorrhea-galactorrhea, Cushing's disease and isolated tumoral syndrome. Acta Neuropathol (Berl) 77:320–328
Pearse AG, Takor T (1979) Embryology of the diffuse neuroendocrine system and its relationship to the common peptides. Fed Proc 38:2288–2294
Serebrin R, Robertson DM (1984) Ganglioneuroma arising in the pituitary fossa: a twenty year follow-up. J Neurol Neurosurg Psychiatry 47:97–98
Swift PG, Bloom JR, Harris F (1975) Watery diarrhoea and ganglioneuroma with secretion of vasoactive intestinal peptide. Arch Dis Child 50:896–899
Voorhess ML (1980) Functioning tumors. Am J Dis Child 134:14–15
Willis RA (1967) Pathology of tumors, 4th edn. Butterworth, London, pp 857–885

Pituitary Gland in the Human Growth-Releasing Factor Transgenic Mouse

R. Yoshiyuki Osamura

Introduction

Transgenic animals (usually mice) are produced by the introduction of a foreign gene in a segment of DNA into an isolated ovum, followed by transfer of the ovum into the oviduct or uterus of a surrogate female mouse. Some of these altered ova survive, resulting in viable young with the foreign gene stably integrated into the host's genome. The foreign gene is carried from generation to generation in viable offspring, and selection can be made for phenotypic effects of the gene. The affected mice can be raised to adulthood and produce offspring carrying this transferred gene or genes. Mutant forms of normal genes can be produced and special strains of mice may be developed for study of the effects of foreign genes. The transgenic murine model used in our studies reported here was developed by others (Mayo et al. 1988) by the introduction of the gene controlling human growth releasing factor (hGRF) into a line of mice. These transgenic mice (TgM) have been studied at several institutes including ours. This report describes the characteristics of the pituitary glands in these mice (hGRF TgM), with special emphasis on their functional differentiation (Osamura et al. 1993).

It has been reported that hGRF mRNA is expressed in various organs, including the pituitary gland, pancreas, liver, and testis. Among these the pituitary gland has been investigated most extensively, especially in relation to tumorigenesis (Osamura et al. 1993; Stefaneanu et al. 1989; Lloyd et al. 1992; Helseth et al. 1992).

Genesis of hGRF Transgenic Mice

Whole genomic hGRF is constructed with the promoter of metalothionein in the upstream region (Mayo et al. 1988). These TgM, which gain more body weight, have been demonstrated to have higher serum levels of hGRF and growth hormone (hGH). These serum levels vary from mouse to mouse. Northern blotting has demonstrated hGRF mRNA not only in the pituitary gland but also in the liver, pancreas, and testes (Mayo et al. 1988). These grossly overweight TgM usually die by the age of 1 year due to renal failure resulting from glomerulonephritis. In certain long-lived male hGRF transgenic mice it has been reported that the pituitary glands may contain adenomas (Osamura et al. 1993; Stefaneanu et al. 1989; Lloyd et al. 1992; Helseth et al. 1992).

Morphologic Changes in the Pituitary Glands of hGRF Transgenic Mice

Pituitary glands are enlarged and hyperplastic in 6-, 8-, and 10-month-old male and female TgM. In 10-month-old male TgM a few discrete adenomatous nodules develop. In the nonadenomatous pituitary gland and in the pituitary glands of the younger TgM a severe hyperplasia of acidophilic

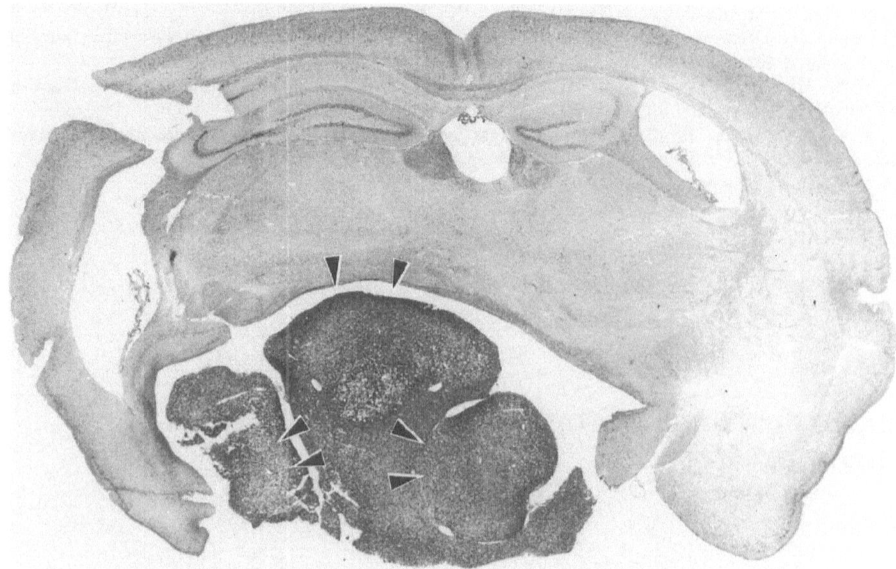

Fig. 118. Enlarged pituitary gland in hGRF transgenic mouse. *Arrow heads* indicate adenomas. H&E, ×40

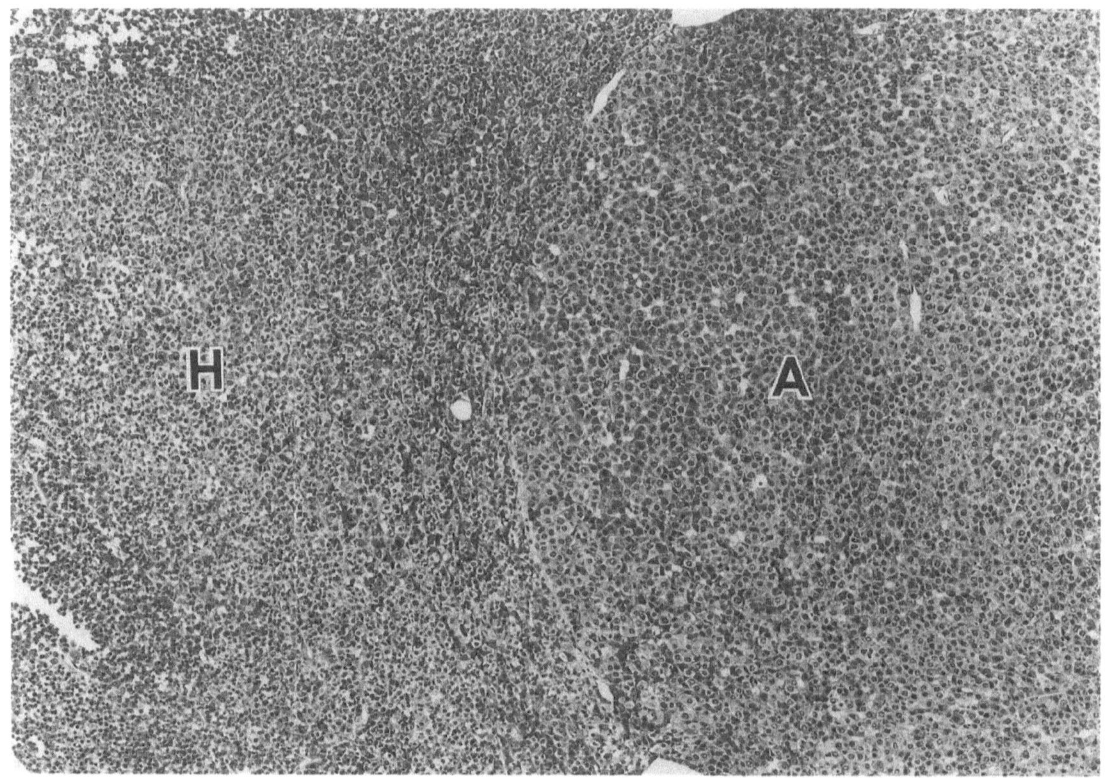

Fig. 119. Pituitary gland in hGRF transgenic mouse. Note hyperplasia (*H*) and adenoma (*A*). H&E, ×200

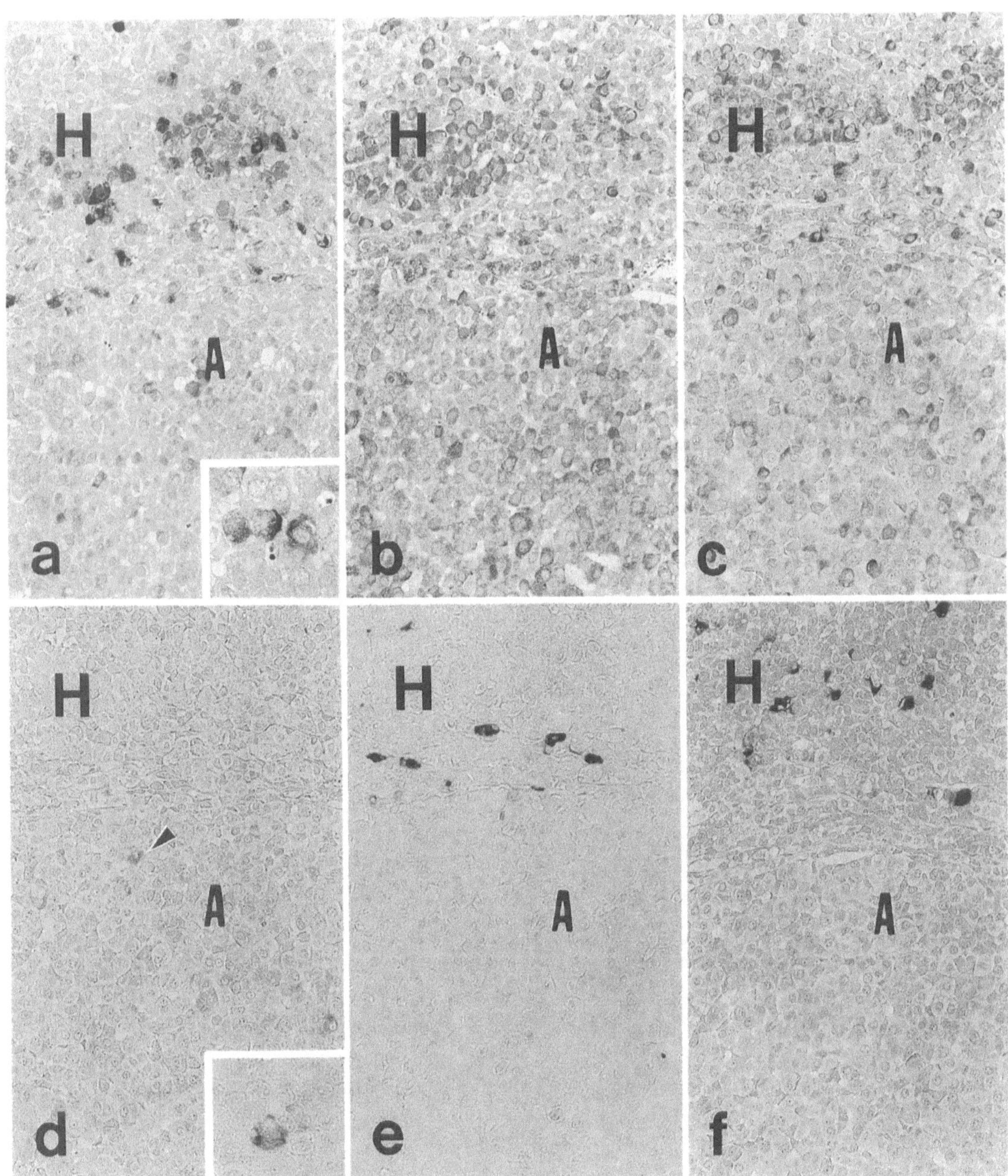

Fig. 120a,b. Immunohistochemical staining for various hormones or subunits in hyperplastic (*H*) and adenomatous (*A*) pituitary gland. **a** Human growth releasing factor (*hGRF*). **b** Growth hormone (*GH*). **c** Prolactin (*PRL*). **d** Thyroid-stimulating hormone (*TSH*). **e** α-Subunit. **f** Adrenocorticotropic hormone (*ACTH*). In hyperplasia and adenoma somatomammotrophic cells containing hGRF, GH and PRL are evident. Adenoma cells lack immunoreactivity for α-subunit and ACTH. ×200

cells occurred (Figs. 118, 119). Immunohistochemically the hyperplastic pituitary glands contained many cells which were positive for growth hormone (GH), prolactin (PRL), and hGRF. These hyperplastic cells are somatomammotrophs, probably under the regulation of an autocrine mechanism. The adenomatous nodules in 10-month-old male hGRF TgM were composed of larger and more uniform (monotonous) cells with decreased acidophilic cytoplasm. Immunohistochemically, most of these adenoma cells were positive for GH, PRL, and thyroid stimulating hormone (TSH) β-subunit (SU) as well as hGRF. Other hormones, including ACTH α-SU, follicle stimulating hormone (FSH) β-SU, and luteinizing hormone (LH) β-SU, were negative. In most tumor cells GH, PRL, and hGRF were colocalized in the cytoplasm. TSH β-SU appeared to be present in the neoplastic somatomammotrophs (Fig. 120). Under the electron microscope the adenoma cells were seen to contain scattered small secretory granules containing both GH and PRL (Fig. 121). These results suggest that the adenoma in hGRF TgM is similar to the human somatomammotroph cell adenoma (Osamura et al. 1993). In the 8-month-old male hGRF TgM a few tiny nodular areas showed similar histologic features to those in the above adenomas, and the appearance of TSH β-SU in these nodules was considered to be a marker of neoplastic transformation.

Transcriptional Factor pit-1 and Its Role in the Functional Differentiation of the hGRF TgM Pituitary Adenomas

Pit-1 protein consists of 291 amino acids and is a nuclear binding protein. It has a segment of 60 amino acids, which is similar to that of the homeodomain of *Drosophila* and shares extremely high homology among various species including the rat, mouse, and human. Simmons et al. (1990) reported that pit-1 protein is expressed immunohistochemically in GH, PRL, and TSH β-SU cells in the developing rat pituitary gland, although pit-1 mRNA is present in most of the anterior pituitary cells. In our studies the pituitary gland of a 10-month-old male hGRF TgM expressed pit-1 protein in the nuclei of not only the adenoma cells but also in the hyperplastic somatomammotrophs. The staining of pit-1 was more intense in the adenoma cells. These findings suggest that pit-1

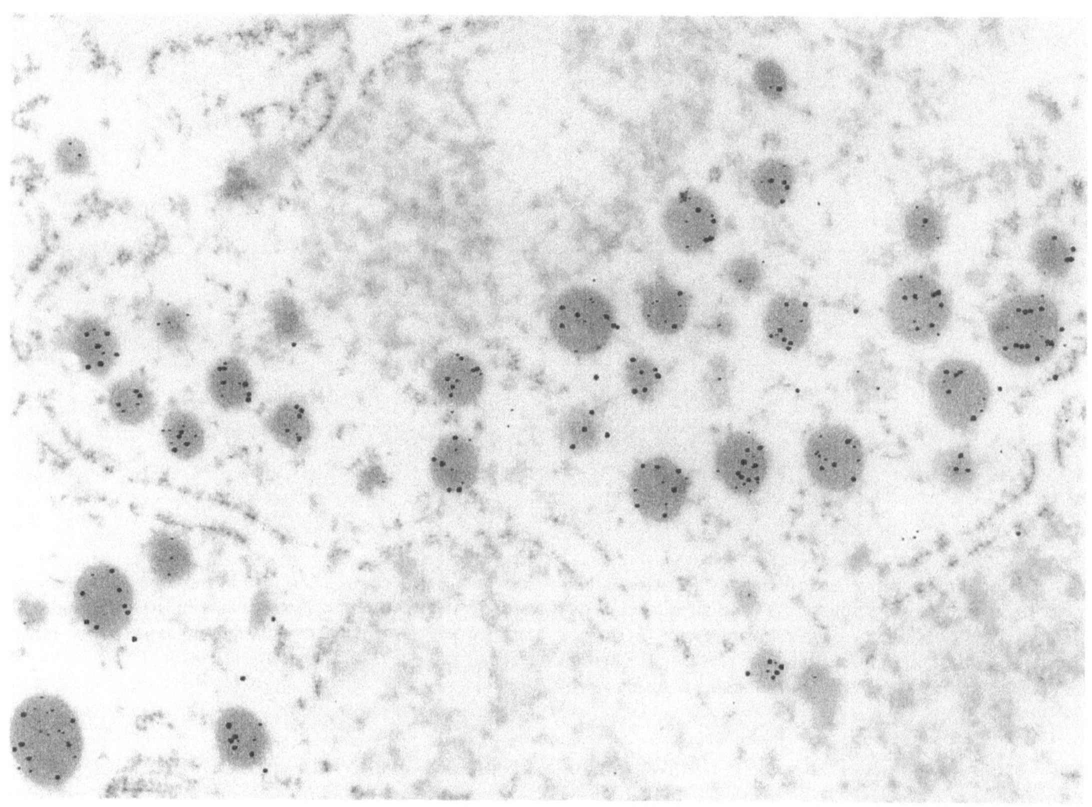

Fig. 121. Immunoelectron microscopic observation of growth hormone (*GH*) and prolactin (*PRL*) in a tumor cell. Note colocalization of GH and PRL in some of the same secretory granules. Postembedding method. Size of gold particles: GH, 20 nm; PRL, 10 nm. ×55 000

protein may play a role in the functional differentiation toward somatomammotrophs (GH plus PRL) in both adenoma and hyperplasia. Some additional factors may be involved in the appearance of TSH β-SU in the adenoma cells (Osamura et al. 1993).

References

Helseth A, Siegal GP, Haug E, Bautch VL (1992) Transgenic mice that develop pituitary tumors. A model for Cushing's disease. Am J Pathol 140:1071-1080

Lloyd RV, Jin L, Chang A, Kulig E, Camper SA, Ross BD, Downs TR, Frohman LA (1992) Morphologic effects of hGRH gene expression on the pituitary, liver, and pancreas of MT-hGRH transgenic mice. An in situ hybridization analysis. Am J Pathol 141:895-906

Mayo KE, Hammer RE, Swanson LW, Brinster RL, Rosenfeld, MG, Evans RM (1988) Dramatic pituitary hyperplasia in transgenic mice expressing a human growth hormone-releasing factor gene. Mol Endocrinol 2:606-612

Osamura RY, et al. (1993) Immunohistochemical expression of pit-1 protein in pituitary glands of human GRF transgenic mice. Its relationship with hormonal expressions. Endocr J 40:133-139

Simmons DM, Voss JW, Ingraham HA, Holloway JH, Broide RS, Rosenfeld NG, Swanson LW (1990) Pituitary cell phenotypes involve cell-specific pit-1 mRNA translation and synergistic interactions with other classes of transcription factors. Genes Dev 4:695-711

Stefaneanu L, Kovacs K, Horvath E, Asa SL, Losinski NE, Billestrup N, Price J, Vale W (1989) Adenohypophysial changes in mice transgenic for human growth hormone-releasing factor: a histological, immunocytochemical and electron microscopic investigation. Endocrinology 125: 2710-2718

Cysts, Pituitary, Rat, Mouse, and Hamster

William W. Carlton and Christian L. Gries

Gross Appearance

Cysts of the craniopharyngeal duct in rodents are usually microscopic. A few large cysts enlarge the gland and may appear as blisterlike lesions filled with mucoid-colloid material.

Microscopic Features

Epithelial-lined cysts have been described in the pituitary gland of the rat (Opper 1940; Lansdown and Grasso 1971) and the mouse (Blumenthal 1955). The cysts may be found either confined to the pars distalis, especially in the periphery of the anterior lobe, or joined to the lumen of Rathke's cleft. Most of the cysts are microscopic, lie within the anterior lobe, contain a mucoproteinaceous material, are lined by ciliated, cuboidal to columnar epithelium, and are simple tubular or multilocular in form (Fig. 122). Ciliated cells are not distributed continuously around the walls of the cysts but are often interspersed with nonciliated flat cells and with swollen, spherical cells having mucinous cytoplasm. The epithelium has single, basal, and round nuclei.

A cystic lesion in the region of the pars nervosa of a rat has been described (Lansdown and Grasso 1971). This rare lesion consisted of a large cyst surrounded by a cluster of smaller cysts. A single- or double-layered, cuboidal to columnar, aciliate epithelium lined the cysts, which were filled with a PAS-positive mucoproteinaceous material. A thin connective tissue sheath surrounded the cysts̈

Rathke's cleft (hypophyseal) cysts are found most often between the pars distalis and pars intermedia in the region of the hypophyseal cleft but may occur either in the pars intermedia or the pars distalis near the cleft. The distal wall of these cysts is composed of cells of the pars distalis, and the proximal wall is composed of cells of the pars intermedia. Such cysts may contain either a colloidlike proteinaceous material, blood, or breakdown products of blood pigments (Figs. 123, 124).

Differential Diagnosis

The location and histologic features of craniopharyngeal cysts are sufficient for diagnosis. A cyst with extensive squamous metaplasia must be differentiated from the rare craniopharyngioma.

Biologic Features

In the development of the pituitary gland the adenohypophysis arises from Rathke's pouch, a dorsal evagination of the posterior nasopharynx (stomodeum). The neurohypophysis arises from the infundibulum, a ventral process of the floor of the diencephalon. The proximal wall of Rathke's pouch touching the saccus infundibuli differentiates into the pars intermedia, and the distal wall forms the pars distalis. The hypophyseal cleft is the residual lumen of the original pouch persisting between these two lobes. The portion of Rathke's pouch connected with the roof of the buccal cavity constricts into the craniopharyngeal stalk.

Cysts of the craniopharyngeal duct located in the anterior lobe are not common in rodents, but an incidence of 10% was reported in one study of Wistar strain rats (Opper 1940). Rathke's cleft cysts are more common.

Most of the intrasellar cysts arising from the craniopharyngeal duct produce no clinical disease, and the cysts are incidental findings at histopathologic examination of the pituitary gland.

Cysts of the craniopharyngeal duct may be site of origin of craniopharyngioma, but this is a rare occurrence (Capen 1993; Jubb 1962).

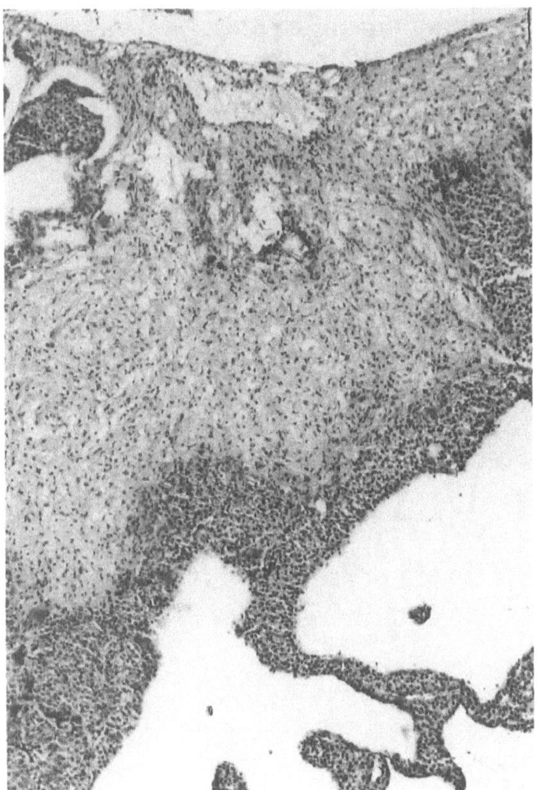

Fig. 122. Multilocular pituitary cysts, F334 rat. H&E, ×64

Comparison with Other Species

Persistence of remnants of the craniopharyngeal duct is rare in domestic animals except for the dog (Rao and Bhat 1971; Capen 1993; Oghiso et al. 1982; Benjamin 1981). Portions of either end of the duct may persist and serve as a site for the development of cysts. Cystic distention and persistence of the intrasellar portion of the craniopharyngeal duct (Rathke's cleft) is congenital and common in some breeds of dogs such as the German shepherd, and some cysts are large enough to produce clinical signs of hypopituitarism including dwarfism, cachexia, diabetes insipidus, genital atrophy, and obesity (Anderson and Capen 1978; Muller and Jones 1973; Allan et al. 1978; Capen 1993). Remnants of the oropharyngeal portion give rise to the pharyngeal hypophysis, a cystic structure in the dorsal wall of the pharynx. The pharyngeal hypophysis in the dog is tubular and lined by ciliated columnar epithelium (McGrath 1974). It may be continuous with a multilocular cyst containing colloid and cellular debris and lined by either squamous, cuboidal, or columnar epithelium.

Remnants of the intrasellar portion of the duct may develop into cysts which may be single, multiple, unilocular, or multilocular, and are most commonly located at the periphery of the pars distalis and in the pars tuberalis. These intrasellar cysts are common in brachycephalic breeds of dogs, contain a mucinous material, vary greatly in size, and are lined by either ciliated cuboidal or columnar epithelium. The large cysts push out the periphery and cause herniation of the capsule of the pituitary gland. In the rat the pharyngeal hypophysis is a tubular diverticulum of the pharyngeal mucosa with a well-defined fibrous wall and is lined by ciliated columnar epithelial cells (McGrath 1974).

Pituitary gland cysts have been reported in nonhuman primates including *Macaca sinica*, gorilla (*Gorilla gorilla gorilla*), and chimpanzee (*Pan troglodytes*) (Anderson and Capen 1978; Rao and Bhat 1971), and were the most common finding in the anterior lobe of baboons (McConnell et al. 1974). A ciliated cuboidal to columnar epithelium or squamous epithelium lined these cysts, which contained a mucinous material.

Suprasellar and intrasellar cysts have been described in human patients (Russell and Rubinstein 1972; Diengdoh and Scott 1983). The suprasellar cysts are epidermoid in type, are found principally in children and adolescents, and originate from small nests of squamous cells that represent remnants of Rathke's pouch. Intrasellar cysts are rare, generally macroscopic, and have fluid or inspissated contents. The cysts may be lined, in part, by a cuboidal, sometimes ciliated epithelium. The cyst lining of a Rathke's cleft cyst in electron micrographs has been described as composed of three types of cells: (a) ciliated columnar cells with secretory granules, (b) nonciliated cells with secretory granules, and (c) epidermoid (or prickle) cells. The latter group of cells included both squamous epithelial cells forming squames and irregularly shaped prickle cells lying on the basement membrane (Diengdoh and Scott 1983).

Most of the pituitary gland cysts in humans are clinically silent. However, some large cysts cause compression atrophy of adjacent structures and produce clinical signs and symptoms including cachexia and diabetes insipidus suggestive of either a neoplasm of the pituitary gland or of hypopituitarism.

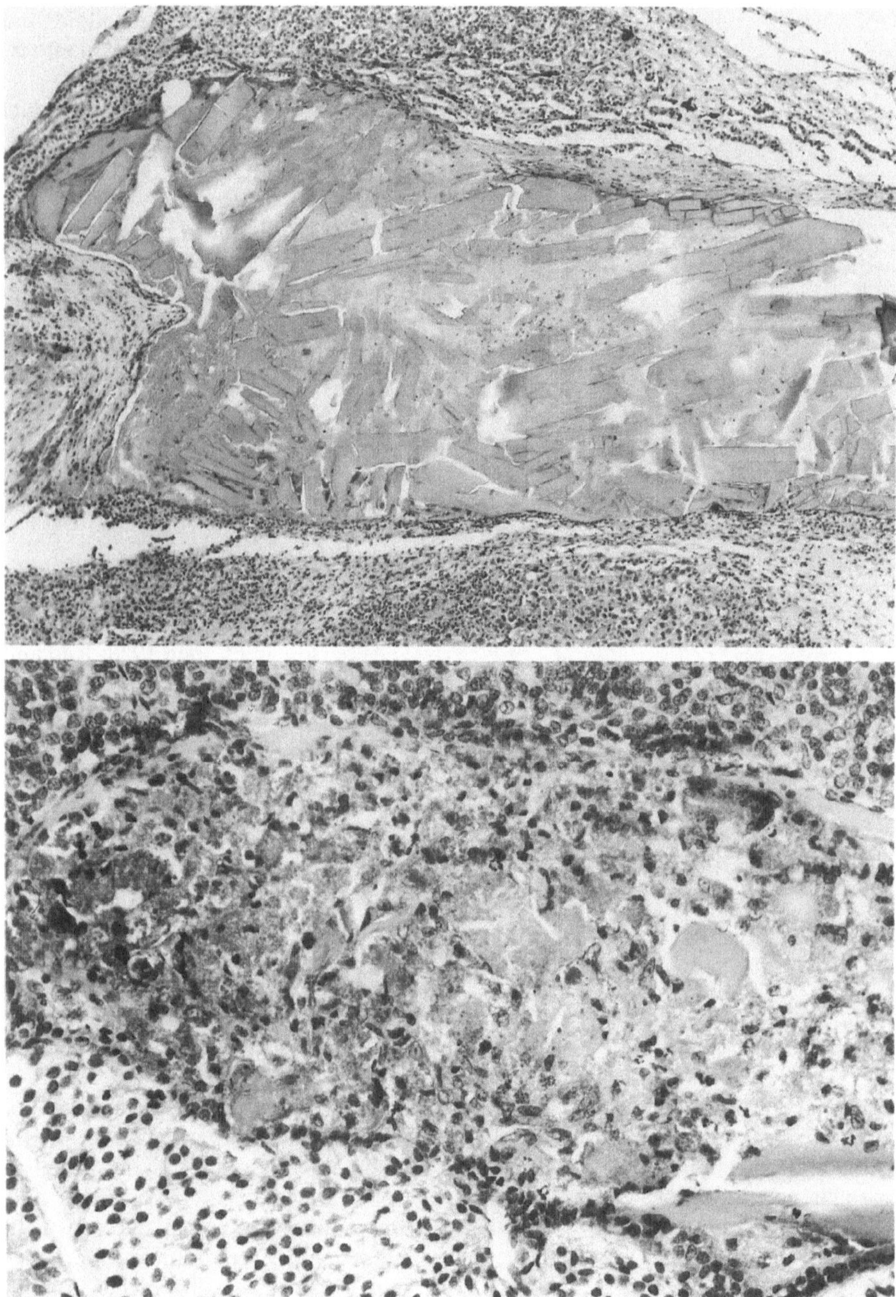

Fig. 123. (*above*) Rathke's cleft cyst filled with proteinaceous fluid and hemoglobulin crystals, F334 Rat. H&E, ×64

Fig. 124. (*below*) Small Rathke's cleft cyst filled with macrophages and debris, F334 Rat. H&E, ×224

References

Allan GS, Huxtable CRR, Howlett CR, Baxter RC, Duff B, Farrow BRH (1978) Pituitary dwarfism in German shepherd dogs. J Small Anim Pract 19:711–727

Anderson MP, Capen CC (1978) The endocrine system. In: Benirschke K, Garner FM, Jones TC (eds) Pathology of laboratory animals, vol I. Springer, Berlin Heidelberg New York, pp 423–508

Benjamin M (1981) Cysts (large follicles) and colloid in pituitary glands. Gen Comp Endocrinol 45:425–445

Blumenthal HT (1955) Aging processes in the endocrine glands of various strains of normal mice: relationship of hypophyseal activity to aging changes in other glands. J Gerontol 10:253–267

Capen CC (1993) The endocrine glands. In: Jubb KVF, Kennedy PC, Palmer N (eds) Pathology of domestic animals, vol III, 4th edn. Academic, San Diego, pp 275–277

Diengdoh IV, Scott T (1983) Electron-microscopical study of a Rathke's cleft cyst. Acta Neuropathol (Berl) 60:14–18

Jubb KV (1962) The hypophysis. In: Innes JRM, Saunders LZ (eds) Comparative neuropathology. Academic Press, New York, pp 245–266

Lansdown AB, Grasso P (1971) Histological observations on a Ratlike's cleft abnormality in a laboratory rat. J Comp Pathol 81:141–144

McConnell EE, Basson PA, de Vos V, Myers BJ, Kuntz RE (1974) A survey of diseases among 100 free-ranging baboons (Papio ursinus) from the Kruger National Park. Onderstepoort J Vet Res 41:97–167

McGrath P (1974) The pharyngeal hypophysis in some laboratory animals. J Anat 117:95–115

Muller GH, Jones SR (1973) Pituitary dwarfism and alopecia in a German shepherd with a cystic Rathke's cleft. J Am Anim Hosp Assoc 9:567–572

Oghiso Y, Fukuda S, Jida H (1982) Histopathological studies on distribution of spontaneous lesions and age changes in the beagle. Jpn J Vet Sci 44:941–950

Opper L (1940) Incidence and morphology of epithelial cysts in the anterior lobe of the hypophysis of the rat. Anat Rec 76:135–143

Rao RR, Bhat NG (1971) Incidence of cysts in pars distalis of mongrel dogs. Indian Vet J 48:128–133

Russell DS, Rubinstein LJ (1989) Pathology of tumours of the nervous system, 5th edn. Williams and Wilkins, Baltimore

Inflammation, Pituitary Gland: Rat, Mouse, and Hamster

William W. Carlton and Christian L. Gries

Gross Appearance

Inflammatory cell infiltrations of the pituitary gland, by extension from the meninges, usually produce no gross alterations; pituitary gland involvement in these cases is detected by histopathologic examination. Severe, suppurative inflammation leading to abscess formation may produce enlargement and distortion of the gland, however.

Microscopic Features

Neutrophilic and lymphocytic infiltrations may involve the meninges and pituitary gland. Inflammatory cells are found within the sinusoids and between parenchymal cells. Suppurative foci may have associated parenchymal cell necrosis, but vascular thrombosis and infarction are rare in the pituitary gland of laboratory rodents.

Differential Diagnosis

In cases of leukemic lymphosarcoma of the rat and mouse, infiltrates of neoplastic cells are occasionally seen in the pituitary gland as well as in the cerebral meninges. Usually these neoplastic infiltrates are more extensive than those seen with the more rarely occurring lymphocytic inflammatory infiltrations. These lesions may be differentiated by cytopathologic and/or immunohistochemical methods. Special stains for bacteria, such as the tissue Gram stain and silver stains, could be useful in differentiating among bacterial causes of inflammation of the pituitary gland.

Biologic Features

Inflammatory diseases of the pituitary gland in laboratory rodents are rare, and none are specific. The few cases of suppurative and lymphocytic infiltrations seen in the pituitary gland most commonly represent extensions to the pituitary gland from meningitis established by penetration of otitis interna or from a sinusitis due to extension of a periodontitis. No reports are presently available to indicate that acute inflammation of the pituitary occurs at all commonly in laboratory rodents during the course of septicemias.

Comparison with Other Species

Inflammations of the pituitary gland are quite common in domestic animals. Those in the neurohypophysis are associated with either meningitis or encephalitis. Both the anterior and posterior lobes are affected by suppurative inflammations in bacteremic diseases in which bacterial embolism is common. Bacterial embolisms from suppurative processes in other organs, such as the uterus and reticulum, are known sources of suppurative pituitary gland inflammations in ruminants. These lesions, particularly in ruminants and swine, have been associated with infections by *Actinobacillys pyogenes*; however, other bacteria have also been isolated from such lesions (Jubb et al. 1993).

In human patients acute inflammation of the pituitary gland occurs in the course of septicemia or pyemia and has been seen in cases of suppurative infections of the urinary tract. The pituitary gland, especially the anterior lobe, can develop acute inflammatory lesions as a result of extension from suppurative meningitis and infiltrative lesions of the hypothalamus (Kelly 1989). Diffuse lymphocytic infiltration of the anterior pituitary gland has been described in patients with autoimmune hypophysitis (Kelly 1989). Granulomatous inflammations of the pituitary gland are sometimes found in patients with sarcoidosis, tuberculosis, syphilis, or mycotic infections, but such cases are considered rare (Wright and Symmers 1966).

References

Kelly WN (ed) (1989) Textbook of internal medicine. Lippincott, Philadelphia

Jubb KVF, Kennedy PC, Palmer N (1993) Pathology of domestic animals, 4th edn, vol I. Academic Press, San Diego

Wright GP, Symmers WS (1966) Systemic pathology, vol II. Elsevier, New York

Cystoid Degeneration Due to Diethylstilbestrol, Anterior Pituitary, Mouse

Alexander M. Cameron and Winslow G. Sheldon

Gross Appearance

This lesion is not grossly recognizable.

Microscopic Features

Cystoid degeneration of the anterior pituitary gland is seen in H- and E-stained sections as irregular foci in which parenchymal cells are absent. The alterations are usually of moderate size and number (Figs. 125,126), although the lesions vary from a few relatively small (Fig. 127) to multiple and relatively large foci. Individual lesions generally vary from about 50 to 150 μm in their greatest dimension. The foci of cell loss are generally lined by normal appearing cells of the anterior pituitary (Fig. 127). The spaces usually contain finely granular eosinophilic material occasionally including erythrocytes. Cellular remnants are present in some spaces. This lesion may be seen in anterior pituitary glands that are otherwise morphologically normal, or in association with hyperplastic or neoplastic proliferations.

Ultrastructure

In affected areas, the spaces from which cells have been lost usually contain fine, granular material interspersed with a few secretory granules and degenerated mitochondria. Some spaces also contain other fragments of degenerated cells. Cells adjacent to the cystoid areas are often more electron lucent than more distant cells. In some instances, the changes include disrupted plasma membranes with occasional extrusion of cell organelles, swollen mitochondria with loss of cristae, separation of rough endoplasmic reticulum profiles, dilated Golgi, and modest numbers of secretory granules (Figs. 128, 129).

Differential Diagnosis

Pituitary cysts, focal necrosis, and vascular congestion resemble cystoid degeneration but may be differentiated without difficulty. Pituitary cysts have regular outlines, are usually lined by simple squamous to columnar epithelium which is often

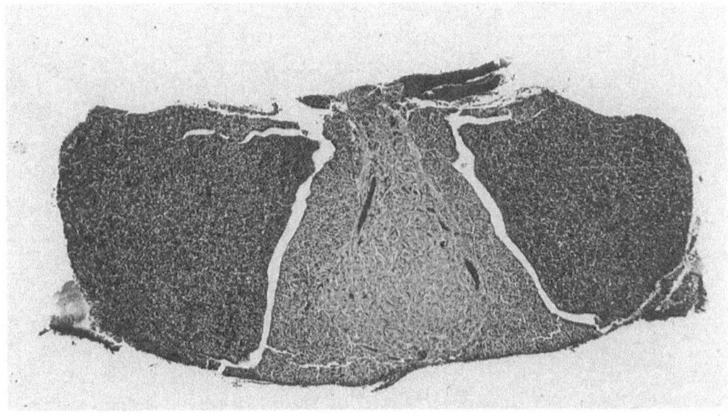

Fig. 125. Normal mouse pituitary. H&E, ×50

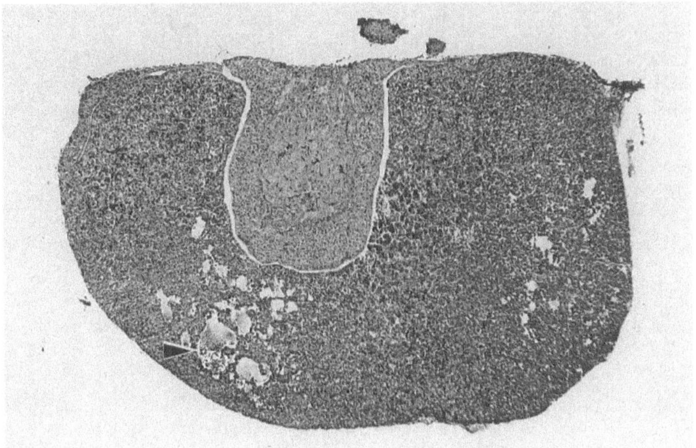

Fig. 126. Mouse pituitary with several areas of cystoid degeneration of the pars distalis (*arrowhead*). H&E, ×50

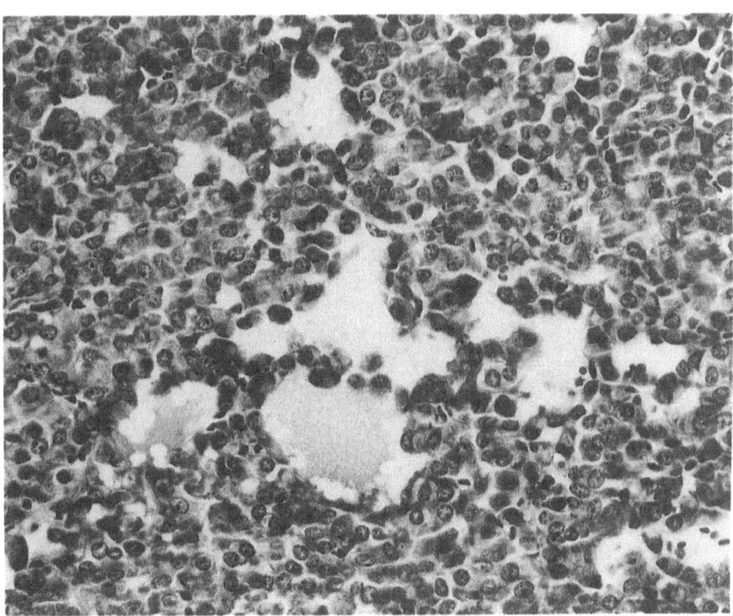

Fig. 127. Cystoid degeneration of the anterior pituitary. Spaces contain finely granular material and occasionally cellular remnants. Note that lining cells are parenchymal cells of the pars distalis. H&E, ×275

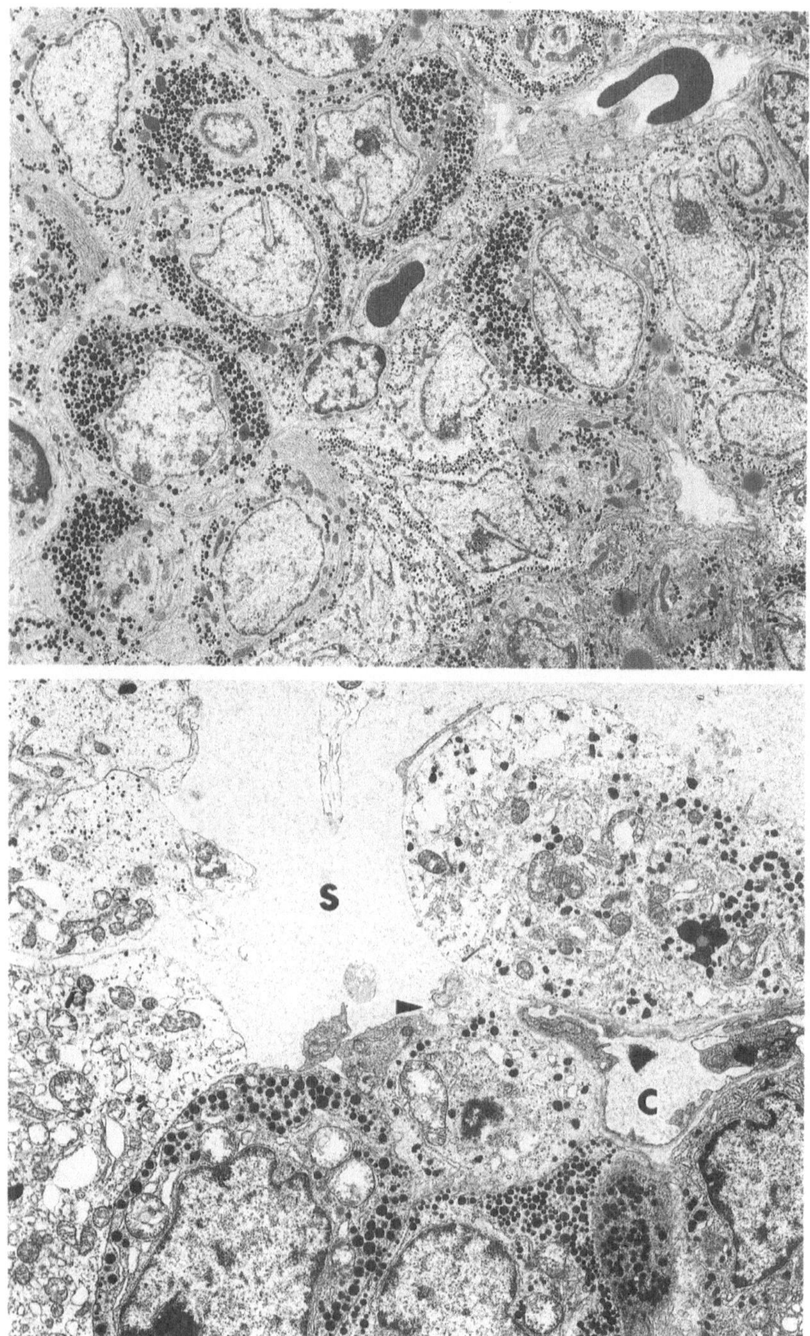

Fig. 128. (*above*) Electron micrograph of normal mouse anterior pituitary, ×2000

Fig. 129. (*below*) Area of cystoid degeneration (*S*) of anterior pituitary. Most cells adjacent to the space are more electron-lucent than cells more distant from the space. Spaces contain granular material, organelles, and other larger cellular remnants. Apparent lysis of cell (*arrow* head), capillary (*C*), TEM ×6000

ciliated, and generally contain homogeneous eosinophilic material (Anderson and Capen 1978). The lesions of cystoid degeneration have irregular outlines, are lined only by surviving parenchymal cells and usually contain fine, granular, lightly staining eosionophilic material and/or erythrocytes.

Focal necrosis is recognized by the presence of necrotic cells, cellular debris, and/or hemorrhage in or about areas of cell damage. Necrotic cellular debris is not a prominent feature of cystoid degeneration, however, focal necrosis remains a possible precursor.

In vascular congestion, excessive amounts of blood are surrounded by endothelium. The spaces found in cystoid degeneration are not lined by endothelial cells, although some cystoid lesions do contain erythrocytes.

Biologic Features

Virgin C3H/H_EN MTV+ female mice fed 320 or 640 parts per billion of diethylstilbestrol (DES) for different periods of time during an 18 month study developed cystoid degeneration of the pituitary gland. The frequency of the lesion was increased by the larger dosage and earlier or longer postnatal exposure to DES (Figs. 130, 137) and was seen rarely in control mice. The lesion was also reported in C3H/H_EJ MTV+ mice exposed to DES (Andrews et al. 1980). A similar lesion has been reported in association with pituitary neoplasms in untreated C57BL/6J mice (Schechter et al. 1981).

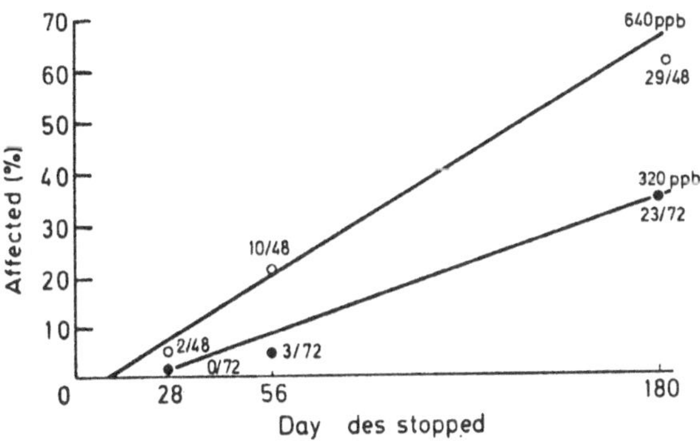

Fig. 130. Cystoid degeneration of the pituitary in mice; the effects of dose of DES and of the age when exposure was discontinued. Day 0 is weaning age, 21 days. *ppb*, parts per billion DES fed in diet

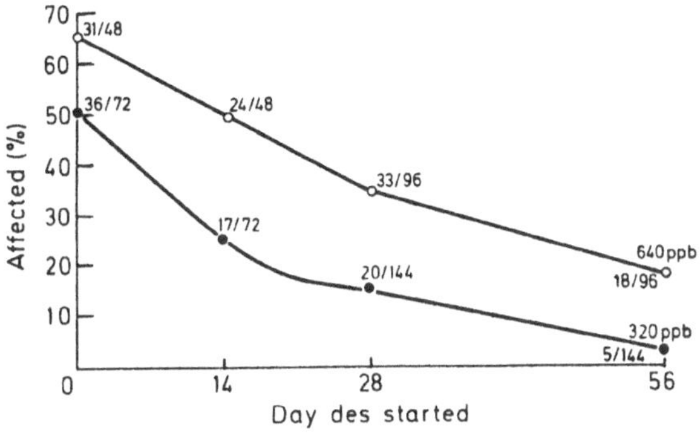

Fig. 131. Cystoid degeneration of the pituitary in mice; the effects of dose of DES and of the age when treatment was begun. Day 0 is weaning age, 21 days. *ppb*, parts per billion DES fed in diet

Comparison with Other Species

Although certain lesions have been attributed to exposure to DES in rodents (Highman et al. 1980; Vorherr et al. 1979), other animals (McMartin et al. 1978), and humans (Bibbo et al. 1977; Ulfelder 1976; Robboy et al. 1977), no similar pituitary lesion induced by DES has been described in rodents (Anderson and Capen 1978; Russfield 1967), other laboratory animals (Anderson and Capen 1978), or man (Horvath and Kovacs 1980).

References

Anderson MP, Capen CC (1978) The endocrine system. In: Benirschke K, Garner FM, Jones TC (eds) Pathology of laboratory animals. Springer, Berlin Heidelberg New York, chap 6

Andrews AM, Cameron AM, Townsend JW, Sheldon WG (1980) Cystoid degeneration of mouse pituitary-ultrastructural study. In: Bailey GW (ed) 38th Ann Proc Electron Microscopy Soc Amer San Francisco, California

Bibbo M, Gill WB, Azizi F, Blough R, Faug VS, Rosenfield RL, Schmacher GFB, Sleeper K, Sonek MG, Wied GL (1977) Follow-up study of male and female offspring of DES-exposed mothers. Obstet Gynecol 49:1–8

Frith CH, Ward JM (1988) Color atlas of neoplastic and non-neoplastic lesions in aging mice. Elsevier, Amsterdam

Highman B, Greenman DL, Norvell MJ, Farmer J, Shellenberger TE (1980) Neoplastic and preneoplastic lesions induced in female C3H mice by diets containing diethylstilbestrol or 17-estradiol. J Environ Pathol Toxicol 4:81–95

Horvath E, Kovacs K (1980) Pathology of the pituitary gland. In: Ezrin C, Horvath E, Kaufman B, Kovacs K, Weiss MH (eds) Pituitary diseases. CRC Press, Boca Raton, Florida, chap 1

McMartin KE, Kennedy KA, Greenspan P, Alam SN, Greiner P, Yam J (1978) Diethylstilbestrol: a review of its toxicity and use as a growth promotant in food-producing animals. J Environ Pathol Toxicol 1:279–313

Robboy SJ, Scully RE, Welch WR, Herbst AL (1977) Intrauterine diethylstilbestrol exposure and its consequences. Arch Pathol Lab Med 101:1–5

Russfield AB (1967) Pathology of the endocrine glands, ovary and testis of rats and mice. In: Cotchin E, Roe FJC (eds) Pathology of laboratory rats and mice. Blackwell Scientific, Oxford, chap 14

Schechter JE, Felicio LS, Nelson JF, Finch CE (1981) Pituitary tumorigenesis in aging female C57BL/6L mice: A light and electron microscopic study. Anat Rec 199:423–432

Ulfelder H (1976) The stilbestrol-adenosis-carcinoma syndrome. Cancer [Suppl] 38:426–431

Vorherr H, Messer RH, Vorherr UF, Jordan SW, Kornfeld M (1979) Teratogenesis and carcinogenesis in rat offspring after transplacental and transmammary exposure to diethylstilbestrol. Biochem Pharmacol 28:1865–1877

Craniopharyngeal Derivatives in the Neurohypophysis, Rat and Hamster

Eberhard Karbe and Heinrich Ernst

Synonyms. Aberrant craniopharyngeal structures in the neurohypophysis.

Gross Appearance

This pathologic entity is generally too small to be recognized macroscopically at necropsy.

Microscopic Features

The lesion may be located anywhere within the neurohypophysis or the adjacent pars intermedia. In the rat the lesion consists of simple epithelium, including cuboidal to columnar cells, which may be ciliated, goblet cells, and form tubular and/or acinar structures with similarities to salivary glands, as well as stratified squamous epithelium, all arranged in a haphazardous manner, forming cysts containing mucous and/or cellular debris (Figs. 132–137).

In parts of the neurohypophysis, especially toward the pars intermedia, smaller cells lacking epithelial characteristics may form irregular clusters (Figs. 134–136). These less differentiated cells have similarities to pars intermedia cells. However, they are not identical and appear more primitive with their smaller amount of cytoplasm, which does not react with PAS.

This pathologic entity may be associated with relatively large cysts lined by simple or ciliated epithelium, or goblet cells. These cysts are located within or adjacent to the neurohypophysis, outside the pituitary, or between the neurohypophysis and the pars intermedia.

Immunohistochemical staining indicates the presence of cytokeratin, characteristic for epithelia, especially in the stratified squamous portion of the lesions. Hormones or precursors characteristic for the adenohypophysis so far have not been found in the rat (Schaetti et al. 1994); however, investigations on squamous cell nests in the human pars tuberalis suggest that these structures may derive from hormone-producing cells of the adenohypophysis (Sumi et al. 1993).

Mitotic figures are not generally seen within these craniopharyngeal lesions. Single-cell necrosis occurs. Compression of the surrounding neurohypophysial tissue is absent or, at most, minimal in some areas. On a particular section of the neurohypophysis the lesion may occupy most of the plane cut (Fig. 132). The presence or proportion of the various differentiated cell types varies among cases. Any cell type including the undifferentiated (Fig. 135) or the tubular (Fig. 136) may predominate.

Craniopharyngeal derivatives in the neurohypophysis can also occur in the Syrian hamster. The case presented here in a 28-month-old female (Figs. 138, 139) is probably the first to be published. The lesion consists of differentiated acinar structures similar to salivary glands located within the neurohypophysis. Neither mitotic

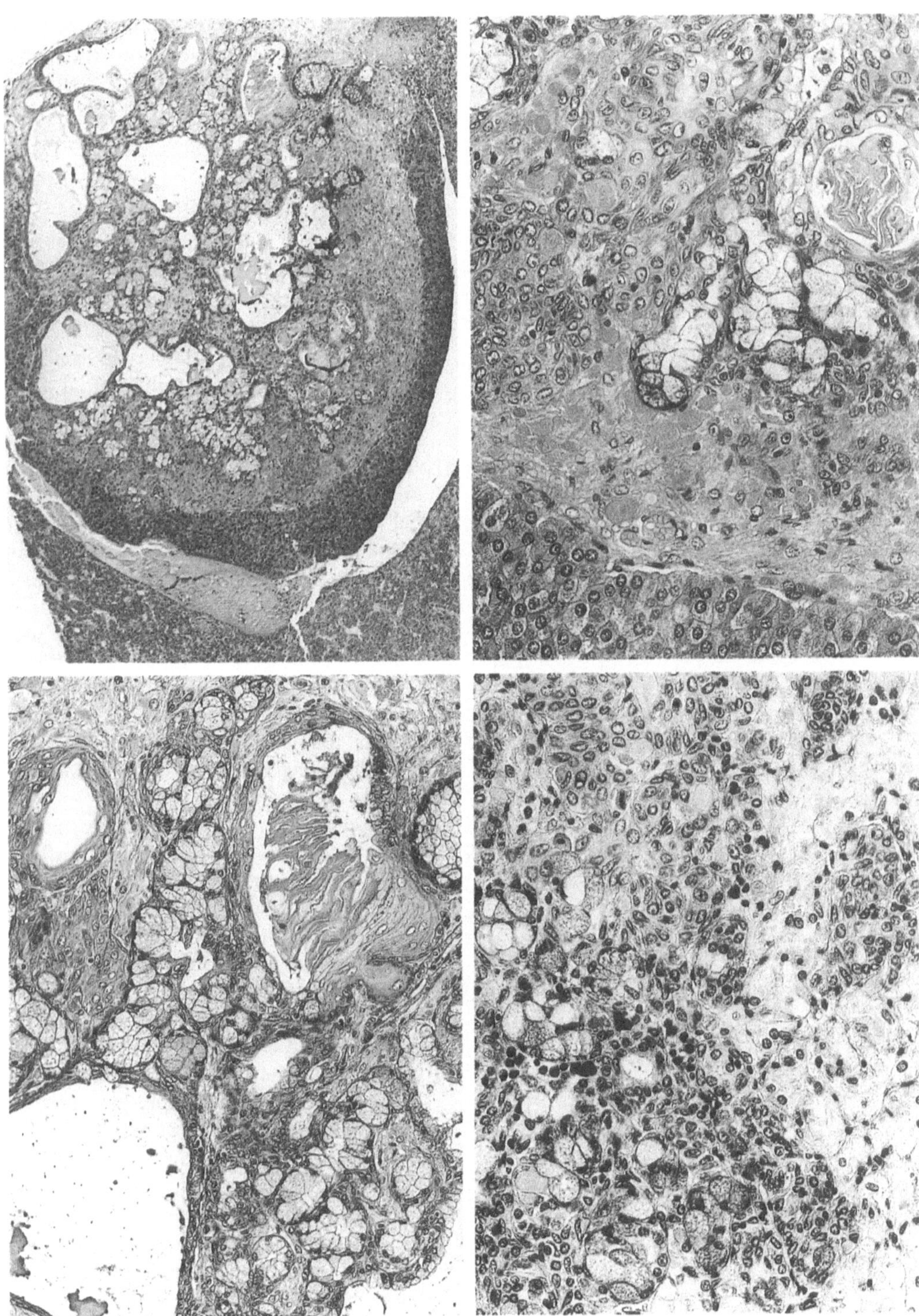

Fig. 132. (*upper left*) Male Wistar rat, 11 weeks old. Various epithelial structures within the neurohypophysis. H&E, ×40

Fig. 133. (*lower left*) Detail of Fig. 132 with mucinous glandular structures, epidermoid and stratified squamous epithelium. H&E, ×120

Fig. 134. (*upper right*) High magnification of Fig. 132. Note in addition to epithelial structures, less differentiated cells towards pars intermedia (*bottom*). H&E, ×230

Fig. 135. (*lower right*) Wistar rat, female, 23 weeks old. Note clusters of less differentiated cells with glandular cells in neurohypophysis. H&E, ×200

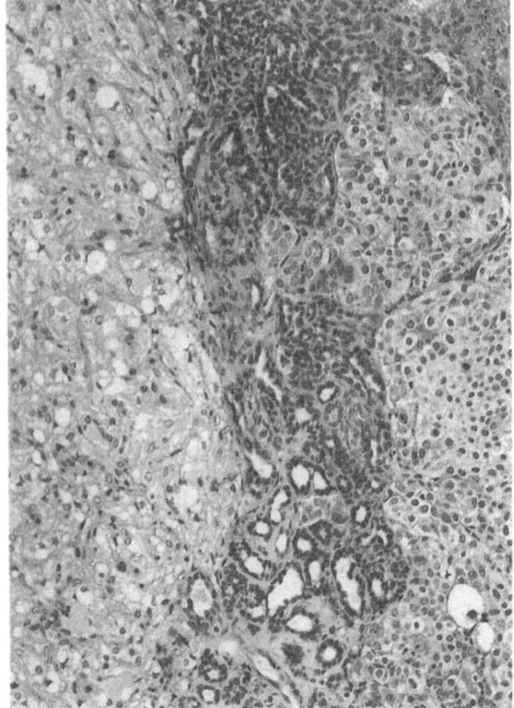

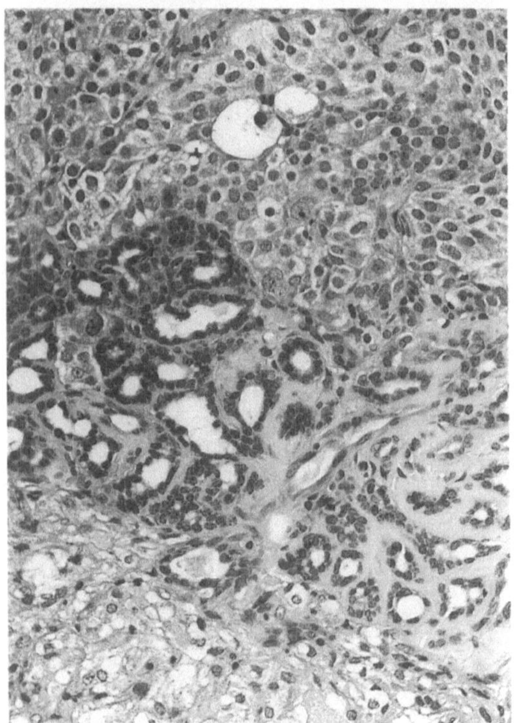

Fig. 136. (*above*) Wistar rat, female, 22 months old. Solid and tubular structures between pars intermedia and neurohypophysis extending into pars intermedia. H&E, ×120

Fig. 137. (*below*) High magnification of Fig. 136. Note presence of fibrous tissue between tubular structures. H&E, ×200

figures nor compression can be seen. Such acinar structures are observed in the rat intermingled with other less differentiated epithelial components and therefore are considered part of this entity.

Differential Diagnosis

Nonneoplastic craniopharyngeal tissue in the neurohypophysis is most easily confused with craniopharyngioma, known to occur rarely in rats (Fitzgerald et al. 1971; Heinrichs et al. 1990) and mice (Heider 1986). The differential diagnosis of the craniopharyngioma has been published with the WHO diagnostic criteria (Karbe et al. 1994). As in other animals the tumor has been described in rat and mouse as a stratified squamous epithelial type and not as the adamantinoma type seen in man. The craniopharyngioma in rats and mice is dominated histopathologically by cells forming a stratified squamous epithelium, while nonneoplastic craniopharyngeal derivatives within the neurohypophysis in the rat are usually more complex, as described above, and may even lack the stratified squamous component. Craniopharyngiomas are usually closely associated with the neurohypophysis but appear to be located mainly outside the pituitary.

Craniopharyngeal cysts are lined by a mostly single layer of cuboidal to columnar, partly ciliated, epithelium, including goblet cells, and lack solid epithelial components. They may be multiple and located within the neurohypophysis (Lansdown and Grasso 1971). In man they can become large enough to form multicystic lesions leading to clinical signs (Berge and Eriksson 1967).

Although diffuse hyperplasia of the pars intermedia may be severe enough to lead to the "infiltration" of the neurohypophysis, such cells are uniform and obviously projections of the pars intermedia within the adjacent neurohypophysis. "Basophil invasion," described as a common change in man after puberty, consists of ACTH-positive cells of the pars anterior "infiltrating" the pars nervosa (Scheithauer 1991). To our knowledge, no report of this change in rats has been published. Cells can be recognized as pars anterior cells, especially with immunohistochemical methods.

Metastases or systemic tumors growing in the neurohypophysis must be differentiated.

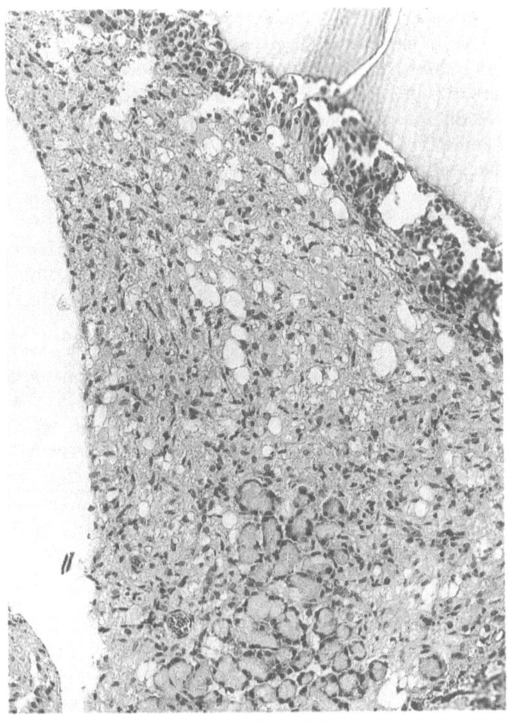

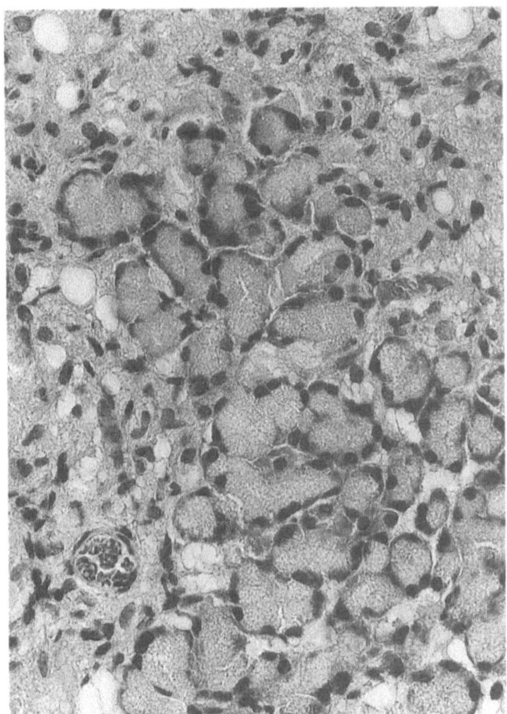

Fig. 138. (*above*) Male Syrian hamster, 28 months old. Neurophypophysis with glandular tissue. H&E, ×120

Fig. 139. (*below*) Detail of Fig. 138. Note well-differentiated acini mimicking salivary gland. H&E, ×350

Biologic Features

The craniopharyngeal derivatives within the neurohypophysis described here and not considered to be neoplastic do not cause clinical signs and do not appear to produce hormones. They are incidental findings causing diagnostic problems. Most cases have been observed in rats about 2 years of age (Schaetti et al. 1994). However, we also found these lesions in a Wistar rat as young as 11 weeks. It is difficult to conceive that the lesions develop from pluripotent cells of the adenohypophysis and spread into the neurohypophysis within weeks after birth. In addition, there does not appear to be a relationship between the amount of craniopharyngeal tissue observed and the age of the animal. Also, the common association with craniopharyngeal cysts suggests a congenital background. Therefore this entity should be considered as a developmental aberration that can no longer be induced after birth. It may be important to know whether such a rare lesion is found in toxicity studies in treated animals only.

Etiology. The etiology of this lesion is unknown.

Frequency. Craniopharyngeal derivatives described here within the neurohypophysis appear to be quite rare since they were not reported before MacKenzie and Boorman (1990), who observed them in Fischer rats. Recently we observed these lesions in more than 17 rats of two Wistar and two Sprague-Dawley substrains in five laboratories in Germany, Italy, and Switzerland, indicating a widespread but rather rare occurrence (Schaetti et al. 1994).

Comparison with Other Species

These craniopharyngeal derivatives occur within the neurohypophysis of rat and hamster but have probably not been described in nonrodent animal species (apart from cysts (as their pituitaries are investigated in small numbers by comparison. In man acinar structures (Scheithauer 1991) and squamous epithelial cell nests (Kovacs and Horvath 1986) have been described in the literature as having no clinical relevance except when giving rise to large cysts or craniopharyngiomas.

References

Berge T, Eriksson S (1967) Cystic pituitary tumour developed from Rathke's cleft. Acta Pathol Microbiol Scand 71: 321–327

Fitzgerald JE, Schardein JL, Kaump DH (1971) Several uncommon pituitary tumors in the rat. Lab Anim Sci 21(4): 581–584

Heider K (1986) Spontaneous craniopharyngioma in a mouse. Vet Pathol 23:522–523

Heinrichs M, Baumgartner W, Durchfeld B (1990) Kraniopharyngeom bei einer Ratte: ein Fallbericht. 39th meeting of the Europäischen Gesellschaft für Veterinärpathologie, Aachen. Berl Munch Tierarztl Wochenschr 103: 430

Karbe E et al (1994) International classification of rodent tumours. I. The rat, vol 6. Endocrine system. Pituitary gland. International Agency for Research on Cancer, Lyon, pp 1–11 (IARC scientific publication no 122)

Kovacs K, Horvath E (1986) Tumors of the pituitary gland. Atlas of tumor pathology, second series, fascicle 21. Armed Forces Institute of Pathology, Washington DC

Lansdown AB, Grasso P (1971) Histological observations on a Rathke's cleft abnormality in a laboratory rat. J Comp Pathol 81:141–144

MacKenzie WF, Boorman GA (1990) Pituitary gland. In: Boorman GA et al (eds) Pathology of the Fischer rat. Academic, San Diego, pp 485–500

Schaetti P, Argentino-Storino A, Mirea D, Popp A, Heinrichs M, Karbe E (1994) Craniopharyngeal structures within the neurohypophysis of rats of four different strains. Exp Tox Pathol (in press)

Scheithauer BW (1991) The hypothalamus and neurohypophysis. In: Kovacs K (ed) Functional endocrine pathology. Blackwell Scientific Publications, St Louis, pp 170–244

Sumi T, Stefeneanu L, Kovacs K (1993) Squamous-cell nests in the pars tuberalis of the human pituitary: immunocytochemical and in situ hybridization studies. Endocr Pathol 4:155–161

Hypothalamus

Stereotaxic Map, Cytoarchitectonic and Neurochemical Summary of the Hypothalamic Nuclei, Rat

Miklós Palkovits

Introduction and Guide to the Stereotaxic Atlas

The topographical anatomy of the hypothalamic nuclei has been the subject of many fine books (Clark Le Gros 1938; Diepen 1962; Haymaker et al. 1969), book chapters (Bleier et al. 1979; Swanson 1987), atlases (Massopust 1961; de Groot 1963; König and Klippel 1963; Albe-Fessard 1966; Szentágothai et al. 1968; Pellegrino et al. 1979; Paxinos and Watson 1982; Swanson 1992), and review articles (Gurdjian 1927; Krieg 1932). (For additional references, see Palkovits 1983). Most of the maps contain coronal sections through the hypothalamus, but relatively few of them show comprehensive series of horizontal (Simson et al. 1981; Paxinos and Watson 1982) or sagittal (Paxinos and Watson 1982) planes.

In this chapter the topography of hypothalamic nuclei is summarized and illustrated in 18 coronal (frontal) and 15 sagittal sections. Series of 10-µm thick sections were obtained from brains of rats weighing 200 ± 10 g (Wistar CFY strain), and stained with Luxol fast blue cresyl violet. Sections were photographed under a microscope ("a" panels in Figs. 144–176) and outlines of major nuclei and bundles were drawn ("b" panels) from every 30th coronal and 15th sagittal section.

The major regions of the hypothalamus, including the preoptic region and the mamillary body, are illustrated in a coordinate system in millimeter scales (Figs. 140–142). The frontal zero plane lies in the bregma level. The bregma is the point of the surface of the skull at the junction of the coronal and sagittal sutures. This is a well-defined external-internal landmark: a vertical plane which corresponds to the bregma outside on the skull and to the decussation of the anterior commissure inside the brain. This plane is perpendicular to the surface of the brain if the head is fixed in a 5° nose-down position in a stereotaxic apparatus (König and Klippel 1963). In adult rats (200 ± 10 g) the bregma level is 7.2 mm rostral to the interauricular line, which is also a useful landmark for determining rostrocaudal coordinates. Distances from the bregma (0 µm) level are indicated in µm (P, posterior to the bregma). The sagittal zero plane is the midline. The vertical coordinates start from the dorsal surface of the brain, which corresponds to the zero horizontal level. The hypothalamus is present in 18 consecutive coronal sections, with 300 µm between the neighboring sections (Figs. 140–142).

Macroscopic Distribution of the Hypothalamic Regions

The hypothalamus may be divided into three major regions: anterior, middle, and posterior. Although the preoptic region and the mamillary body are treated separately from the hypothalamus by a number of authors, mainly for functional reasons, in the present work we follow the earlier anatomical classifications, i.e., these areas are also detailed.

The *preoptic area* lies between frontal planes 300 µm rostral and 600 µm caudal to the bregma. Dorsally it reaches to the anterior commissure and the bed nucleus of the stria terminalis. Ventrally the preoptic area is separated from the olfactory tubercle by the diagonal band. Caudally it passes into the anterior hypothalamus. This area can be divided into medial and lateral parts (Fig. 140). The cell-dense medial preoptic area contains the preoptic nuclei, while the lateral is occupied by the fibers and intrinsic cells of the medial forebrain bundle.

The *rostral* border of the hypothalamus is approximately 0.6 mm behind the bregma level. The *anterior hypothalamus* extends caudally as far as the caudal edge of the optic chiasm. About 40% of the total hypothalamus (preoptic area and mamillary body are excluded) belongs to the anterior hypothalamus. It can be divided by a vertical section through the fornix into medial and lateral parts (Fig. 140).

The *middle hypothalamus* starts from the caudal edge of the optic chiasm, rostrally, and ends at the level of the separation of the pituitary stalk, caudally. A vertical cut through the fornix and mamillothalamic tract divides it into medial and lateral parts. The medial one can be further

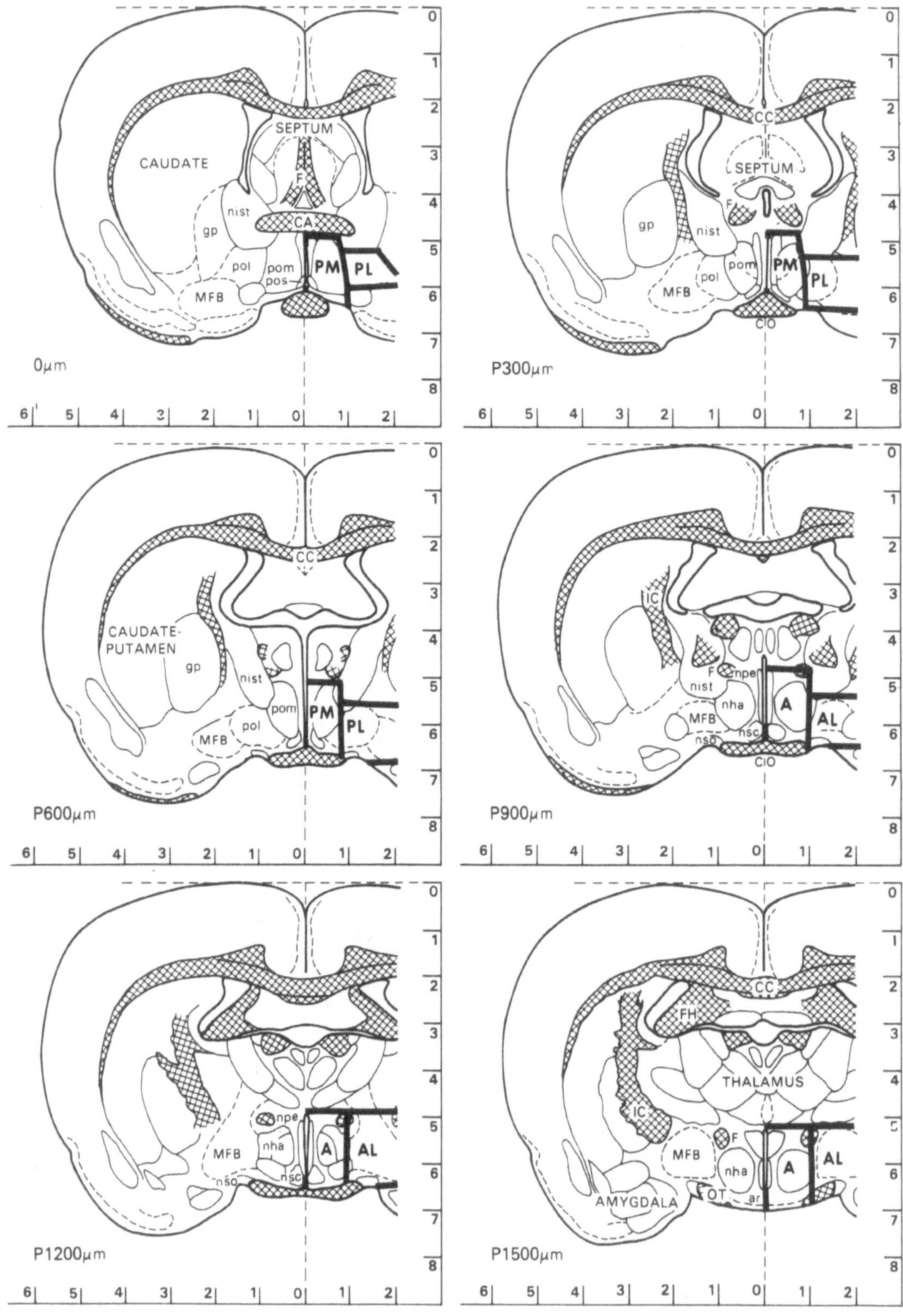
SEPTUM
CAUDATE
F
nist
gp
CA
pol
pom
pos
PM
PL
MFB
0μm
CC
SEPTUM
F
gp
nist
pom
PM
pol
PL
MFB
CIO
P300μm
CC
CAUDATE-PUTAMEN
gp
nist
pom
PM
PL
pol
MFB
P600μm
IC
F
npe
nist
nha
A
AL
MFB
nsc
nso
CIO
P900μm
npe
nha
A
AL
MFB
nso
nsc
P1200μm
CC
FH
THALAMUS
IC
F
MFB
nha
A
AL
AMYGDALA
OT
ar
P1500μm

divided by a horizontal cut bisecting the third ventricle into mediobasal and dorsal parts (Fig. 141).

The *posterior hypothalamus* is relatively small, constituting only 20% of the total hypothalamus. It is bounded by an imaginary plane extending from the posterior commissure to the mamillary body. The medial portion of this region contains the premamillary and posterior hypothalamic nuclei, as well as cells around the *inframamillary* recess, while the lateral portion is practically equal with the territory of the medial forebrain bundle (Fig. 142).

The *mamillary body* is recognizable by the ellipsoid arrangement of cells and fiber systems between frontal planes 4.2 and 5.3 mm caudal to the bregma and occupies a ventral territory of the diencephalon between the posterior hypothalamus and mesencephalon. Medial and lateral mamillary nuclei have been generally recognized (Fig. 142).

◀

Fig. 140. Hypothalamus, anterior. Drawings of serial (300 µm between consecutive sections) coronal (frontal) sections of adult rat forebrain. 0 µm = Bregma level (*P*, posterior to the bregma). Coordinates are in millimeter scales. *Right, heavy lines*, major hypothalamic areas. *PM*, medial preoptic region; *PL*, lateral preoptic region (between 0–P600 µ) and lateral posterior hypothalamus (betwene P3900–P4800 µ); *A*, medial anterior hypothalamus; *AL*, lateral anterior hypothalamus; *MD*, medial dorsal hypothalamus; *MB*, medial basal hypothalamus; *L*, lateral region of the middle part of the hypothalamus; *P*, medial posterior hypothalamus; *PL*, lateral posterior hypothalamus. Abbreviations for hypothalamic nuclei and major bundles: *ar*, retrochiasmatic area; *CA*, anterior commissure; *CC*, corpus callosum; *CO*, optic chiasm; *F*, fornix; *FH*, fimbria hippocampi; *FMT*, mamillothalamic tract; *gp*, globus pallidus; *IC*, internal capsule; *la*, ventromedial nucleus, pars lateralis anterior; *ma*, ventromedial nucleus, pars medialis anterior; *me*, median eminence; *MFB*, medial forebrain bundle; *na*, arcuate nucleus; *ndm*, dorsomedial nucleus; *nha*, anterior hypothalamic nucleus; *nhp*, posterior hypothalamic nucleus; *nist*, bed nucleus of the stria terminalis; *nme*, medial mamillary nucleus, pars medianus; *nml*, lateral mamillary nucleus; *nmm*, medial mamillary nucleus, pars medialis; *nmx*, medial mamillary nucleus, pars lateralis; *npe*, periventricular nucleus; *npf*, perifornical nucleus; *npmd*, dorsal premamillary nucleus; *npmv*, ventral premamillary nucleus; *npv*, paraventricular nucleus; *nsc*, suprachiasmatic nucleus; *nsu*, supramamillary nucleus; *nvm*, ventromedial nucleus; *nvma*, anterior ventromedial nucleus; *OT*, optic tract; *pol*, lateral preoptic area; *pom*, medial preoptic nucleus; *pop*, periventricular preoptic nucleus; *pos*, suprachiasmatic preoptic nucleus; *SN*, substatia nigra

Nuclear Pattern of the Rat Hypothalamus

Detailed literary data regarding the cytoarchitecture of the hypothalamus can be found for mammals (Palkovits 1983). In the rat the nuclear pattern of the hypothalamus was described almost 50 years ago by Gurdjian (1927) and Krieg (1932), and not much can be added to those earlier accounts. A comprehensive review of the hypothalamus in most vertebrates has been given by Diepen (1962) and by Crosby and Showers (1969). A detailed description of the cytoarchitecture of the hypothalamus is beyond the scope of this chapter. Only the following brief remarks are added to the map. The rostrocaudal extensions of the hypothalamic nuclei are shown in Fig. 143. (Nucleus is used here in the neuroanatomic sense, meaning a collection of neurons, not to be confused with that component of a cell.)

The hypothalamic nuclei can also be recognized on frozen or unstained sections and removed individually by the microdissection technique for neurochemical measurements. For a guide of this procedure, see Palkovits and Brownstein (1988).

Preoptic Region

The *medial preoptic nucleus* (pom) is an oval cell group located lateral to the periventricular cell layers. According to the size and density of the cells, it can be divided into medial and lateral subdivisions.

The *periventricular preoptic nucleus* (pop) consists of small cells which occupy the wall of the anterior end of the third ventricle (between frontal planes 0.4 mm rostral and 0.6 mm caudal to the bregma). The central part of this nucleus (0.2 mm rostral to 0.2 mm caudal to the bregma) is densely packed by cells, which along the lamina terminalis can be followed upwards over the anterior commissure. This group of cells is referred to as *median preoptic nucleus*.

The *suprachiasmatic preoptic nucleus* (pos) is densely packed group of small cells immediately dorsal to the optic chiasm, on both sides of the third ventricle. Caudally the nucleus merges with the hypothalamic suprachiasmatic nucleus.

The *lateral preoptic area* (pol) consists of rather diffuse cell masses lateral to the medial preoptic nucleus. The major ventrolateral portion of this area corresponds to the medial forebrain bundle.

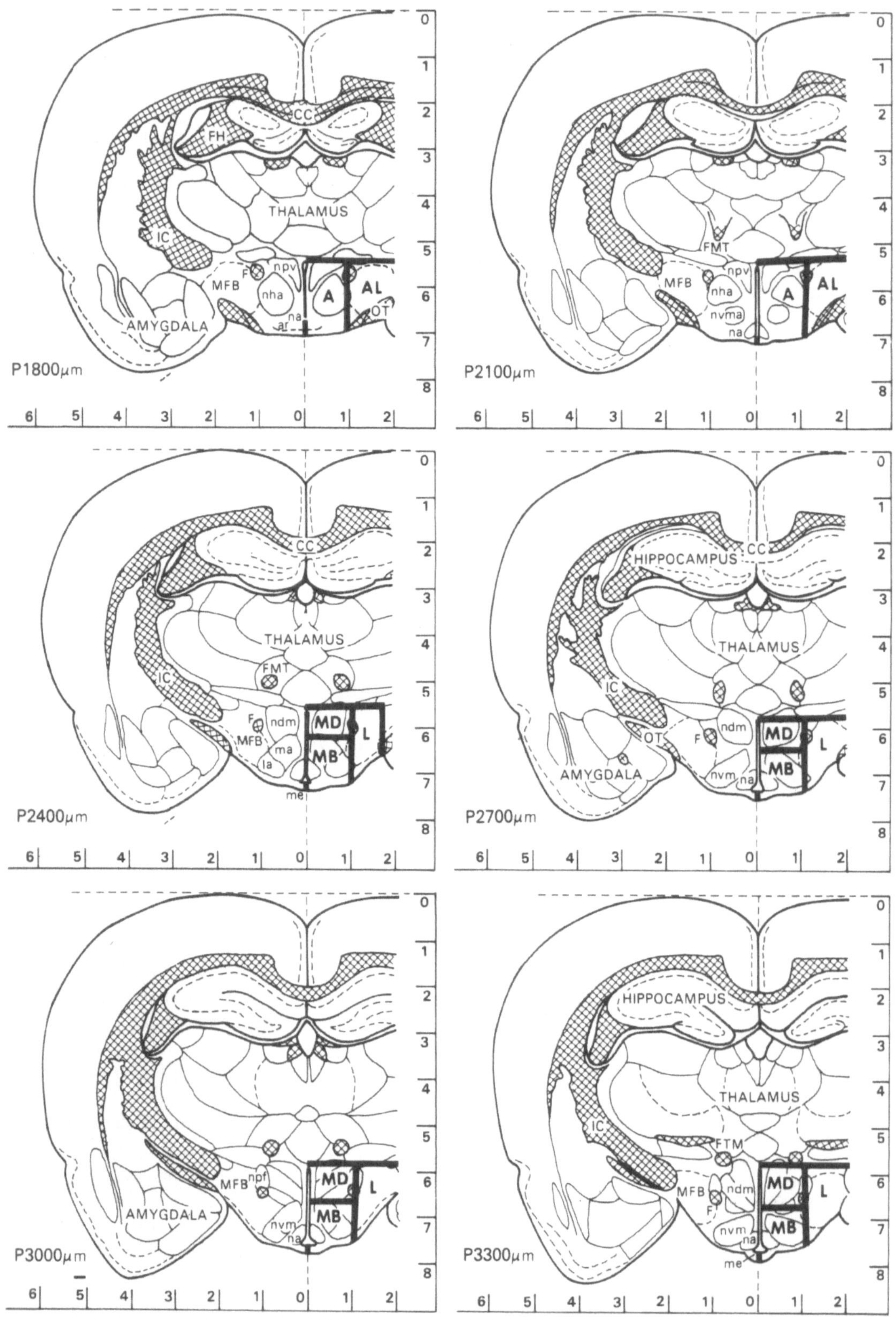

Fig. 141. Hypothalamus, middle. Drawings of serial (300 µm between consecutive sections) coronal (frontal) sections of adult rat forebrain. 0 µm = Bregma level (*P*, posterior to the bregma). Coordinates are in millimeter scales. *Right*, *heavy lines*, major hypothalamic areas. Abbreviations, see Fig. 140

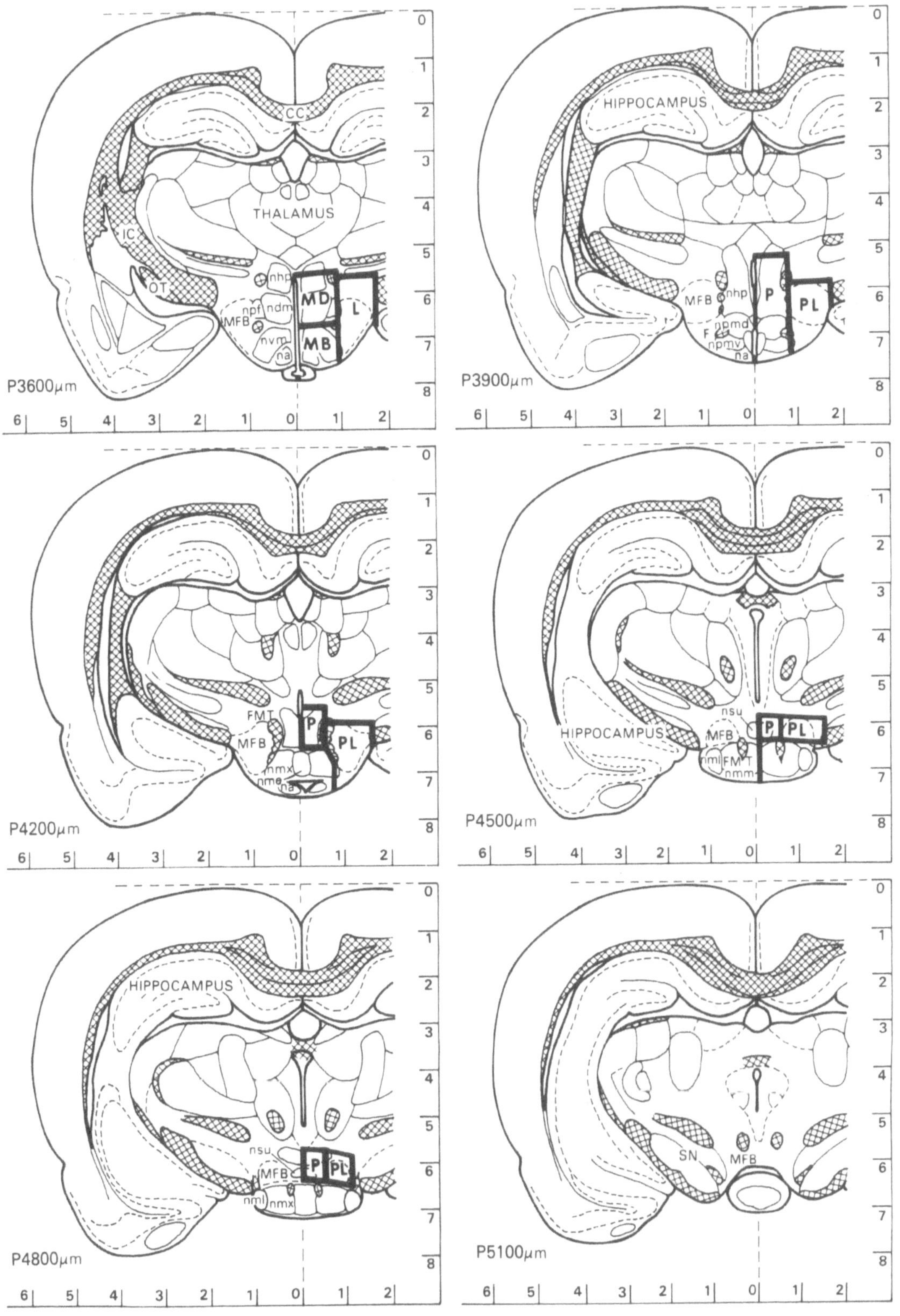

Fig. 142. Hypothalamus, posterior. Drawings of serial (300 μm between consecutive sections) coronal (frontal) sections of adult rat forebrain. 0 μm = Bregma level (*P*, posterior to the bregma). Coordinates are in millimeter scales. *Right*, *heavy lines*, major hypothalamic areas. Abbreviations, see Fig. 140

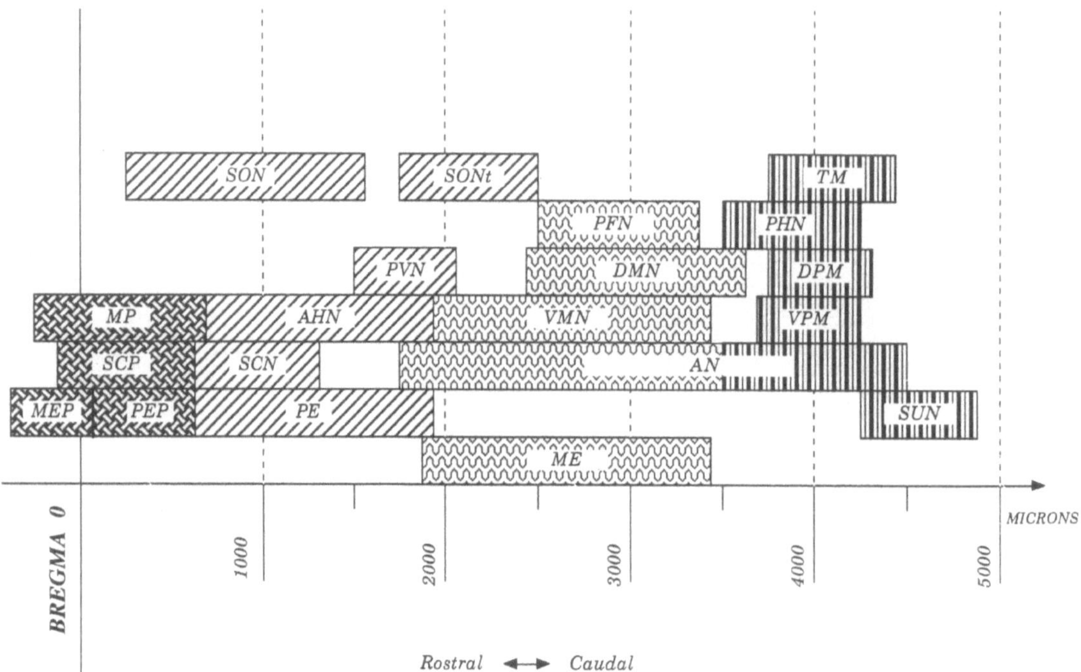

Fig. 143. Rostrocaudal extension of the hypothalamic nuclei of adult (200 ± 10 g) rats. Distances from the bregma (zero) level are given in micrometers. ▩, Preoptic area; ▨, anterior hypothalamus; ▩, middle hypothalamus; ▥, posterior hypothalamus (premamillary region). *AHN*, Anterior hypothalamic nucleus; *AN*, arcuate nucleus; *DMN*, dorsomedial nucleus; *DPM*, dorsal premamillary nucleus; *ME*, median eminence; *MEP*, median preoptic nucleus; *MP*, medial preoptic nucleus; *PE*, periventricular nucleus; *PEP*, preoptic periventricular nucleus; *PFN*, perifornical nucleus; *PHN*, posterior hypothalamic nucleus; *PVN*, paraventricular nucleus; *SCN*, suprachiasmatic nucleus; *SCP*, preoptic suprachiasmatic nucleus; *SON*, supraoptic nucleus; *SONt*, tuberal part of the supraoptic nucleus; *SUN*, supramamillary nucleus; *TM*, tuberomamillary nucleus; *VMN*, ventromedial nucleus; *VPM*, ventral premamillary nucleus

Anterior Hypothalamus

The *periventricular nucleus* (npe) is comprised of a narrow band of cells lying along the third ventricle between the preoptic region and the rostral third of the middle hypothalamus. A small group of the relatively large cells is embedded in the periventricular gray beside the upper part of the third ventricle. This cell group is called the *magnocellular periventricular nucleus* (npm) (synonym: anterior magnocellular paraventricular nucleus.)
The *suprachiasmatic nucleus* (nsc) is found beside the third ventricle immediately above the optic chiasm. Caudally it becomes the retrochiasmatic area.
The *anterior hypothalamic nucleus* (nha) is one of the largest hypothalamic nuclei and consists of four subdivisions (dorsal, ventral, medial, and caudal). It occupies the major portion of the anterior medial hypothalamus.
The *supraoptic nucleus* (nso) extends mainly along the dorsolateral border of the optic chiasm. It contains exclusively large, so-called magnocellular neurosecretory cells.
The *paraventricular nucleus* (npv) is located at the border of the anterior and medial-dorsal hypothalamus, dorsally, immediately beside the top of the third ventricle. Magnocellular and five parvocellular subdivisions can be recognized.
The lateral hypothalamic area corresponds to the *medial forebrain bundle* (mfb) and its intrinsic cells in this region. Rostrally it is continuous with the lateral preoptic area.

Middle Hypothalamus

The *retrochiasmatic area* (ar) is not a nucleus in the cytoarchitectonic sense. It occupies a territory between the optic chiasm and median eminence at the base of the hypothalamus on either side of

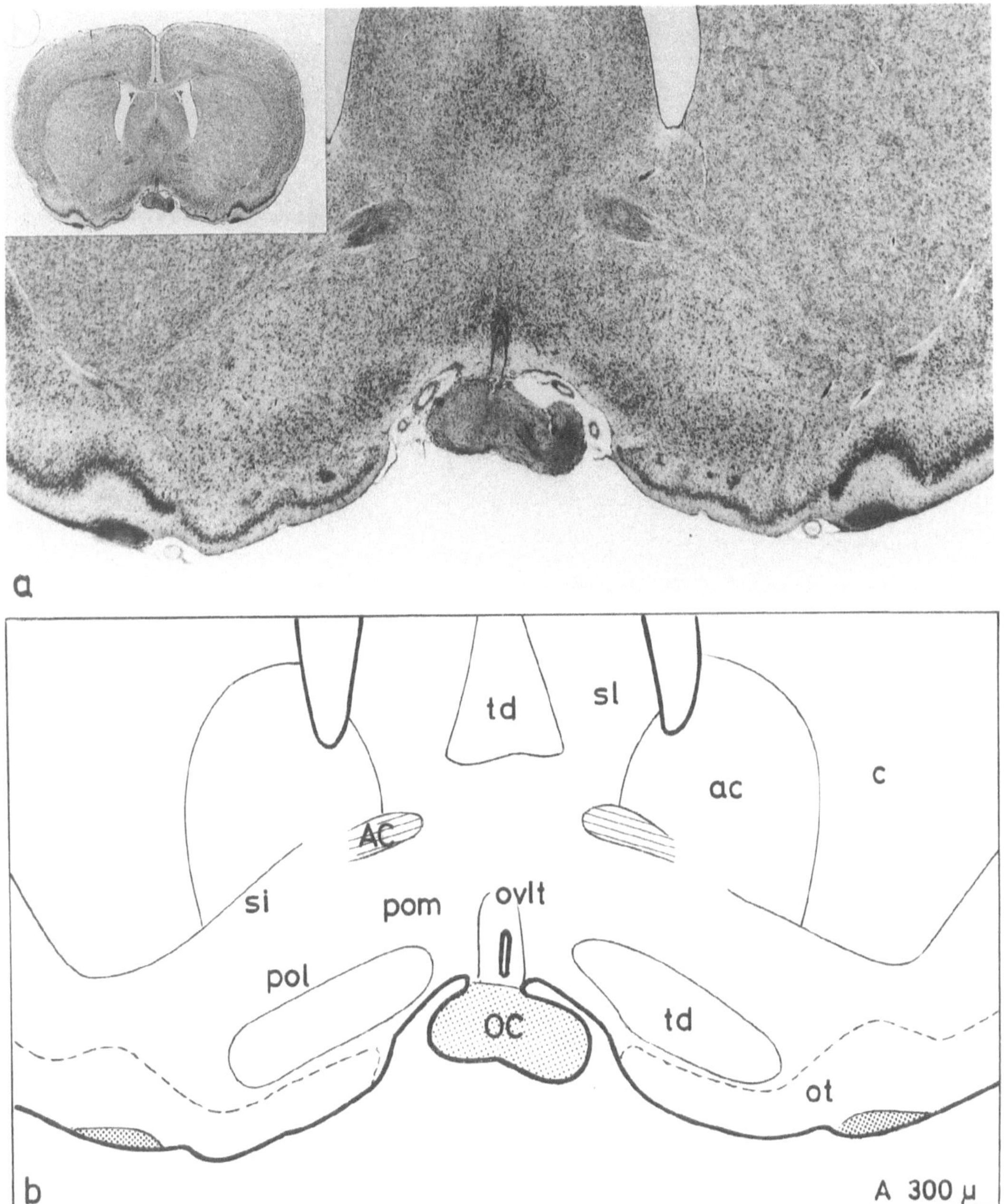

Fig. 144a,b. Coronal sections (Figs. 144–161) of the hypothalamus from the preoptic area to the mamillary. Sections were taken from equal distances (300 µm) rostral (*A*, anterior) and caudal (*P*, posterior) to the bregma (zero) level. Rats, 200 ± 10 g body weight. α Luxol fast blue cresyl violet staining, ×15. *Inserts*, the whole coronal section. **b** Schematic drawings corresponding to **a,** with demarcation of the hypothalmic nuclei. *a*, Arcuate nucleus; *aa*, anterior amygdaloid area; *ac*, accumbens nucleus; *AC*, anterior commissure; *c*, caudate nucleus; *CC*, crus cerebri; *cp*, caudate-putamen; *CP*, posterior commissure; *dm*, dorsomedial nucleus; *F*, fornix; *FR*, fasciculus retroflexus; *ha*, anterior hypothalamic nucleus; *HI*, hippocampus; H_l, Forel's *Hl* field; *IC*, internal capsule; *1h*, lateral hypothalamic area; *LM*, medial lemniscus; *lon*, nucleus of the lateral olfactory tract; *1s* lateral septal nucleus; *LV*, lateral ventricle; *me*, median eminence; *MFB*, medial forebrain bundle; *ml*, lateral mamillary nucleus; *mm*, medial parts of the medial mamillary nucleus; *mp*, posterior mamillary nucleus; *mrca*, medial retrochiasmatic area; *MT*, mamillothalamic tract; *MTe*, mamillotegmental tract; *mx*, median part of the medial mamillary nucleus; *nist*, bed nucleus of the stria terminalis; *OC*, optic chiasm; *ot*, olfactory tubercle; *OT*, optic tract; *ovlt*, organum vasculosum laminae terminalis; *pe*, periventricular nucleus; *peth*, periventricular thalamic nucleus; *pf*, perifornical nucleus; *ph*, posterior hypothalamic nucleus; *pmd*, dorsal premamillary nucleus; *pmv*, ventral premamillary nucleus; *pol*, lateral preoptic area; *pom*, medial preoptic nucleus; *pop*, periventricular preoptic nucleus; *pos*, suprachiasmatic preoptic nucleus; *pv*, paraventricular nucleus; *s*, pituitary stalk; *sc*, surprachiasmatic nucleus; *sfo*, subfornical organ; *si*, substantia innominata; *sm*, supramamillary nucleus; *SM*, stria medullaris; *sn*, substantia nigra, *so*, supraoptic nucleus; *sut*, subthalamic nucleus; *td*, diagonal band of Broca; *vm*, ventromedial nucleus; *vma*, anterior ventromedial nucleus; *vta*, ventral tegmental area; *zi*, zona incerta

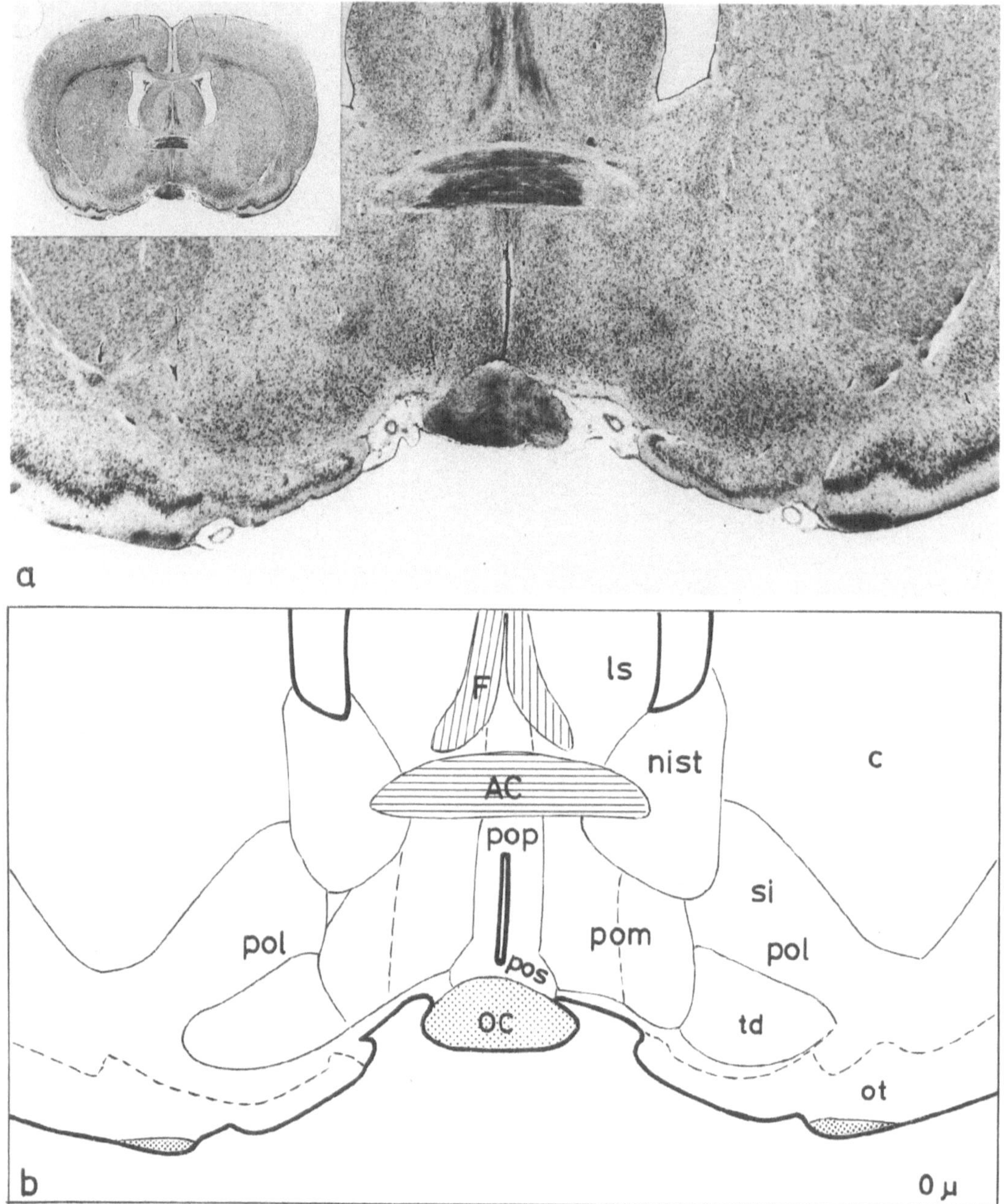

Fig. 145a,b. Coronal sections (Figs. 144–161) of the hypothalamus from the preoptic area to the mamillary. Sections were taken from equal distances (300 µm) rostral (*A*, anterior) and caudal (*P*, posterior) to the bregma (zero) level. Rats, 200 ± 10 g body weight. **a** Luxol fast blue cresyl violet staining, ×15. *Inserts*, the whole coronal section. **b** Schematic drawings corresponding to **a**, with demarcation of the hypothalmic nuclei. Abbreviations, see Fig. 144

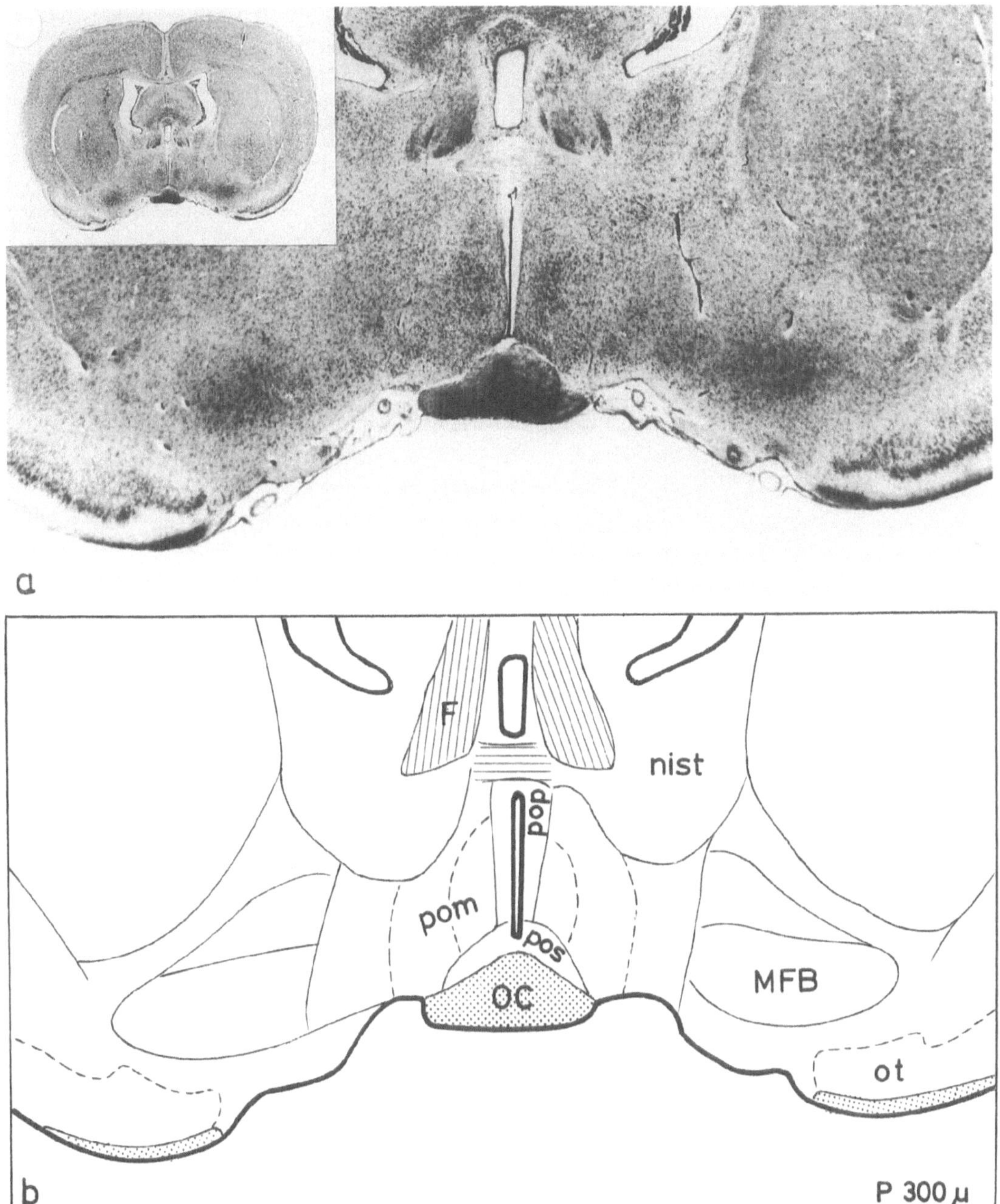

Fig. 146a,b. Coronal sections (Figs. 144–161) of the hypothalamus from the preoptic area to mamillary. Sections were taken from equal distances (300 µm) rostral (*A*, anterior) and caudal (*P*, posterior) to the bregma (zero) level. Rats, 200 ± 10 g body weight. **a** Luxol fast blue cresyl violet staining, ×15. *Inserts*, the whole coronal section. **b** Schematic drawings corresponding to **a**, with demarcation of the hypothalmic nuclei. Abbreviations, see Fig. 144

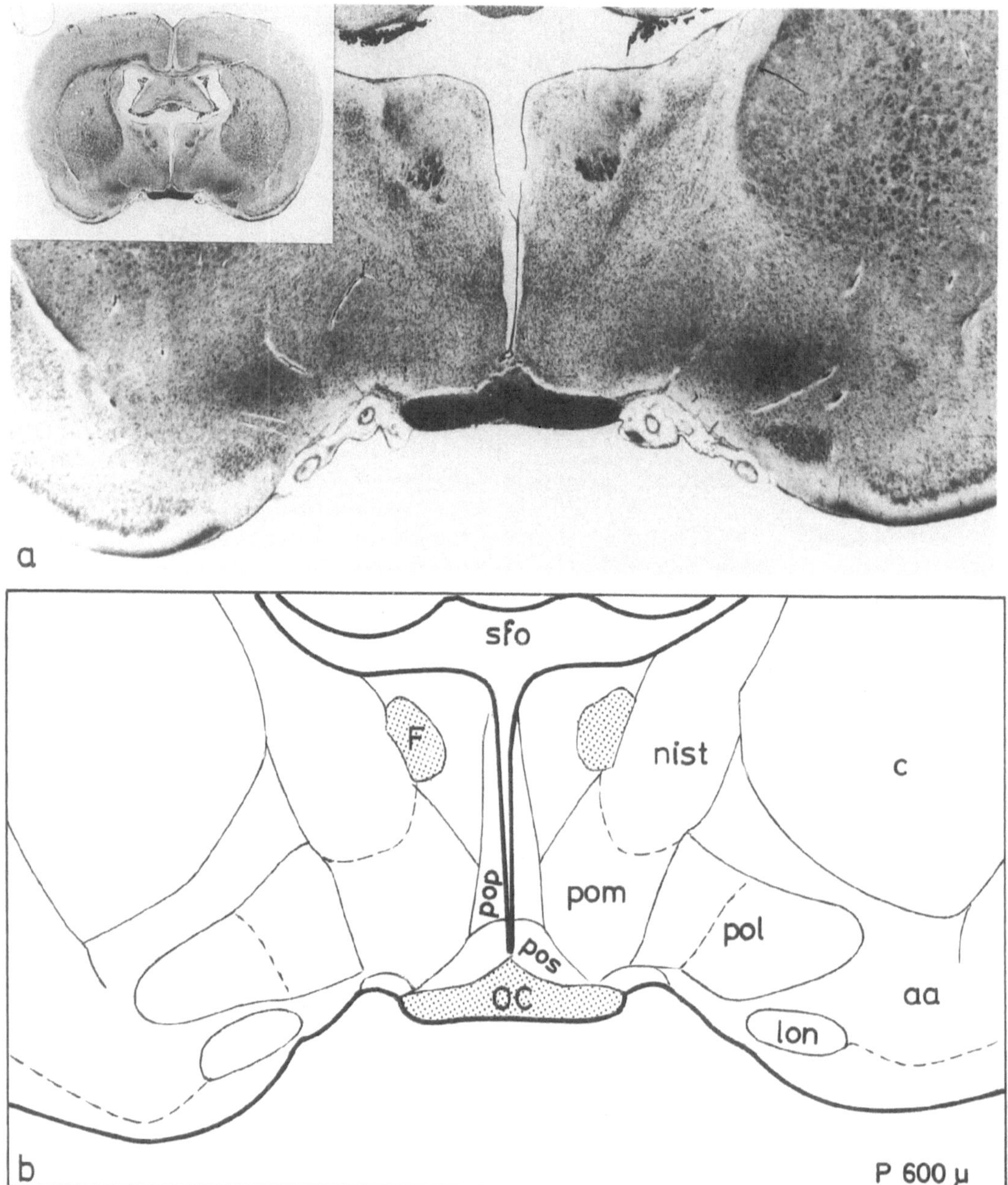

Fig. 147a,b. Coronal sections (Figs. 144–161) of the hypothalamus from the preoptic area to the mamillary. Sections were taken from equal distances (300 µm) rostral (*A*, anterior) and caudal (*P*, posterior) to the bregma (zero) level. Rats, 200 ± 10 g body weight. **a** Luxol fast blue cresyl violet staining, ×15. *Inserts*, the whole coronal section. **b** Schematic drawings corresponding to **a**, with demarcation of the hypothalmic nuclei. Abbreviations, see Fig. 144

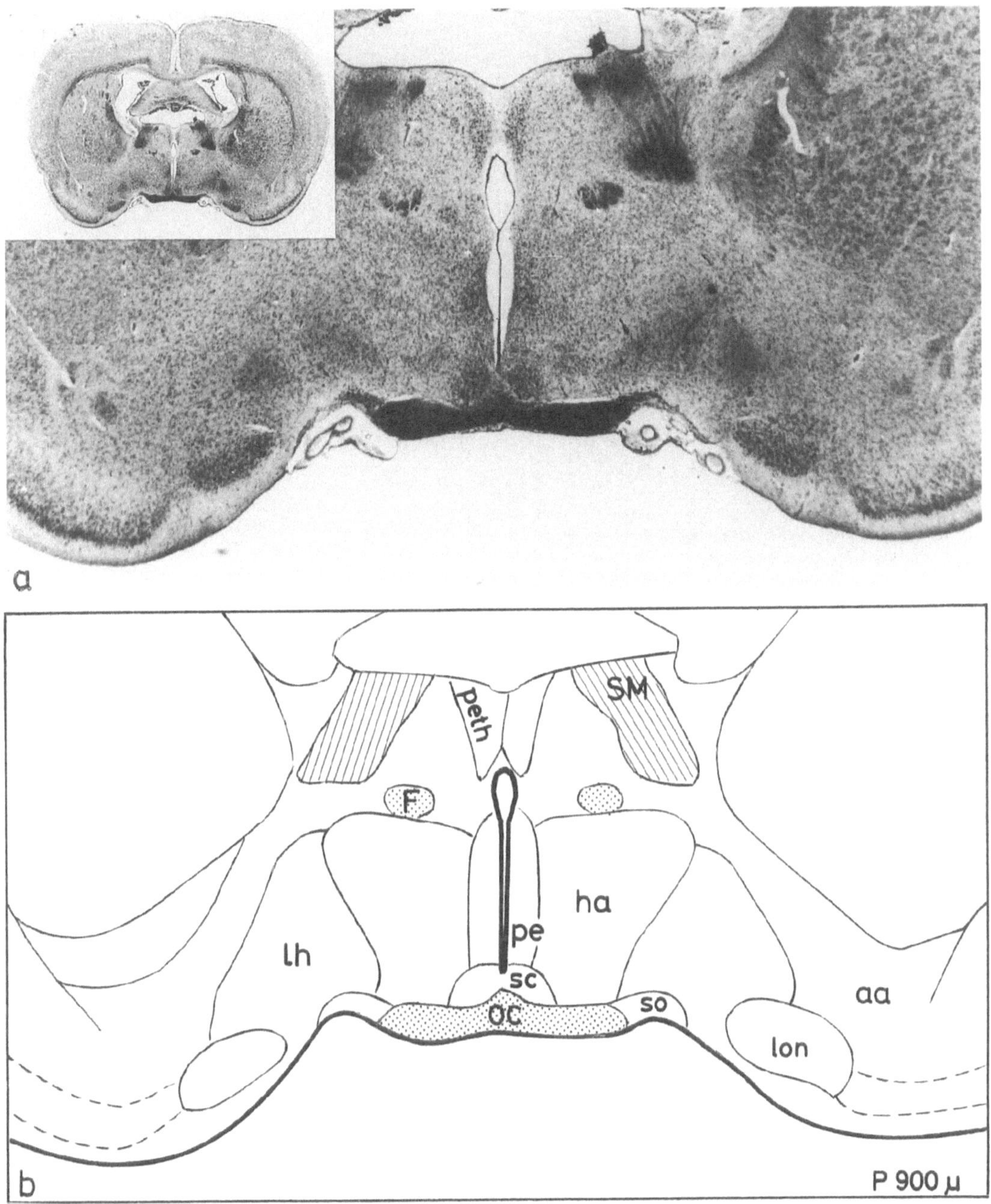

Fig. 148a,b. Coronal sections (Figs. 144–161) of the hypothalamus from the preoptic area ot the mamillary. Sections were taken from equal distances (300 μm) rostral (*A*, anterior) and caudal (*P*, posterior) to the bregma (zero) level. Rats, 200 ± 10 g body weight. **a** Luxol fast blue cresyl violet staining – 15. *Inserts*, the whole coronal section. **b** Schematic drawings corresponding to **a**, with demarcation of the hypothalmic nuclei. Abbreviations, see Fig. 144

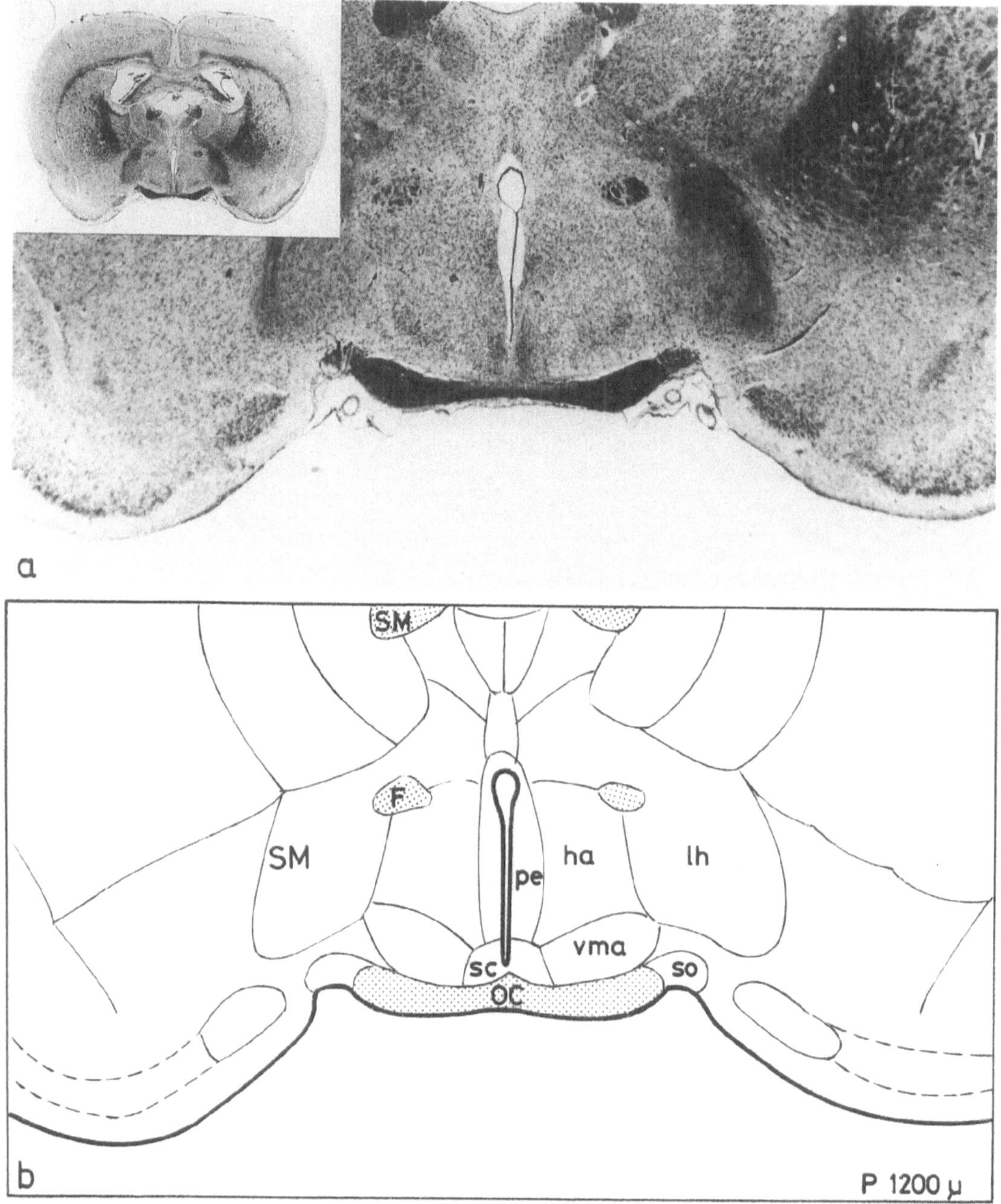

Fig. 149a,b. Coronal sections (Figs. 144–161) of the hypothalamus from the preoptic area to the mamillary. Sections were taken from equal distances (300 μm) rostral (*A*, anterior) and caudal (*P*, posterior) to the bregma (zero) level. Rats, 200 ± 10 g body weight. **a** Luxol fast blue cresyl violet staining, ×15. *Inserts*, the whole coronal section. **b** Schematic drawings corresponding to **a**, with demarcation of the hypothalmic nuclei. Abbreviations, see Fig. 144

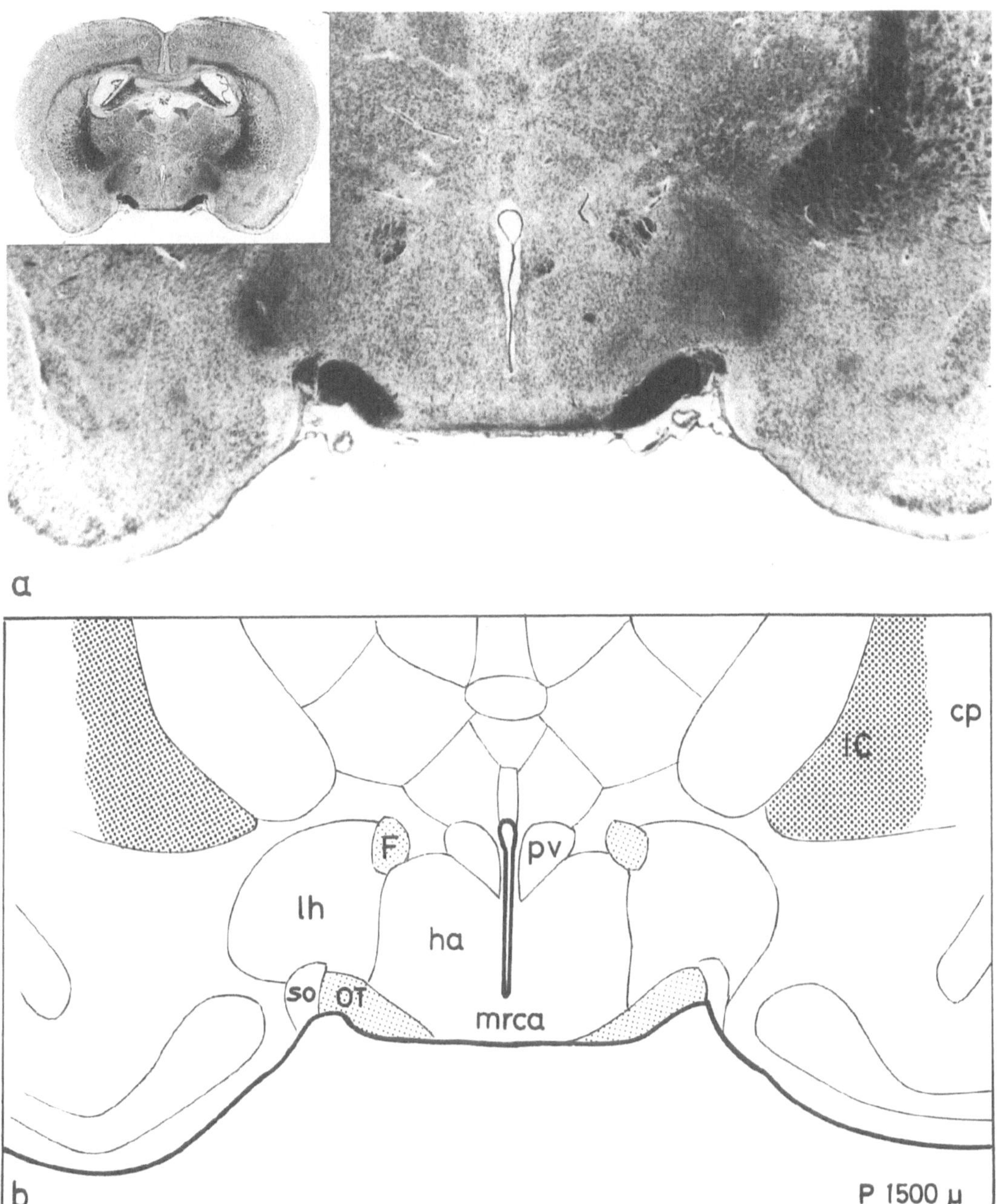

Fig. 150a,b. Coronal sections (Figs. 144–161) of the hypothalamus from the preoptic area to the mamillary. Sections were taken from equal distances (300 µm) rostral (*A*, anterior) and caudal (*P*, posterior) to the bregma (zero) level. Rats, 200 ± 10 g body weight. **a** Luxol fast blue cresyl violet staining, ×15. *Inserts*, the whole coronal section. **b** Schematic drawings corresponding to **a**, with demarcation of the hypothalmic nuclei. Abbreviations, see Fig. 144

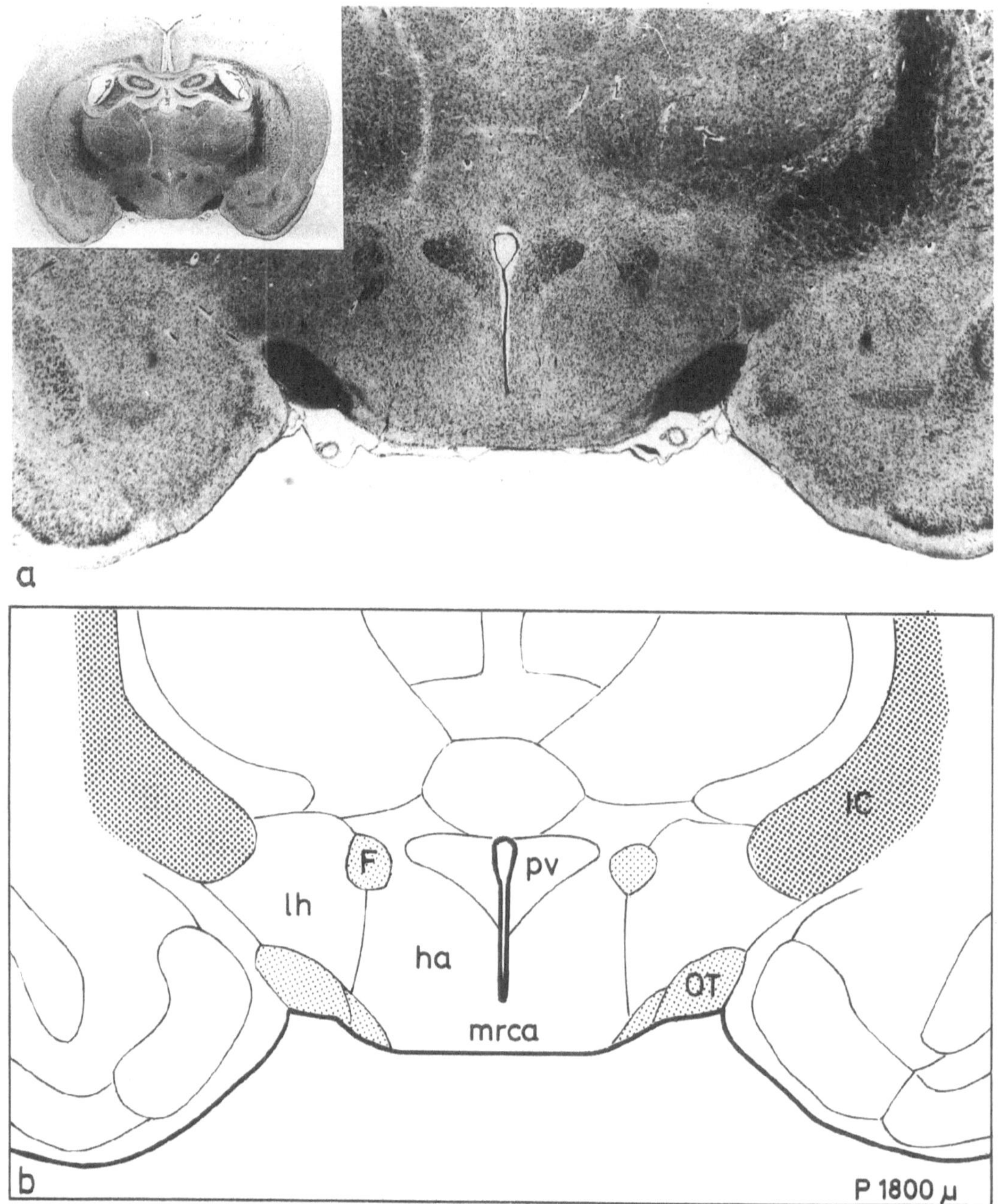

Fig. 151a,b. Coronal sections (Figs. 144–161) of the hypothalamus from the preoptic area to the mamillary. Sections were taken from equal distances (300 μm) rostral (*A*, anterior) and caudal (*P*, posterior) to the bregma (zero) level. Rats, 200 ± 10 g body weight. **a** Luxol fast blue cresyl violet staining, ×15. *Inserts*, the whole coronal section. **b** Schematic drawings corresponding to **a**, with demarcation of the hypothalmic nuclei. Abbreviations, see Fig. 144

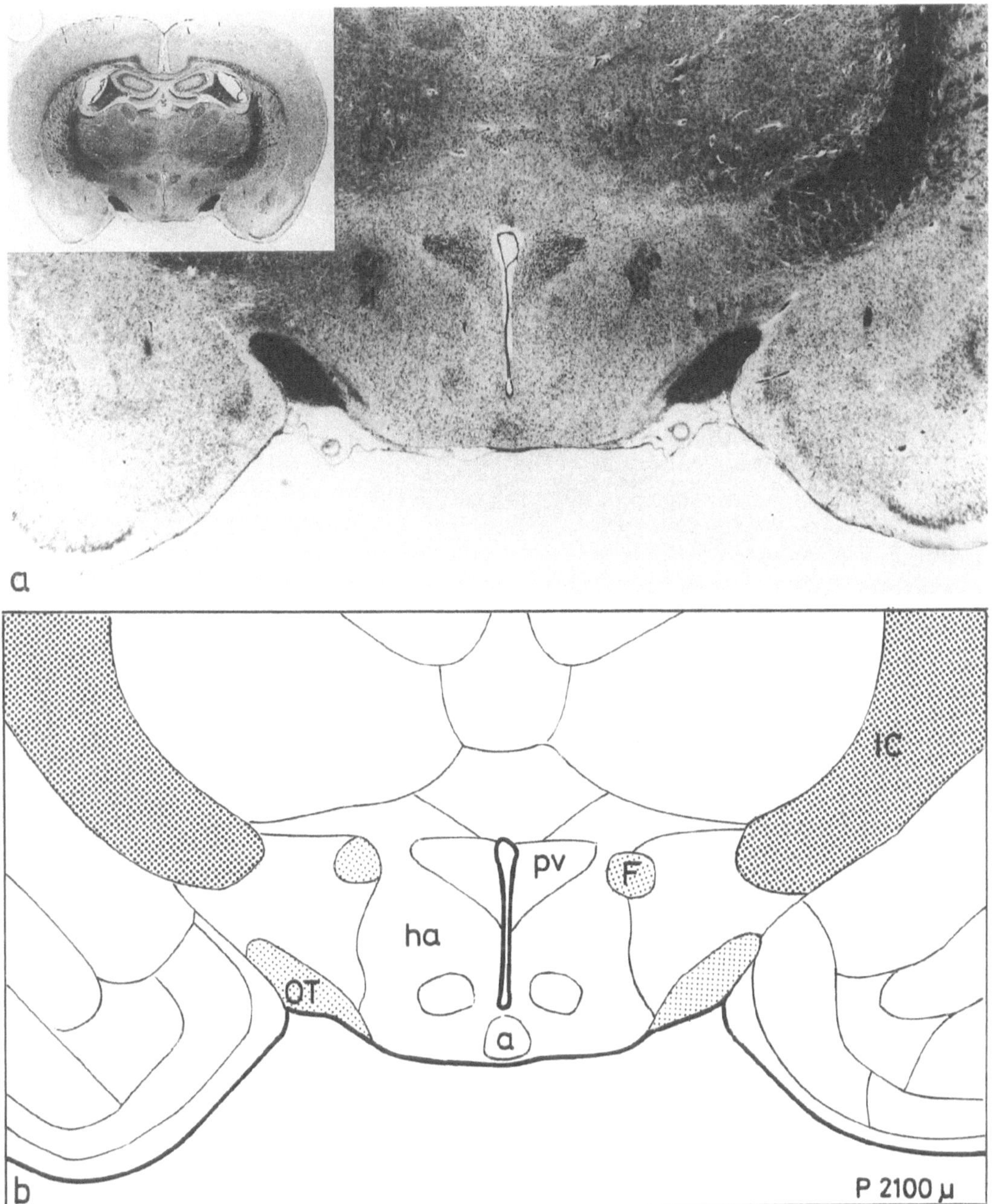

Fig. 152a,b. Coronal sections (Figs. 144–161) of the hypothalamus from the preoptic area to the mamillary. Sections were taken from equal distances (300 µm) rostral (*A*, anterior) and caudal (*P*, posterior) to the bregma (zero) level. Rats, 200 ± 10 g body weight. **a** Luxol fast blue cresyl violet staining, ×15. *Inserts*, the whole coronal section. **b** Schematic drawings corresponding to **a**, with demarcation of the hypothalmic nuclei. Abbreviations, see Fig. 144

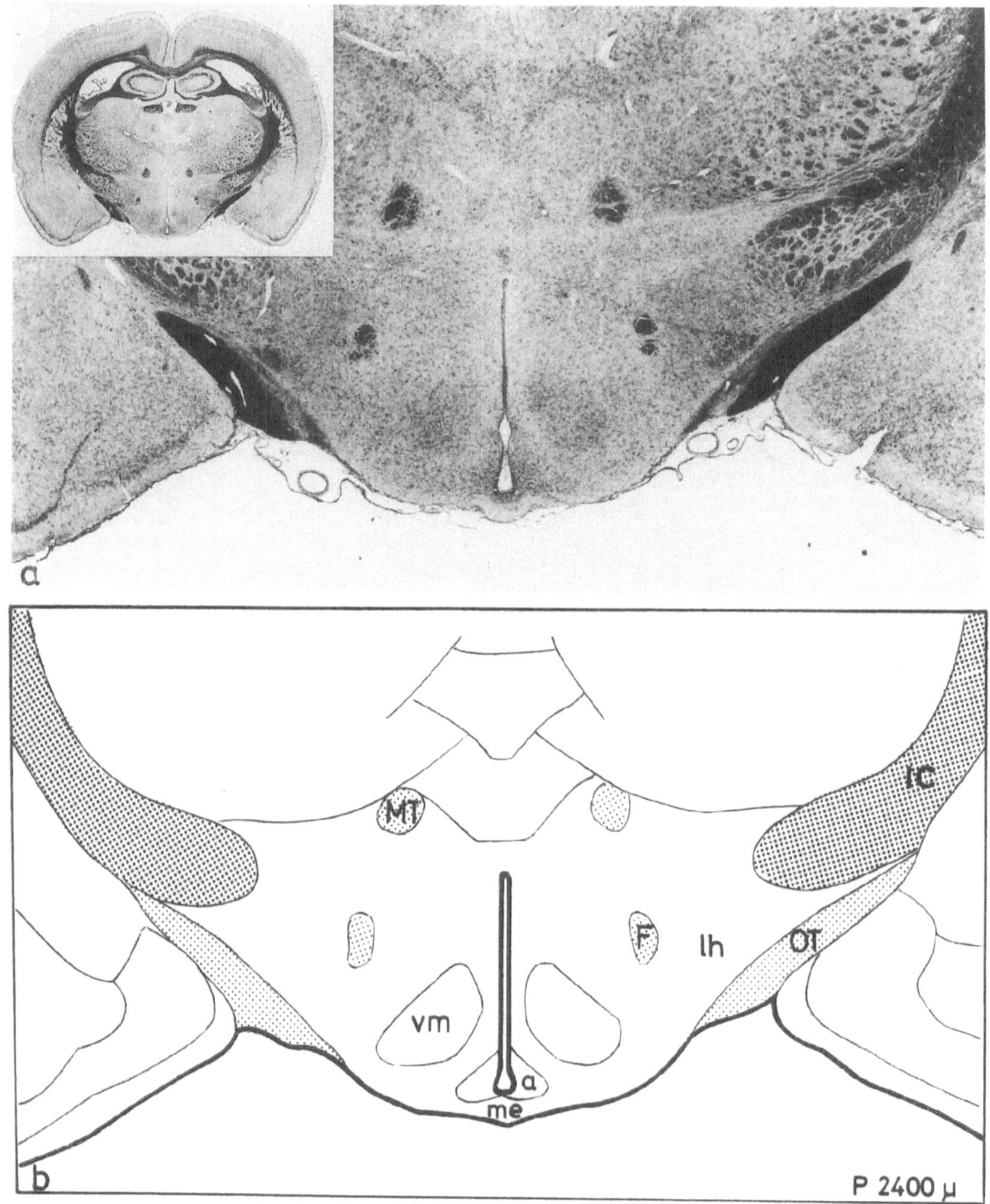

Fig. 153a,b. Coronal sections (Figs. 144–161) of the hypothalamus from the preoptic area to the mamillary. Sections were taken from equal distances (300 μm) rostral (*A*, anterior) and caudal (*P*, posterior) to the bregma (zero) level. Rats, 200 ± 10 g body weight. **a** Luxol fast blue cresyl violet staining, ×15. *Inserts*, the whole coronal section. **b** Schematic drawings corresponding to **a**, with demarcation of the hypothalmic nuclei. Abbreviations, see Fig. 144

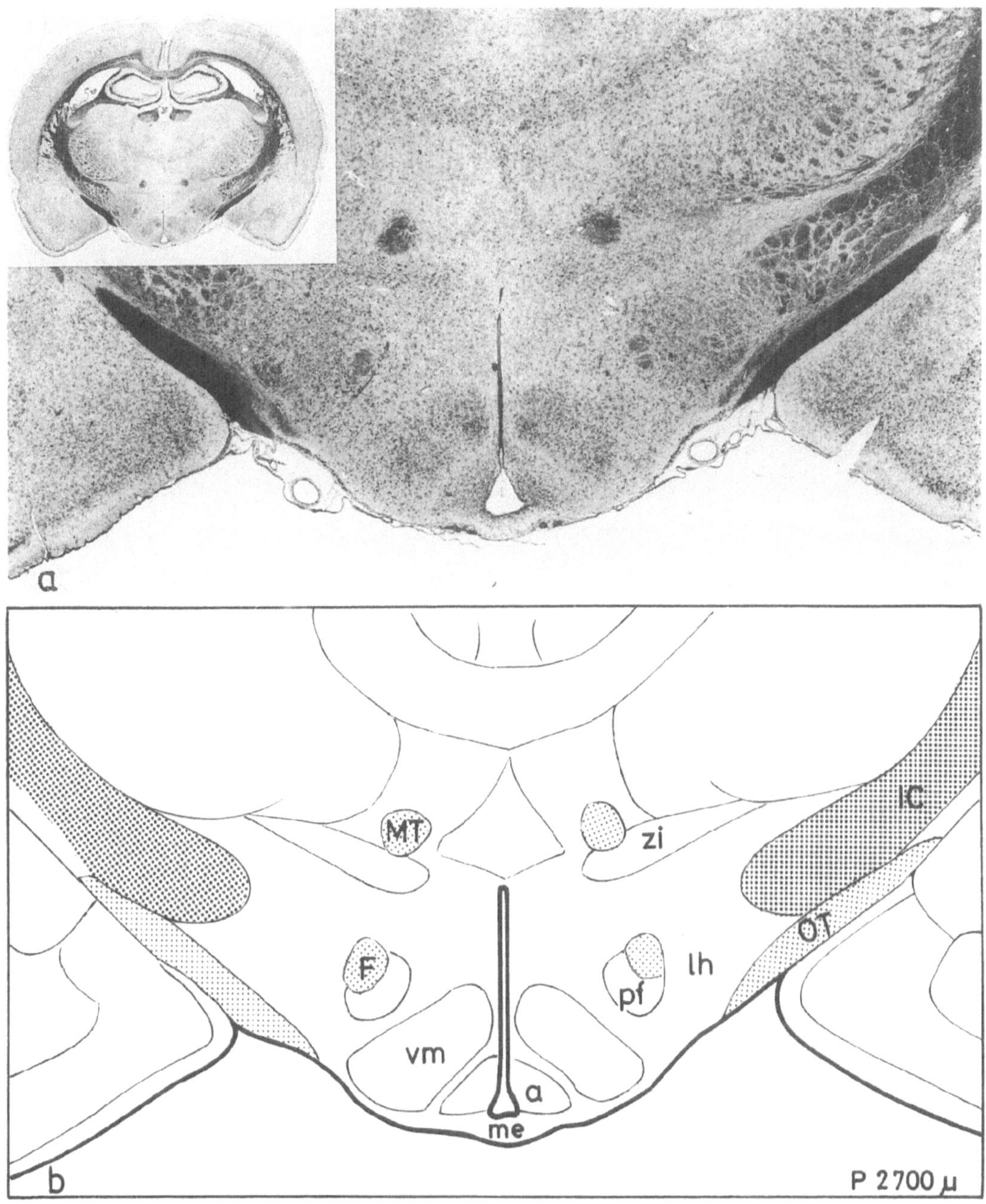

Fig. 154a,b. Coronal sections (Figs. 144–161) of the hypothalamus from the preoptic area to the mamillary. Sections were taken from equal distances (300 µm) rostral (*A*, anterior) and caudal (*P*, posterior) to the bregma (zero) level. Rats, 200 ± 10 g body weight. **a** Luxol fast blue cresyl violet staining, ×15. *Inserts*, the whole coronal section. **b** Schematic drawings corresponding to **a**, with demarcation of the hypothalmic nuclei. Abbreviations, see Fig. 144

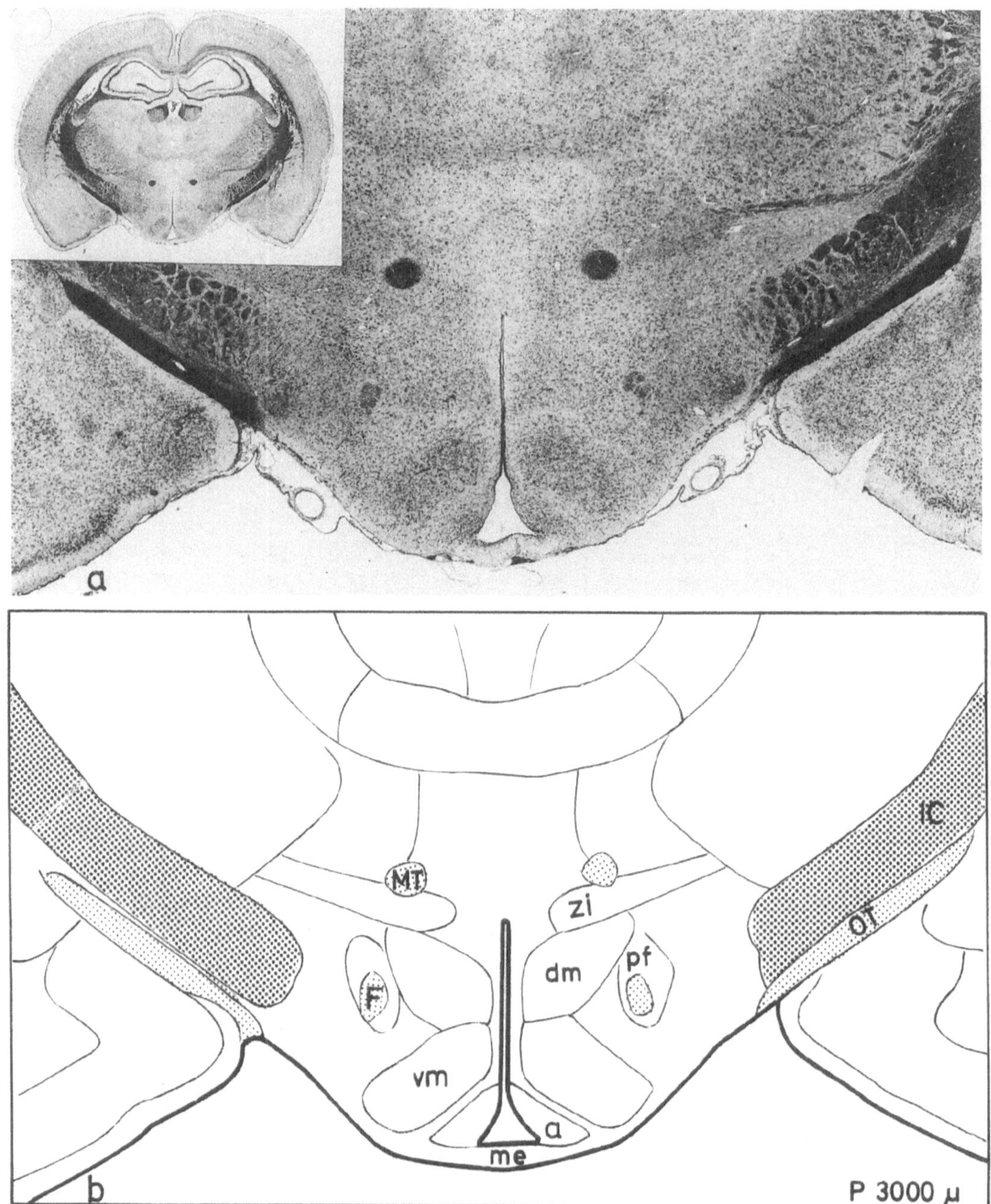

Fig. 155a,b. Coronal sections (Figs. 144–161) of the hypothalamus from the preoptic area to the mamillary. Sections were taken from equal distances (300 μm) rostral (*A*, anterior) and caudal (*P*, posterior) to the bregma (zero) level. Rats, 200 ± 10 g body weight. **a** Luxol fast blue cresyl violet staining, ×15. *Inserts*, the whole coronal section. **b** Schematic drawings corresponding to **a**, with demarcation of the hypothalmic nuclei. Abbreviations, see Fig. 144

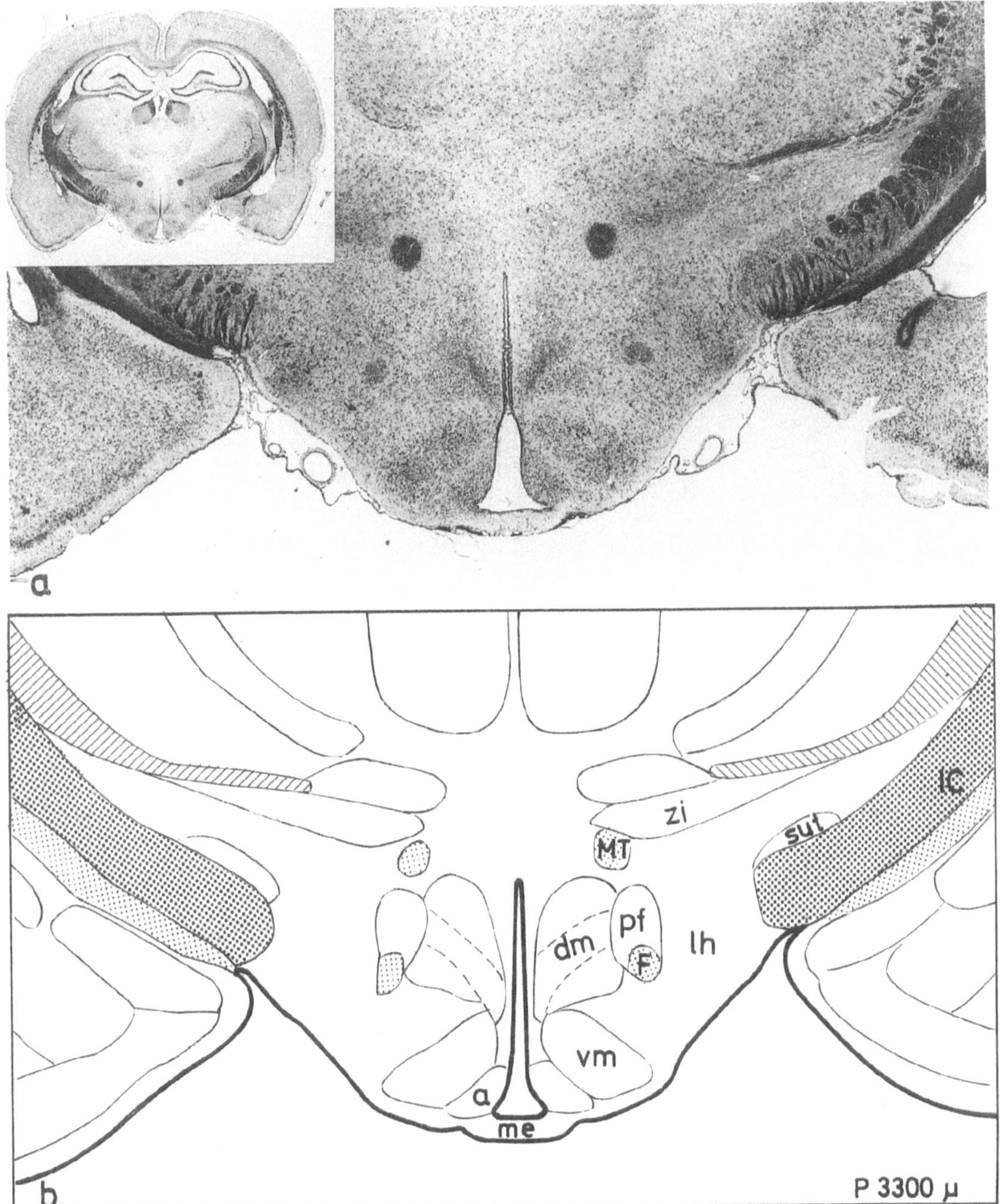

Fig. 156a,b. Coronal sections (Figs. 144–161) of the hypothalamus from the preoptic area to the mamillary. Sections were taken from equal distances (300 μm) rostral (*A*, anterior) and caudal (*P*, posterior) to the bregma (zero) level. Rats, 200 ± 10 g body weight. **a** Luxol fast blue cresyl violet staining, ×15. *Inserts*, the whole coronal section. **b** Schematic drawings corresponding to **a**, with demarcation of the hypothalmic nuclei. Abbreviations, see Fig. 144

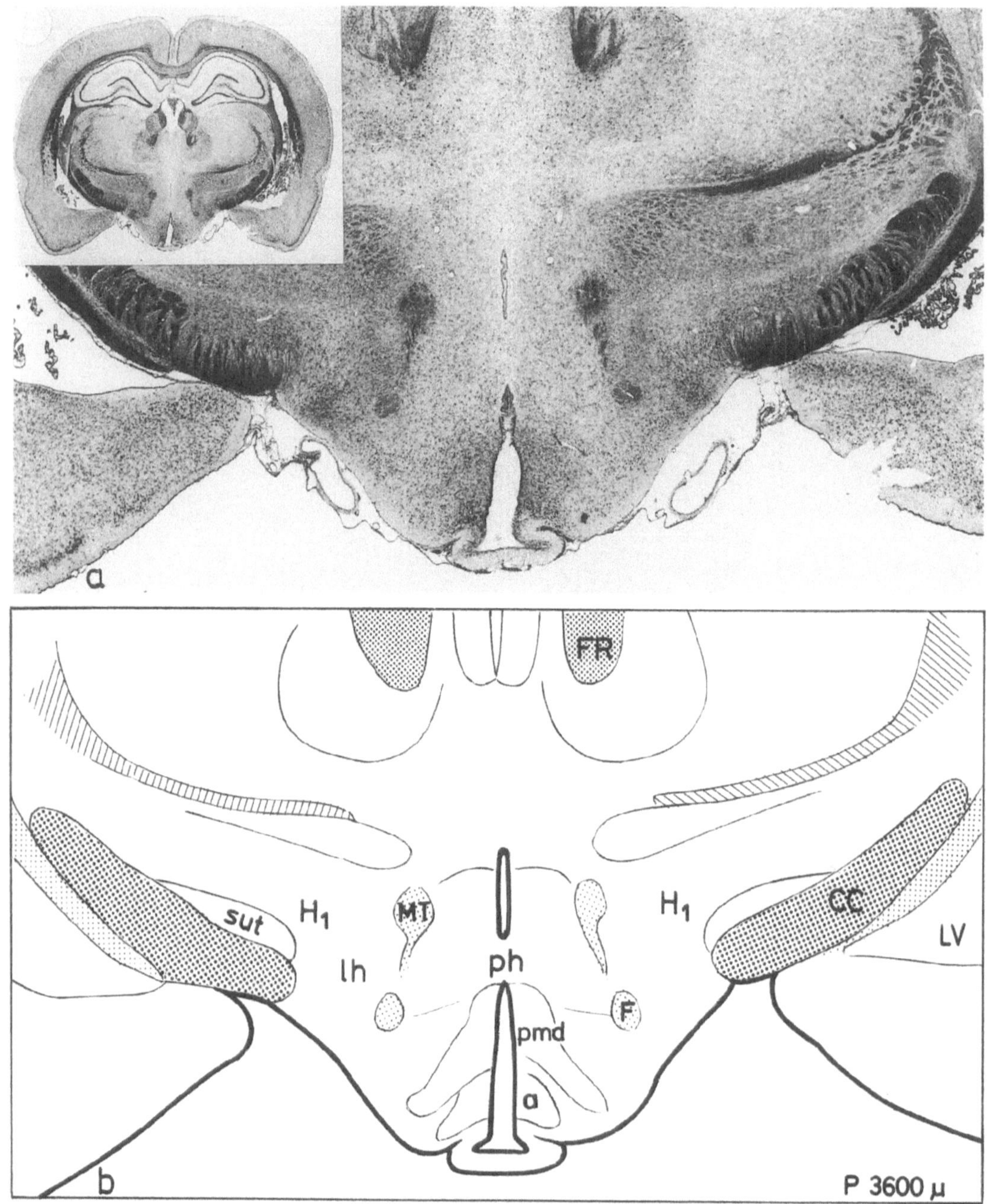

Fig. 157a,b. Coronal sections (Figs. 144–161) of the hypothalamus from the preoptic area to the mamillary. Sections were taken from equal distances (300 μm) rostral (*A*, anterior) and caudal (*P*, posterior) to the bregma (zero) level. Rats, 200 ± 10 g body weight. **a** Luxol fast blue cresyl violet staining, ×15. *Inserts*, the whole coronal section. **b** Schematic drawings corresponding to **a**, with demarcation of the hypothalmic nuclei. Abbreviations, see Fig. 144

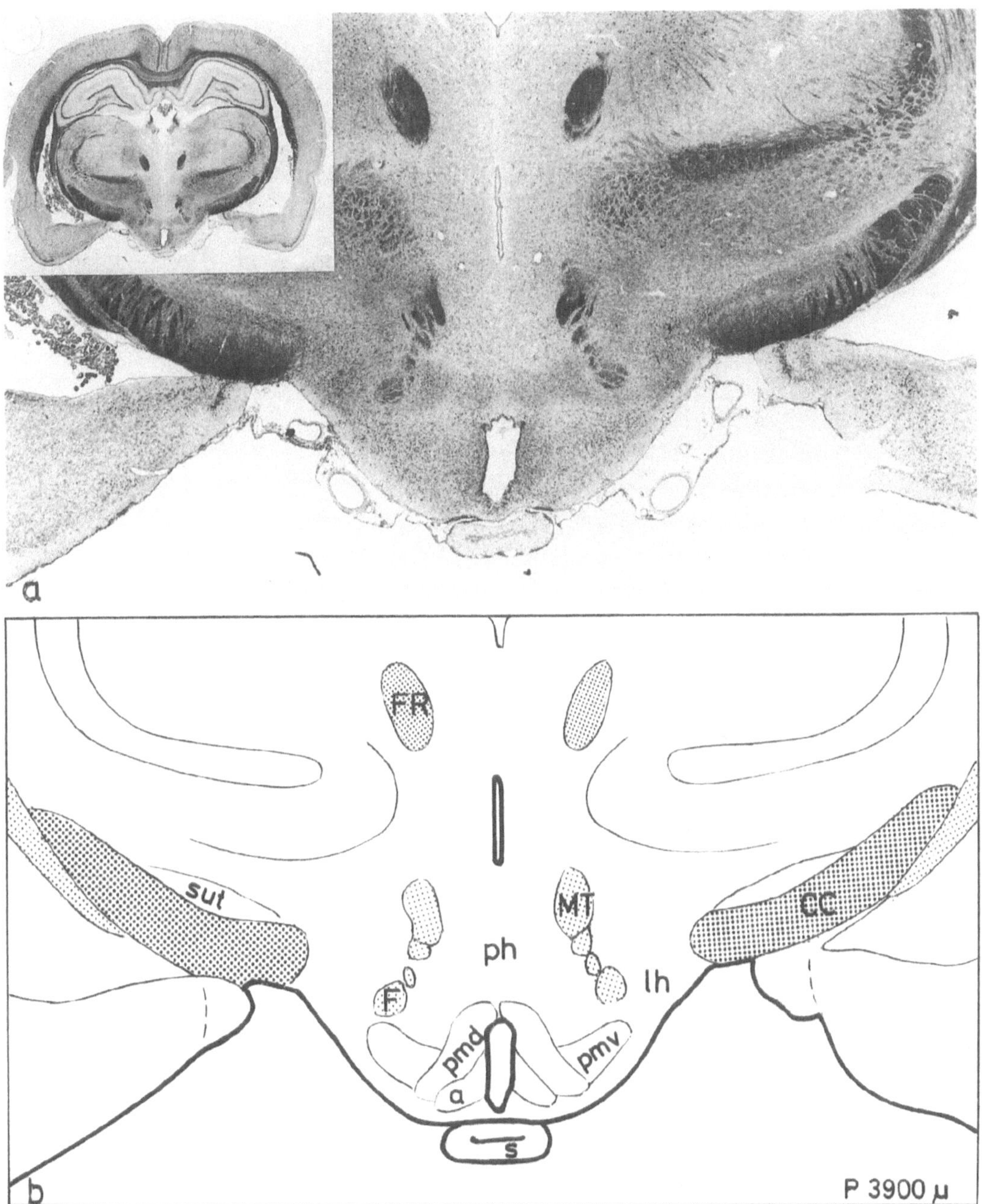

Fig. 158a,b. Coronal sections (Figs. 144–161) of the hypothalamus from the preoptic area to the mamillary. Sections were taken from equal distances (300 µm) rostral (*A*, anterior) and caudal (*P*, posterior) to the bregma (zero) level. Rats, 200 ± 10 g body weight. **a** Luxol fast blue cresyl violet staining, ×15. *Inserts*, the whole coronal section. **b** Schematic drawings corresponding to **a**, with demarcation of the hypothalmic nuclei. Abbreviations, see Fig. 144

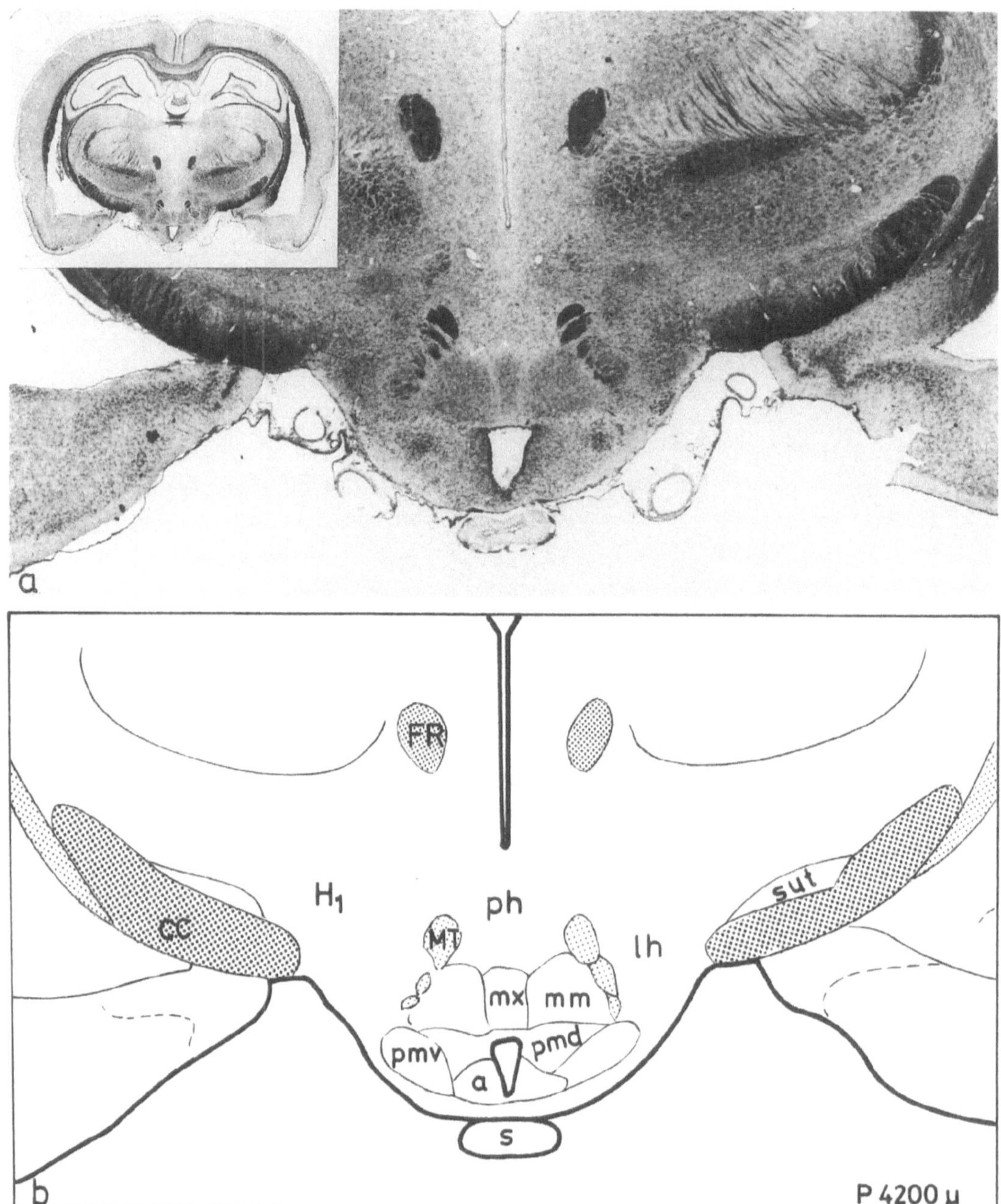

Fig. 159a,b. Coronal sections (Figs. 144–161) of the hypothalamus from the preoptic area to the mamillary. Sections were taken from equal distances (300 μm) rostral (*A*, anterior) and caudal (*P*, posterior) to the bregma (zero) level. Rats, 200 ± 10 g body weight. **a** Luxol fast blue cresyl violet staining, ×15. *Inserts*, the whole coronal section. **b** Schematic drawings corresponding to **a**, with demarcation of the hypothalmic nuclei. Abbreviations, see Fig. 144

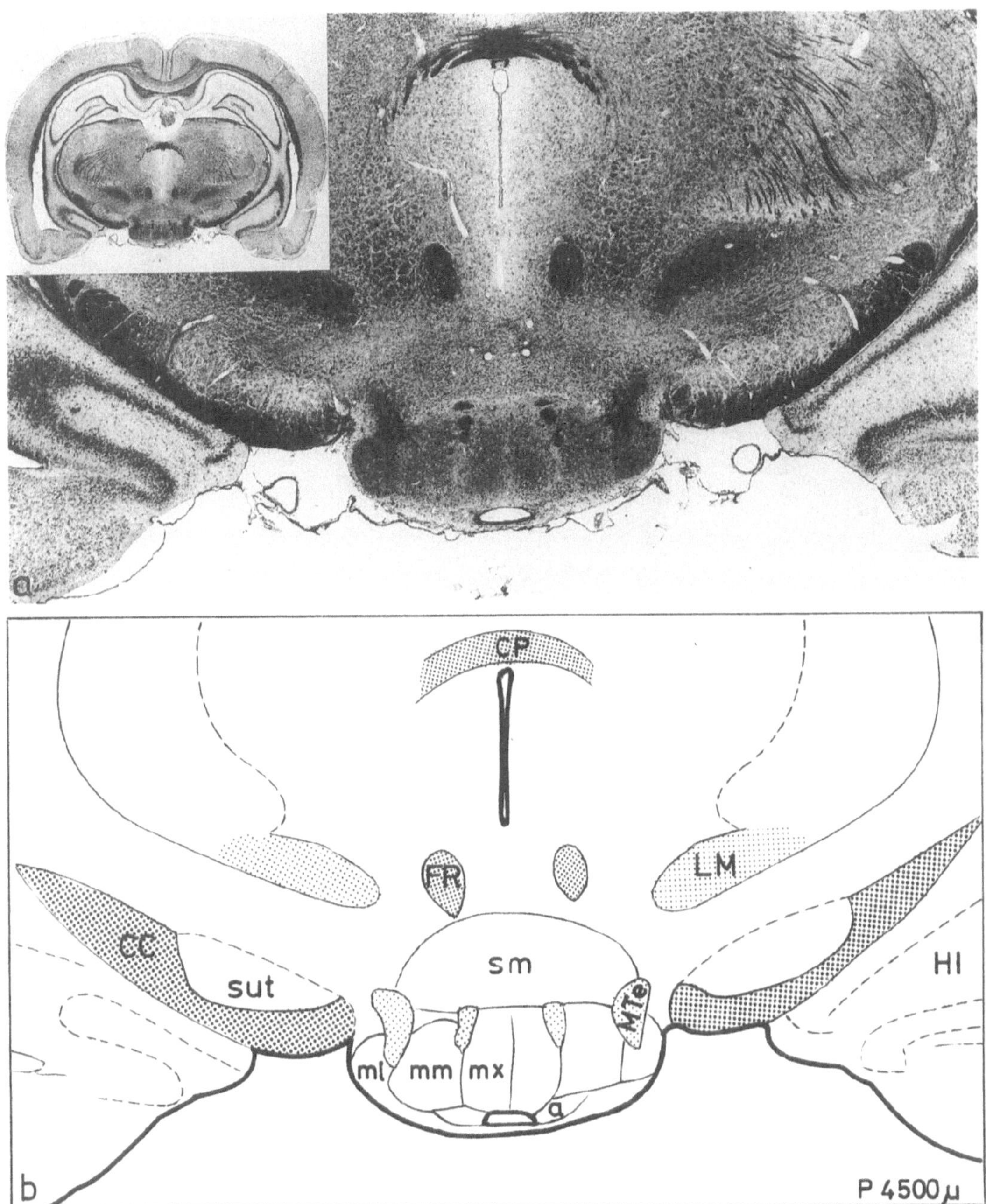

Fig. 160a,b. Coronal sections (Figs. 144–161) of the hypothalamus from the preoptic area to the mamillary. Sections were taken from equal distances (300 µm) rostral (*A*, anterior) and caudal (*P*, posterior) to the bregma (zero) level. Rats, 200 ± 10 g body weight. **a** Luxol fast blue cresyl violet staining, ×15. *Inserts*, the whole coronal section. **b** Schematic drawings corresponding to **a**, with demarcation of the hypothalmic nuclei. Abbreviations, see Fig. 144

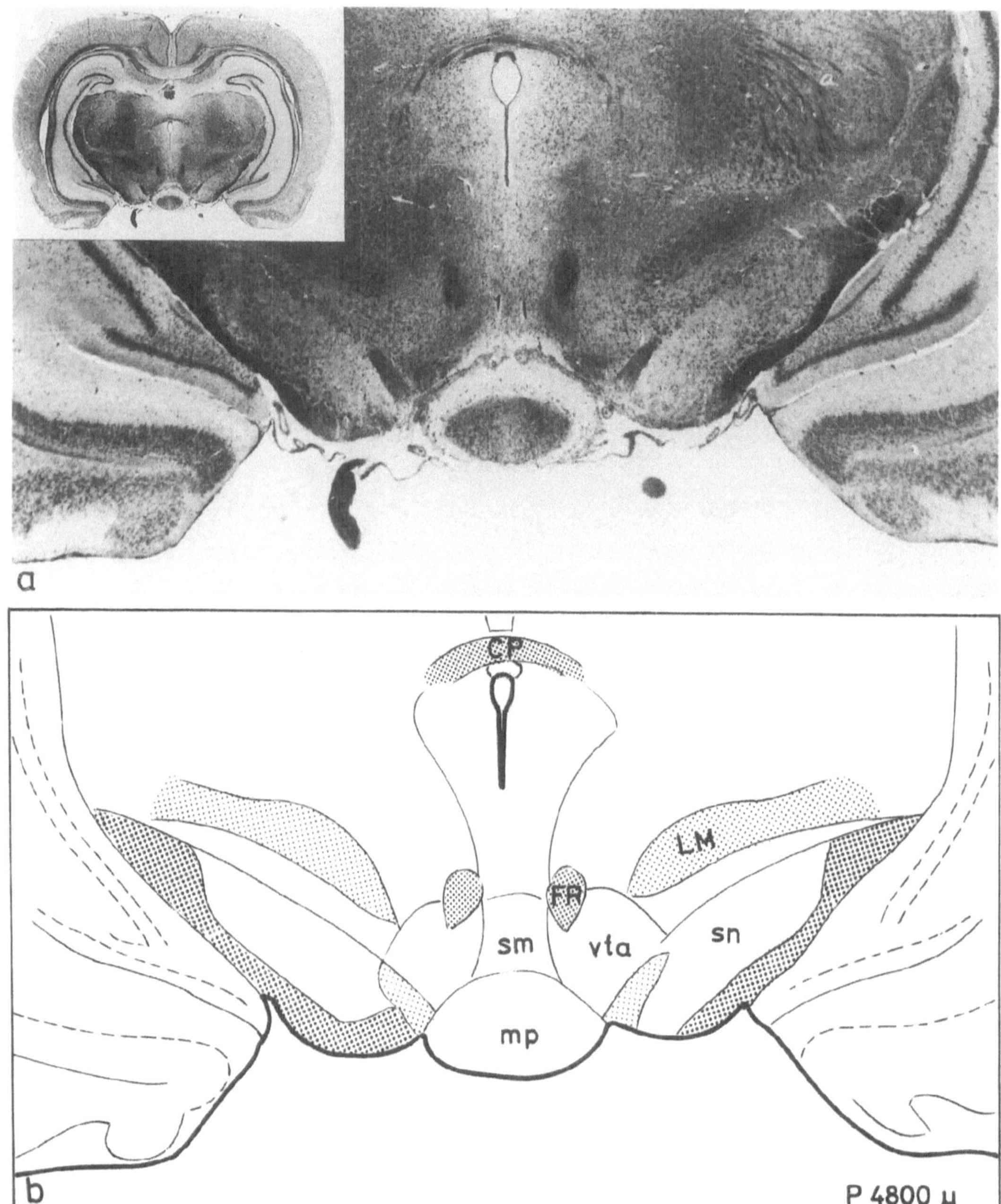

Fig. 161a,b. Coronal sections (Figs. 144–161) of the hypothalamus from the preoptic area to the mamillary. Sections were taken from equal distances (300 μm) rostral (*A*, anterior) and caudal (*P*, posterior) to the bregma (zero) level. Rats, 200 ± 10 g body weight. **a** Luxol fast blue cresyl violet staining, ×15. *Inserts*, the whole coronal section. **b** Schematic drawings corresponding to **a**, with demarcation of the hypothalmic nuclei. Abbreviations, see Fig. 144

Fig. 162a,b. Sagittal sections (Figs. 162–176) of the hypothalamus from the midline at equal distances (150 μm), latterally. Rats, 200 ± 10 g body weight. **a** Luxol fast blue cresyl violet staining, ×15. *Inserts*, the whole sagittal section. **b** Schematic drawings corresponding to **a**, with demarcation of the hypothalmic nuclei. *dg*, Dentate gyrus; *DS*, supramamillary decussations; *hab*, habenula; h_2, Forel's H_2 field; *pml*, lateral part of the tuberomamillary nucleus; *rth*, reticular thalamic nucleus; *S*, supraoptic decussations; *Th*, thalamus; *III.*, third ventricle. Other abbreviations, see Fig. 144 ▶

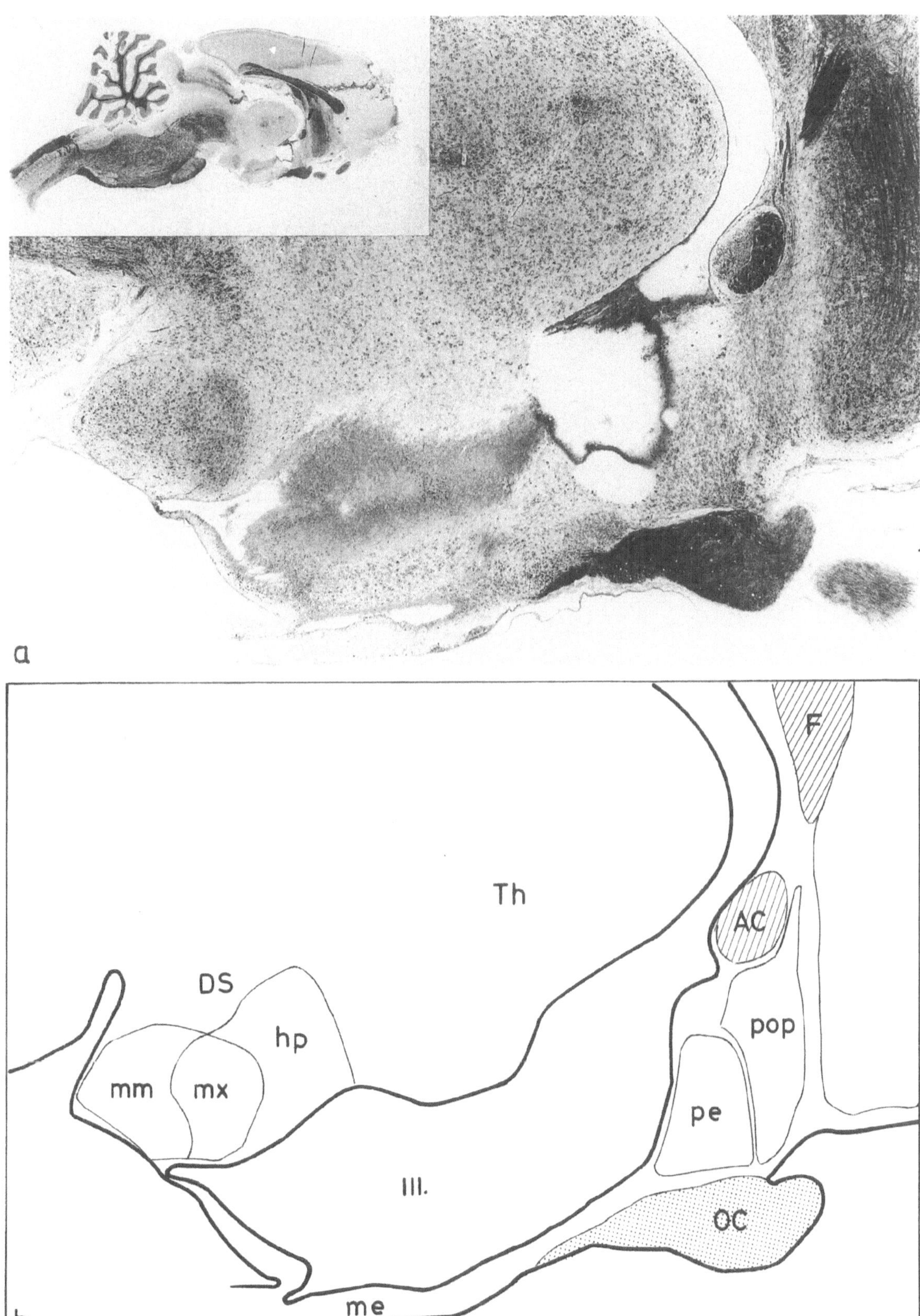
a
b
F
Th
AC
DS
hp
pop
mm
mx
pe
III.
OC
me

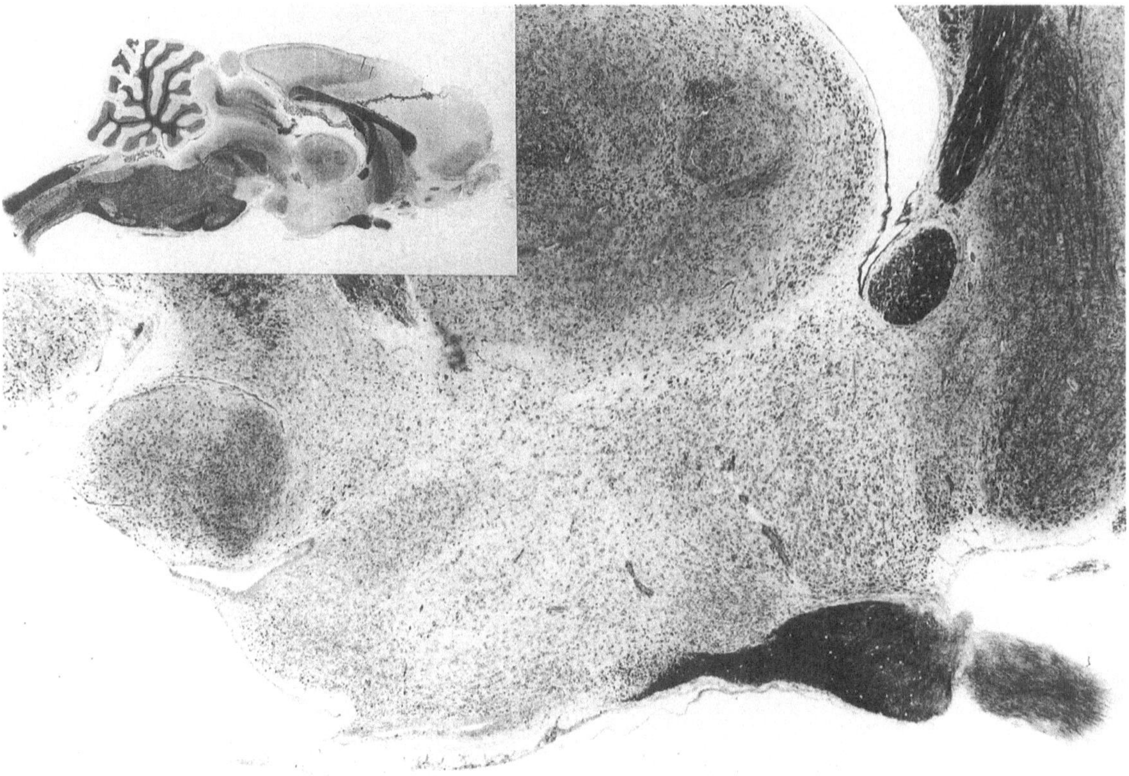

a

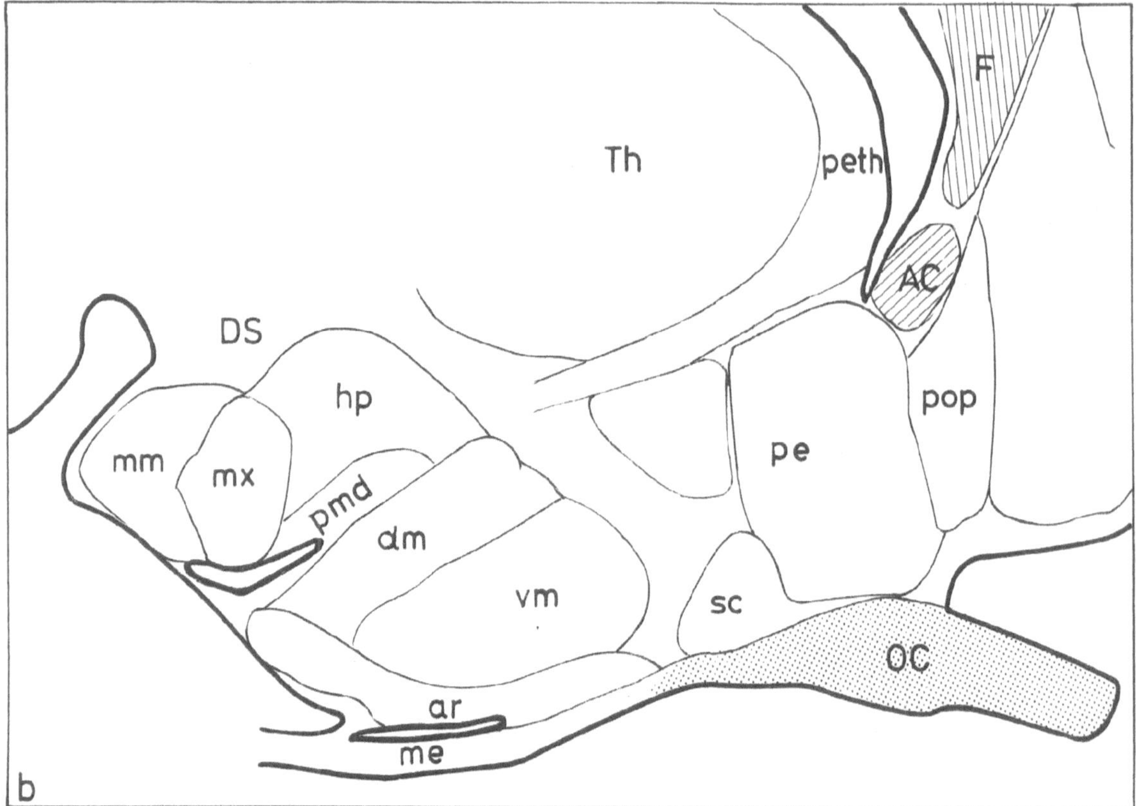

Fig. 163a,b. Sagittal sections (Figs. 162–176) of the hypothalamus from the midline at equal distances (150 µm), latterally. Rats, 200 ± 10 g body weight. **a** Luxol fast blue cresyl violet staining, ×15. *Inserts*, the whole sagittal section. **b** Schematic drawings corresponding to **a**, with demarcation of the hypothalmic nuclei. *dg*, Dentate gyrus; *DS*, supramamillary decussations; *hab*, habenula; h_2, Forel's H_2 field; *pml*, lateral part of the tuberomamillary nucleus; *rth*, reticular thalamic nucleus; *S*, supraoptic decussations; *Th*, thalamus; *III.*, third ventricle. Other abbreviations, see Fig. 144

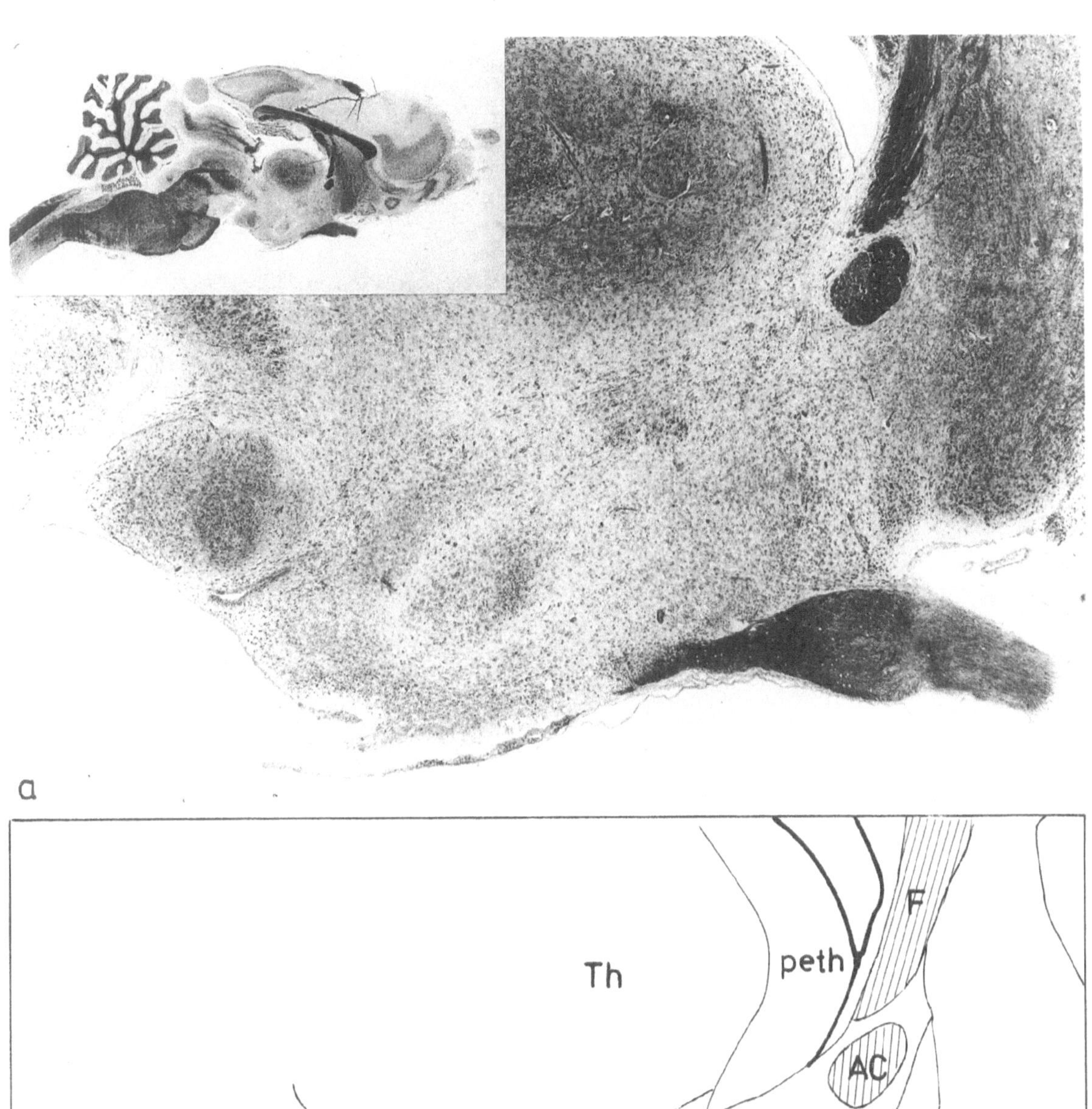

Fig. 164a,b. Sagittal sections (Figs. 162–176) of the hypothalamus from the midline at equal distances (150 μm), latterally. Rats, 200 ± 10 g body weight. **a** Luxol fast blue cresyl violet staining, ×15. *Inserts*, the whole sagittal section. **b** Schematic drawings corresponding to **a**, with demarcation of the hypothalmic nuclei. *dg*, Dentate gyrus; *DS*, supramamillary decussations; *hab*, habenula; H_2, Forel's H_2 field; *pml*, lateral part of the tuberomamillary nucleus; *rth*, reticular thalamic nucleus; *S*, supraoptic decussations; *Th*, thalamus; *III.*, third ventricle. Other abbreviations, see Fig. 144

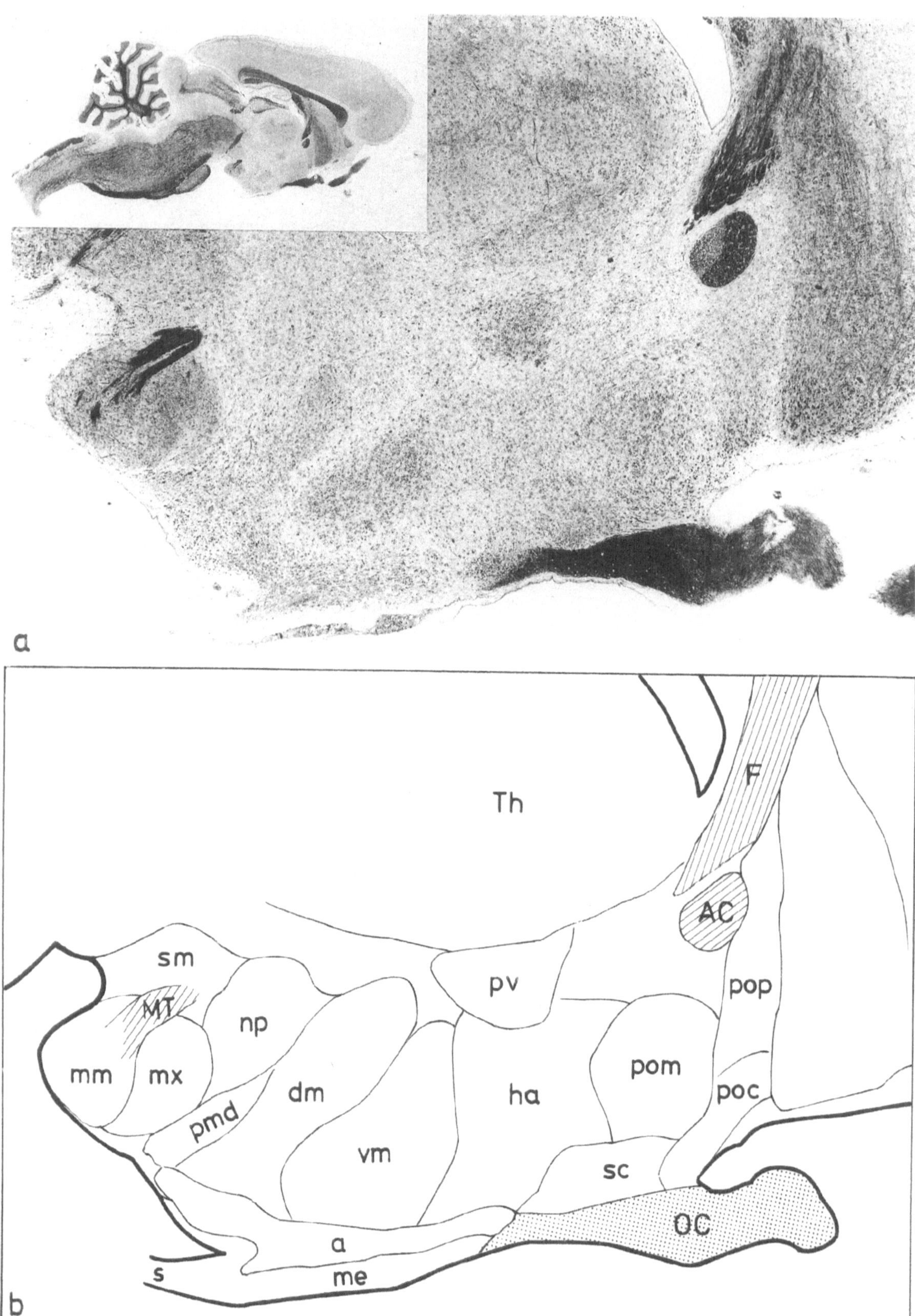

Fig. 165a,b. Sagittal sections (Figs. 162–176) of the hypothalamus from the midline at equal distances (150 µm), latterally. Rats, 200 ± 10 g body weight. **a** Luxol fast blue cresyl violet staining, ×15. *Inserts*, the whole sagittal section. **b** Schematic drawings corresponding to **a**, with demarcation of the hypothalmic nuclei. *dg*, Dentate gyrus; *DS*, supramamillary decussations; *hab*, habenula; H_2, Forel's H_2 field; *pml*, lateral part of the tuberomamillary nucleus; *rth*, reticular thalamic nucleus; *S*, supraoptic decussations; *Th*, thalamus; *III.*, third ventricle. Other abbreviations, see Fig. 144

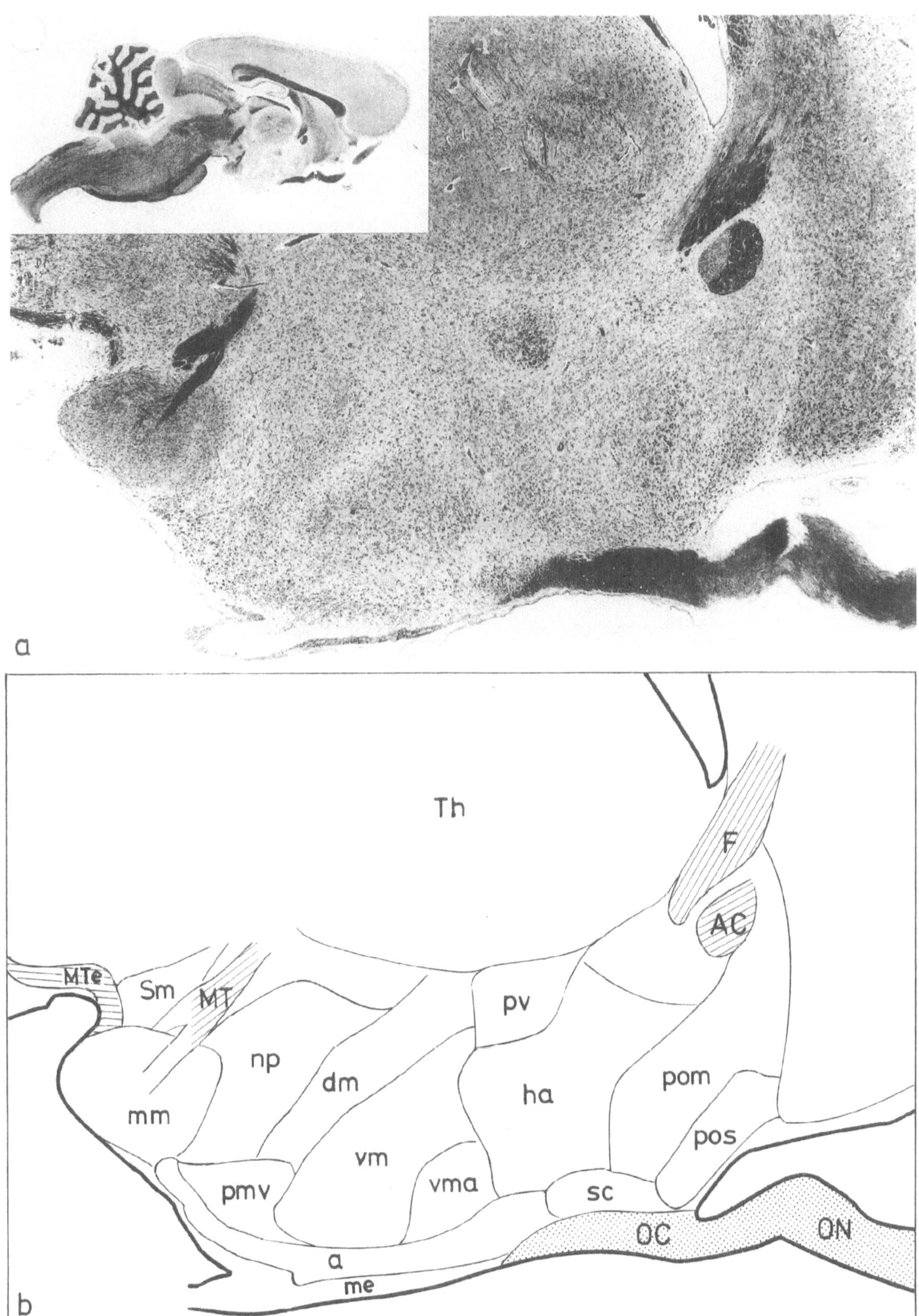

Fig. 166a,b. Sagittal sections (Figs. 162–176) of the hypothalamus from the midline at equal distances (150 μm), latterally. Rats, 200 ± 10 g body weight. **a** Luxol fast blue cresyl violet staining, ×15. *Inserts*, the whole sagittal section. **b** Schematic drawings corresponding to **a**, with demarcation of the hypothalmic nuclei. *dg*, Dentate gyrus; *DS*, supramamillary decussations; *hab*, habenula; H_2, Forel's H_2 field; *pml*, lateral part of the tuberomamillary nucleus; *rth*, reticular thalamic nucleus; *S*, supraoptic decussations; *Th*, thalamus; *III.*, third ventricle. Other abbreviations, see Fig. 144

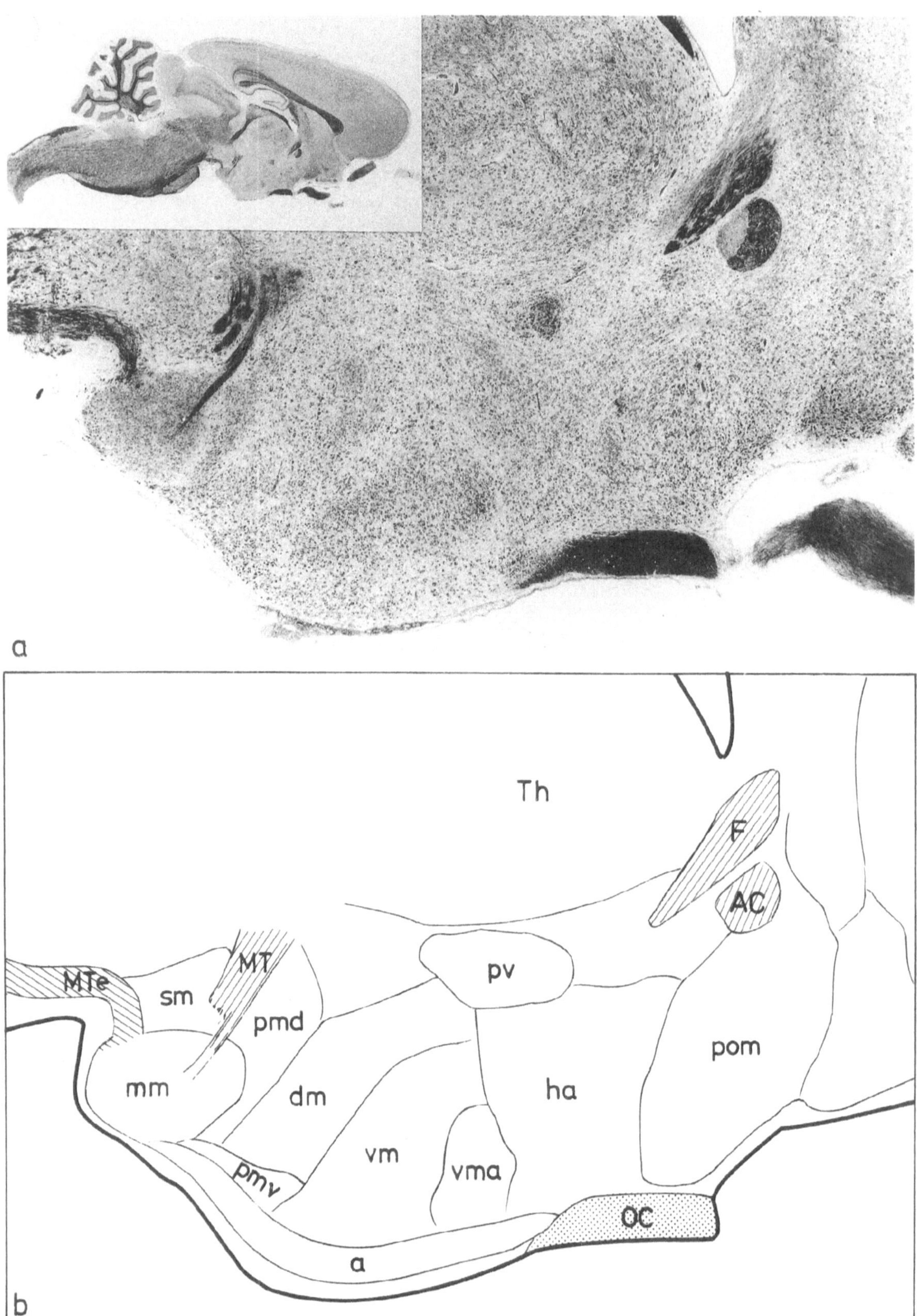

Fig. 167a,b. Sagittal sections (Figs. 162–176) of the hypothalamus from the midline at equal distances (150 µm), latterally. Rats, 200 ± 10 g body weight. **a** Luxol fast blue cresyl violet staining, ×15. *Inserts*, the whole sagittal section. **b** Schematic drawings corresponding to **a**, with demarcation of the hypothalmic nuclei. *dg*, Dentate gyrus; *DS*, supramamillary decussations; *hab*, habenula; H_2, Forel's H_2 field; *pml*, lateral part of the tuberomamillary nucleus; *rth*, reticular thalamic nucleus; *S*, supraoptic decussations; *Th*, thalamus; *III.*, third ventricle. Other abbreviations, see Fig. 144

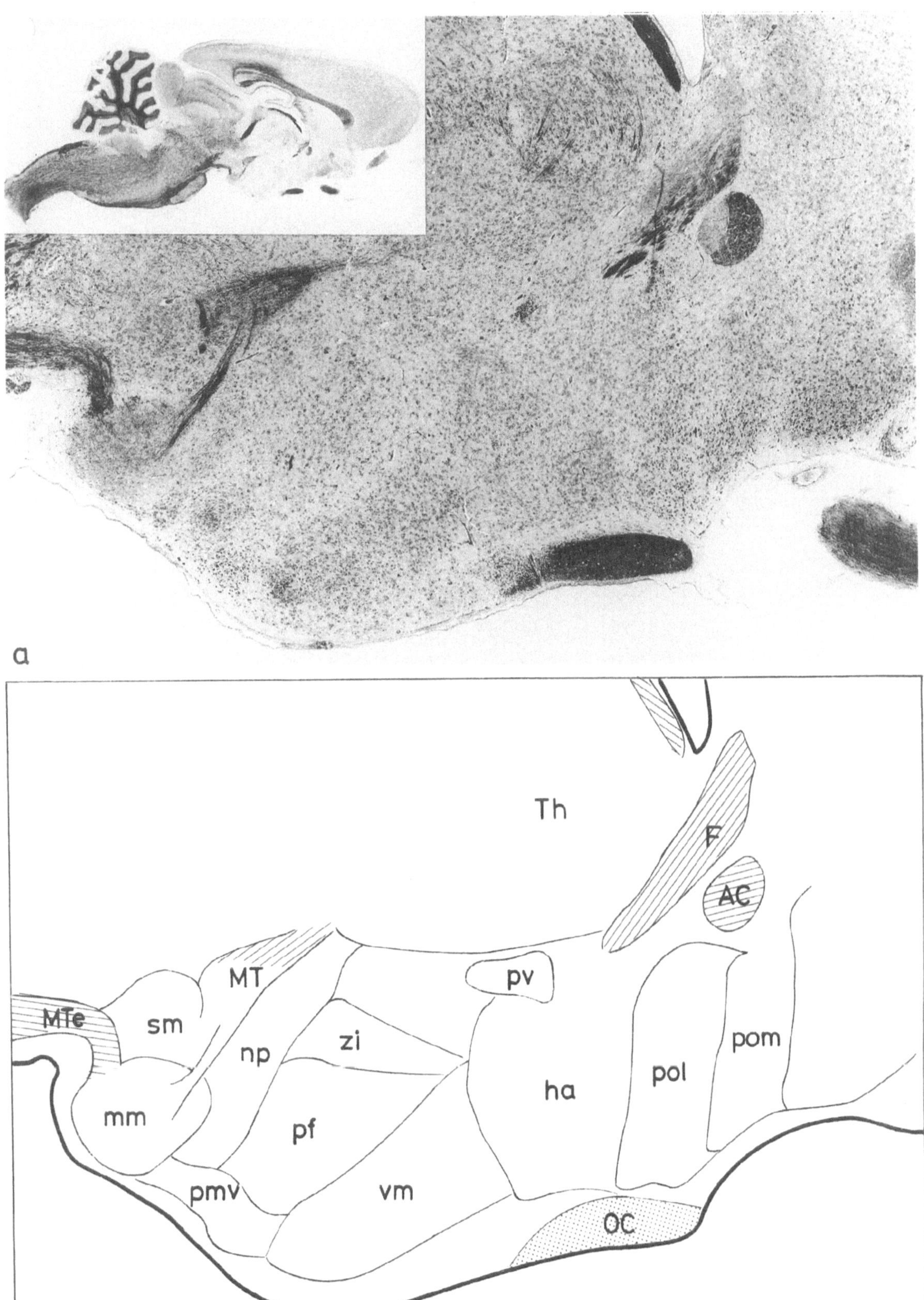

Fig. 168a,b. Sagittal sections (Figs. 162–176) of the hypothalamus from the midline at equal distances (150 μm), latterally. Rats, 200 ± 10 g body weight. **a** Luxol fast blue cresyl violet staining, ×15. *Inserts*, the whole sagittal section. **b** Schematic drawings corresponding to **a**, with demarcation of the hypothalmic nuclei. *dg*, Dentate gyrus; *DS*, supramamillary decussations; *hab*, habenula; H_2, Forel's H_2 field; *pml*, lateral part of the tuberomamillary nucleus; *rth*, reticular thalamic nucleus; *S*, supraoptic decussations; *Th*, thalamus; *III.*, third ventricle. Other abbreviations, see Fig. 144

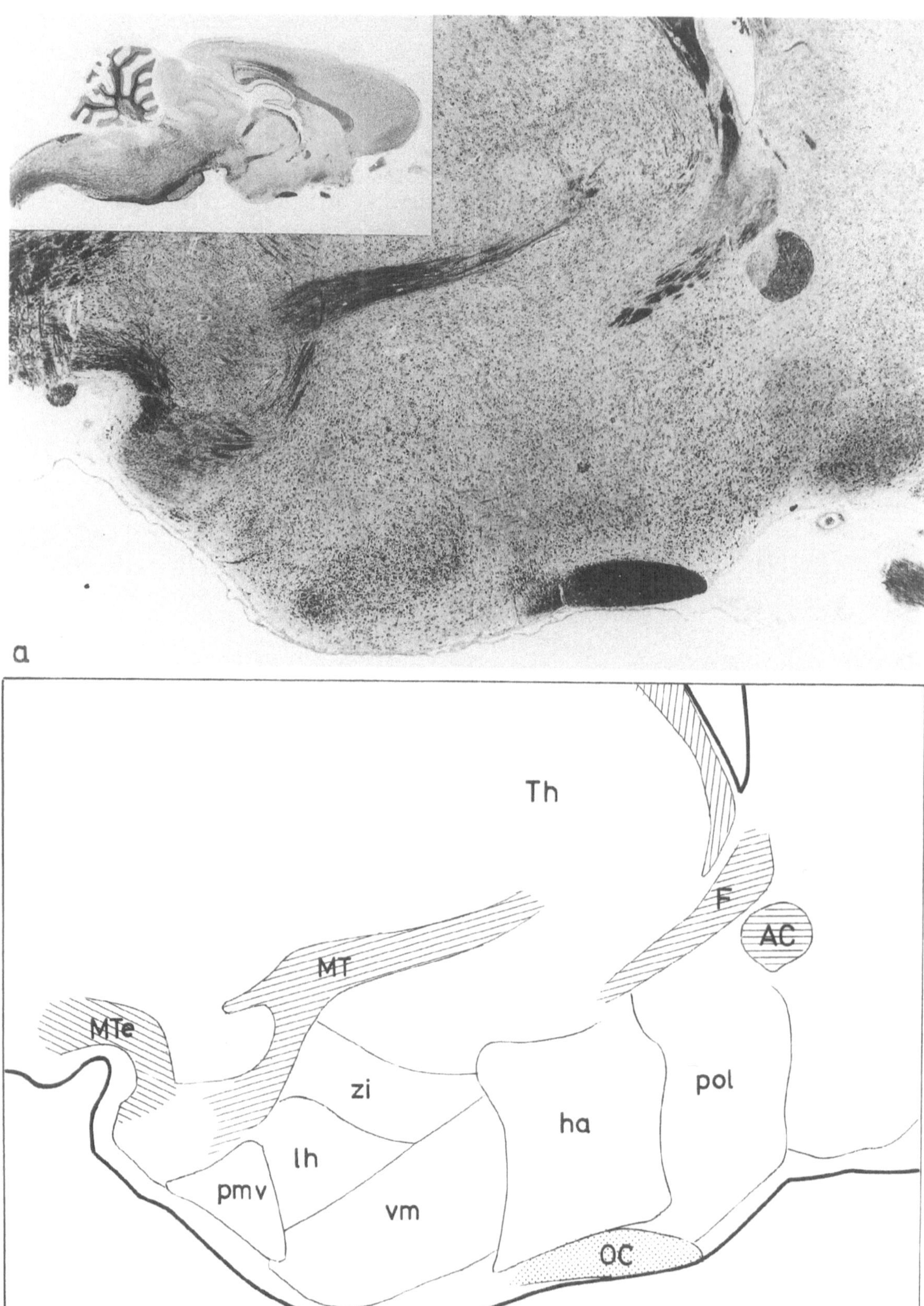

Fig. 167a,b. Sagittal sections (Figs. 162–176) of the hypothalamus from the midline at equal distances (150 μm), latterally. Rats, 200 ± 10 g body weight. **a** Luxol fast blue cresyl violet staining, ×15. *Inserts*, the whole sagittal section. **b** Schematic drawings corresponding to **a**, with demarcation of the hypothalmic nuclei. *dg*, Dentate gyrus; *DS*, supramamillary decussations; *hab*, habenula; H_2, Forel's H_2 field; *pml*, lateral part of the tuberomamillary nucleus; *rth*, reticular thalamic nucleus; *S*, supraoptic decussations; *Th*, thalamus; *III.*, third ventricle. Other abbreviations, see Fig. 144

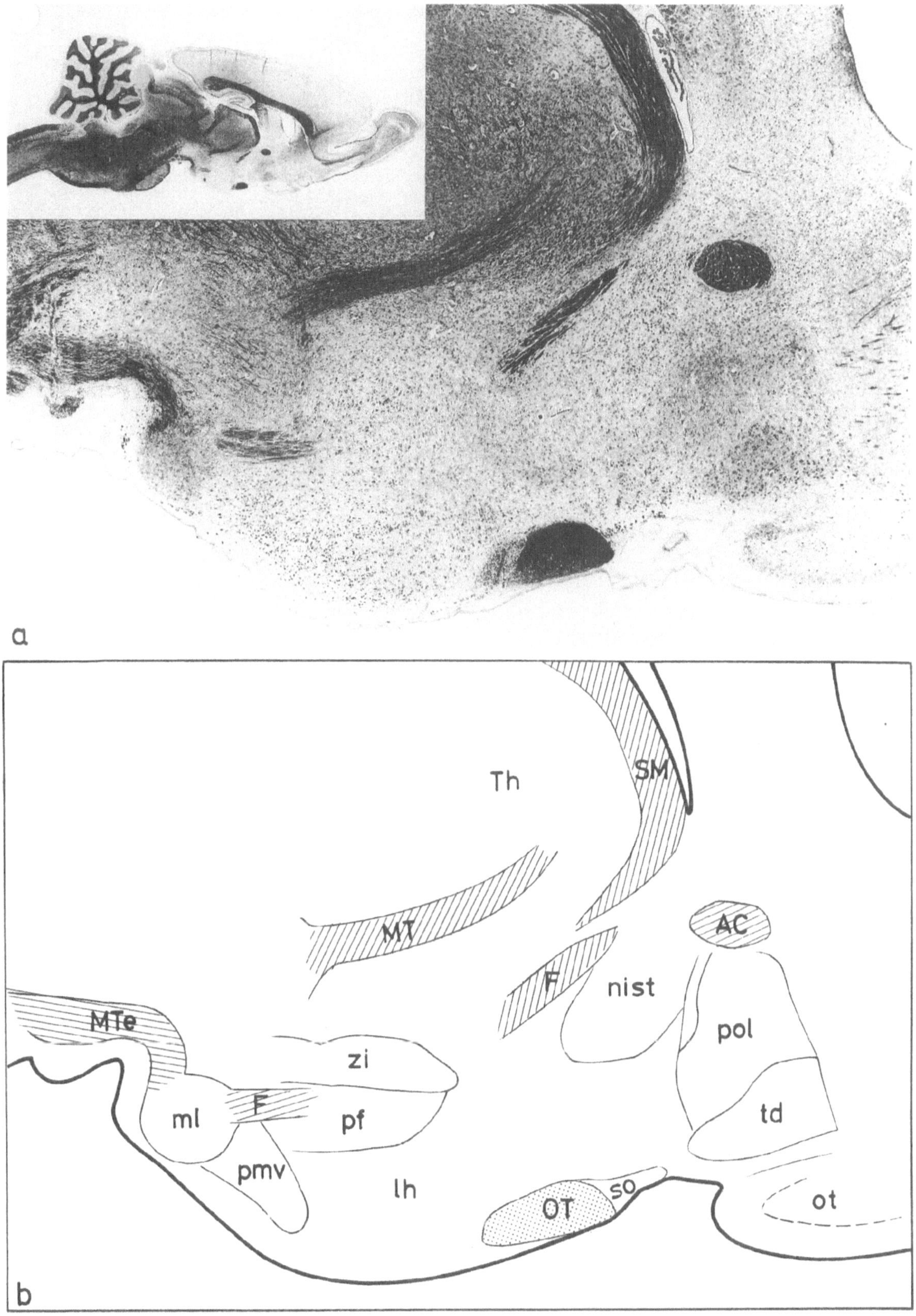

a

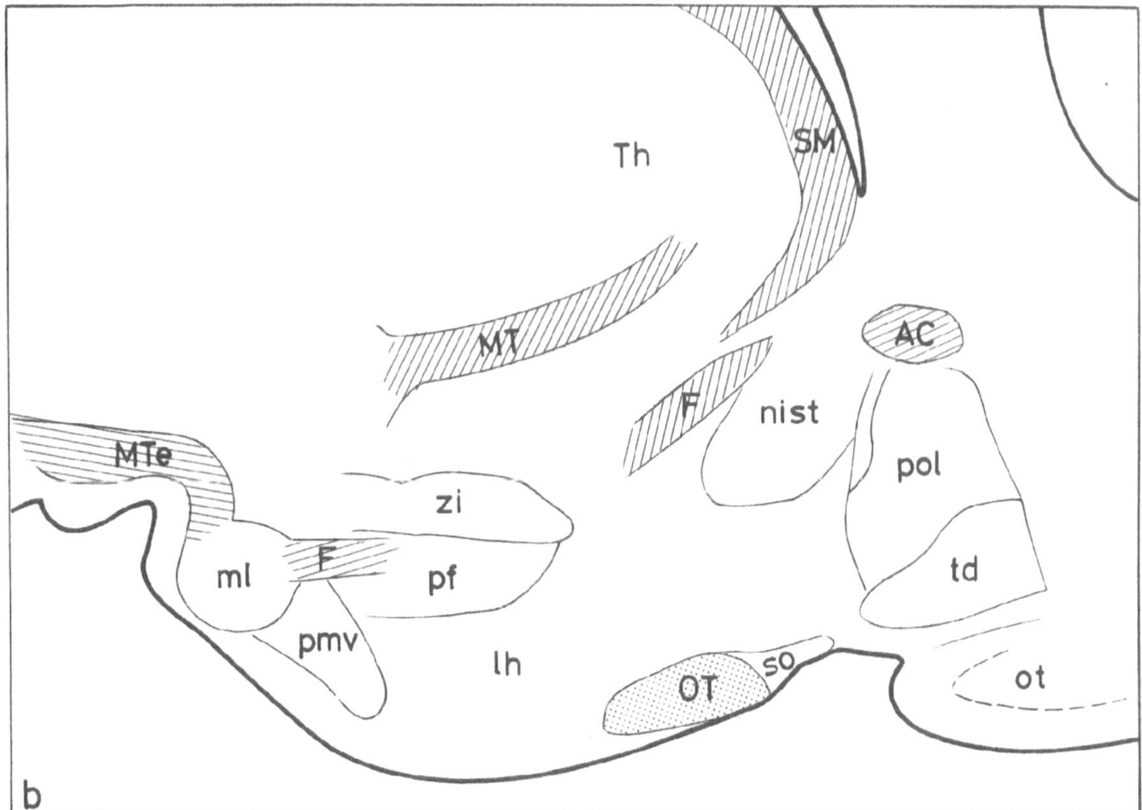

Fig. 168a,b. Sagittal sections (Figs. 162–176) of the hypothalamus from the midline at equal distances (150 μm), latterally. Rats, 200 ± 10 g body weight. **a** Luxol fast blue cresyl violet staining, ×15. *Inserts*, the whole sagittal section. **b** Schematic drawings corresponding to **a**, with demarcation of the hypothalmic nuclei. *dg*, Dentate gyrus; *DS*, supramamillary decussations; *hab*, habenula; H_2, Forel's H_2 field; *pml*, lateral part of the tuberomamillary nucleus; *rth*, reticular thalamic nucleus; *S*, supraoptic decussations; *Th*, thalamus; *III.*, third ventricle. Other abbreviations, see Fig. 144

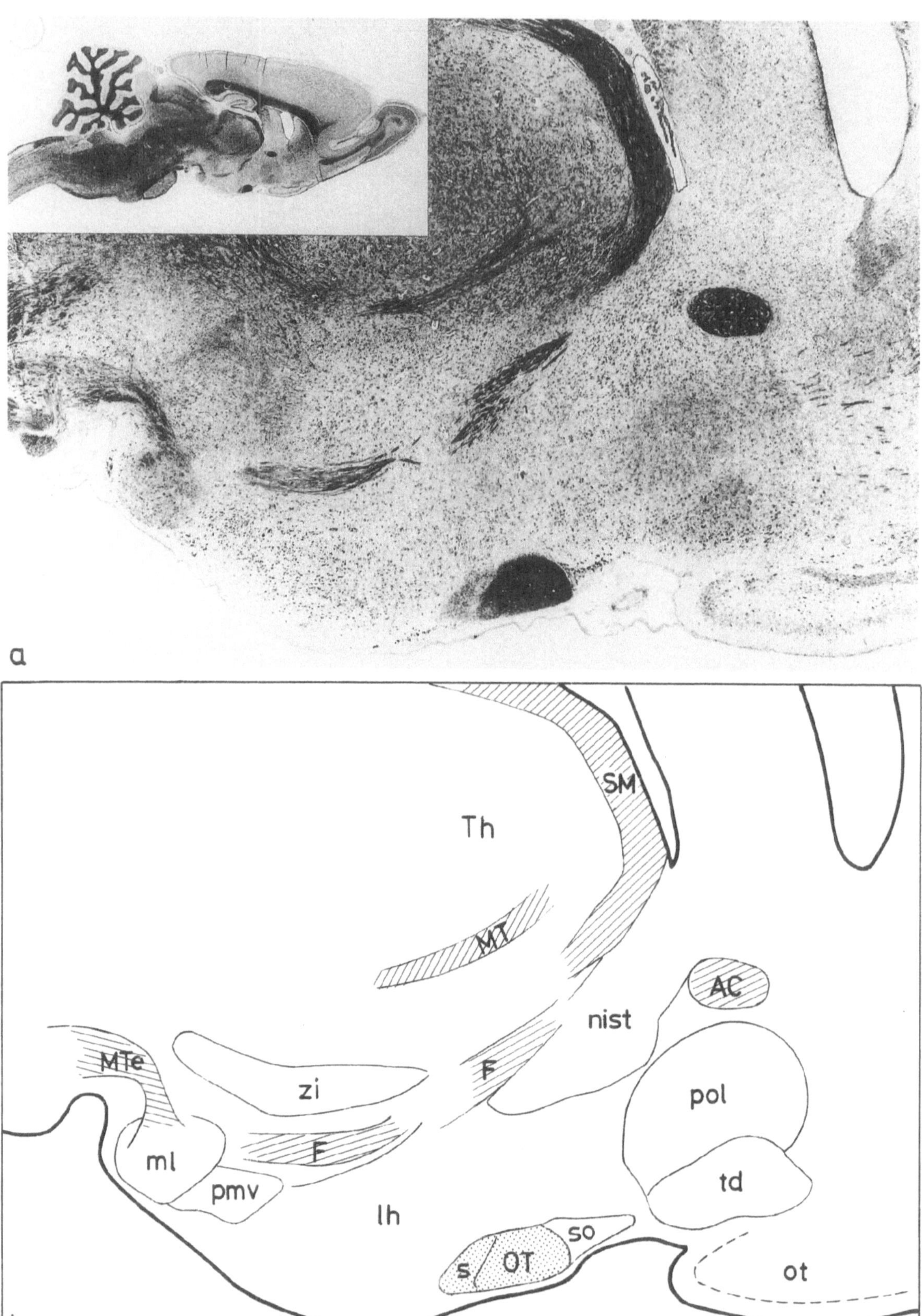

Fig. 171a,b. Sagittal sections (Figs. 162–176) of the hypothalamus from the midline at equal distances (150 μm), latterally. Rats, 200 ± 10 g body weight. **a** Luxol fast blue cresyl violet staining, ×15. *Inserts*, the whole sagittal section. **b** Schematic drawings corresponding to **a**, with demarcation of the hypothalmic nuclei. *dg*, Dentate gyrus; *DS*, supramamillary decussations; *hab*, habenula; H_2, Forel's H_2 field; *pml*, lateral part of the tuberomamillary nucleus; *rth*, reticular thalamic nucleus; *S*, supraoptic decussations; *Th*, thalamus; *III.*, third ventricle. Other abbreviations, see Fig. 144

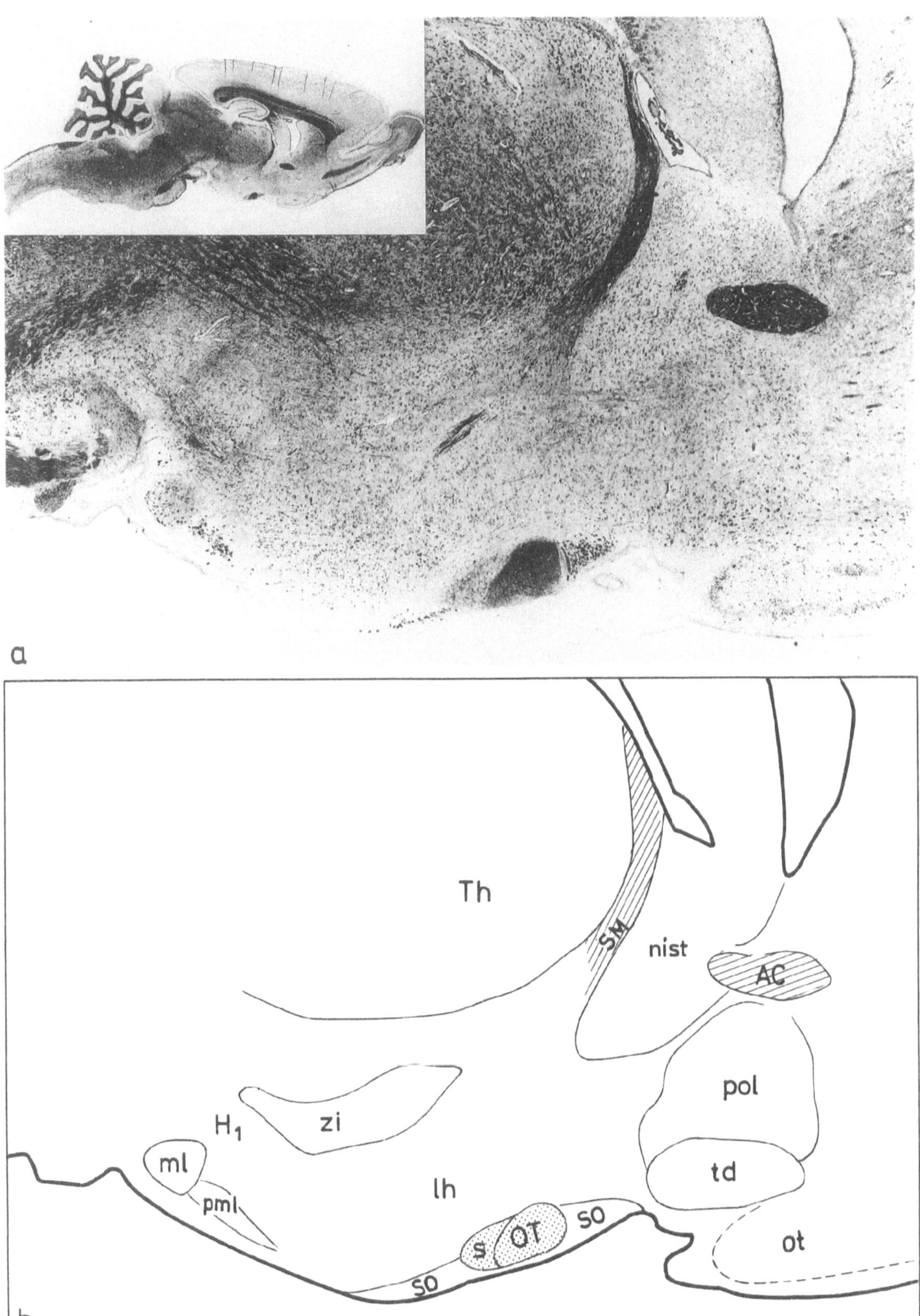

Fig. 172a,b. Sagittal sections (Figs. 162–176) of the hypothalamus from the midline at equal distances (150 µm), latterally. Rats, 200 ± 10 g body weight. **a** Luxol fast blue cresyl violet staining, ×15. *Inserts*, the whole sagittal section. **b** Schematic drawings corresponding to **a**, with demarcation of the hypothalmic nuclei. *dg*, Dentate gyrus; *DS*, supramamillary decussations; *hab*, habenula; H_2, Forel's H_2 field; *pml*, lateral part of the tuberomamillary nucleus; *rth*, reticular thalamic nucleus; *S*, supraoptic decussations; *Th*, thalamus; *III.*, third ventricle. Other abbreviations, see Fig. 144

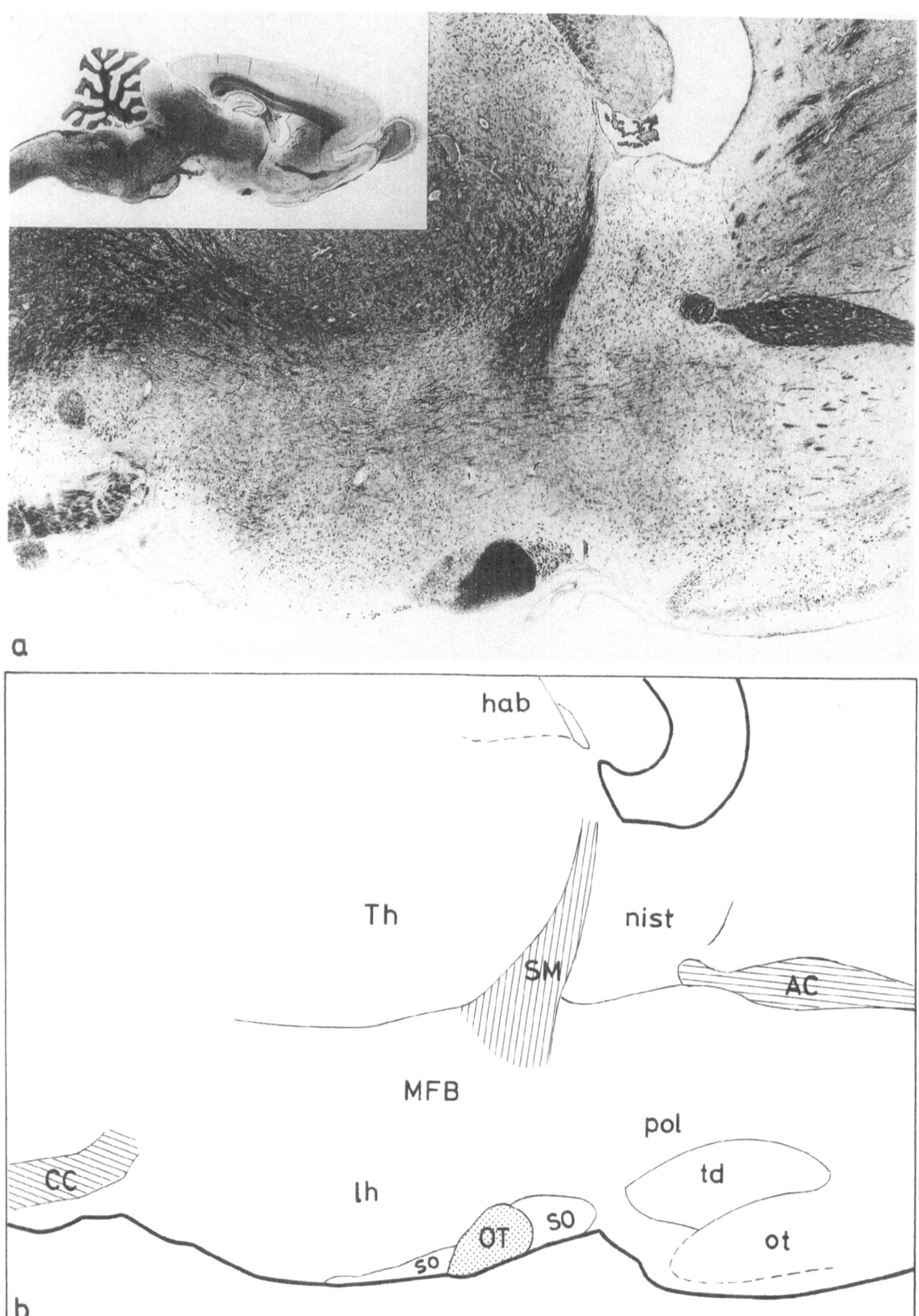

Fig. 173a,b. Sagittal sections (Figs. 162–176) of the hypothalamus from the midline at equal distances (150 µm), latterally. Rats, 200 ± 10 g body weight. **a** Luxol fast blue cresyl violet staining, ×15. *Inserts*, the whole sagittal section. **b** Schematic drawings corresponding to **a**, with demarcation of the hypothalmic nuclei. *dg*, Dentate gyrus; *DS*, supramamillary decussations; *hab*, habenula; H_2, Forel's H_2 field; *pml*, lateral part of the tuberomamillary nucleus; *rth*, reticular thalamic nucleus; *S*, supraoptic decussations; *Th*, thalamus; *III.*, third ventricle. Other abbreviations, see Fig. 144

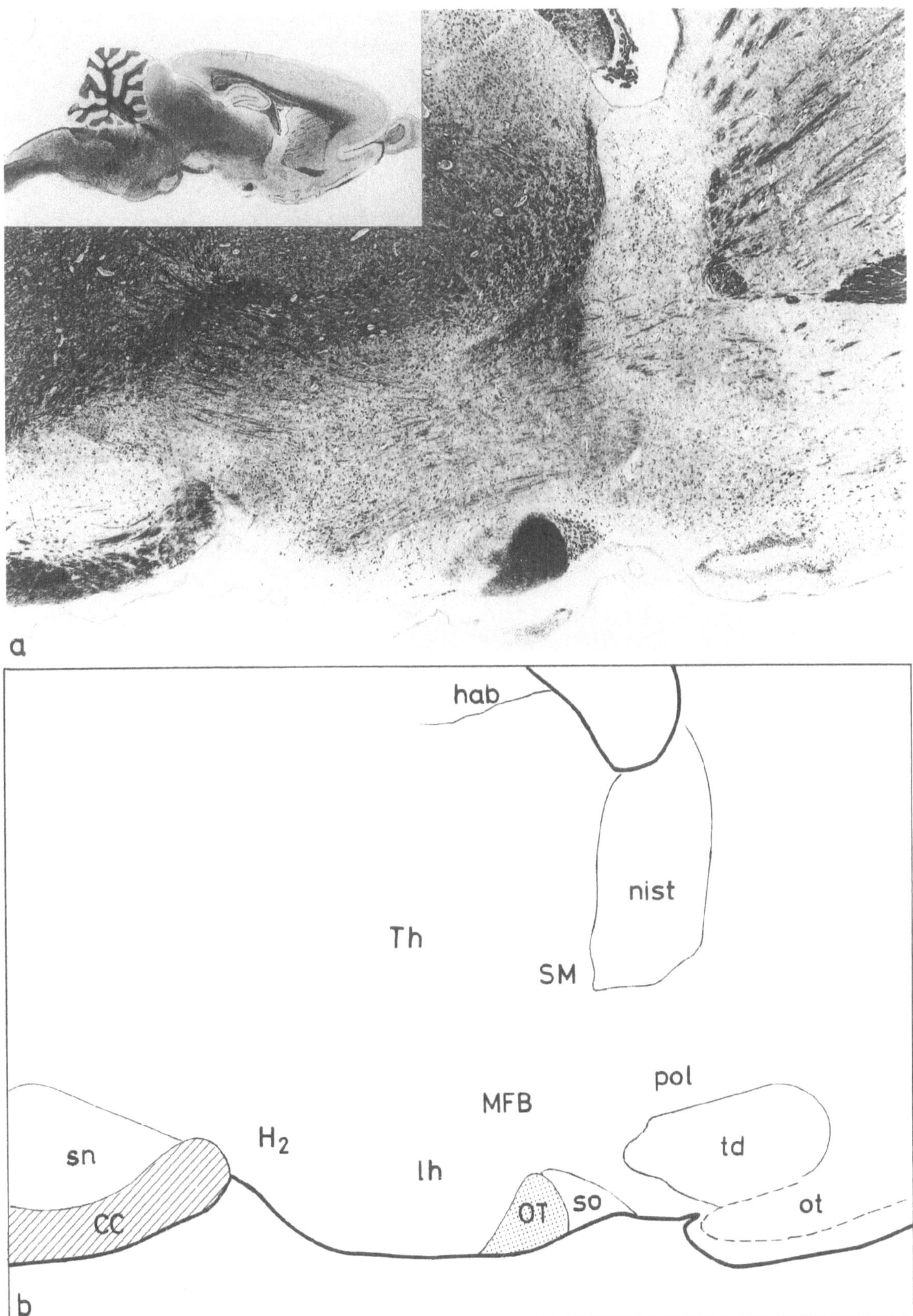

Fig. 174a,b. Sagittal sections (Figs. 162–176) of the hypothalamus from the midline at equal distances (150 μm), laterally. Rats, 200 ± 10 g body weight. **a** Luxol fast blue cresyl violet staining, ×15. *Inserts*, the whole sagittal section. **b** Schematic drawings corresponding to **a**, with demarcation of the hypothalmic nuclei. *dg*, Dentate gyrus; *DS*, supramamillary decussations; *hab*, habenula; H_2, Forel's H_2 field; *pml*, lateral part of the tuberomamillary nucleus; *rth*, reticular thalamic nucleus; *S*, supraoptic decussations; *Th*, thalamus; *III.*, third ventricle. Other abbreviations, see Fig. 144

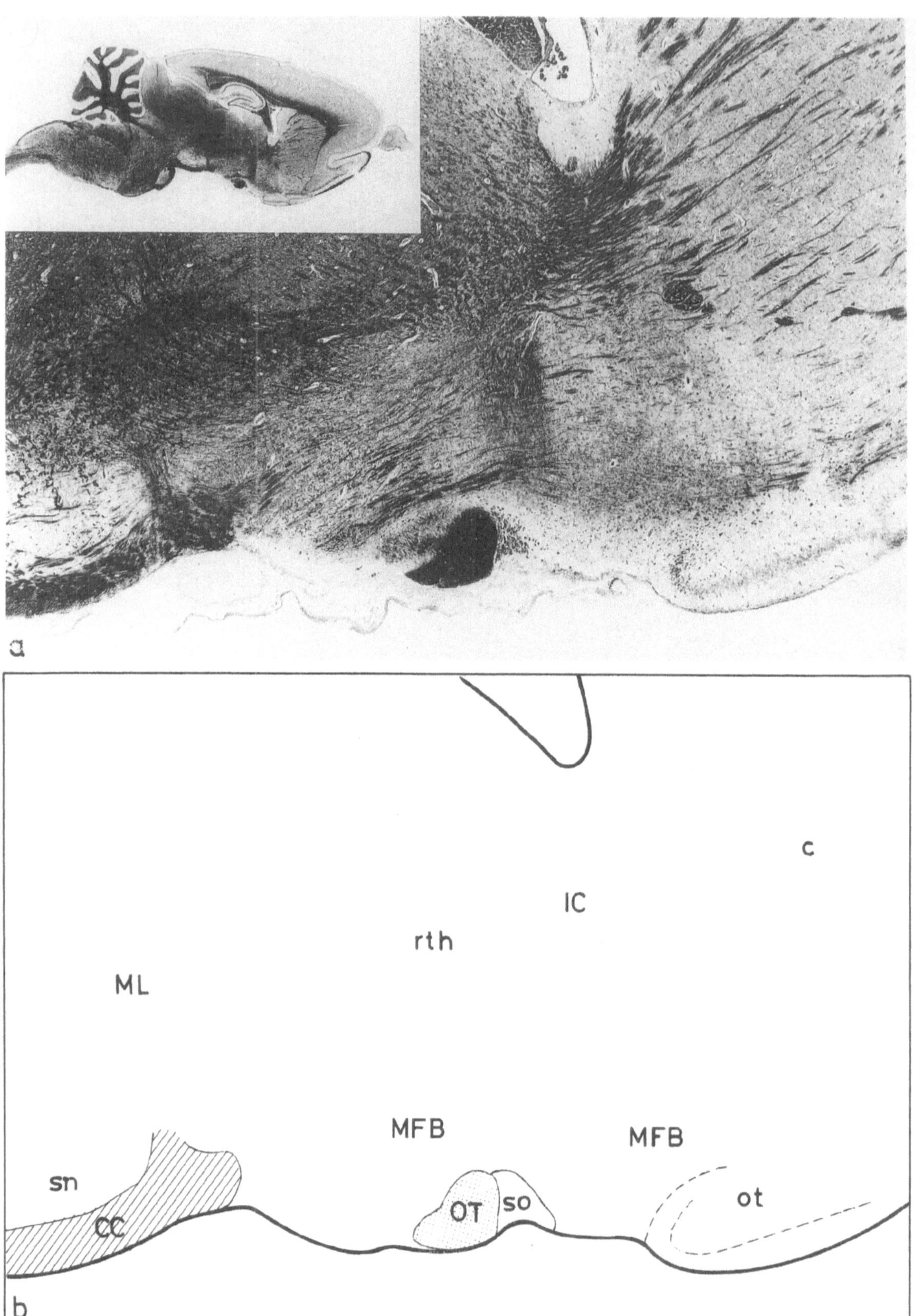

Fig. 175a,b. Sagittal sections (Figs. 162–176) of the hypothalamus from the midline at equal distances (150 µm), laterally. Rats, 200 ± 10 g body weight. **a** Luxol fast blue cresyl violet staining, ×15. *Inserts*, the whole sagittal section. **b** Schematic drawings corresponding to **a**, with demarcation of the hypothalmic nuclei. *dg*, Dentate gyrus; *DS*, supramamillary decussations; *hab*, habenula; h_2, Forel's H_2 field; *pml*, lateral part of the tuberomamillary nucleus; *rth*, reticular thalamic nucleus; *S*, supraoptic decussations; *Th*, thalamus; *III.*, third ventricle. Other abbreviations, see Fig. 144

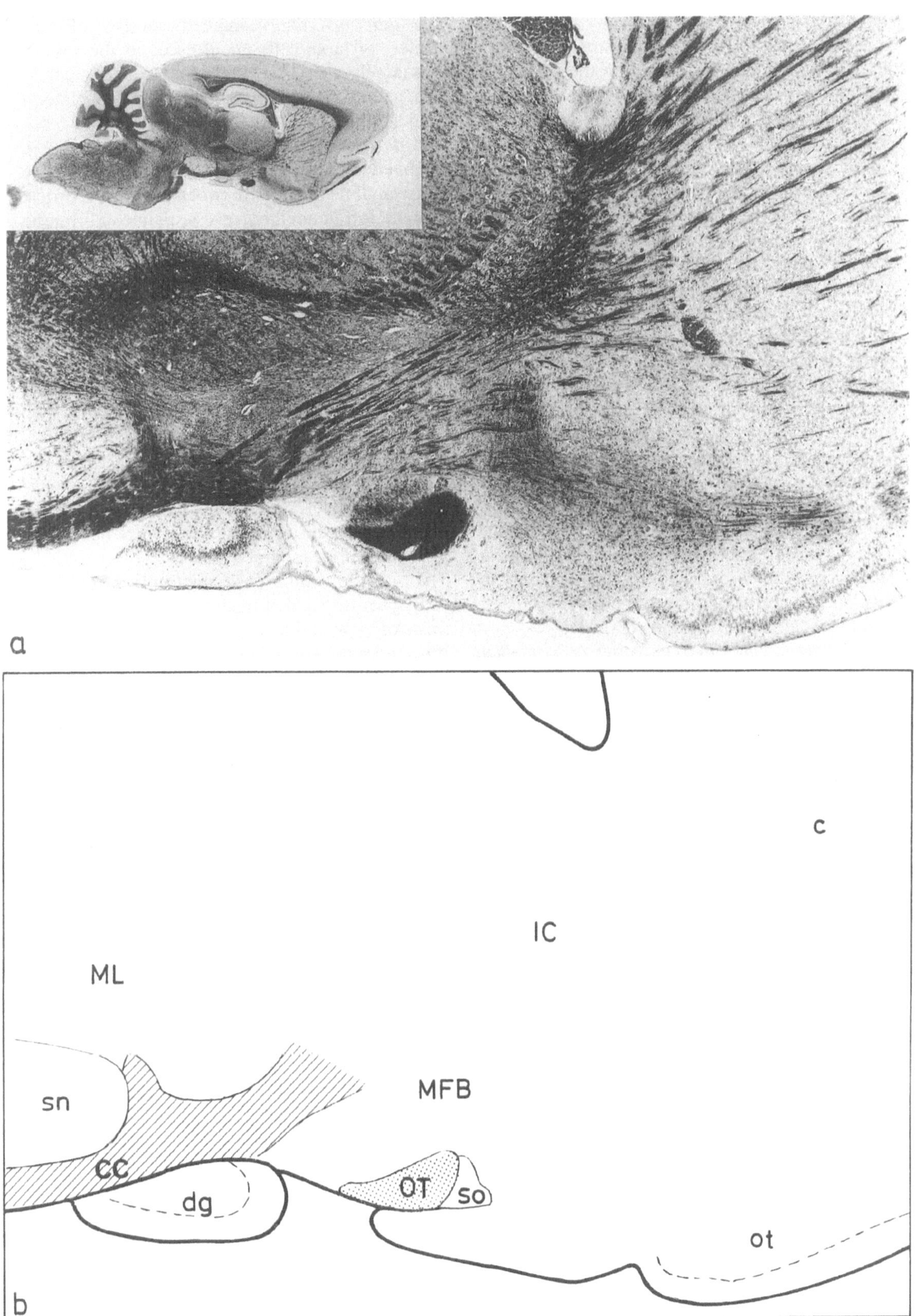

Fig. 176a,b. Sagittal sections (Figs. 162–176) of the hypothalamus from the midline at equal distances (150 μm), latterally. Rats, 200 ± 10 g body weight. **a** Luxol fast blue cresyl violet staining, ×15. *Inserts*, the whole sagittal section. **b** Schematic drawings corresponding to **a**, with demfrcation of the hypothalmic nuclei. *dg*, Dentate gyrus; *DS*, supramamillary decussations; *hab*, habenula; H_2, Forel's H_2 field; *pml*, lateral part of the tuberomamillary nucleus; *rth*, reticular thalamic nucleus; *S*, supraoptic decussations; *Th*, thalamus; *III.*, third ventricle. Other abbreviations, see Fig. 144

the midline. It has been subdivided into medial and lateral parts. The latter consists of fibers in the lateral hypothalamus between the optic tract and the fibers of the mfb.

A small, dense cell group with medium-size neurons is readily recognized between the caudal subdivision of the anterior hypothalamic and ventromedial nucleus, immediately above the ar. This is called the *anterior ventromedial nucleus* (nvma).

The *arcuate* (infundibular) *nucleus* (na) is located in the medial basal hypothalamus surrounding the most ventral portion of the third ventricle and inframamillary recess. Rostrocaudally five subdivisions can be demarcated. The first three belong to the middle and the caudal two to the posterior hypothalamus. The first subdivision is unpaired, lying in the midline under the third ventricle at the rostral beginning of the median eminence.

The *ventromedial nucleus* (nvm) occupies the major part of the medial-basal hypothalamus. Three major subdivisions (medial, central, lateral) can be recognized, which may be subdivided into further groups of cells. The nucleus is surrounded by a cell-poor area.

The *paraventricular nucleus* (npv) is located at the border of the anterior and medial-dorsal hypothalamus, dorsally, immediately beside the top of the third ventricle. Magnocellular and parvocellular subdivisions can be recognized.

The cell-dense *dorsomedial nucleus* (ndm) is made up of three subdivisions (dorsal, central, ventral). It borders the dorsal half of the third ventricle in the middle portion of the hypothalamus and extends caudally to the posterior hypothalamus.

The *perifornical nucleus* (npf) is comprised of a group of medium-large cells lying dorsal and lateral to the fornix, between frontal planes 3.0 and 3.5 mm behind the bregma.

Posterior Hypothalamus

In the rat five nuclei are recognized in the premamillary region. The *dorsal premamillary nucleus* (npmd) lies immediately caudal to the dorsomedial and the *ventral premamillary nucleus* (npmv) caudal to the ventromedial nucleus. They are fairly well distinguished from the mamillary nuclei by cell size and density.

The *tuberomamillary nucleus* consists of four clusters of large cells mainly around the ventral premamillary nucleus. Its largest (tuberal) part is also called "caudal magnocellular" or "lateral premamillary" nucleus.

The *posterior hypothalamic nucleus* (nhp) is a relatively diffuse group of cells which fill the entire midline territory between the third ventricle and the inframamillary recess, delineated by the mamillothalamic tract bilaterally.

The *supramamillary nucleus* (nsu) is formed by cells located among the fibers of the supramamillary decussations, immediately dorsal to the mamillary body.

Mamillary Body

The *medial mamillary nucleus* (nmm), which has four subdivisions (median, medial, lateral, posterior), occupies the major part of the mamillary body. Its posterior subdivision has been also recognized as a separate nucleus.

The *lateral mamillary nucleus* (nml) differs basically from the medial nucleus, from a cytological point of view and as regards neural connections. It occupies the entire lateral part of the mamillary body.

Neurochemical Summary

The development of biochemical microassays has made it possible to detect concentrations of "classical neurotransmitters" [γ-aminobutyric acid (GABA), acetylcholine, biogenic amines] and neuropeptides in the individual hypothalamic nuclei. The chemical characterization of neurons in the brain by immunocytochemistry is providing a rapidly growing body of information. Both biochemical and immunocytochemical studies have shown that all the above substances are distributed in almost all brain regions. The hypothalamus is generally rich or very rich in these substances; abundant fiber networks and nerve terminals for most of them can be visualized everywhere. Literature on their mapping and topography is widespread, and a survey of it is not possible here (for references, see Börklund and Hökfelt 1984, 1985; Börklund et al. 1984, 1990; Palkovits and Brownstein 1985; Palkovits 1988a,b).

Biochemical data are summarized in Table 4, and the immunocytochemical orservations – density

Table 4. Concentrations of neurcpeptides (μg/mg protein) in rat hypothalamic nuclei

Nuclei	Substances																									
	LHRH	TRH	CRF	SOM	GRF	VP	OX	ACTH	α-MSH	β-END	m-ENK	l-ENK	Dyn A_{1-8}	Dyn B	α-neo-END	β-neo-END	Substance P	NPY	CCK	VIP	PHI-27	Bombesin	Galanin	Neurotensin	ANF	CGRP
Medial preoptic	0.4	1.9	0.6	10.4		0.5	2.6	0.3	4.9	0.5	11.0	0.4	0.4	0.4	0.5	0.2	4.4	93.4	1.1	1.0	0.2	2.1	13.5	2.3	0.2	0.3
Periventric. preoptic						1.8																		1.7	0.4	0.7
Lateral preoptic	0.3		0.4	8.4		–	–		2.9		6.4	0.5	1.1	0.9	1.2	0.3	3.3	53.7	1.7	0.4	0.3	1.4		2.5		
Periventricular	–	4.2	0.6	23.7	–	13.1	–	0.6	7.2	1.7	1.9	0.4	0.4	0.4	0.5	0.3	3.3	129.7	2.9	0.6	4.9	2.0	15.7	1.7	0.3	
Suprachiasmatic	1.4	1.8	0.5	8.0	–	23.0	–	0.5	5.8	0.9	4.8	0.3	0.4	0.5	0.5	0.3	1.9	194.0	1.7	9.2	12.0			1.3		
Anterior hypoth.	0.3	0.8	0.4	8.6	1.3		8.4	0.3	5.1	0.5	7.2	0.5	0.5	0.6	0.6	0.3	3.2	104.4	1.6	1.1	0.8	1.8	8.7			0.7
Supraoptic	–	0.8	<0.3	3.2	–	52.9	59.8	0.1	3.2	0.1		0.2	0.3	0.2	0.2	0.2	1.6	53.7	1.8	1.0	0.3				0.1	
Paraventricular	0.2	2.6	0.6	4.4	–	38.3	56.6	0.5	4.7	0.8	6.4	0.4	0.3	0.5	0.5	0.3	3.1	244.7	1.7	0.6	1.4	2.5	11.3		0.2	1.6
Arcuate	10.3	3.9	1.5	44.6	3.5	4.0	23.3	0.8	8.1	1.8	3.0	0.4	0.5	0.4	0.4	0.3	2.5	244.2	2.6	1.3	0.5	3.8	12.3	0.1	0.2	1.2
Median eminence	210.6	38.4	39.3	309.1	32.3	261.2	223.0	1.1	11.5	1.4	2.7	0.3	0.4	0.6	0.6	0.4	1.0	182.1	2.3	1.5	–	1.5	17.0	3.4	0.2	1.1
Ventromedial	0.6	6.0	0.3	14.6	1.4	–	–	0.3	5.3	0.9	5.4	0.4	0.4	0.5	0.4	0.3	2.5		3.0	1.0	–	2.6	12.0	1.7		0.3
Dorsomedial	0.2	3.9	0.6	5.4	1.2	–	–	0.4	5.9	1.2	3.3	0.5	0.5	0.5	0.5	0.4	3.5	160.2	2.9	1.0	0.3	2.1	16.3			0.9
Perifornical	–	2.0	0.4	3.8		2.8		0.2	4.4	0.4		0.3	0.4	0.4	0.2	0.3	2.9								0.1	
Lateral hypoth.	–	0.9	0.5	4.2				0.5	5.4	0.3	9.2	0.3	0.3	0.3	0.4	0.2	2.7	42.3	1.0			2.0	9.3		0.1	0.3
Ventral premamil.	–	1.3	<0.3	17.3	–			0.4	5.5	0.7	4.0	0.4	0.6	0.3	0.3	0.2	1.7		1.6							
Dorsal premamil.	–	1.5	<0.3	4.3				0.3	7.9	0.4	0.7	0.4	0.4	0.3	0.4	0.3	3.3									
Posterior hypothal.	–	1.8	0.3	3.8	–		–	0.2	3.9	0.3	0.8	0.3	0.3	0.3	0.3	0.2	2.8	81.1	1.3	0.9	–			0.3		
Reference	1,2	3	4	5,6	7	8–10	11	12	12	12	13	14	15	16	17	18	19	20	21	22	23	24	25	26		27

1, Selmanoff et al. 1980; 2, Palkovits et al. 1974; 3, Brownstein et al. 1974; 4, Palkovits et al. 1985; 5, Kobayashi et al. 1977; 6, Brownstein et al. 1975; 7, Kita et al. 1985; 8, George and Jabobowitz 1975; 9, Zerbe and Palkovits 1984; 10, Bahner et al. 1990; 11, George et al. 1976; 12, Mezey et al. 1985; 13, Dupont et al. 1980; 14, Zamir et al. 1985; 15, Zamir et al. 1984a; 16, Zamir et al. 1984b; 17, Zamir et al. 1984c; 18, Zamir et al. 1984d; 19, Brownstein et al. 1976; 20, Chronwall et al. 1985; 21, Beinfeld and Palkovits 1981; 22, Rosténe et al. 1982; 23, Beinfeld et al. 1984; 24, Moody et al. 1981; 25, Skofitsch and Jacobowitz 1986; 26, Kobayashi et al. 1977; 27, Skofitsch and Jacobowitz 1985.

Table 5. Neuropeptide-containing neuronal perikarya in rat hypothalamic nuclei

Nuclei	Substances																							
	LHRH	TRH	CRF	Somatostatin	GRF	Vasopressin	Oxytocin	ACTH	α-MSH	β-END	Enkephalins	Dynorphins	Neo-endorphins	Substance P	NPY	CCK	VIP	PHI-27	Bombesin	Galanin	Neurotensin	Angiotensin II	ANF	CGRP
Medial preoptic	+++	+	++						+		++	++		+	++	++			+	++	++	+	+	+
Periventric. preoptic	+	+		++							++			+	+	+				++	++	++	+++	++
Lateral preoptic	+	+	+	+							+			+	+					+	+	+		
Periventricular		+	+	+++	+						+	+			+	+++				++	++	+	+++	+
Suprachiasmatic			+	+		++					+	+		+			+++	+++	+			++	+	
Anterior hypoth.	+	+		+							+				+	+			+	+	+		+	+
Supraoptic			+	+		+++	+++				+	++	+			+				++	+	+++		
Paraventricular		+++	+++	+	+	+++	+++				++	++	+	+	++	++	+	+	++	++	+	+++	+	+
Arcuate		+		++	+++			+++	+++	+++	++	++		++	+++		+			+	++	+	+	+
Median eminence																								
Ventromedial				++							+	+		++	++					+		+	+	
Dorsomedial		+		+	+				++		++	+		+	++	+				+++	+	+	+	+
Perifornical		+	+	+	+				+		++	++		+						+	+	+++	+	++
Lateral hypoth.		+	+	+	+				++		+	++	+	+	+		+			+++	++	+	+	++
Ventral premamil.				+					++	++	++	++	+		+						+			+ +
Dorsal premamil.			+	+								+			+						++			
Posterior Hth.												+			+	+					+	+	+	+

+++, High number; ++, moderate number; +, few immunoreactive cells. References, see Palkovits 1988a,b.

of chemically identified cells and nerve terminals – in Tables 5 and 6, respectively. (These are summarized without critical remarks on the specificity of the assays used.)

GABA. The hypothalamic distribution of GABA is based on its biochemical measurements (Banay-Schwartz et al. 1989a) and on the biochemistry (Tappaz et al. 1977; Brownstein and Palkovits 1984) and immunohistochemistry (Mugnaini and Oertel 1985) of its rate-limiting enzyme, glutamic acid decarboxylase. GABA is present throughout the hypothalamus, mainly in nerve terminals and few cell bodies. The concentration of GABA and its enzyme activity have been found to be moderate except in the preoptic and paraventricular nuclei, where they exceed the hypothalamic levels. *Aspartate* has been found in fairly uneven distribution in the hypothalamic nuclei: very high concentration in the medial preoptic nucleus *versus* very low in the posterior hypothalamus and in the median eminence (Banay-Schwartz et al. 1989a). The hypothalamus is relatively poor in *glutamate*, especially its lateral area (Banay-Schwartz et al. 1989b). A fairly high variation (8:1 ratio) has been measured in *taurine* contents of the hypothalamic nuclei: the highest in the anterior and the lowest in the posterior hypothalamic nuclei (Banay-Schwartz et al. 1989b). Relatively high *glycine* levels were found in the medial preoptic nucleus and in the medial-basal hypothalamus, while moderate or low elsewhere in the hypothalamus (Banay-Schwartz et al. 1989b).

Acetylcholine. The topographical distribution of the cholinergic perikarya and fiber has been studied in the hypothalamus by choline acetyltransferase immunohistochemistry (Armstrong et al. 1983; Satoh et al. 1983), acetylcholinesterase stainings (Jacobowitz and Palkovits 1974; Satoh et al. 1983), and biochemical determination of the concentrations of choline acetyltransferase in individual hypothalamic nuclei (Brownstein and Palkovits 1984). In general, the hypothalamus is very poor in acetylcholine. Cholinergic neurons may occur in the lateral area of the posterior hypothalamus, and occasionally in the paraventricular, arcuate, and premamillary nuclei.

Biogenic Amines. The neurons containing *dopamine*, *noradrenaline*, and *adrenaline* were the first to be visualized by the histofluorescence technique and were were later confirmed by immunofluorescence of tyrosine hydroxylase, dopamine-β-hydroxylase, and phenylethanolamine *N*-methyltransferase. For summary and references, see Björklund and Hökfelt 1984, 1985). *Serotonin*- and *histamine*-containing perikarya, fibers, and nerve terminals have been visualized in the hypothalamus by immunohistochemistry (Steinbusch 1984; Steinbusch and Mulder 1984). The concentrations of biogenic amines and their related enzyme have been measured by biochemical microassays in microdissected hypothalamic nuclei (Brownstein and Palkovits 1984). The distribution of biogenic amines in the hypothalamus has some regularities: (a) in general, the hypothalamus is rich in biogenic amines, which are present in each of the nuclei but in different densities and concentrations (Palkovits 1983); (b) only dopamine (in the arcuate and preoptic periventricular nuclei) and histamine (in the tuberomamillary nucleus) synthesizing neurons are present in the hypothalamus, while noradrenaline-, adrenaline, and serotonin-containing perikarya are located in the lower brainstem (midbrain, pons, medulla oblongata); (c) several well-defined aminergic projections ascend from the lower brainstem to the hypothalamus with a certain overlap in their innervation patterns.

Neuropeptides. So far 23 neuropeptides have been identified and localized in rat hypothalamic nuclei by radioimmunoassays (Table 4) and immunohistochemistry (Tables 5, 6; Björklund et al. 1984, 1990; Palkovits 1988a,b). A group of these peptides is constituted by the so-called *hypothalamic neuropeptides*, which regulate anterior pituitary functions (releasing or inhibiting hormones such as luteinizing hormone releasing hormone, thyrotropin-releasing hormone, corticotropin-releasing factor, growth hormone releasing factor, and somatostatin) or are stored in the posterior lobe (vasopressin, oxytocin). Since they have been identified in almost all brain areas, their terminology does not exclusively relate to their topography. Generally their concentrations and densities are highest in the hypothalamus, particularly in the median eminence (Tables 4, 6). So-called *pituitary peptides* (the opiomelanocortin family: β-endorphin, adrenocorticotropic hormone, α-melanocyte-stimulating hormone; and growth hormone, thyrotropin and prolactin) are all present in the rat hypothalamus (and many

Table 6. Neuropeptide-containing nerve fibers and terminals in hypothalamic nuclei

Nuclei	Substances																							
	LHRH	TRH	CRF	Somatostatin	GRF	Vasopressin	Oxytocin	ACTH	α-MSH	β-END	Enkephalins	Dynorphins	Neo-endorphins	Substance P	NPY	CCK	VIP	PHI-27	Bombesin	Galanin	Neurotensin	Angiotensin II	ANF	CGRP
Medial preoptic	+	+	++	++	+	+		+	++	+	+	+		++	++	++	+		++	++	+	+	+	+
Periventric. preoptic		+	+	++	++	++		+	+	++	+	+		+	++	+	+			++	++	++	++	++
Lateral preoptic	+	+	+	+		+		+	+	+	+	++	++	+	+	+				++	+	+	+	
Periventricular	+	+	+	+	++	++		++	++	++	+	++		+	+	++	+			++	++	++	++	+
Suprachiasmatic		+		+		+			+	+	+	+		+	+	+	++	++	++			++	+	+
Anterior hypoth.	+	+		+	+		+	+	++	+	+	+	+	+	+	+	+		++	+	+	+	+	+
Supraoptic				+		++	++		+	+	+	+	+	+	+	+				+		+++	+	+
Paraventricular			++	+	+	++	++	+	+	+	++	++	+	+	+++	+		+	++	++	++	++	+	+
Arcuate	+	+	+	+	++	+		+	+	+	++	++		+	+++	++	+		++	++	+	+	+	+
Median eminence	+++	+++	+++	+++	+++	+++	+++	+	+	+	+	++	+	+	+	+	++	++		++	+++	+++	+	+
Ventromedial				++				+	+	+	+	++		+	++	++	+		+		+		+	+
Dorsomedial		+	+	+	+	+		++	++	++	++	+		+	++	+++	+		+	++	+	+	+	+
Perifornical		+	+	+	+			+	+	+	+	+		+	+					+	+	+	+	+
Lateral hypoth.		++	+	++	+	+		+	+	+	+	+	+	+	+	+	+		+	++	+	++	+	+
Ventral premamil.	+	+		+	+	+		+	+	+	++	+		+	++	+	+		+	+			+	+
Dorsal premamil.		+		+		+		+		+	++	+		+	+	++				++	+	+		
Posterior Hth.		+	+	+		+		+			+	+		+	+	++	+	+	+	+	+	+		+

+++, Dense; ++, moderate networks; +, scattered immunoreactive fibers. References, see Palkovits 1988a,b.

other brain areas) in lower concentrations than in the pituitary gland. Their origin in the brain is supported by their invariable presence after hypophysectomy. Opiomelanocortins (derived from a common precursor molecule, 31-kDa pro-opiocortin) are present in the same neurons, mainly in the arcuate and ventral premamillary nuclei. *Opioid peptides* (other than β-endorphin) such as Met- and Leu-enkephalin, Met-enkephalin-Arg-Phe, Met-enkephalin-Arg-Gly-Leu, dynorphin A, dynorphin$_{1-8}$, dynorphin B, α-neo-endorphin, β-neoendorphin are all present in the central nervous system in individual distribution pattern. Their concentrations in the hypothalamic, especially in the preoptic nuclei exceed the brain average (Table 5). The so-called brain-born *gastrointestinal peptides* – substance P, neuropeptide Y, cholecystokinin, vasoactive intestinal polypeptide, peptide histidine isoleucine amide 27 peptide, bombesin, galanin, and calcitonin gene-related peptide – are all present in the hypothalamus in variable concentrations and densities (Tables 4–6). Several *other neuropeptides* such as neurotensin, atrial natriuretic peptide, and angiotensin II are also widely distributed in the hypothalamus in relation to their perikaryonal and terminal locations (Tables 5, 6).

In trying to synthesize in topographical terms the chemically identified neurons in the hypothalamus it is evident that we can hardly find any homogenous cell group containing only one substance. Certain hypothalamic nuclei contain 10–14 types of cells, differing in their chemical characters (Tables 5, 6). In many cases the coexistence of various substances within the same neurons has become evident. None of the hypothalamic cell groups receive only one kind of chemical input; nerve terminals with a number of different neurotransmitters and neuropeptides are present in each nucleus (Tables 4–6). Some hypothalamic nuclei contain certain substances in higher concentrations than do other cell groups (Table 4), but it would be unrealistic to regard an anatomical unit (nucleus) as the center of production of a single type of physiologically active substance. The same applies to neuronal connections (pathways) with respect to the transport of a neurohormone or a neurotransmitter.

Within the hypothalamus the highest levels of many substances investigated are contained by the median eminence (Table 4). Perikarya are practically absent here; neurotransmitters and neuropeptides occur in axons and axonal varicosities. Among the cell groups of the hypothalamus the arcuate nucleus contains particularly numerous, chemically identifiable types of cells and nerve terminals (Table 6). Several types of cells have been visualized in the periventricular, supraoptic, paraventricular, dorsomedial, and perifornical nuclei (Table 5).

Although a great number of substances have been verified in the hypothalamic nuclei chemically and immunocytochemically, a fairly high number of hypothalamic neurons and nerve terminals have not yet been identified chemically.

References

Albe-Fessard D, Denise G (1966) Atlas stéréotaxique du diencéphale du rat blanc. CNRS, Paris

Armstrong DK, Saper CB, Levey AI, Wainer BH, Terry RD (1983) Distribution of cholinergic neurons in rat brain: demonstrated by the immunocytochemical localization of choline acetyltransferase. J Comp Neurol 216:53–68

Bahner U, Geiger H, Palkovits M, Gander D, Michel J, Heidland A (1990) Atrial natriuretic peptides in brain nuclei of rats with inherited diabetes insipidus (Brattleboro rat). Neurobiology 51:721–727

Banay-Schwartz M, Laitha A, Palkovits M (1989a) Changes with aging in the levels of amino acids in rat CNS structural elements. I. Glutamate and related amino acids. Neurochem Res 14:555–562

Banay-Schwartz M, Laitha A, Palkovits M (1989b) Changes with aging in the levels of amino acids in rat CNS structural elements. II. Taurine and small neutral amino acids. Neurochem Res 14:563–570

Beinfeld MC, Palkovits N (1981) Distribution of cholecystokinin (CCK) in the hypothalamus and limbic system of the rat. Neuropeptides 2:123–129

Beinfeld MC, Korchak DM, Roth BL, O'Donohue TL (1984) The distribution and chromatographic characterization of PHI (peptide histidine isoleucine amide)-27-like peptides in rat and porcine brain. J Neurosci 4:2681–2688

Björklund A, Hökfelt T (eds) (1984) Handbook of chemical neuroanatomy, vol 2. Elsevier, Amsterdam, p 463

Björklund A, Hökfelt T (eds) (1985) Handbook of chemical neuroanatomy, vol 4, part I. Elsevier, Amsterdam, p 638

Björklund A, Hökfelt T, Kuhar MJ (eds) (1984) Handbook of chemical neuroanatomy, vol 3, part II. Elsevier, Amsterdam, p 435

Björklund A, Hökfelt T, Kuhar NJ (eds) (1990) Handbook of chemical neuroanatomy, vol 9, part II. Elsevier, Amsterdam, p 549

Bleier R, Cohn P, Siggelkow IR (1979) A cytoarchitectonic atlas of the hypothalamus and hypothalamic third ventricle of the rat. In: PJ Morganer J Panksepp (eds) Handbook of the hypothalamus, vol 1. Dekker, New York, pp 137–220

Brownstein MJ, Palkovits N (1984) Catecholamines, serotonin, acetylcholine, and IT-aminobutyric acid in the rat brain: biochemical studies. In: Björklund A, Hökfelt T (eds) Handbook of chemical neuroanatomy, vol 2, part I. Elsevier, Amsterdam, chap II, pp 23–54

Brownstein MJ, Saavedra JN, Palkovits M, Axelrod J (1974) Histamine content of hypothalamic nuclei of the rat. Brain Res 77:151–156

Brownstein MJ, Arimura A, Sato H, Schally AV, Kizer JS (1975) The regional distribution of somatostatin in the rat brain. Endocrinology 96:1456–1461

Brownstein MJ, Mroz EA, Kizer JS, Palkovits M, Leeman SE (1976) Regional distribution of substance P in the brain of the rat. Brain Res 116:299–305

Chronwall BM, DiMaggio DA, Massari VJ, Pickel VM, Ruggiero DA, O'Donohue TL (1985) The anatomy of neuropeptide Y-containing neurons in rat brain. Neuroscience 15:1159–1181

Clark Le Gros WE (1938) Morphological aspects of the hypothalamus. In: Clark Le Gros WE, Beattie J, Riddoch G, Dott NM (eds) The hypothalamus. Oliver and Boyd, Edinburgh, pp 43–50

Crosby EC, Showers MJC (1969) Comparative anatomy of the preoptic and hypothalamic areas. In: Haymaker W, Anderson E, Nauta WJH (eds) The hypothalamus. Thomas, Springfield, pp 61–135

De Groot J (1963) The rat forebrain in stereotaxic coordinates. North Holland, Amsterdam

Diepen R (1962) Der Hypothalamus. In: Bargmann W (ed) Handbuch der mikroskopischen Anatomie des Menschen, vol IV/7. Springer, Berlin Göttingen Heidelberg

Dupont A, Lepine J, Lanelier P, Mérand Y, Rouleau D, Vaudry H, Gros C, Barden N (1980) Differential distribution of β-endorphin and enkephalins in rat and bovine brain. Regul Pept 1:43–52

George JM, Jacobowitz DK (1975) Localization of vasopressin in discrete areas of the rat hypothalamus. Brain Res 93: 363–366

George JM, Staples S, Marks BM (1976) Oxytocin content of microdissected areas of rat hypothalamus. Endocrinology 98:1430–1433

Gurdjian ES (1927) The diencephalon of the albino rat. Studies of the brain of the rat. II. J Comp Neurol 43:1–114

Haymaker W, Anderson E, Nauta WJH (eds) (1969) The hypothalamus. Thomas, Springfield

Jacobowitz DM, Palkovits M (1974) Topographic atlas of catecholamine and acetylcholinesterase-containing neurons in the rat brain. I. Forebrain (telencephalon, diencephalon). J Comp Neurol 157:13–28

Kita T, Chihara K. Abe H, Hinamitani N, Kaii H, Kodama H, Kashio Y, Okimura Y, Fujita T, Ling N (1985) Regional distribution of rat growth hormone releasing factor-like imunoreactivity in rat hypothalamus. Endocrinology 116: 259–262

Kobayashi RM, Brown M, Vale W (1977) Regional distribution of neurotensin and somatostatin in rat brain. Brain Res 126:584–588

König JFR, Klippel RA (1963) The rat brain: a stereotaxis atlas of the forebrain and lower parts of the brain stem. Williams and Wilkins, Baltimore

Krieg WJS (1932) The hypothalamus of the albino rat. J Comp Neurol 55:19–89

Massopust LC Jr (1961) Stereotaxic atlases. A diencephalon of the rat. In: Sheer DE (ed) Electrical stimulation of the brain. University of Texas Press, Austin

Mezey E, Kiss JZ, Mueller GP, Eskay R, O'Donohue TL, Palkovits K (1985) Distribution of the pro-opiomelanocortin derived peptides, adrenocorticotrope hormone, α-melanocyte-stimulating hormone and β-endorphin (ACTH, α-MSH, β-END) in the rat hypothalamus. Brain Res 328: 341–347

Moody TW, O'Donohue TL, Jacobowitz DM (1981) Biochemical localization and characterization of bombesin-like peptides in discrete regions of rat brain. Peptides 2:75–79

Mugnaini E, Oertel WR (1985) An atlas of the distribution of GABAergic neurons and terminals in the rat CNS as revealed by GAD imunohistochemistry. In: Björklund A, Hökfelt T (eds) Handbook of chemical neuroanatomy, vol 4, part J. Elsevier, Amsterdam, chap 10, pp 436–608

Palkovits H (1983) Stereotaxic map, cytoarchitectonic and neurochemical summary of the hypothalamic nuclei, rat. In: Jones TC, Mohr U, Hunt RD (eds) Endocrine system, monographs on pathology of laboratory animals. Springer, Berlin Heidelberg New York, pp 316–331

Palkovits M (1988a) Neuropeptides in the brain. In: Martini L, Ganons WF (eds) Frontiers in neuroendocrinology, vol 10. Raven, New York, pp 1–44

Palkovits M (1988b) Distribution of neuropeptides in brain: a review of biochemical and imunohistochemimical studies. In: Negro-Vilar A, Conn PM (eds) Peptide hormones: effects and mechanisms of action, vol 1. CRC, Boca Raton, pp 3–67

Palkovits M, Brownstein MJ (1985) Distribution of neuropeptides in the central nervous system using biochemical micromethods. In: Björklund A, Hökfelt T (eds) Handbook of chemical neuroanatomy, vol 4, part 1. Elsevier, Amsterdam, pp 1–71

Palkovits M, Brownstein NJ (1988) Maps and guide to microdissection of the rat brain. Elsevier, New York

Palkovits M, Arimura A, Brownstein M, Schally AV, Saavedra JN (1974) Luteinizing hormone-releasing homone (LH-RH) content of the hypothalamic nuclei in rat. Endocrinology 96:554–558

Palkovits M, Brownstein M, Vale W (1985) Distribution of corticotropin-releasing factor in rat brain. Fed Proc 44: 215–219

Paxinos G, Watson C (1982) The rat brain in stereotaxic coordinates. Academic, Sydney

Pellegrino LJ, Pellegrino AS, Cushman AJ (1979) A stereotaxic atlas of the rat brain, 2nd edn. Plenum, New York

Rosténe (Rotsztejn) WH, Léránth C, Maletti M, Mezey E, Besson J, Eiden LE, Rosselin G, Palkovits K (1982) Distribution of vasoactive intestinal peptide (VIP) following various brain transections in the rat by radioimmunoassay and electronmicro seopic immunocytochemistry. Neuropeptides 2:337–350

Satoh K, Armstrong DM, Fibiger HC (1983) A comparison of the distribution of central cholinergic neurons as demonstrated by acetylcholinesterase pharmacohistochemistry and choline acetyltransferase immunohistochemistry. Brain Res Bull 11:693–720

Selmanoff MK, Wise PM, Barraclough CA (1980) Regional distribution of luteinizing hormone-releasing hormone (LH-RH) in rat brain determined by microdissection and radioimmunoassay. Brain Res 192:421–432

Simson EL, Jones AP, Gold RM (1981) Horizontal stereotaxic atlas of the albino rat brain. Brain Res Bull 6:297–326

Skofitsch G, Jacobowitz DH (1985) Quantitative distribution of calcitonin gene-related peptide in the rat central nervous system. Peptides 6:1069–1073

Skofitsch G, Jacobowitz DM (1986) Quantitative distribution of galanin-like immunoreactivity in the rat central nervous system. Peptides 7:609–613

Steinbusch HWM (1984) Serotonin-immunoreactive neurons and their projections in the CNS. In: Björklund A, Hökfelt T, Kuhar MJ (eds) Handbook of chemical neuroanatomy, vol 3, part II. Elsevier, Amsterdam, pp 68–125

Steinbusch HWM, Mulder AH (1984) Immunohistochemical localization of histamine in neurons and mast cells in the rat brain. In: Björklund A, Hökfelt T, Kuhar MJ (eds) Handbook of chemical neuroanatomy, vol 3, part II. Elsevier, Amsterdam, pp 126–140

Swanson LW (1987) The hypothalamus. In: Björklund A, Hökfelt T, Swanson LW (eds) Handbook of chemical neuroanatomy, vol 5, part I, Elsevier, Amsterdam, pp 1–124

Swanson LW (1992) Brain maps: structure of the rat brain. Elsevier, Amsterdam

Szentágothai J, Flerkó B, Ness B, Halász B (1968) Hypothalamic control of the anterior pituitary. An experimental-morphological study. Akadémiai Kiadó, Budapest

Tappaz KL, Brownstein MJ, Kopin IJ (1977) Glutamate decarboxylase (GAD) and γ-aminobutyric acid (GABA) in discrete nuclei of hypothalamus and substantia nigra. Brain Res 125:109–121

Zamir N, Palkovits M, Brownstein MJ (1984a) Distribution of immunoreactive dynorphin A_{1-8} in discrete nuclei of the rat brain: comparison with dynorphin A. Brain Res 307:61–68

Zamir N, Palkovits M, Weber E, Nezey E, Brownstein MJ (1984b) A dynorphinergic pathway of Leu-enkephalin production in rat substantia nigra. Nature 307:643–645

Zamir N, Palkovits M, Brownstein MJ (1984c) The distribution of immunoreactive β-neo-endorphin in the central nervous system of the rat. J Neurosci 4:1240–1247

Zamir N, Palkovits M, Brownstein MJ (1984d) Distribution of immunoreactive β-neo-endorphin in discrete areas of the rat brain and pituitary gland: comparison with α-neo-endorphin. J Neurosci 4:1248–1252

Zamir N, Palkovits M, Brownstein MJ (1985) Distribution of immunoreactive Met-enkephalin-Arg^6-Gly^7-Leu^8 and Leu-enkephalin in discrete regions of the rat brain. Brain Res 326:1–8

Zerbe RL, Palkovits M (1984) Changes in the vasopressin content of discrete brain regions in response to stimuli for vasopressin secretion. Neuroendocrinology 38:285–289

Study of Pathologic Lesions in the Hypothalamic-Pituitary System, Rat

Giovanni L. Rossi, Gilberto E. Bestetti, and Claude E. Boujon

Neuroendocrinological studies on rodent models frequently suggest a functionally and structurally impaired hypothalamic-pituitary system. It is of primary importance to have adequate techniques for sucessful morphological and functional studies of lesions in the central nervous system of laboratory animals. Over several years we have developed and employed the techniques described here for morphological and immunocytochemical study of the lesions and for the in vitro assessment of functional neuroendocrine disturbances.

In particular, for the structural investigations of the rat hypothalamus we gave special attention to (a) method of fixation (Rossi 1975), (b) dissection of tissues (Bestetti and Rossi 1980), and (c) further processing (Rossi and Bestetti 1981; Bestetti et al. 1987). Among the functional in vitro techniques we recently developed and applied (d) a method to assay morphology and function of the mediobasal hypothalamus (Boujon et al. 1987) and (e) a method to assay the secretory function of isolated pituitary cells by reverse hemolytic plaque (Rossi et al. 1989). Both methods permit a reduction in the number of animals needed for an experiment and replacement of in vivo by in vitro investigations. Use of these methods (Boujon et al. 1987; Rossi et al. 1989; Bestetti et al. 1989) enables us to assess, in vitro in the same animal, both structure and function of the hypothalamus and hypophysis to identify multiple neuroendocrinological disturbances (Bestetti and Rossi 1988, 1990; Rossi and Bestetti 1990).

Method of Fixation

Perfusion fixation is the method of choice for most tissues, including those of the brain. We use an inexpensive perfusion system of simple construction which offers several advantages (Rossi 1975). It is suitable for rats of any age as well as for newborn swine, young dogs, rabbits, mice, and Chinese hamsters. The apparatus consists of pressurized containers for solutions, devices for pressurization and for measuring pressure, vinyl tubing, and needles and catheters to deliver solutions into the vascular bed (Fig. 177).

The system is schematized in Fig. 178. Two 1-l glass bottles with airtight screw stoppers contain the solutions. The first holds the rinsing fluid, the

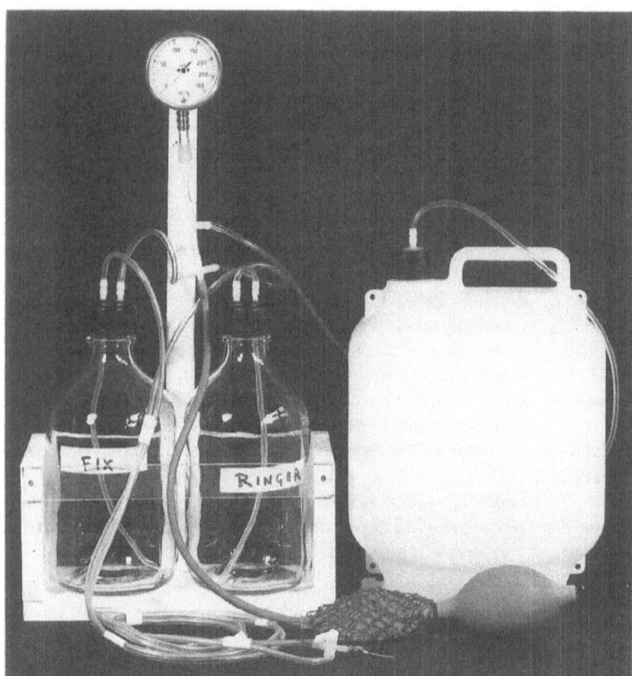

Fig. 177. Perfusion system apparatus

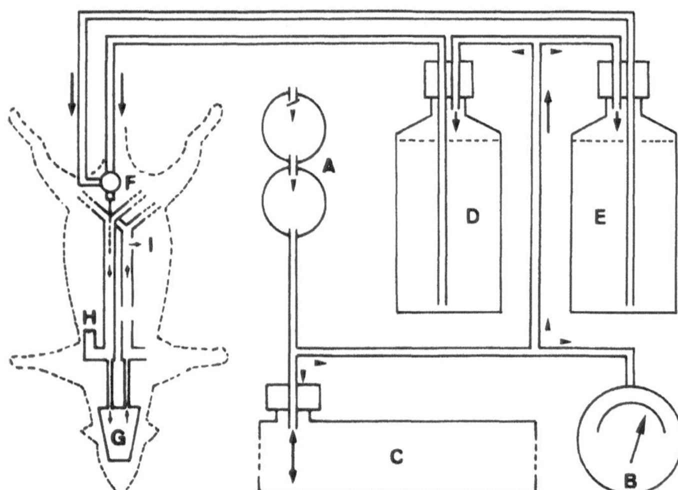

Fig. 178. Diagram of perfusion system. *A*, Rubber bulb syringe; *B*, manometer; *C*, pressurized buffer tank; *D*, bottle for Ringer's solution; *E*, bottle for fixative solution; *F*, three-way stopcock; *G*, brain with incoming carotis and outgoing jugularis; *H*, aortic semilunar valves; *I*, opening of abdominal cava

second the fixative. Each stopper is pierced by two holes (4 mm in diameter); two PVC connectors are inserted through these and cemented in place by araldite. One connector joins by mean of vinyl tubing the air space of each bottle with the pressure system. This consists of (a) a rubber bulb syringe, (b) a manometer, and (c) a 5-l plastic container as buffer tank. The second connector joins lengths of vinyl tubing, extending to the bottom of the bottles with lengths of this tubing (about 150 cm) connected at their outer ends to two arms of a three-way plastic stopcock. The third arm carries the needle with catheter for entering the abdominal aorta. Needles and catheters differ in outside diameter, depending on animal size. For adult rats we employ a truncated no. 1 hypodermic needle fitted with a 10-mm-long polyethylene microtube (PE90), tip cut at 45° (Fig. 179).

For operation one bottle is filled with Ringer's solution (pH 7.4), containing 0.1% procainhydrochloride and 0.0032% heparin, with which we

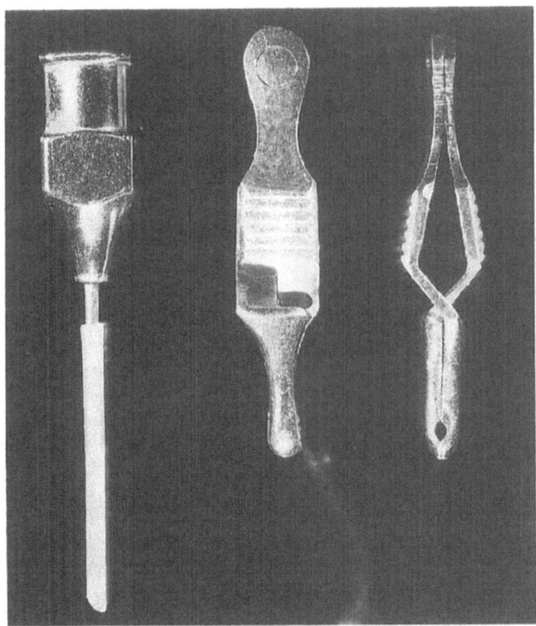

Fig. 179. Apparatus used to study lesions in rat hypothalamus. *Left*, perfusion needle and catheter; *center, right*, lateral and frontal view, respectively, of grooved clamp

rinse the blood out of the vascular system. The second bottle is filled with the fixative solution, consisting of 2% paraformaldehyde, 1.5% glutaraldehyde phosphate buffered to pH 7.4. Stoppers are screwed on tightly; the system is pressurized and freed of air bubbles by manipulation of the three-way stopcock. Afterwards the stopcock is turned to an intermediate position to prevent further loss of solutions, and pressure is raised to physiological level (adult rat 110–120 mmHg). Solutions are used at room temperature.

Under intraperitoneal ketamine hydrochloride anesthesia (20 mg $0.4\,ml^{-1}$ $100\,g^{-1}$ body wt.) the abdomen is opened, and viscera displaced until the aorta, and venae cavae are visible caudally from renal arteries. Then the aortic bifurcation is freed with rounded tipped forceps and the aorta closed with a rounded edged surgical clamp just caudal to the renal arteries. Subsequently the aorta is incised with fine scissors at the bifurcation and entered with the catheter to the level of the surgical clamp. The needle is then locked in place by means of a small grooved clamp (Fig. 179, center and right) and the surgical clamp at the renal arteries level is removed, thus reestablishing circulation. With the three-way stopcock correctly positioned, the Ringer's solution is admitted into the aorta at a pressure barely above physiological level to ensure flow against aortic blood pressure and to maintain the semilunar valves in closed position (Fig. 178, *H*). As the Ringer's solution starts to flow, the vena cava is cut open (Fig. 178, *I*), and rinsing is completed within 60 s. By repositioning of the stopcock the fixative solution is admitted, and fixation is achieved within 10 min. During this time a constant pressure is maintained. All organs, except lungs and those caudal to the point of needle insertion, are perfused. In particular, the fluids reach the brain via carotid arteries and leave via jugular veins (Fig. 178, *G*), thus assuring complete perfusion.

Subsequently the head skin is incised, the skull partially opened by small bone cutters avoiding damage to brain tissue. The head remains in the fixative solution for at least an additional 4 h.

Dissection of Tissues

Opening of the upper skull completed, the brain is gently lifted and removed from the head. During this operation the pituitary is held in

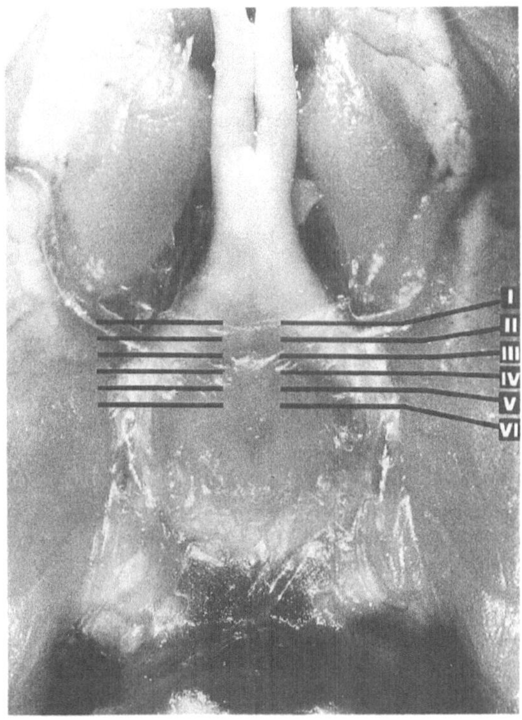

Fig. 180. Ventral view of brain with hypothalamic region. *Lines I–IV*, hypothalamic levels considered

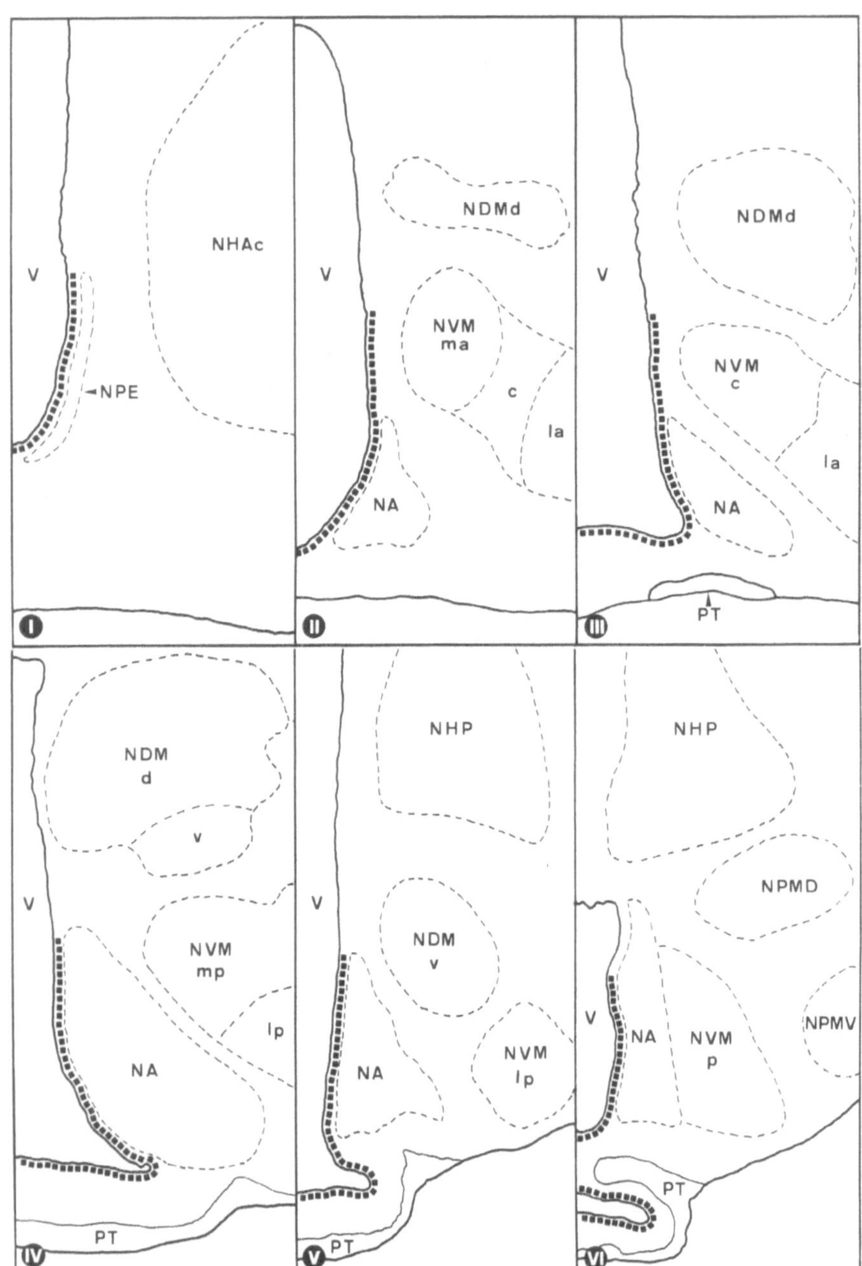

Fig. 181. Diagram of frontal sections through the hypothalamic region. *Section numbering I–VI*, in fronto-occipital direction. *NA*, Nucleus arcuatus; *NDMd*, nucleus dorsomedialis, pars dorsalis; *NDMv*, nucleus dorsomedialis, pars ventralis; *NHAc*, nucleus hypothalamicus anterior, pars caudalis; *NHP*, nucleus hypothalamicus posterior; *NPE*, nucleus periventricularis hypothalami; *NPMD*, nucleus premamillaris dorsalis; *NPMV*, nucleus premamillaris ventralis; *NVMc*, nucleus ventromedialis, pars centralis; *MVMla*, nucleus ventromedialis, pars lateralis anterior; *MVMlp*, nucleus ventromedialis, pars lateralis posterior; *MVMma*, nucleus ventromedialis, pars medialis anterior; *MVMmp*, nucleus ventromedialis, pars medialis posterior; *MVMp*, nucleus ventromedialis, pars posterior; *PT*, pars tuberalis hypophysis; *V*, third ventricle; heavy line, tanycytes. ×160 (Nomenclature according to Palkovits 1975)

position by the basal meninges. Consequently the pituitary stalk is disrupted at some distance from the infundibulum. During the dissection the tissue must be repeatedly moistened with fixative to avoid desiccation. The brain is placed on its dorsal surface under a stereomicroscope (5×)

with the hypothalamic region exposed (Fig. 180). A series of frontal sections is cut with a razor blade, free hand, perpendicular to the dorsal surface. The first section should be caudal to the optic chiasm, at the beginning of tractus opticus (Fig. 180, level 1), the last just after the beginning of the pituitary stalk (Fig. 180, level VI). In rats of about 250 g body wt. six sections can be obtained spaced at 400–500 μm. A block about 5 × 5 mm containing hypothalamus and median eminence is then cut from the basal portion of each section and numbered I–VI in fronto-occipital direction. In these six blocks we find a representative sample of most hypothalamic nuclei (Fig. 181; see also Palkovits 1975; and p. 121, this volume).

Processing of Tissues

Blocks used for morphological studies are postfixed in 2% OsO_4 solution (pH 7.4) for 2 h. Blocks used for immunohistochemistry are not postfixed. After dehydration in graded acetone tissues are infiltrated and embedded in Spurr's low-viscosity medium.

For light microscopy semithin sections are cut, and stained with toluidine blue, PAS, or other methods. Subsequently thin sections are cut from selected areas of the same blocks, stained for contrast with uranyl acetate and lead citrate, and studied under the electron microscope.

Immunohistochemical localization of releasing hormones and regulatory polypeptides in hypothalamus and median eminence can be performed on semithin and thin sections for light and electron microscopy, respectively. Semithin sections are pretreated with Mayor's reagent (Mayor et al. 1961) to partially remove the polymerized resin. Among others, we have localized luteinizing hormone-releasing hormone (LHRH; Fig. 182a), thyrotropin-releasing hormone (TRH; Fig. 182b), corticotropin-releasing factor (CRF; Fig. 182c), somatostatin (SRIF; Fig. 182d), tyrosine hydroxylase (TH; Fig. 182e), and β-endorphin (β-END; Fig. 182f). The primary antibodies were rabbit anti-synthetic LHRH (Bio-Makor, Rehovot, Israel) diluted 1:400, 1 h incubation, rabbit anti-rat TRH 1:1000 and rabbit anti-rat CRF 1:400 (both provided by C. Oliver, Université d'Aix-Marseille, France), overnight incubation, rat anti-human SRIF (DAKO, Carpinteria, CA) 1:200, 1 h incubation, rat anti-bovine TH (Eugene Tech International, Ramsey, NJ) used at the original dilution, overnight incubation, and rabbit anti-human β-END (UCB-Bioproducts, Braine L'Alleud, Belgium) 1:200, 1 h incubation. The link serum for peroxidase-antiperoxidase (PAP) reaction (Sternberger et al. 1970) was diluted 1:20, the PAP complex 1:100, 1 h incubation, the alkaline phosphatase conjugate (Bestetti et al. 1987) 1:60 to 1:100, 1 h incubation. For specificity control primary antisera were substituted with normal rabbit serum or were preadsorbed with the specific antigen.

Reagents

Glutaraldehyde-Paraformaldehyde Fixative

Solutions (stock)

1. Potassium phosphate-buffer (concentrated)
   - KH_2PO_4 0.4 *M* 54.44 g/1000 ml H_2O, 18 parts
   - $K_2HOP_4 \cdot 3H_2O$ 0.4 *M* 91.29 g/1000 ml H_2O, 82 parts
   - pH 7.4
   - To be diluted 1:10 before use
2. Glutaraldehyde 25% (as commercially available)
3. Paraformaldehyde 15%
   - Paraformaldehyde 15 g
   - H_2O dest. 100 ml
   - Heat but do not boil (60°–70°C) and stir constantly; add paraformaldehyde slowly
   - Add 1 ml 1 *N* NaOH while stirring to help clear solution; cool solution with running cold water
4. $CaCl_2$ 1%
   - Fixative
   - Solution 1 (diluted 1:10!), 820 ml
   - Solution 2, 80 ml
   - Solution 3, 100 ml
   - Solution 4, 3 ml
   - pH 7.2–7.4

Buffer Solution for Tissue Rinsing

Solutions (Stock)

1. Buffer
   - 2,4,6-trimethylpyridin ($C_8H_{11}N$), 2.66 ml
   - 1 *N* HCl, 9.00 ml
   - H_2O dest. ad., 100.00 ml
   - pH 7.4
2. NaCl 3.4%
   - Ready-to-use buffer
   - Solution 1, 88.00 ml
   - Solution 2, 12.00 ml

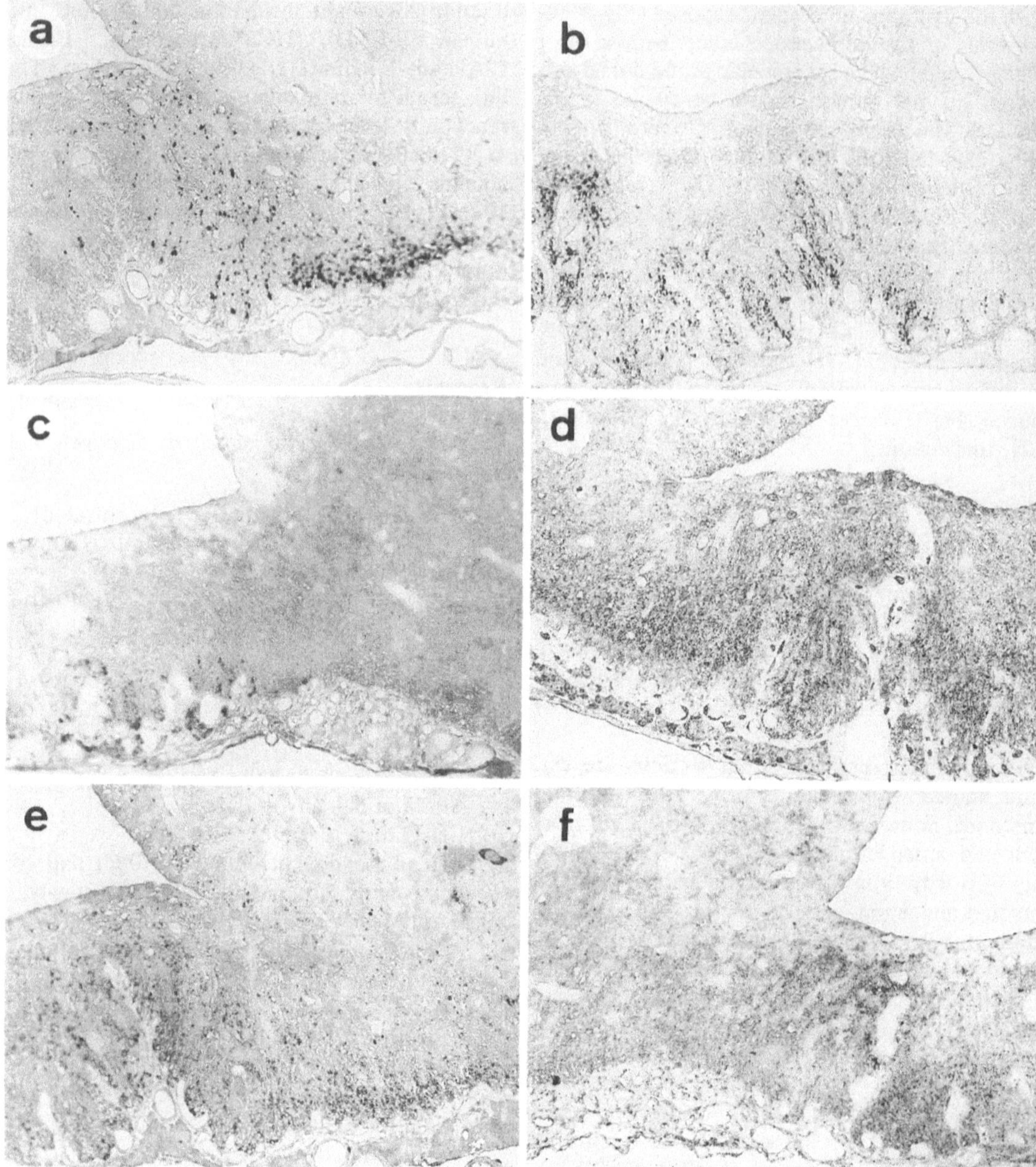

Fig. 182. Immunohistochemical Localization of LHRH (**a**), TRH (**b**), CRF (**c**), SRIF (**d**), TH (**e**), and β-END (**f**) in sections taken at level III. Semithin sections. PAP or alkaline phosphatase reaction. ×330

Osmium Tetroxide Fixative (2%)
Solutions (stock)

1. Buffer
   - 2,4,6-trimethylpyridin ($C_8H_{11}N$), 2.66 ml
   - 1 *N* HCl, 9.00 ml
   - H_2O dest. ad., 100.00 ml
   - pH 7.4
2. NaCl 3.4%
3. Diluting solution for osmium
   - Solution 1 6.0 ml Solution 2 4.0 ml 4. OsO_4 4%
   - Fixative
   - Solution 3, 1 part
   - Solution 4, 1 part

Mayor's. Cut 2.5 g metallic sodium into cubes 1/8 in. or less on a side and drop piece into 25 ml methyl alcohol in a hood or well-ventilated area (exothermic reaction, danger of fire!). Solution of the sodium to form sodium methoxide is more rapid at 50°–60°C. During the process the level of solution must be maintained at 25 ml by adding alcohol to compensate for evaporation. When sodium is dissolved, add an equal volume of benzene. After a phase boundary is seen, addi-

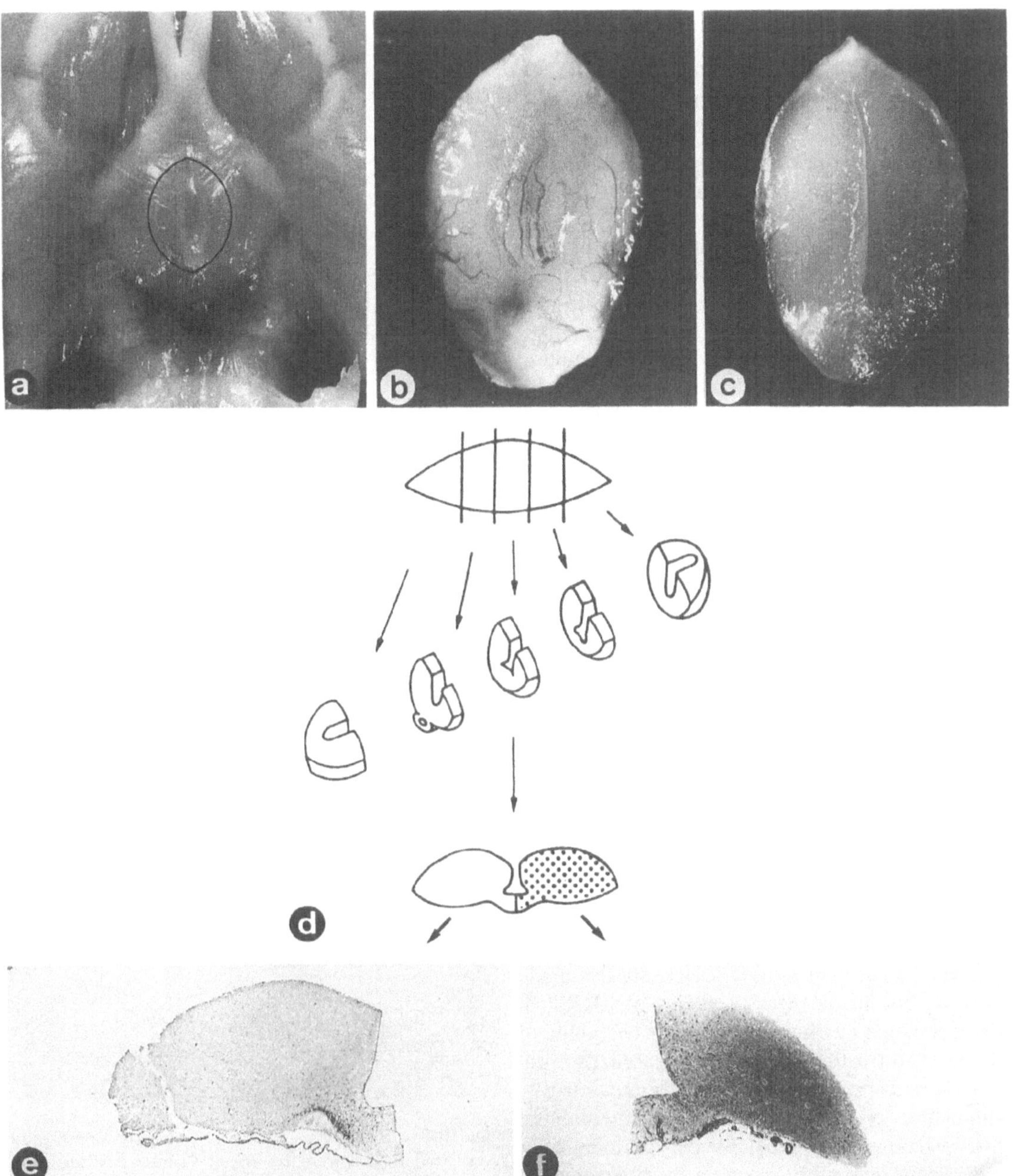

Fig. 183a–f. Hypothalamus isolation. **a** Ventral view of the brain with the limits of the specimen. **b** Ventral view of the specimen. **c** Dorsal view of the specimen. **d** Three-dimensional drawing of the hypothalamic sections. **e,f** Semithin sections. **e** Left half not postfixed, anti-LHRH, alkaline phosphatase method. **f** Right half postifxed, toluidine blue staining, ×53 (Boujon et al. 1987)

tional methyl alcohol must be added until the resulting mixture is clear. Store the stock solution in a dark bottle and use it as solvent for cured epoxy resins diluted in a mixture of methyl alcohol/benzene 50:50.

Suggested Dilution for Semithin Sections

- Mayor's solution, 1 part
- Methyl alcohol/benzene, 1 part
- Apply for 15 min

Method to Assay the Morphology and Function of the Mediobasal Hypothalamus

The techniques of explant preparation, in vitro incubation, and further processing are extensively described by Boujon et al. (1987) and Bestetti et al. 1989 (Figs. 183, 184).
After decapitation of the rat the mediobasal hypothalamus is isolated under a stereomicroscope, put in a flask containing 0.5 ml HEPES-buffered Locke's medium, gassed by 5 ml/min O_2/CO_2 (95%/5%), and shaken in a water bath at 37°C. After a 10-min washing the medium is changed twice at an interval of 20 min. After the in vitro incubation the tissue is determined by light and electron-microscopic analysis to be satisfactorily preserved. Microtubing which connected syringes to the tissue vial is used to withdraw medium samples or add stimulatory, inhibitory, or fixative solutions. Hormones are then measured in the medium by radioimmunoassay, and morphometric and densitometric measurements are made on tissue sections.

Data Obtained by This Method. As an example of results obtained by this method we summarize the data of a study (Boujon et al. 1987) on the in vitro LHRH release from the mediobasal hypothalamus of 3-month-old male Sprague-Dawley rats and subsequent morphological studies made on the same tissue. Measurements of LHRH in the incubation medium, 30 min after beginning of the in vitro treatment, indicate a stabilized basal LHRH secretion and a markedly increased K^+-stimulated LHRH release from the mediobasal hypothalamus (Fig. 185). By conventional light microscopy on semithin sections the tissue may be seen to be free of artifacts (Fig. 186a). By light-microscopic immunohistochemistry LHRH and other releasing factors may be demonstrated (Fig. 186b,c). Electron-microscopic study of the same

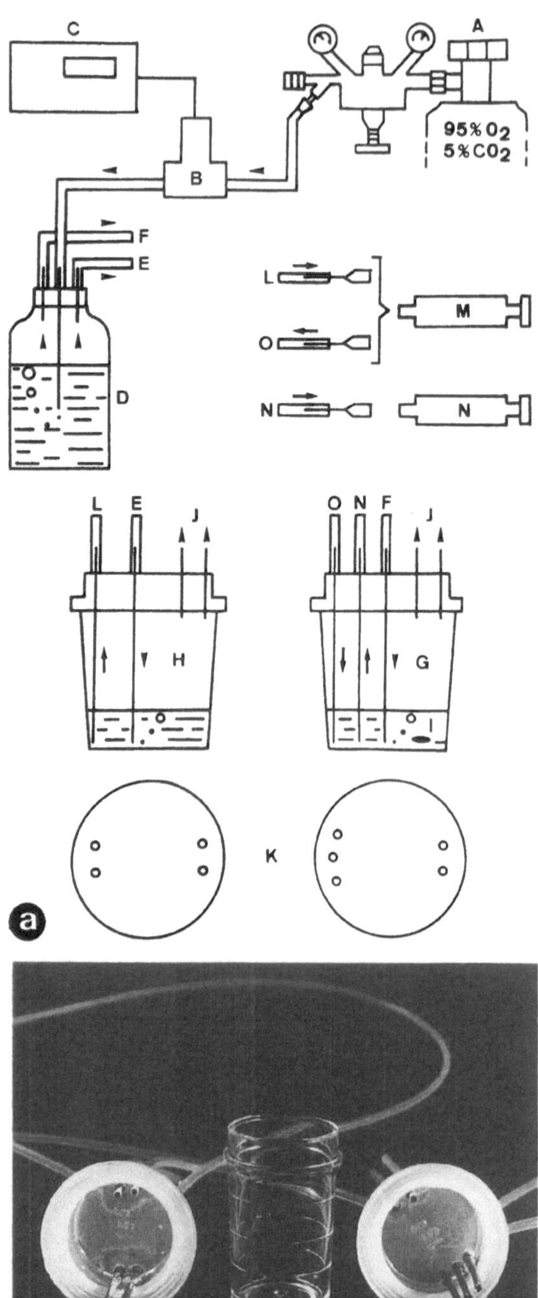

Fig. 184. **a** Incubation system. *A*, Gas bottle and pressure regulator; *B*, mass flow controller; *C*, mass flow reader; *D*, humidification bottle; *E,F*, tubes to the chambers; *G*, incubation chamber; *H*, medium reserve chamber; *I*, hypothalamic specimen; *J*, gas outlet; *K*, position of the needle segments in the stopper; *L,M,N,O*, silicon capillaries and syringes. **b** Stopper of the medium reserve chamber (*left*), incubation chamber (*middle*), and stopper of the incubation chamber (*right*). (Boujon et al. 1987)

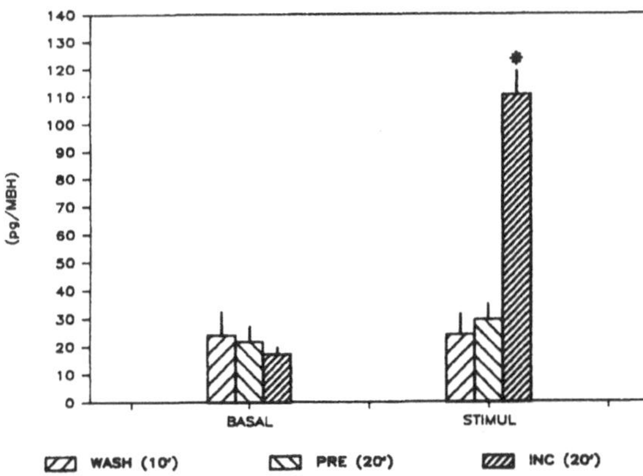

Fig. 185. LHRH secretion from the in vitro incubated mediobasal hypothalamus. $*p < 0.001$ vs. preincubation medium of experiment (*stimul*) and incubation medium of experiment (*basal*). In the incubation medium of experiment *stimul* the K^+ concertration was raised to 61.6 m*M*.

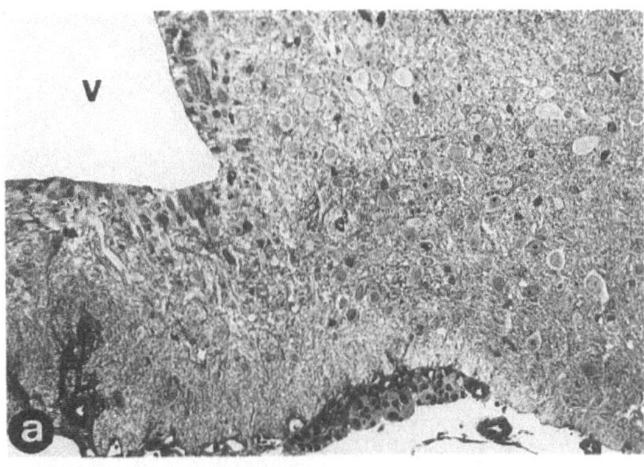

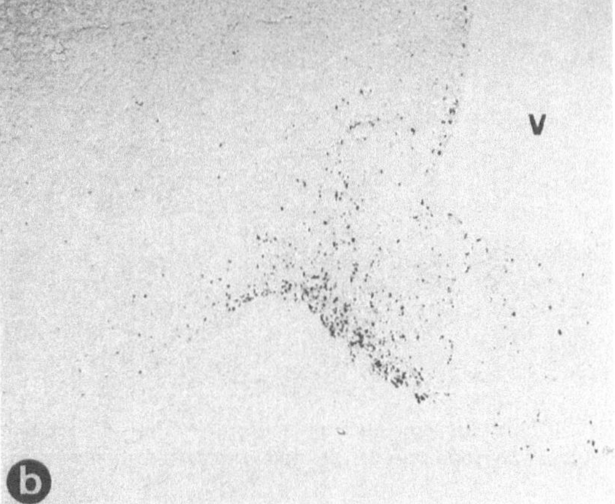

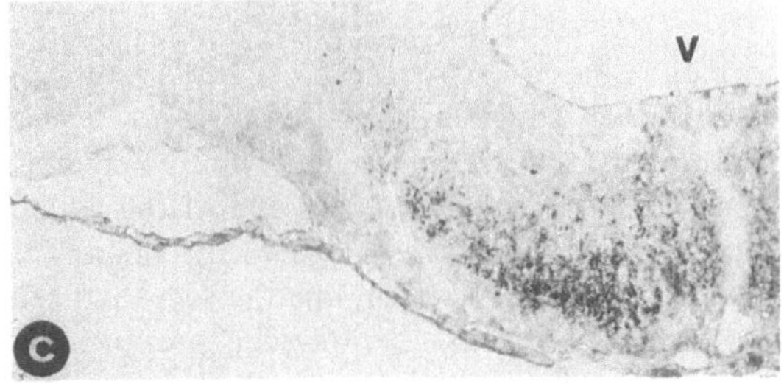

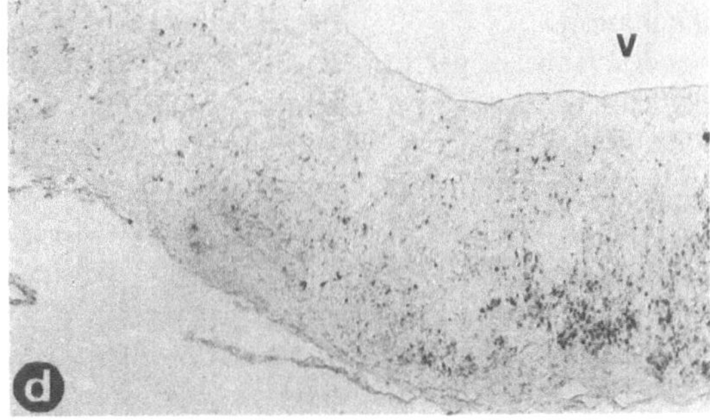

Fig. 186. a Postfixed tissue, semithin section, toluidine blue staining. **b–d** Not postfixed tissue, semithin sections. **b** Anti-LHRH alkaline phosphatase method. **c** Anti-SRIF PAP method. **d** Anti-TRH alkaline phosphatase method. *v*, Third ventricle. ×210. (Boujon et al. 1987)

median eminence explant permits identification of neurons and secretory granules in axon cross-sections (Fig. 187a,b). Moreover, LHRH granules may be labeled by the immunogold method (Fig. 187c). Our hypothalamic model is useful to make combined functional and morphological in vitro studies of the isolated mediobasal hypothalamus. This method warrants the two conditions: (a) the tissue must be well preserved, free of morphological artifacts and functionally unimpaired until the end of the in vitro incubation, and (b) the tissue must be processed for morphology in optimal settings.

Method to Assay the Secretory Function of Isolated Pituitary Cells by Reverse Hemolytic Plaque

The technique of the reverse hemolytic plaque assay is described by Rossi et al. (1989) and Bestetti et al. (1989). After decapitation the pituitary gland is isolated and the posterior lobe removed under a stereomicroscope and discarded. The adenohypophyseal tissue is fragmented, trypsinized for 1 h, centrifuged twice, and resuspended in saline. After cell viability is assessed, equal amounts of the final cell suspension and of protein A-coupled sheep erythrocytes are put into an observation chamber and incubated for 1 h at 37°C to allow the formation of a monolayer. After adding the antibodies (e.g., 50 µl antiluteinizing

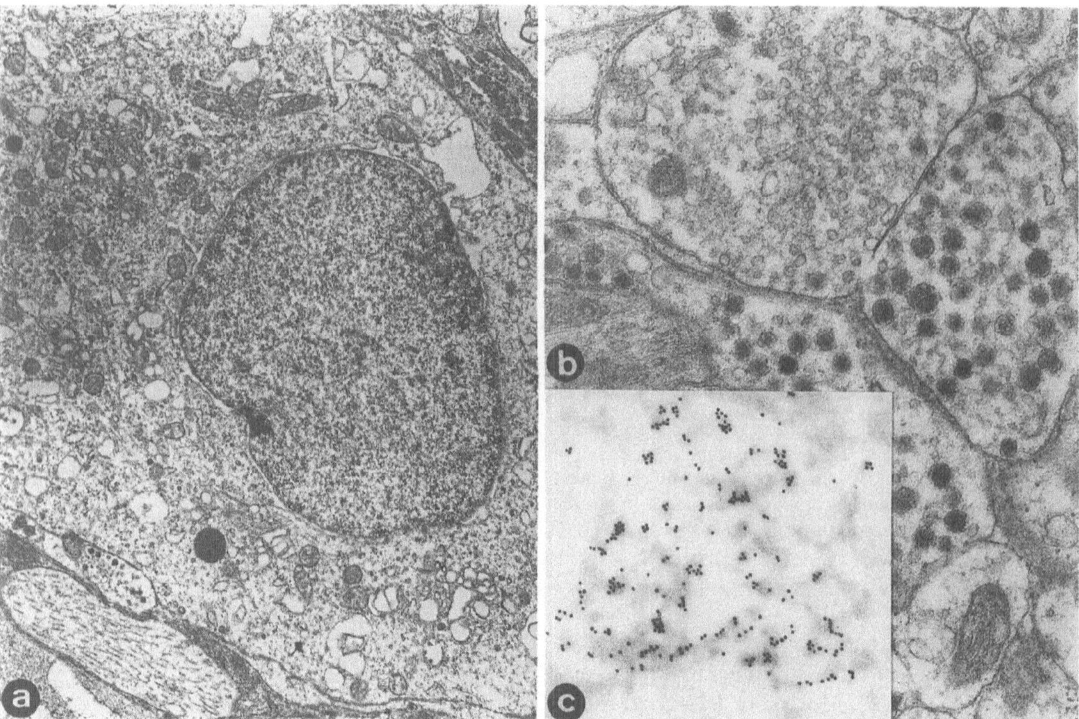

Fig. 187. a Arcuate nucleus neuron. ×8360. **b** Median eminence neuropil with vesicle- and granule-containing axons. ×27 060. **c** Intraaxonal granules positive to anti-LHRH, colloidal gold method. ×27 060. (Boujon et al. 1987)

hormone diluted 1:200 with 1.8% NaCl solution) the chamber is further incubated for 2 h.

The combination of antigen [e.g., luteinizing hormone (LH)] secreted by a cell and of the added antibody, and complement causes the hemolysis of the erythrocytes surrounding the secreting cell (Fig. 188). The area of hemolysis is proportional to the amount of antigen secreted during the incubation.

Several tests are performed to establish the specificity of the assay, for example, the stimulation with releasing factors. Three hours after adding LHRH (10^{-10}) into the chamber the secretion of luteinizing hormone is increased ($p < 0.05$) by almost 60% (Fig. 189a,b).

Data Obtained by This Method. After incubation with the antibodies the slide-chamber complex may be immersed and kept overnight in fixative solution, the cover glasses removed, and the cells stained immunocytochemically by the PAP method for the various hormones to be studied (Fig. 189c,d). Measurements are made of the area of immunoreactive plaque-forming and non-

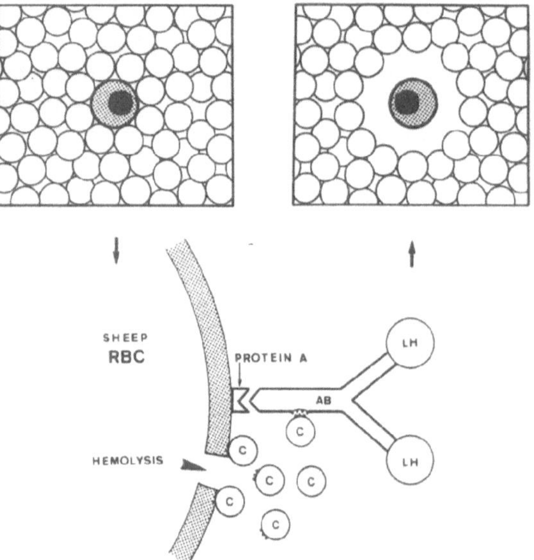

Fig. 188. Schematic drawing of the plaque formation. *Above*, a pituitary cell in an erythrocyte monolayer before (*left*) and after (*right*) the hemolytic plaque formation. *AB*, Rabbit anti-LH antibody; *c*, complement. (Bestetti et al. 1989)

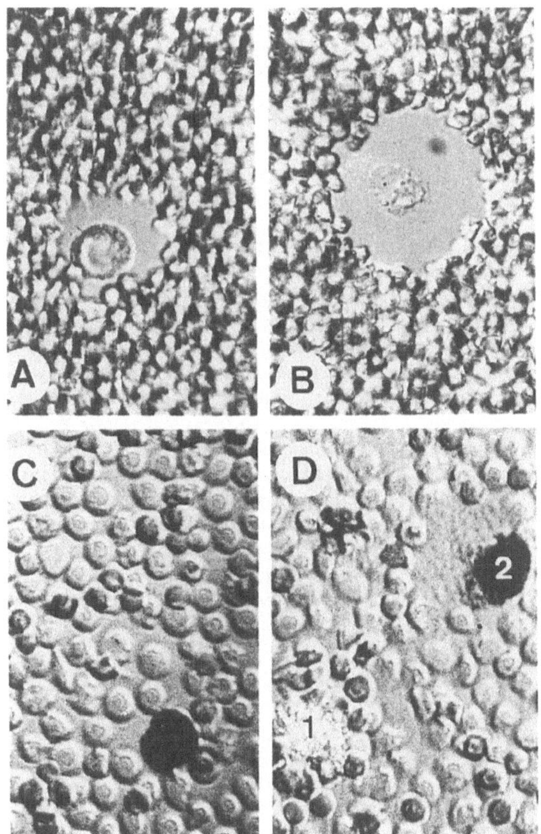

Fig. 189. Example of an LH-plaque in basal conditions (**a**) and after LHRH stimulation (**b**). Fresh preparations, interference-contrast microscopy. ×1000. LH plaques after immunocytochemistry: a labeled but non-plaque-forming cell (**c**), an unlabeled cell (**d**, *1*), and a plaque-forming cell (**d**, *2*). ×1300. (Rossi and Bestetti 1990)

plaque-forming cells and the plaque area. The ratio of immunoreactive plaque-forming to non plaque-forming cells is calculated. After cell reembedding (Rossi et al. 1979) hormone immunogold-labeling may also be performed for electron-microscopic studies (Fig. 190a,b).

Acknowledgements. This research was supported in part by the Swiss National Science Foundation (grants 3.034-0.84, 3.028-0.87, 3.659-0.87), Swiss Federal Veterinary Board (Bundesamt für Veterinärwesen, Grant 014.89.4), and Berne University Foundation for Research Promotion (Hochschulstiftung, grants 11.6.1985, 23.3.1986, 26.6.1987, 15.6.1988, 13.6.1989).

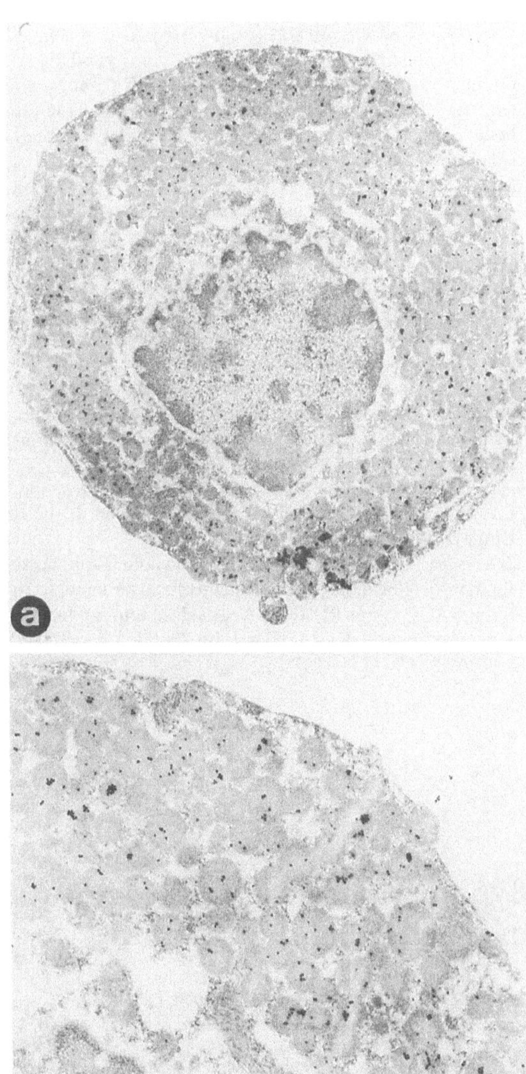

Fig. 190. Electron-microscopic immunogold anti-LH labeling of a plaque-forming cell after embedding. TEM; **a**, ×6000; **b**, ×13 500

References

Bestetti GE, Rossi GL (1980) Hypothalamic lesions in rats with longterm streptozotocin-induced diabetes mellitus. Acta Neuropathol (Berl) 52:119–127

Bestetti GE, Rossi GL (1988) Neuroendocrine changes in experimentally diabetic rats. In: Shafrir E, Renold AE (eds) Frontiers in diabetes research. Lessons from animal diabetes. II. Libbey, London, pp 444–452

Bestetti GE, Rossi GL (1990) Effect of diabetes on functional and morphological complications in the hypothalamo-pituitary system of diabetic rodent models. A pathogenetic overview. In: Shafrir E, Renold AE (eds) Frontiers in diabetes research. Lessons from animal diabetes III. Libbey, London, pp 466–470

Bestetti GE, Junker U, Locatelli V, Rossi GL (1987) Continuous subtherapeutic insulin counteracts hypothalamo-pituitary-gonadal alterations in diabetic rats. Diabetes 36: 1315–1319

Bestetti GE, Boujon CE, Tontis K, Forster U, Grimm S, Rossi GL (1989) Méthodes alternatives: développement et utilisation de deux modèles "in vitro" pour des études endocriniennes. Schweiz Arch Tierheilkd 131:537–545

Boujon CE, Bestetti GE, Raymond MJ, Rossi GL (1987) A model for combined morphological and functional investigations on the isolated mediobasal rat hypothalamus. Neuroendocrinology 45:311–317

Mayor HD, Hampton JC, Rosario B (1961) A simple method for removing the resin from epoxy-embedded tissue. J Biophysiol Biochem Cytol 9:909–910

Palkovits M (1975) Isolated removal of hypothalamic nuclei for neuroendocrinological and neurochemical studies. In: Stumpf WE, Grant LD (eds) Anatomical neuroendocrinology: proceedings. Karger, Basel, pp 72–80

Rossi GL (1975) Simple apparatus for perfusion fixation for electron microscopy. Experientia 31:998–1000

Rossi GL, Bestetti G (1981) Morphological changes in the hypothalamic-hypophyseal-gonadal axis of male rats after twelve months of streptozotocin-induced diabetes. Diabetologia 21:476–481

Rossi GL, Bestetti GE (1990) In vitro assessment of functional and morphological complications in the hypothalamo-pituitary system of diabetic rodent models. In: Shafrir E, Renold AE (eds) Frontiers in diabetes research. Lessons from animal diabetes. III. Libbey, London, pp 471–474

Rossi GL, Luginbühl H, Probst D (1979) A method for ultrastructural study of lesions found in conventional histological sections. Virchows Arch [A] 350:216–224

Rossi GL, Bestetti GE, Tontis DK, Varini M (1989) Reverse hemolytic plaque assay study of luteinizing and follicle-stimulating hormone and thyrotropin secretion in diabetic rat pituitary glands. Diabetes 38:1301–1306

Sternberger LA, Hardy PH Jr, Cuculis JJ, Meyer HG (1970) The unlabeled antibody enzyme method of immunohistochemistry: preparation and properties of soluble antigen-antibody complex (horseradish peroxidase-antihorseradish peroxidase) and its use in identification of spirochetes. J Histochem Cytochem 18:315–333

Hypothalamic-Pituitary Lesions Associated with Diabetes and Aging, Rat

Gilberto E. Bestetti and Giovanni L. Rossi

Introduction

Numerous studies demonstrate that changes in the mediobasal hypothalamus are common in several animal models for diabetes mellitus (Bestetti et al. 1990; Bestetti and Rossi 1988) and aging (Bestetti et al. 1991; Rossi et al. 1992). The alterations in the mediobasal hypothalamus are associated with multiple dysfunctions of the anterior pituitary gland and of its target organs. These neuroendocrinopathies are not only diabetes- or aging-associated disorders but possibly a main component of each of the two conditions (Bestetti et al. 1990; Bestetti and Rossi 1988). We summarize here the results of some of our recent studies on the neuroendocrinopathies of old rats and streptozotocin-induced diabetic rats (Bestetti and Rossi 1982, 1988).

Material and Methods

The diabetes studies were performed on male streptozotocin-diabetic (Wistar and Sprague-Dawley) and corresponding control rats. Diabetes lasted 1 month. Three- and 23-month old female Long-Evans rats were used for the aging studies. Some experiments were terminated by whole body perfusion and the tissues processed for morphological study, as described previously (Rossi and Bestetti 1983; Bestetti et al. 1987a). In other experiments in vivo or in vitro tests were performed (Boujon et al. 1987; Bestetti et al. 1985, 1989a; Rossi et al. 1989), or tissues were homogenated for plasma hormone determination by radioimmunoassay (Bestetti et al. 1985, 1987) or fluorimetric immunoassay (Bestetti et al. 1989b). For in vitro studies the animals were decapitated, and the tissue was processed as described previously (Bestetti et al. 1985, 1987b; see p. 42, this volume).

Results

Hypothalamic-Pituitary-Gonadal Axis in Streptozotocin-Diabetic Rats. Hypothalamus. Striking light- and electron-microscopic degenerative changes were seen in the arcuate nucleus, median eminence, and tanycytes (Bestetti and Rossi 1980). In particular, vacuoles were observed by light microscopy (Fig. 191A,B), which by electron microscopy were seen as swollen, degenerate axon cross-sections (Bestetti et al. 1985; Bestetti and Rossi 1980; Fig. 191C–G). Since these alterations occurred in a region of the median eminence rich in neurosecretory axons, and our rats had macroscopically visible testicular atrophy, we assumed that the two changes were causally related. This assumption was confirmed by the following immunocytochemical findings: (a) intra-axonal luteinizing hormone releasing hormone (LHRH) accumulation in degenerate axons in the median eminence, by light microscopy, and (b) abnormal morphology of LHRH granules in normal axons, by electron microscopy (Rossi and Bestetti 1981). Furthermore, the plasma luteinizing hormone response to naloxone-stimulated endogenous LHRH secretion was lower in diabetic than in control rats (Bestetti et al. 1985). This reduced LHRH secretion is possibly caused by lesions in the median eminence with consequent accumulation of morphologically abnormal LHRH (Rossi and Bestetti 1981). Comparable findings were obtained by functional and morphological studies of the in vitro LHRH release from the mediobasal hypothalamus of diabetic and control animals (Bestetti et al. 1989). In fact the measurement of LHRH in the incubation medium showed a markedly reduced K^+-stimulated LHRH release from the mediobasal hypothalamus of streptozotocin-diabetic rats (Fig. 192A). The light-microscopic immunodensitometry performed on tissue sections from explants from the median eminence indicated that the amount of labeled LHRH (total immunoreactivity) was reduced in axon cross-sections of diabetic compared with control rats and that after K^+ stimulation the total immunoreactivity was lower in control and increased in diabetic rats (Fig. 192B). The electron microscopic study of the same explants of the

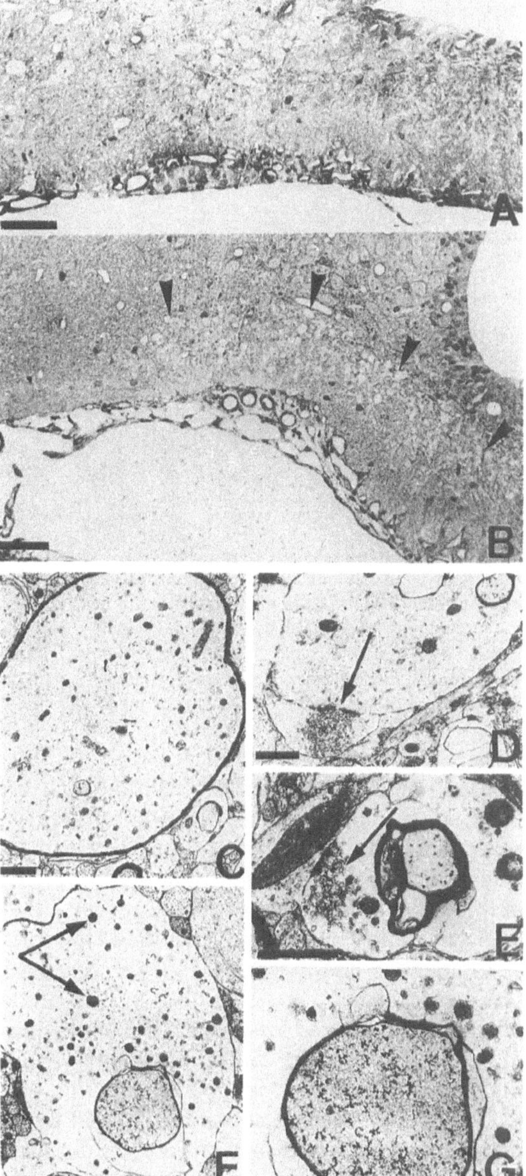

Fig. 191. Semithin section of the mediobasal hypothalamus (*MBA*) of a control (**A**) and STZ-diabetic (**B**) rat. **B** Several vacuoles can be observed in the middle layer of the median eminence. ×300; *bar*, 50 µm. Electron micrographs of the ME of a diabetic rat (**C–G**). Swollen myelinated axon cross-section (**C**); swollen unmyelinated axon cross-sections carry post- (**C**) and presynaptic (**D**) structures, neurosecretory granules (**E**, *arrow*), and glycogen-containing bodies (**F,G**) **C,D,F**, ×7000; **E**, ×13000; **G**, ×16000; *bar*, 1 µm). (**A,B** From Bestetti and Rossi 1990; **C–G** from Bestetti et al. 1985)

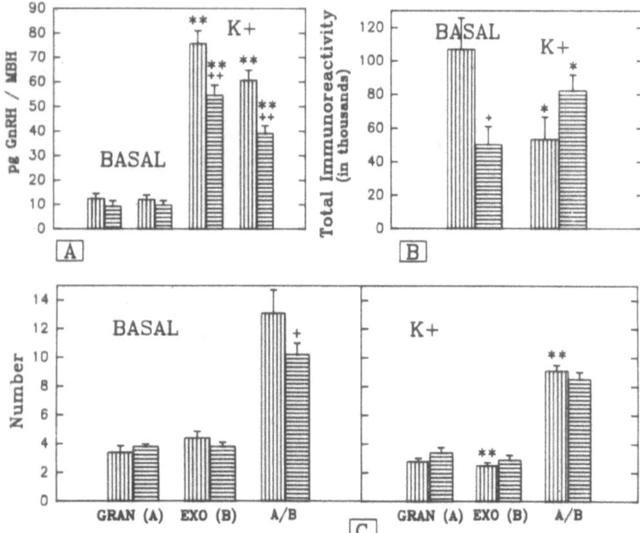

Fig. 192A–C. Results of a study on gonadotropin-releasing hormone (*GNRH*) secretion after incubation in basal or high K^+ medium of mediobasal hypothalamus (*MBA*) explants from control (*horizontal hatch*) and diabetic (*vertical hatch*) male rats. **A** GNRH secretion during two consecutive incubation periods in each medium. **B** Densitometrical study of immunoreactive GNRH in the median eminence. **C** Electron-microscopic morphometry on axon cross-sections from the median eminence, as seen in Fig. 193. *GRAN (A)*, Number of secretory granules; *EXO (B)*, number of exocytoses (×10); *A/B*, ratio of A to B. (From Rossi and Bestetti 1990)

median eminence permitted identification of secretory granules and exocytoses in axon cross-sections. The morphometric study of the electron-microscopic images obtained from the lower part of the explants of median eminence revealed that after incubation under basal conditions the ratio of number of secretory granules to exocytoses was reduced in diabetic rats (Fig. 192C). This study pointed out that the releasable LHRH pool seems to be exhausted in the control mediobasal hypothalamus because of long-term stimulation, and to be reduced in the diabetic mediobasal hypothalamus because of diabetes. To ascertain whether not only the LHRH secretion but also the synthesis of this polypeptide is affected by diabetes we studied the neuroendocrinologically important yet relatively poorly described preoptic area, the preoptic medial nucleus with its sexually dimorphic area, and the suprachiasmatic nucleus in particular (Bestetti et al. 1987a). The neurons of these nuclei were atrophic in diabetic animals. We therefore concluded that in addition to a defective secretion the LHRH synthesis and regulation could also be impaired by diabetes and thus be responsible for the pituitary disorders, testicular atrophy, and lack of preovulatory luteinizing hormone surges (Bestetti et al. 1987a).

Pituitary Gland. The pituitary gonadotropes were atrophic, degenerate, or hyperplastic (Bestetti et al. 1985; Rossi and Bestetti 1981; Pitton et al. 1987). By means of the reverse hemolytic plaque assay (Rossi et al. 1989) the luteinizing hormone and follicle-stimulating hormone secreting cells of diabetic rats released less hormone and were less numerous than the corresponding cells of control rats. By comparing the areas of diabetic plaques and cells expressed as percentage of the corresponding control means we found that the plaque area was more severely reduced than the cell area (Fig. 193). Despite the smaller but more numerous immunoreactive gonadotropes the plasma luteinizing and follicle-stimulating hormone levels were therefore reduced.

Testis. The reduced cross-section surface of testicular seminiferous tubules (Pitton et al. 1987) and the less numerous and degenerate Leydig's cells (Rossi and Bestetti 1981) may possibly be consequent to the pituitary lesions. The Leydig's cell changes are responsible for the low testosterone secretion (Bestetti et al. 1987a). The gonadal axis changes can be prevented by subtherapeutic doses of insulin; thus these impairments appear to be consequent to the fall of insulin below a critical plasma level and are not

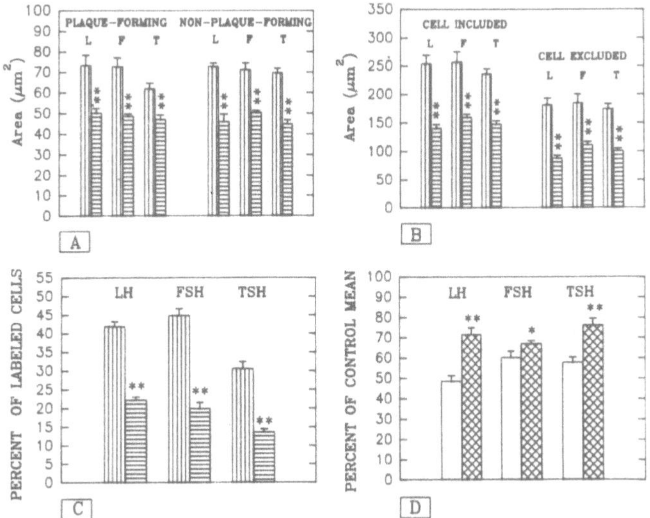

Fig. 193A–D. Morphometrical data of RHPA on pituitary cells from control (*horizontal hatch*) and STZ-diabetic (*vertical hatch*) male rats. The area of LH, FSH, and TSH immunoreactive plaque-forming and non-plaque-forming cells (**A**), the areas of the plaques (**B**), and the number of plaque-forming cells per hundred labeled cells (**C**) are reduced in diabetic rats. The percentage of control mean of diabetic plaque area (*empty bars*) is lower than the percentage of control mean of diabetic cell area (*cross-hatched bars*; **D**). (From Rossi and Bestetti 1990)

due to streptozotocin toxicity (Paz and Homonnai 1979; Bestetti et al. 1987b).

Hypothalamic-Pituitary-Thyroid Axis in Streptozotocin-Induced Diabetic Rats. Hypothalamus. Axonal lesions but no thyrotropin-releasing hormone (TRH) accumulation was observed in the median eminence region, site of axons containing thyrotropin releasing hormone (Bestetti et al. 1987a). Hypothyroidism, possibly of central origin, however, has been described in diabetic rats (Bestetti et al. 1987a,b). Consequently we also studied functional and morphological aspects of the in vitro TRH release from the isolated mediobasal hypothalamus in diabetic and control animals and demonstrated impaired TRH secretion (Bestetti et al. 1989). The measurement of TRH in the incubation medium showed a significantly reduced basal TRH release from the mediobasal hypothalamus of streptozotocin-induced diabetic rats during both basal incubations (Fig. 194). In depolarizing conditions the release of TRH was reduced during the second incubation in control and in diabetic rats during both incubations (Fig. 194A). Despite the reduced release the amount of labeled THR (total immunoreactivity) in axon cross-sections was higher in the stimulated diabetic mediobasal hypothalamus compared with both stimulated control and basal diabetic mediobasal hypothalamus by immunodensitometry (Fig. 194B). In addition, the stimulated diabetic mediobasal hypothalamus acquired an increased total area of immunoreactive TRH (Bestetti et al. 1989). This demonstrated impaired in vitro TRH secretion without reduced content of TRH in the diabetic mediobasal hypothalamus. These findings may explained by a possibly K^+-stimulated TRH transport toward the axon terminals not associated with increased release of the hormone. It must be mentioned that our antiserum recognized only mature TRH. "Extended forms" possibly "intermediate in the TRH biosynthesis," demonstrated by Lechan et al. (1987) to be abundant in the median eminence of normal rats, could be present in a large amount in the hypothalamus of diabetic rats. One could therefore speculate that increased "immature" TRH is present in the diabetic mediobasal hypothalamus, and that K^+ induces further processing of these molecules to the mature immunoreactive form. Indeed, in the diabetic hypothalamus the total area of immunoreactive TRH increases after K^+ stimulation. Depolarizing conditions may induce mature TRH immunoreactivity in median eminence regions, which under basal conditions do not contain this immunoreactive hormone.

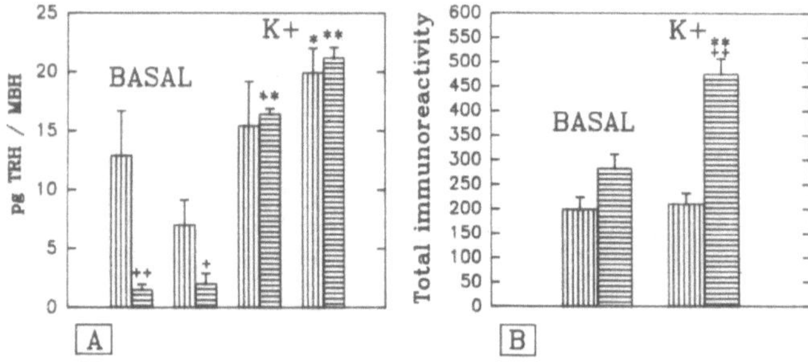

Fig. 194A,B. Results of a study on thyrotropin-releasing hormone (*TRH*) secretion after incubation in basal or high K^+ medium of mediobasal hypothalamus (*MBA*) explants from control (*horizontal hatch*) and STZ-diabetic (*vertical hatch*) male rats. **A** TRH secretion during two consecutive incubation periods in each medium. **B** Densitometrical study of immunoreactive TRH in the median eminence. (From Rossi and Bestetti 1990)

Pituitary Gland. We also investigated by reverse hemolytic plaque assay the thyroid-stimulating hormone release from thyrotropes of control and diabetic rats (Rossi et al. 1989). The results were similar to those obtained from the gonadotropes (Fig. 193). The lower plasma TRH level of diabetic rats (Bestetti et al. 1987c), despite the smaller but more numerous immunoreactive thyrotropes, is therefore due to these changes, which in turn are due to the low TRH secretion.
Thyroid Gland. The low plasma thyroid stimulating hormone levels are responsible for the severe thyroid changes that we found in diabetic rats (Bestetti et al. 1987b): (a) smaller follicles, (b) flattened follicular epithelium, (c) low intracolloidal and intraepithelial thyroglobulin, and in turn (d) low triiodothyronine and thyroxine.

Hypothalamic-Pituitary-Gonadal Axis in Aging Rats. Age-related functional and morphological alterations in the hypothalamic-pituitary-gonadal axis were investigated in old recurrently pseudopregnant female rats. As control animals we used young diestrous rats (Bestetti et al. 1991). The LHRH in the median eminence and mediobasal hypothalamus as well as plasma follicle-stimulating hormone, luteinizing hormone, and progesterone were measured by radioimmunoassay. LHRH in the lateral median eminence as well as pituitary follicle-stimulating hormone and luteinizing hormone were evaluated by morphometry and densitometric immunocytochemistry. Furthermore, by light microscopy we classified and counted the number of ovarian follicles and corpora lutea (Bestetti et al. 1991). The LHRH concentration in the median eminence and mediobasal hypothalamus was similar in old and young rats, whereas in old rats plasma follicle-stimulating hormone was markedly increased, luteinizing hormone was moderately increased, and progesterone was unchanged. The number and the total area and immunoreactivity of LHRH-labeled axon cross-sections in the lateral median eminence were reduced in old rats (Table 7). The number of nucleated follicle-stimulating hormone-labeled cells and the total labeled area and immunoreactivity were almost double in old compared with young animals (Table 8). The measurements of cells labeled with luteinizing hormone were not different between the two groups. In old rats the

Table 7. Number, total area, and total immunoreactivity of LHRH-labeled axon cross-sections in LME of young and old female rats

Group[a]	No. of axons	Total area (μm^2)	Total immunoreactivity[b] ($\times 10^{-3}$)
Young	125.4 ± 8.0	293.9 ± 27.9	31.0 ± 3.0
Old	75.6 ± 4.8*	182.0 ± 16.0*	19.8 ± 1.8*

*$p < 0.01$.
[a] Eight rate per group, three serial sections per rat.
[b] Total immunoreactivity = sum of the products of number of pixels times the corresponding gray level.

Table 8. Number of nucleated FSH-labeled cells and total FSH area and immunoreactivity in one pituitary hemisection of young and old female rats

Group (n = 10)	No. of cells	Total area (μm^2)	Total immunoreactivity[a] ($\times 10^{-4}$)
Young	13.5 ± 3.7	233.0 ± 69.5	14.3 ± 4.4
Old	26.9 ± 2.7**	510.0 ± 72.5**	29.8 ± 4.7*

$^*p < 0.05$. $^{**}p < 0.01$.
[a] Total immunoreactivity = sum of the products of number of pixels times the corresponding gray level.

number of ovarian follicles and corpora lutea was reduced, and atretic follicles were increased in number (Bestetti et al. 1991).

Dopaminergic Axis in Aging Rats. Aging in female rats is also accompanied by hyperprolactinemia, lactotrope hyperplasia, and functional impairment of the hypothalamic tuberoinfundibular dopaminergic neurons. The aim of this morphometric, immunocytochemical, and densitometrical study was to gain a better anatomical knowledge of neurons and axons as well as of lactotropes in old female rats with or without pituitary adenomas, compared with young animals (Rossi et al. 1992). At the hypothalamic level we found that tyrosine hydroxylase-labeled neurons in the arcuate nucleus (Fig. 195) were comparable in young and old rats without adenomas yet their size and thyrosine hydroxylase content were increased in animals with adenomas (Table 9). Also, the thyrosine hydroxylase-labeled axons of the median eminence did not differ significantly between young and old rats without adenomas but were more numerous in the old rats with adenomas (Table 10). Independently from adenomas, both the number of prolactin-labeled structures (Fig. 196) and content of immunoreactive prolactin were increased in pituitaries of old rats; the plasma levels, however, were high only in rats with adenomas (Table 11; Rossi et al. 1992).

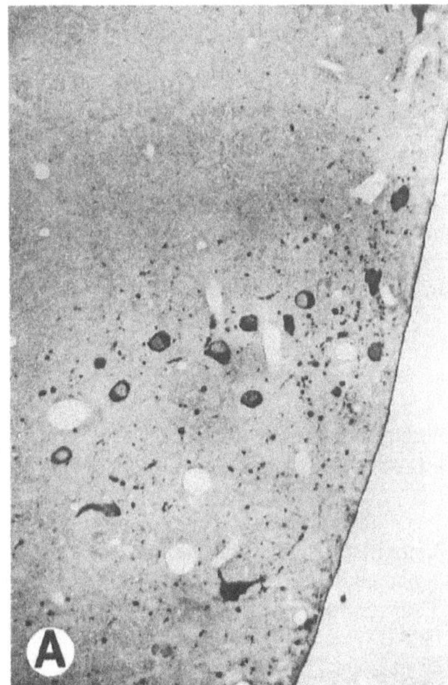

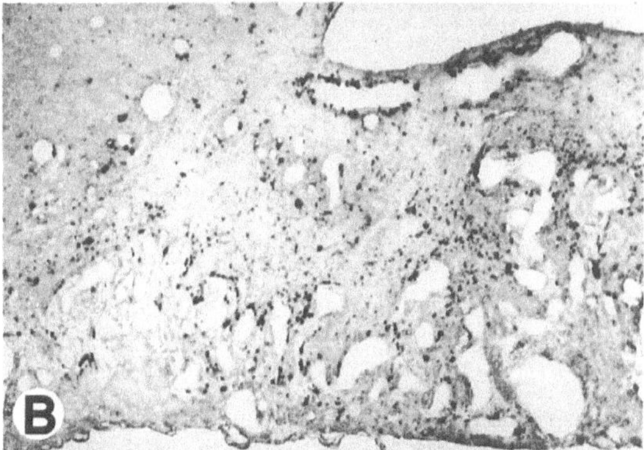

Fig. 195A,B. Mediobasal hypothalamus (*MBA*). **A** Thyroxine (*TH*) labeled neurons in the arcuate nucleus. **B** TH-labeled axon cross-sections in the median eminence. Semithin sections, anti-TH peroxidase anti-peroxidase immunocytochemistry, ×250. (From Rossi et al. 1992)

Conclusions

Although the pathogenesis of the diabetic lesions in mediobasal hypothalamus is still hypothetical, insulin plays an important role at the hypothalamic-pituitary level in streptozotocin-diabetic rats. In these diabetic animals the functional meaning of the lesions in the mediobasal hypo-

Table 9. Effect of age and pituitary adenomas on TH immunoreactivity of arcuate nucleus neurons

Group	Cytoplasm Area (μm^2)	TH Immunoreactivity	
		Per μm^2 cytoplasm	Per neuron ($\times 10^{-3}$)
Young ($n = 10$)	20.42 ± 0.47	870.73 ± 3.01	17.75 ± 0.41
Old NAC ($n = 8$)	22.10 ± 0.70	871.44 ± 3.24	19.36 ± 0.66
Old AC ($n = 7$)	24.41 ± 0.63**,***	882.22 ± 4.06*	21.64 ± 0.60**,***

*$p < 0.05$, **$p < 0.01$ old versus young, ***$p < 0.01$ old AC versus old NAC (Kruskall-Wallis H-test).
Area of perikaryal cytoplasm of TH-labeled nucleated neurons and total immunoreactivity per cytoplasm unit area and per neuron in three cross-sections of the arcuate neucleus of young and old female rats NAC or AC of pituitary adenoma (242 cells from young, 217 cells from old NAC, and 163 from old AC rats were considered).

Table 10. Effect of age and pituitary adenomas on TH immunoreactivity of median eminence axon cross-sections

Group	Number	Total Area (μm^2)	TH Immunoreactivity	
			Total ($\times 10^{-3}$)	Per Axon
Young ($n = 8$)	833 ± 130.8	1190 ± 161.5	806 ± 113.3	1007 ± 141.7
Old NAC ($n = 8$)	728 ± 114.6	975 ± 209.7	668 ± 145.2	960 ± 137.3
Old AC ($n = 7$)	1176 ± 171.3*	1779 ± 323.5	1236 ± 236.3	1132 ± 111.8

*$p < 0.05$ old AC versus old NAC (Mann-Whitney U test).
Number, total area, and immunoreactivity of TH-labeled axon cross-sections in the median eminence of young and old female rats of young and old female rats NAC or AC or pituitary adenoma.

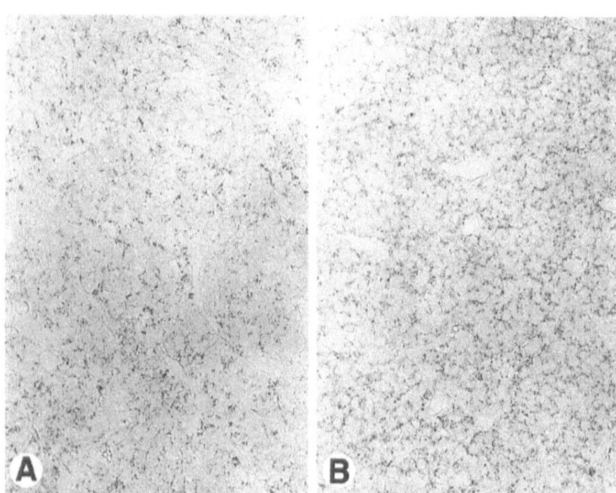

Fig. 196A,B. Pituitary lactotropes. Young rat (**A**) and old rat (**B**) not carrier of adenoma. Semithin sections, anti-prolactin (PRL) alkaline phosphatase immunocytochemistry, ×100. (From Rossi et al. 1992)

Table 11. Effect of age and pituitary adenomas on PRL immunoreactivity of pituitary lactotropes

Group	Number	Total Area (μm^2)	Total PRL Immunoreactivity ($\times 10^{-3}$)
Young ($n = 11$)	7408 ± 385.3	24371 ± 2546.9	2677 ± 291.4
Old NAC ($n = 11$)	11361 ± 262.6*	42634 ± 2940.3*	4714 ± 363.2*
Old AC ($n = 6$)	11104 ± 685.3*	42506 ± 4972.7*	4611 ± 544.7*

* $p < 0.01$ old versus young (Mann-Whitney U test).
Number, total area, and immunoreactivity of PRL-labeled structures in the anterior pituitary gland of young and old female rats NAC or AC of pituitary adenoma.

thalamus has been ascertained in vitro, and pituitary changes are definitely related to the dysfunctions of the mediobasal hypothalamus.

Because of the changes that we found in the Chinese hamster 19, in the streptozotocin rat, and in the fa/fa rat (p. 186, this volume) we conclude that the diabetic neuroendocrinopathy has a crucial pathogenetic impact on the pituitary and target organ changes found in different types of diabetes.

As to the pituitary gland, the changes revealed by reverse hemolytic plaque assay in diabetic animals indicate that several pathogenic mechanisms might be involved in the reduced gonadotropin and thyrotropin release at cellular level: (a) anatomical lesions of organelles involved in glycoprotein hormone synthesis and secretion, possibly due to insulin deficiency, (b) decreased LHRH and TRH receptors on pituitary cells, (c) inadequate LHRH and TRH stimulation, or (d) a combination of these three.

Neuroendocrine lesions occur also in old female rats. Based on our results on the gonadal axis changes in old recurrently pseudopregnant rats we can conclude that the morphological impairment of LHRH axons associated with an increased number of follicle-stimulating hormone gonadotropes and higher plasma levels of follicle-stimulating hormone suggest age-related hypothalamic and pituitary disturbances. These may contribute largely to the complex hormonal disarrangement responsible for the decline of reproductive functions in old female rats. Although insulin secretory disorders may occur also during aging (Reaven et al. 1983), the gonadal axis changes of type 1 diabetic and aged rats are so dissimilar that even a pathogenetic analogy seems improbable.

The data on the prolactin axis support the documented lactotrope hypertrophy and hyperplasia in old female rats. However, these changes are associated with hyperprolactinemia only in animal carriers of adenomas. Also the hypothalamic tuberoinfindubular dopaminergic-neuron changes occur only in hyperprolactinemic animals with prolactinomas.

Acknowledgements. This research was supported in part by the Swiss National Science Foundation (grants 3.034-0.84, 3.028-0.87, 3.659-0.87, 32-28273.90, and 32-29761.90), Swiss Federal Veterinary Board (Bundesamt für Veterinärwesen, grant 014.89.4), and Berne University Foundation for Research Promotion (Hochschulstiftung, grants 11.6.1985, 25.3.1986, 26.6.1987, 15.6.1988, 13.6.1989, and 1990).

References

Bestetti G, Rossi GL (1980) Hypothalamic lesions in rats with longterm streptozotocin-induced diabetes mellitus. A semiquantitative light- and electron-microscopic study. Acta Neuropathol (Berl) 52:119–127

Bestetti GE, Rossi GL (1982) Hypothalamic changes in diabetic Chinese hamsters. A semiquantitative, light and electron microscopic study. Lab Invest 47:516–522

Bestetti GE, Rossi GL (1988) Neuroendocrine changes in experimentally diabetic rats. In: Shafrir E, Renold AE (eds) Frontiers in diabetes research. Lessons from animal diabetes II. Libbey, London, pp 444–452

Bestetti GE, Rossi GL (1990) Effects of diabetes on functional and morphological complications in the hypothalamo-pituitary system of diabetic rodent models. A pathogenesis overview. In: Shafrir E (ed) Frontiers in diabetes research II. Lessons from animal diabetes III. Smith-Gordon, London, pp 466–470

Bestetti GE, Locatelli V, Tirone F, Rossi GL, Müller EE (1985) One month of streptozotocin-diabetes induces dif-

ferent neuroendocrine and morphological alterations in the hypothalamo-pituitary axis of male and female rats. Endocrinology 117:208–216
Bestetti G, Hofer R, Rossi GL (1987a) The preoptic-suprachiasmatic nuclei though morphologically heterogeneous are equally affected by streptozotocin diabetes. Exp Brain Res 66:74–82
Bestetti GE, Junker U, Locatelli V, Rossi GL (1987b) Continuous subtherapeutic insulin counteracts hypothalamopituitary-gonadal alterations in diabetic rats. Diabetes 36: 1315–1319
Bestetti GE, Reymond MJ, Perrin IV, Kniel PC, Lemarchand-Béraud T, Rossi GL (1987c) Thyroid and pituitary secretory disorders in streptozotocin-diabetic rats are associated with severe structural changes of these glands. Virchows Arch [B] 53:69–78
Bestetti GE, Boujon CE, Reymond MJ, Rossi GL (1989a) Functional and morphological changes in mediobasal hypothalamus of streptozocin-induced diabetic rats. In vitro study of LHRH release. Diabetes 38:471–476
Bestetti GE, Reymond MJ, Boujon CE, Lemarchand-Béraud T, Rossi GL (1989b) Functional and morphological aspects of impaired TRH release by mediobasal hypothalamus of STZ-induced diabetic rats. Diabetes 38: 1351–1356
Bestetti, GE, Abramo F, Guillaume-Gentil C, Rohner-Jeanrenaud F, Jeanrenaud B, Rossi GL (1990) Changes in the hypothalamo-pituitary-adrenal axis of genetically obese fa/fa rats: a structural, immonocytochemical, and morphometrical study. Endocrinology 126: 1880–1887
Bestetti GE, Reymond MJ, Blanc F, Boujon CE, Furrer B, Rossi GL (1991) Functional and morphological changes in the hypothalamopituitary-gonadal axis of aged female rats. Biol Reprod 45:221–228
Boujon CE, Bestetti GE, Reymond MJ, Rossi GL (1987) A model for combined morphological and functional investigations on the isolated mediobasal rat hypothalamus. Neuroendocrinology 45:311–317
Lechan RM, Wu P, Jackson IM (1987) Immunocytochemical distribution in rat brain of putative peptides derived from thyrotropin-releasing hormone prohormone. Endocrinology 121:1879–1891
Paz G, Homonnai ZT (1979) Leydig cell function in streptozotocin induced diabetic rats. Experientia 35:1412–1413
Pitton I, Bestetti GE, Rossi GL (1987) The changes in the hypothalamo-pituitary-gonadal axis of streptozotocin-treated male rats depend on age at diabetes onset. Andrologia 19:464–473
Reaven E, Wright D, Mondon CE, Solomon R, Ho H, Reaven GM (1983) Effect of age and diet on insulin secretion and insulin action in the rat. Diabetes 32:175–180
Rossi GL, Bestetti GE (1981) Morphological changes in the hypothalamic-hypophyseal-gonadal axis of male rats after twelve months of streptozotocin-induced diabetes. Diabetologia 21:476–481
Rossi GL, Bestetti GE (1983) Technical aspects in the study of pathologic lesions in the hypothalamus of the rat. In: Jones TC, Mohr U, Hunt RD (eds) Monographs on pathology of laboratory animals, endocrine system. Springer, Berlin Heidelberg New York, pp 311–316
Rossi GL, Bestetti GE (1990) In vitro assessment of functional and morphological complications in the hypothalamo-pituitary system of diabetic rodent models. In: Shafrir E (ed) Frontiers in diabetes research II. Lessons from animals diabetes III. Smith-Gordon, London, pp 471–474
Rossi GL, Bestetti GE, Tontis DK, Varini M (1989) Reverse hemolytic plaque assay study of luteinizing and follicle-stimulating hormone and thyrotropin secretion in diabetic rat pituitary glands. Diabetes 38:1301–1306
Rossi GL, Bestetti GE, Reymond MJ (1992) Tuberoinfundibular dopaminergic neurons and lactotropes in young and old female rats. Neurobiol Aging 13:275–281

Hypothalamic-Pituitary-Adrenal Axis of Genetically Obese fa/fa Rats

Gilberto E. Bestetti, Corinne Guillaume-Gentil, Françoise Rohner-Jeanrenaud, Giovanni L. Rossi, Francesca Abramo, and Bernard Jeanrenaud

Introduction

The genetically obese fa/fa rat, first described by Zucker and Zucker in 1961, is a model of the obesity/type 2 diabetes syndrome. The syndrome is due to an autosomal recessive gene. This animal presents a number of behavioral, metabolic, and endocrine disorders such as hyperphagia, hyperinsulinemia, and hyperlipidemia, all of questionable etiology. Most of these alterations are reversed by adrenalectomy and restored by corticosterone treatment of the adrenalectomized animals. In an attempt to clarify the pathogenesis of the syndrome we investigated morphological and functional aspects of the hypothalamic-pituitary-adrenal axis of obese (fa/fa) and lean (FA/?) rats (Bestetti et al. 1990; Guillaume-Gentil et al. 1990).

Material and Methods

We studied by qualitative light and electron microscopy the median eminence axons and the adrenal gland. Moreover, after immunocytochemical labeling we analyzed densitometrically the axons of the median eminence bearing corticotropin-releasing factor and the cells containing adrenocorticotropic hormone (ACTH) of the anterior pituitary lobe. Plasma corticosterone levels were measured, morning and evening, in a large number of resting lean and obese animals. Putative defects of the hypothalamic-pituitary-adrenal axis were assessed by submitting the animals to various tests of stress and by studying the suppressive effect of dexamethasone on diurnal plasma corticosterone levels.

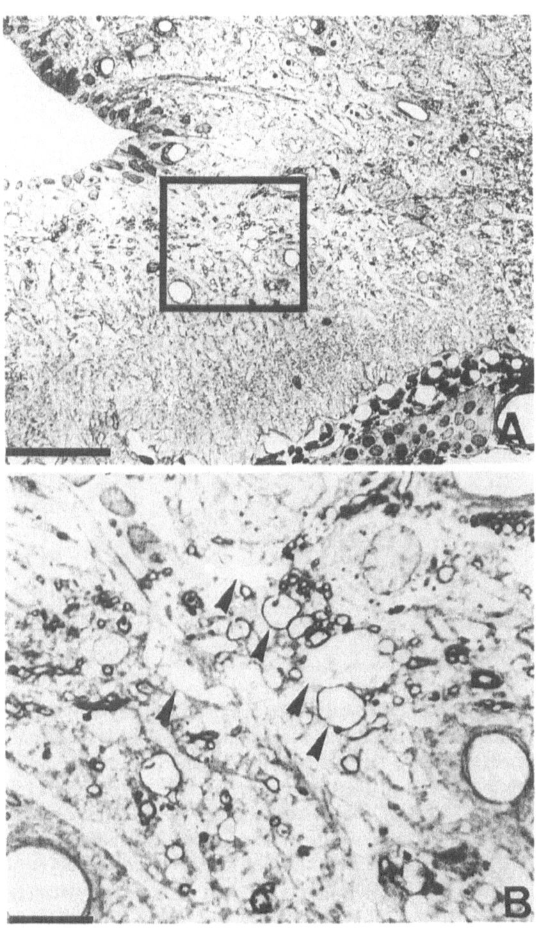

Fig. 197A,B. Mediobasal hypothalamus of an obese rat. **A** Enlarged cellular processes can be observed in the median eminence. ×330; *bar*, 50 µm. **B** Detail of **A**. Note enlarged cellular processes (*arrowheads*). *Bar*, 10 µm. Toluidine blue, ×1320. (From Bestetti et al.1990)

Results and Discussion

Degenerate axon cross-sections were found in the internal layer of the median eminence of obese rats (Figs. 197, 198). In the external layer of the median eminence, remote from the axonal lesions, the content of the immunoreactive corticotropin-releasing factor was increased (Bestetti et al. 1990, Fig. 199). The increased content of this factor in the hypothalamus suggests its increased secretion. The ACTH-labeled anterior pituitary corticotropes of the fa/fa rats were in fact increased in number and were not atrophic (Fig. 200). Further, the ACTH levels in the pituitary as well as in plasma were higher in obese than in lean animals (Bestetti et al. 1990). Basal plasma ACTH (Fig. 201) and both morning and evening corticosterone levels in the blood were higher in obese than in lean rats (Guillaume-Gentile et al. 1990).

The hypothalamic-pituitary-adrenal axis was further investigated using stressful stimuli. Higher ACTH levels were reached in obese than in lean rats when submitted to cold stress (6°C; Fig. 201).

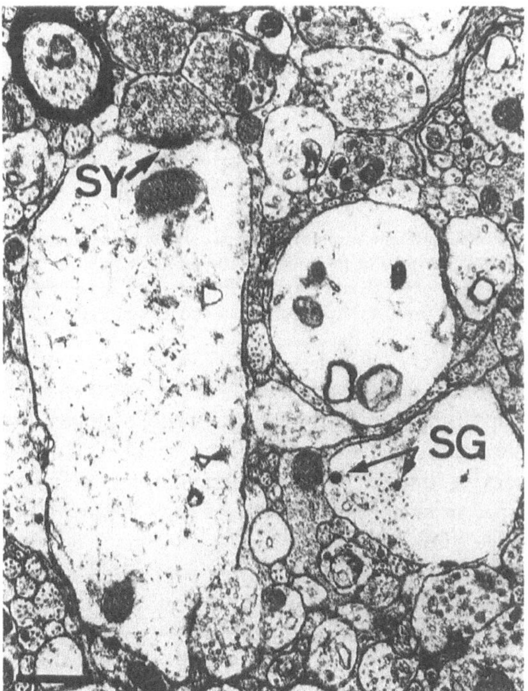

Fig. 198. Median eminence of an obese rat. One dilated and degenerate axon in cross-section contains a synaptic structure (*SY*); another one contains neurosecretory granules (*SG*). *Bar*, 1 µm. TEM, ×12 000. (From Bestetti et al. 1990)

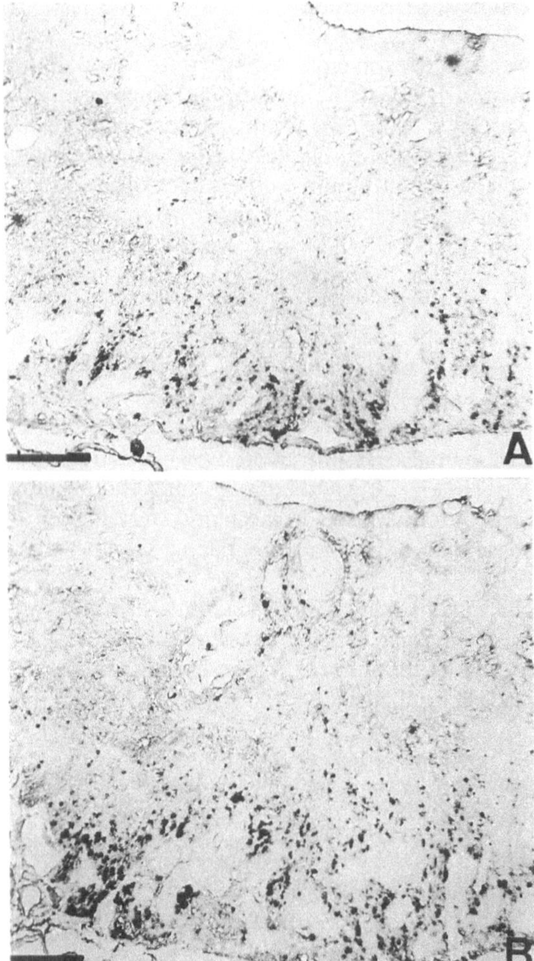

Fig. 199. Immunoreactive corticortropin-releasing factor in semithin sections of the mediobasal hypothalamus of a lean (**A**) and an obese (**B**) rat. In the latter, CRF-labeled axons are more numerous. ×528; *bar*, 20 µm. (From Bestetti et al. 1990)

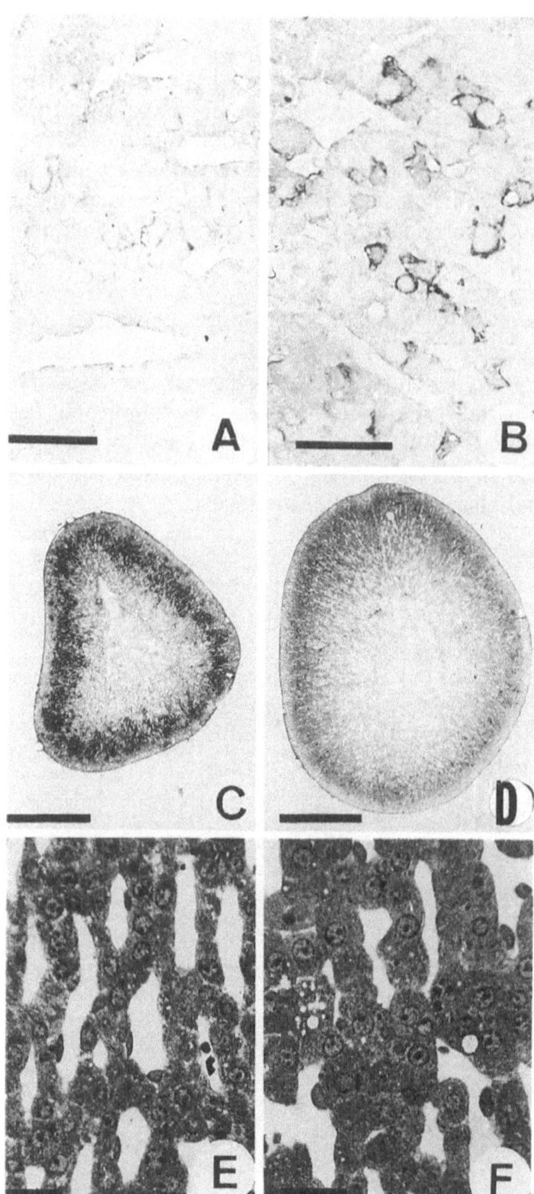

Fig. 200. Immunoreactive adrenocorticotropic hormone in semithin sections of an anterior pituitary lobe of a lean (**A**) and an obese (**B**) rat. The corticotropes are more numerous in the obese (**B**) than in the lean (**A**) rat. ×528; *bar*, 20 µm. Low (**C**,**D**; ×13; *bar*, 1 mm) and high (**E**,**F**; ×528; *bar*, 20 µm) magnifications of semithin section of adrenal glands of a lean (**C**,**E**) and an obese (**D**,**F**) rat. The adrenal cortex is thicker in the obese than in the lean rat. The cells of the zona fasciculata are hypertrophic in the obese rat (**F**). (From Bestetti et al. 1990)

The elevated plasma ACTH levels were in turn responsible for the following adrenal changes: (a) the adrenal glands were larger (Fig. 202) and heavier, and (b) the zona fasciculata, responsible for corticosterone secretion, was hypertrophic (Fig. 200).

These changes account for the hypercorticosteronemia of the obese animals. In fact, plasma corticosterone levels were higher in obese than in lean animals after immobilization (Fig. 200) and ether vapor (Fig. 203) or cold (Figs. 201, 204) stress (6°C). Dexamethasone produced a complete suppression of corticosterone output in both lean and obese rats. During the recovery from such suppression corticosterone levels rose to higher

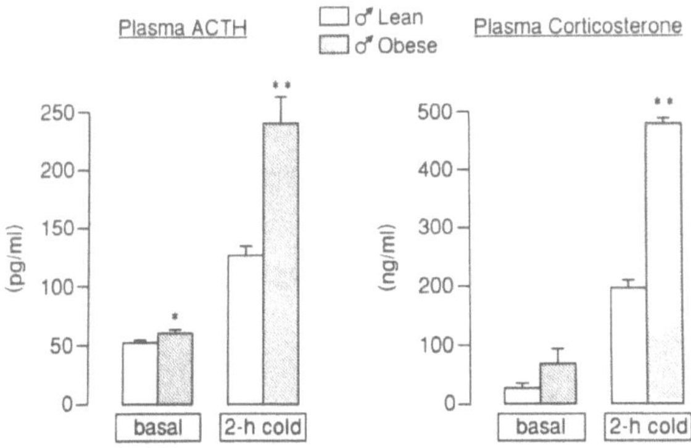

Fig. 201. Pituitary and adrenocortical responses to a 2-h cold exposure (6°C) in 14-week-old lean and obese rats. Each bar is the mean of ten animals. $*p < 0.05$; $**p < 0.001$, lean vs. obese. (From Guillaume-Gentil et al. 1990)

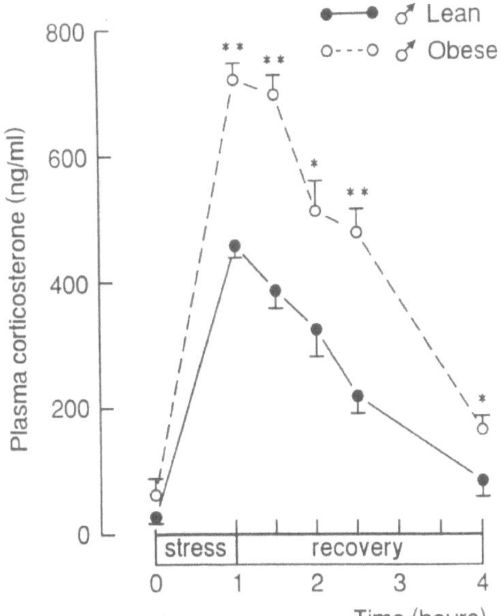

Fig. 202. Plasma corticosterone levels in 15-week-old lean and obese rats submitted to 1-h immobilization stress, followed by a 3-h recovery period. *Point zero*, basal morning levels (0900 hours). Each point is the mean of eight lean or ten obese animals. $*p < 0.05$; $**p < 0.001$, lean vs. obese. (From Guillaume-Gentil et al. 1990)

values in obese than in lean rats (Fig. 205). Based on our results we can conclude that the obesity/type 2 diabetes syndrome of the fa/fa rat is associated with hypothalamic changes leading to hyperactivity of the whole adrenal axis. Alterations also occur in the hypothalamic nuclei controlling glycemia, insulinemia, and circadian corticosterone secretion (Bestetti et al. 1990).

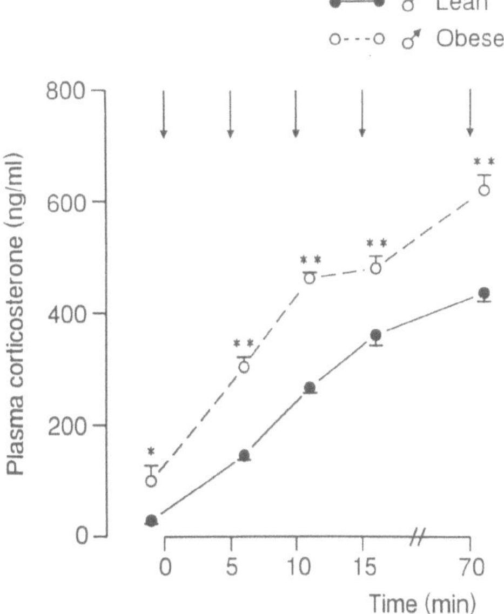

Fig. 203. Plasma corticosterone levels in 14-week-old lean and obese rats submitted to 1-min repeated ether vapor stress. Exposure to ether vapor was carried out at 0, 5, 10, 15, and 70 min. Blood was sampled at −1, 6, 11, 16, and 71 min. *Point zero*, basal morning levels (0900 hours). Each point is the mean of ten animals. $*p < 0.025$; $**p < 0.001$, lean vs. obese. (From Guillaume-Gentil et al. 1990)

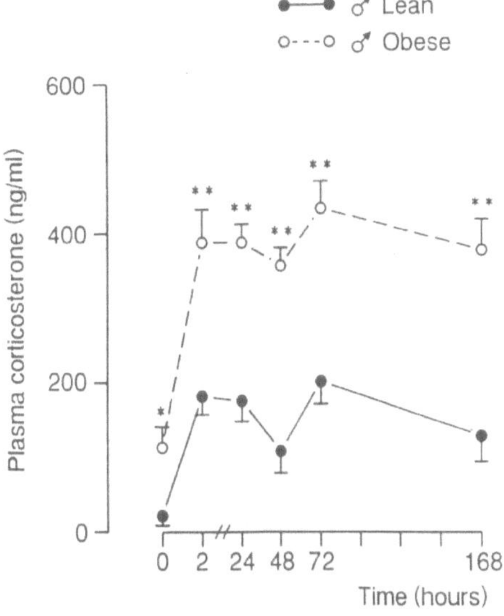

Fig. 204. Plasma corticosterone levels in 12-week-old lean and obese rats submitted to 7-day cold exposure (6°C). *Point zero*, basal morning (0900 hours) values (at 22°C). Except for 2-h point which was collected at 1100 hours, all points refer to morning values (0900 hours) obtained under cold exposure. Each point is the mean of ten animals. $*p < 0.01$; $**p < 0.001$, lean vs. obese. (From Guillaume-Gentil et al. 1990)

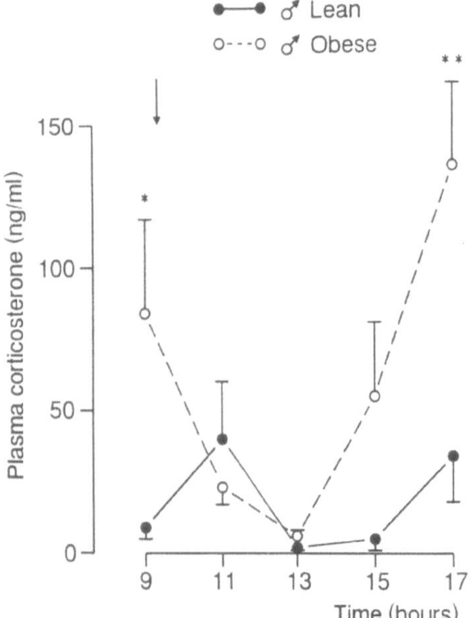

Fig. 205. Dexamethasone suppression of diurnal plasma corticosterone levels in 14-week-old lean and obese rats. Dexamethasone (5 pg/kg BW) was administered i.p. after collection of basal morning samples (0900 hours). Blood was sampled every 2 h until 1700 hours. Each point is the mean of ten animals. $*p < 0.05$; $**p < 0.01$, lean vs. obese. (From Guillaume-Gentil et al. 1990)

The quick recovery of the obese animals from the dexamethasone suppression together with the increased cold-induced ACTH output in obese rats further supports a central origin for the hyperactivity of the hypothalamic-pituitary-adrenal axis of the obese animals. Whatever the precise etiology of the change in the central nervous system may be, it is proposed that the increased activity of the hypothalamic-pituitary-adrenal axis in obese rats and the consequent hypercorticism play a role in the establishment and maintenance of the obesity/type 2 diabetes syndrome in this animal model.

Despite hyperinsulinemia, insulin binding to hypothalamic receptors is decreased (Melnyk 1987), and the hypothalamic insulin content is low in fa/fa rats (Baskin et al. 1985).

Acknowledgements. This research was supported in part by the Swiss National Science Foundation (grants 3.034-0.84, 3.028-0.87, 3.659-0.87, and 32-29761.90), Swiss Federal Veterinary Board (Bundesamt für Veterinäwesen, grant 014.89.4), and Berne University Foundation for Research Promotion (Hochschulstiftung, grants 11.6.1985, 25.3.1986, 26.6.1987, 15.6.1988, 13.6.1989, and 1990).

References

Baskin DG, Stein LJ, Ikeda H, Woods SC, Figlewicz DP, Porte D Jr, Greenwood MRC, Dorsa DM (1985) Genetically obese Zucker rats have abnormally low brain insulin content. Life Sci 36:627–633

Bestetti GE, Abramo F, Guillaume-Gentil C, Rohner-Jeanrenaud F, Jeanrenaud B, Rossi GL (1990) Changes in the hypothalamo-pituitary-adrenal axis of genetically obese fa/fa rats: a structural, immunocytochemical, and morphometrical study. Endocrinology 126:1880–1887

Guillaume-Gentil C, Rohner-Jeanrenaud F, Abramo F, Bestetti GE, Rossi GL, Jeanrenaud B (1990) Abnormal regulation of the hypothalamo-pituitary-adrenal axis in the genetically obese fa/fa rats. Endocrinology 126:1873–1879

Melnyk RB (1987) Decreased binding to hypothalamic insulin receptors in young genetically obese rats. Physiol Behav 40:237–241

Zucker LM, Zucker TF (1961) Fatty, a new mutation in the rat. J Hered 52:275–278

Pineal Gland

Functional Morphology of the Mammalian Pineal Gland

Michal Karasek and Russel J. Reiter

Introduction

The first description of the pineal gland came from Galen (130–200 AD) who named the organ *konareion* (Latin *conarium*) after its shape, similar to that of a pine cone. The pineal was probably already known by Herophilus of Alexandria (325–280 BC), although nothing remains of his writings to document this. According to Galen, Herophilus concluded that the organ is a sphincter which regulates the flow of "pneuma." Galen, on the other hand, believed the cerebellar vermis to be the "pneuma" sphincter and the pineal to be a "gland" that supports the venous network in the brain.

Following Galen there was a long historical hiatus during which virtually nothing new was uncovered in the anatomical sciences. This ended with the first pictorial representation of the pineal in Versalius' anatomical textbook, *De Humani Corporis Fabrica, Libri Septem* (1543). A major revival of interest in the pineal was seen in the seventeenth century when Descartes (1596–1650) regarded the organ (the only unpaired structure in the brain) as the "right hand" of the soul. Parenthetically it should be noted that, contrary to popular opinion, Descartes never described the pineal as the "*seat* of the soul"! While descriptions of the pineal gland were common by anatomists of the eighteenth and early twentieth centuries, it was the discovery of melatonin, the chief pineal hormone, by Lerner and coworkers in 1958 that initiated the modern era of pineal research. The morphology of the mammalian pineal gland has been studied extensively over the past 35 years. This chapter summarizes basic data on pineal gross anatomy, histology, and especially ultrastructure. Additional details related to the history of the pineal gland can be found in a report by Zrenner (1985).

Gross Anatomy

There is considerable variation with respect to pineal form and position in mammals. Vollrath (1979, 1981) classified the pineal gland of mammals according its relationship to the third ventricle of the brain, taking into account the form and position of the pineal tissue. This classification distinguishs proximal (type A), proximo-intermediate (type AB), and proximo-intermedio-distal (type ABC) types. When the bulk of pineal tissue lies close to the third ventricle, the pineal is classified as type A (e.g., the sheep and human). When the pineal is elongated and has a length twice or more its greatest width, it is designated as type AB (e.g., in the cat). Very long, more or less rod-shaped pineals, which reach the cerebellum and lie superficial to the brain surface are classified as type ABC (e.g., in the guinea pig). If any of these parts are greatly reduced in size, the respective upper-case Latin letter is replaced by the corresponding lower-case letter of the Greek alphabet, and if an area is lacking, the corresponding letter is omitted. Hence, type αβC (e.g., in the rat) is elongated structure in which the bulk of pineal tissue has a superficial position and in which the proximal and intermediate parts are greatly reduced in size, whereas type αC (e.g., in the Syrian hamster) consists of small deep pineal and a larger superficial pineal gland (Sheridan and Reiter 1970).

General Histology

The mammalian pineal gland consists of two main cell types: pinealocytes and glial cells. In addition, fibroblasts, plasma cells, mast cells, pigment-containing cells, and nerve cells are occasionally present in some species (Vollrath 1981; Karasek 1983).

The phylogenetic history of the pinealocyte is of particular interest. The mammalian pinealocyte is derived from the neurosensory photoreceptor cell present in the pineal organ of anamniotes, which during evolution loses its outer segment (photoreceptive pole) and thereby also its photoreceptive capacity. Evidence of secretory function is seen early in pineal phylogeny. Hence, in early phylogenetic stages pineal cells seemingly possess both photoreceptor and secretory functions, gradually losing their photoreceptor capacity and becoming exclusively secretory in nature in the mammalian pineal gland (Collin 1971).

Pinealocytes represent the predominant cell type (85%–90% of all cells) in the mammalian pineal (Fig. 206). In hematoxylin and eosin preparations pinealocytes have round, granular nuclei with prominent nucleoli and poorly stained cytoplasm (Fig. 207). With the silver carbonate method of Del Rio-Hortega, pinealocytes appear as cells with one or several processes of variable lengths bearing club-shaped endings.

While a single population of pinealocytes is apparent in the majority of mammalian species, two pinealocyte populations (referred to as pinealocytes I and II) have been found in some mammals. In addition, a distinction is often made between "light" and "dark" pinealocytes, with some authors regarding them as separate cell types. However, since the distinction is based only on a difference in density of the cytoplasm, it seems likely that "light" and "dark" pinealocytes probably reflect differences in the functional stages of the same cell which may be manifested as a differential susceptibility to the fixative (Karasek 1983).

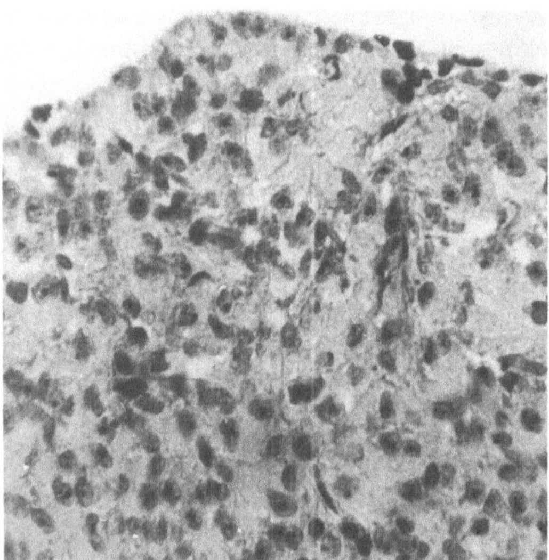

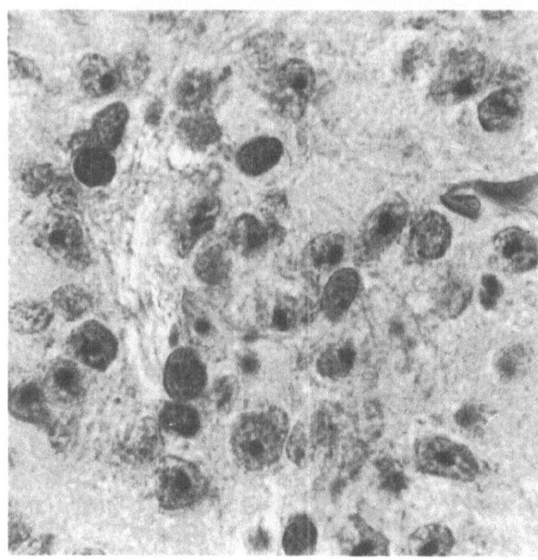

Fig. 206. (*above*) The rat pineal gland. H&E, ×240

Fig. 207. (*below*) The rat pineal gland. The pale nuclei are in pinealocytes; the dark nuclei are associated with glial cells. H&E, ×600

Although glial cells (Fig. 207) are usual components of the mammalian pineal gland, there is some inconsistency in the terminology related to these cells. Because they may differ in some species from the classical astrocytes, some authors prefer to identify them as "interstitial cells." However, fibrous astrocytes are typically present in the majority of species.

Ultrastructure

The description of the ultrastructural features of the mammalian pineal gland presented here is based, for the most part, on the authors' own studies (Karasek 1981, 1983, 1987; Karasek and Reiter 1992). The figures included are representative microphotographs collected over many years of experience investigating the pineal gland of many mammalian species.

Pinealocytes. Ultrastructural features of the pinealocyte are basically similar in all mammals (Figs. 208, 209), although some species differences may be found. Pinealocytes are generally irregularly shaped with a variable number of cytoplasmic processes emerging from their cell bodies.

The pinealocyte nucleus is usually oval or irregular in shape. Cytoplasmic invaginations, varying in number and length from pinealocyte to pinealocyte and from species to species, are characteristic features. In most species the nucleus is characterized by electron-lucent nucleoplasm. A prominent nucleolus is usually present within the pinealocyte nucleus (Figs. 210, 211).

The cytoplasm of the cell body contains the usual organelles (Figs. 209, 212). Mitochondria, showing many variations in shape and size, are present in relatively large numbers in most pinealocytes (Figs. 212, 213). Although mito-

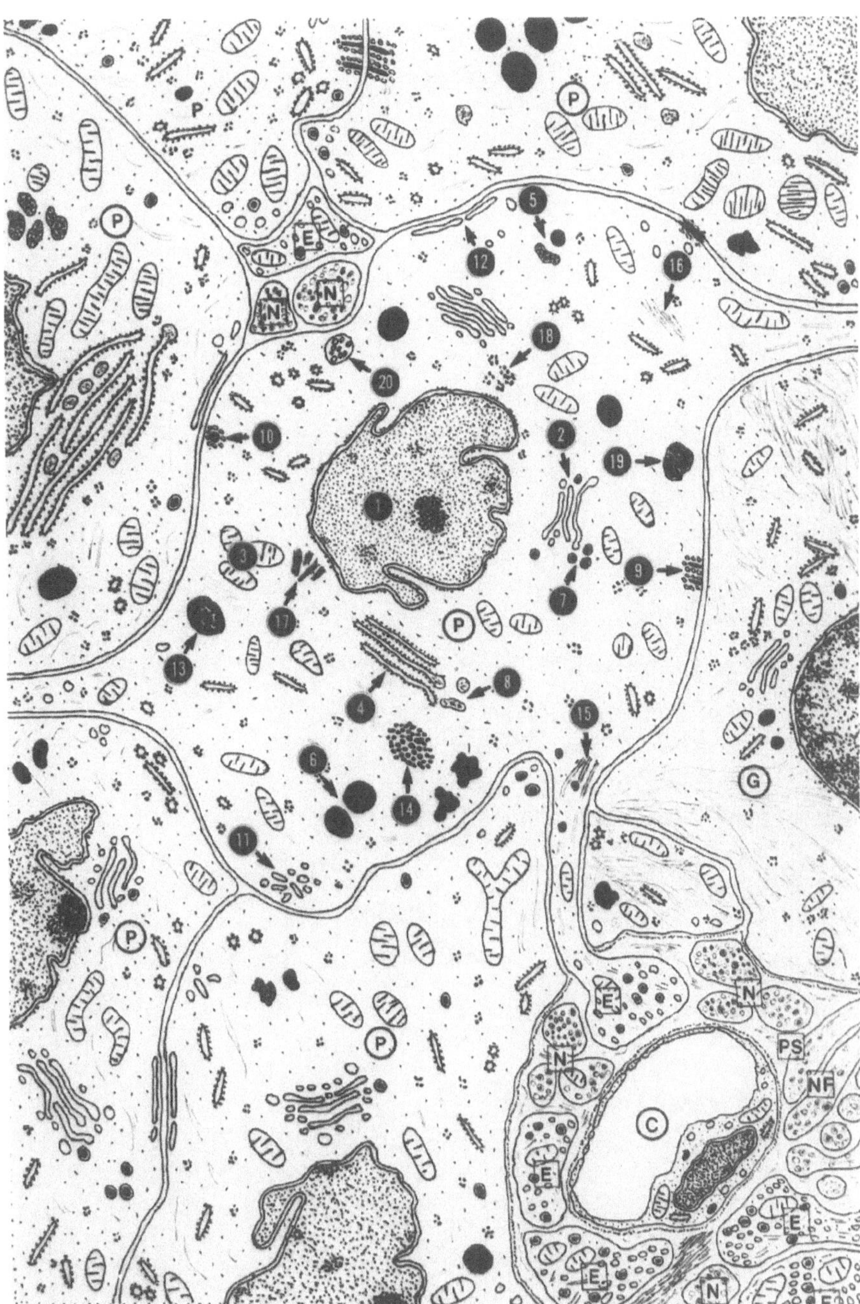

Fig. 208. Generalized architecture of the mammalian pineal gland. *P*, Pinealocyte; *E*, ending of the pinealocyte process; *G*, gilal cell; *C*, capillary surrounded by the pericapillary space (*PS*); *NF*, sympathetic nerve fiber; *N*, sympathetic nerve ending. Within the pinealocyte: *1*, nucleus; *2*, Golgi apparatus; *3*, mitochondria; *4*, granular endoplasmic reticulum; *5*, lysosomes; *6*, lipid droplets; *7*, dense-cored vesicles; *8*, vacuoles with flocculent content; *9*, "synaptic" ribbons; *10*, "synaptic" spherule; *11*, clear vesicles; *12*, subsurface cisternae; *13*, inclusion body; *14*, glycogen particles; *15*, microtubules; *16*, microfilaments; *17*, microtubular sheaves; *18*, polyribosomes; *19*, membrane-bound body; *20*, multivesicular body

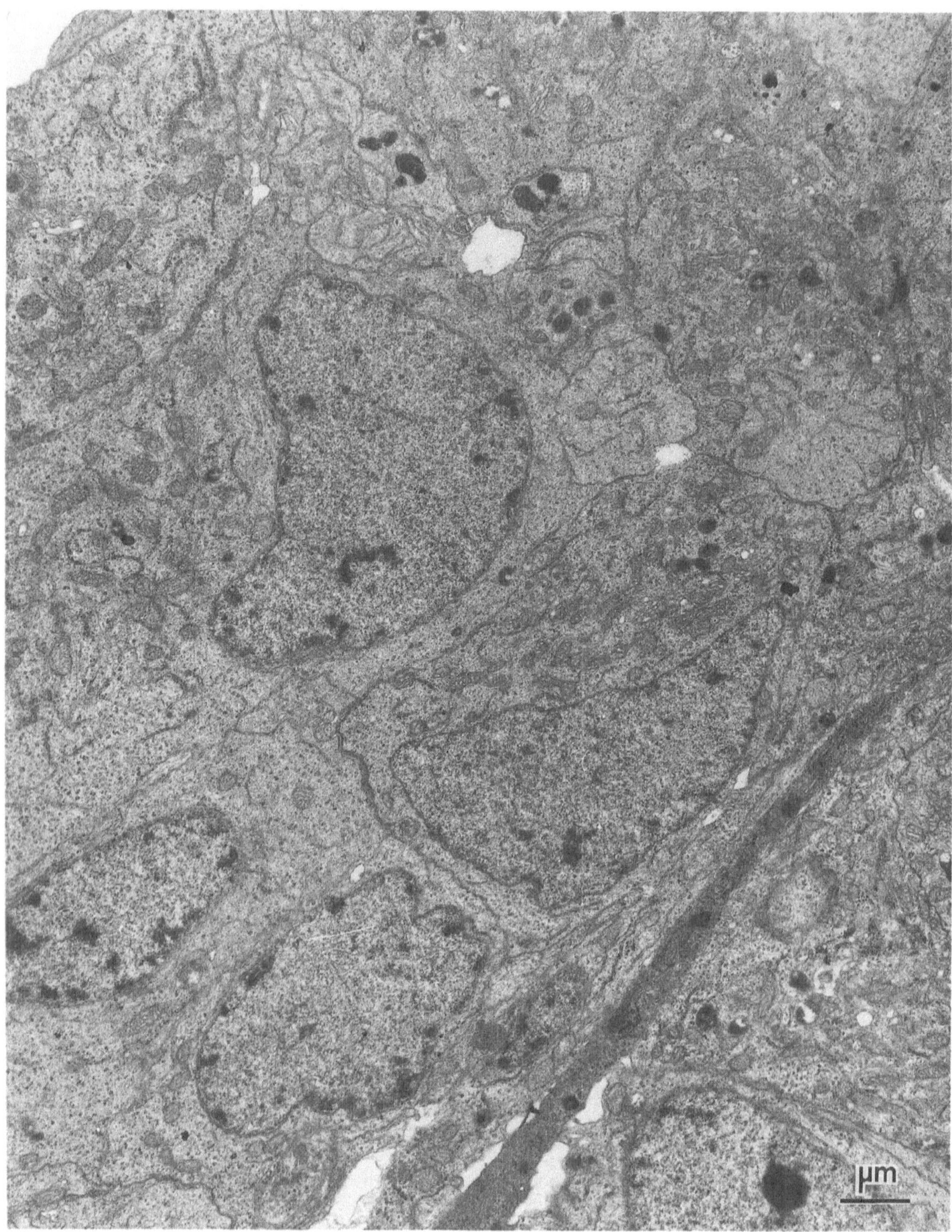

Fig. 209. Pineal parenchyma; Djungarian hamster. Several pinealocytes containing a variety of cytoplasmic organelles are apparent. TEM

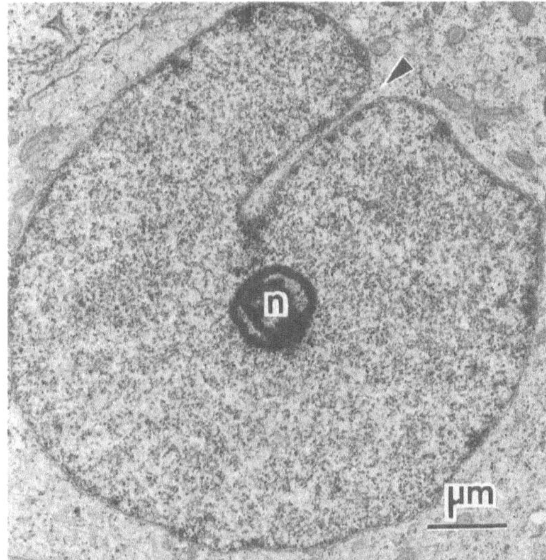

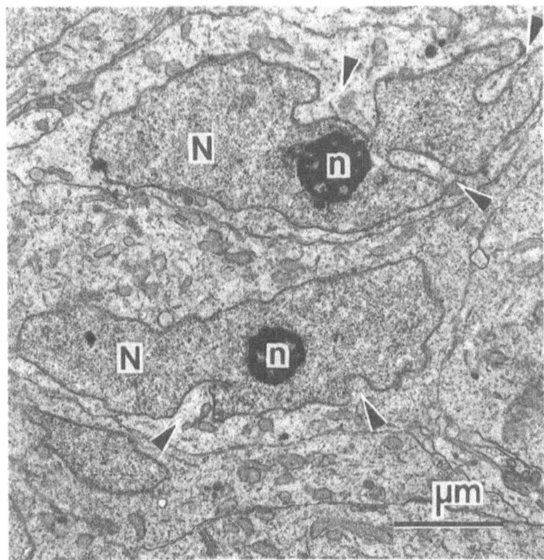

Fig. 210. (*above*) Typical pinealocyte nucleus, brush mouse, with electron-lucent nucleoplasm, deep cytoplasmic invagination (*arrowhead*) and prominent nucleolus (*n*). TEM

Fig. 211. (*below*) Two elongated pinealocyte nuclei, mouse, (*N*) with numerous indentations (*arrowheads*) and prominent nucleoli (*n*). TEM

chondrial profiles have been described as being oval, round, elongated, rod-shaped, arciform, filamentous or branched, typically, oval, round, or elongated mitochondria with a matrix of moderate electron density are present. The average size of a pinealocyte mitochondrium appears to be between 0.5 and 1.5 µm, although "giant" mitochondria of up to 5.8 µm are occasionally seen.

The number of lysosomes in pinealocytes varies widely among species. These structures are spherical or oval in shape, measure 0.2–1.5 µm in diameter, and contain finely granular material of moderate electron density (Fig. 213).

The Golgi apparatus is usually well developed and consists of a system of cisternae which are associated with numerous vesicles of varying diameter (Figs. 212, 214). The majority of the vesicles are clear, although dense-cored vesicles are also present within Golgi profiles or in their vicinity. There is ultrastructural evidence suggesting that the dense-cored vesicles are formed by the Golgi apparatus (Fig. 214). Although the number of dense-cored vesicles varies among species, these structures are usual components of the mammalian pinealocyte. The dense-cored vesicles are observed throughout the perikaryon (Fig. 217) but are especially abundant in the endings of cell processes (Fig. 215).

A moderate amount of granular endoplasmic reticulum is generally present. In the majority of the pinealocytes isolated cisternae of granular endoplasmic reticulum are typically present (Fig. 212), although in some pinealocytes complexes of parallel-oriented cisternae can be found (Fig. 216).

Vacuoles containing flocculent material of moderate electron density are often observed in pinealocytes. Such vacuoles are often associated with cisternae of granular endoplasmic reticulum, but they also can be found throughout the cytoplasm.

Smooth endoplasmic reticulum and clear vesicles are also consistently present in the mammalian pinealocyte (Fig. 217), although in variable amounts. Clear vesicles are scattered throughout the cytoplasm, being most abundant in the endings of pinealocyte processes (Fig. 215).

"Synaptic" ribbons are structures typically present in the mammalian pinealocyte (Fig. 218). These structures consist of an electron-dense rod, measuring 20–60 nm in width and 21.5 µm in length, usually surrounded by a single layer of electron-lucent vesicles, 30–50 nm in diameter. "Synaptic" ribbons lie singly or in groups (ribbon fields), usually in the vicinity of cell membrane. The number of "synaptic" ribbons varies greatly among species, being 30 times more numerous in some species than in others. In addition to "synaptic" ribbons, similar structures, referred to as "synaptic" spherules, are present in some pinealocytes. These structures consist of a spheri-

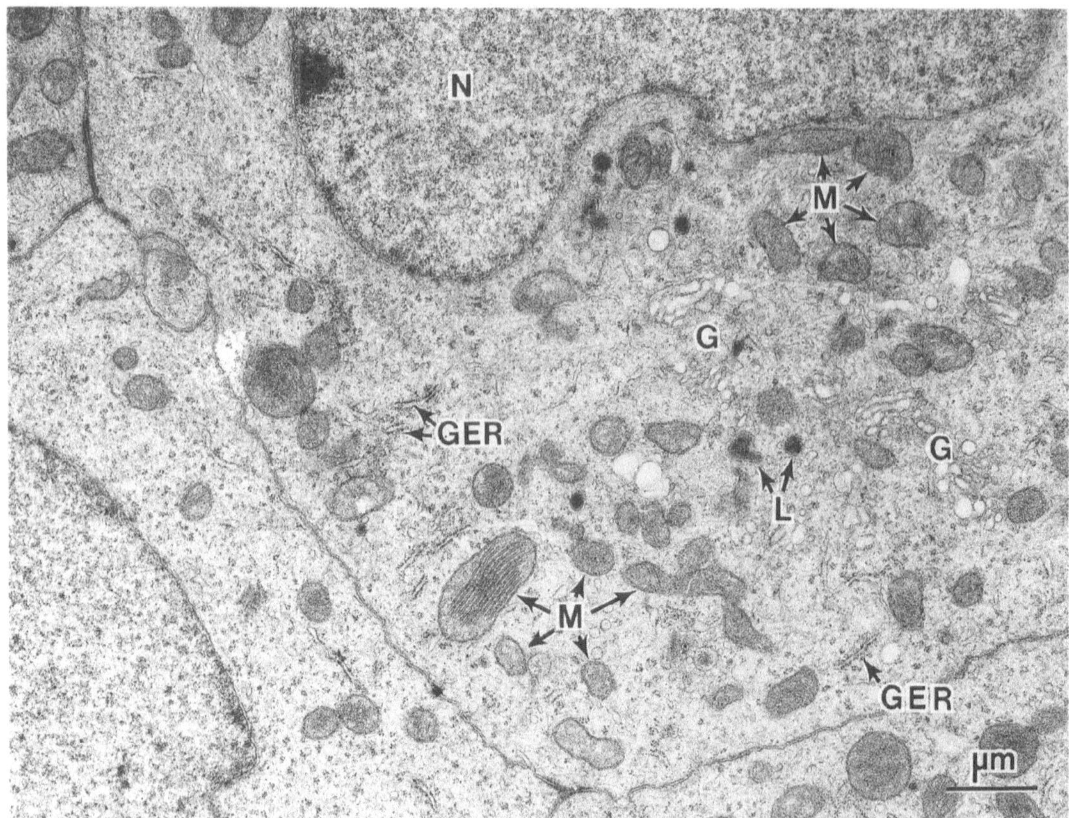

Fig. 212. Portion of a pinealocyte, chipmunk. Note the nucleus (*N*) and cytoplasm containing mitochondria (*M*), Golgi apparatus (*G*), lysosomes (*L*), and isolated cisternae of granular endoplasmic reticulum (*GER*). TEM

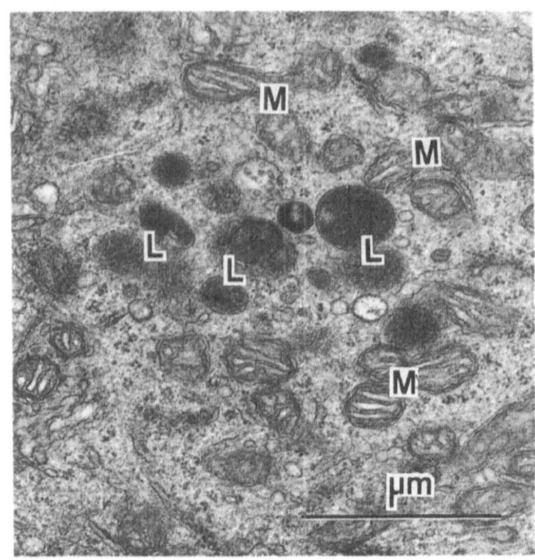

Fig. 213. Pinealocyte Djungarian hamster. Numerous lysosomes (*L*) and mitochondria (*M*) in the cytoplasm. TEM

cal core, 90–180 nm in diameter, surrounded by a layer of electron-lucent vesicles, roughly 30 nm in diameter.

Lipid droplets (Fig. 219) are present in variable numbers in pinealocytes of all mammalian species. Glycogen particles (Fig. 220) are abundant in some species and absent in others. Other cell components of the mammalian pinealocyte include microtubules, microfilaments, microtubular sheaves, multivesicular bodies, subsurface cisternae, cilia, centrioles, and annulate lamellae. Additionally, pigment granules, inclusion bodies, and membrane-bound bodies have been observed.

Ultrastructural Aspects of Pineal Secretion. Although known to be an endocrine gland (Reiter 1991), it has not been possible definitively to link any morphological feature with the secretory processes of the gland. However, on the basis of

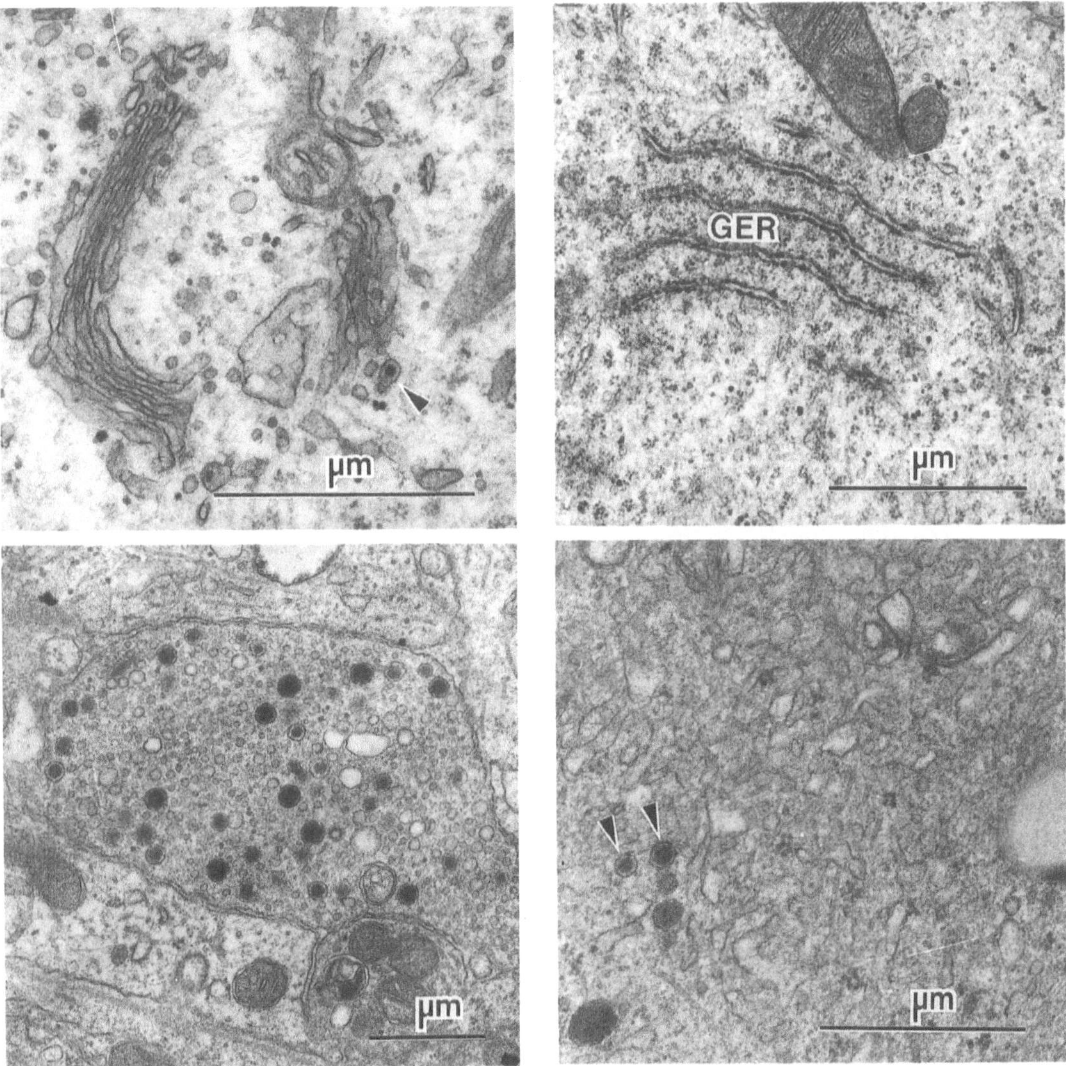

Fig. 214. (*above*) Prominent Golgi apparatus in pinealocyte cytoplasm. *Arrowhead*, the formation of a dense-cored vesicle by the Golgi cisternae. Mouse

Fig. 215. (*below*) Ending of pinealocyte process with numerous dense-cored and clear vesicles. Syrian hamster

Fig. 216. (*above*) Parallel-oriented cisternae of granular endoplasmic reticulum in the pinealocyte cytoplasm. Chipmunk

Fig. 217. (*below*) Vesicular and elongated profiles of smooth endoplasmic reticulum in pinealocyte cytoplasm. *Arrowheads*, dense-cored vesicles. Syrian hamster

ultrastructural studies a few presumed secretory features have been described. There is general agreement that main pineal hormonal product, melatonin, is not stored within the pinealocyte, but rather that it simply diffuses out of the cell after being synthesized. Therefore this process probably cannot be visualized ultrastructurally (Reiter 1981; Karasek 1983). Two different secretory processes which may be involved in protein and/or peptide secretion from the pinealocytes have been defined ultrastructurally (Karasek 1983). The first of these processes, referred to as neurosecretory-like because of its similarity to processes observed in neuroendocrine organs, is characterized by the formation of dense-cored vesicles by the Golgi apparatus and their migration to the inner surface of the limiting membrane of the cell. The second type of pinealocyte secretory process, termed ependymal-like because it resembles that observed in epen-

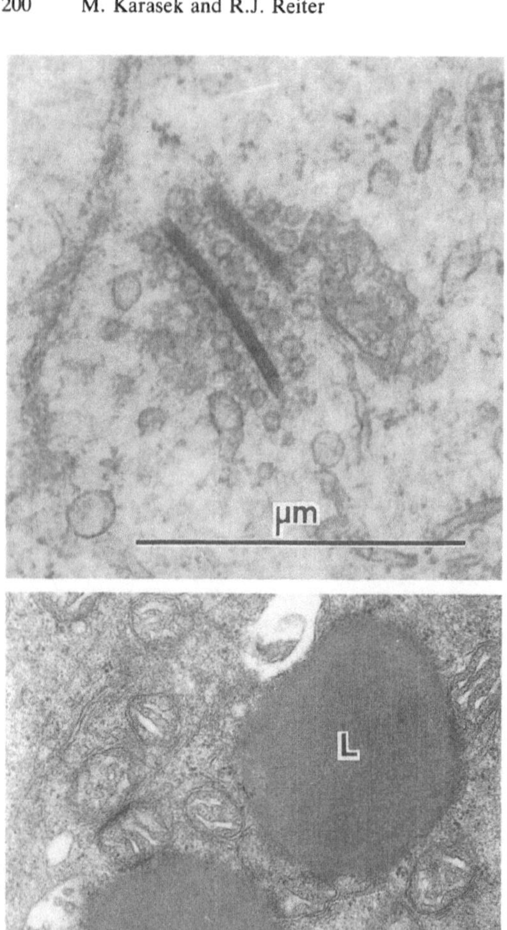

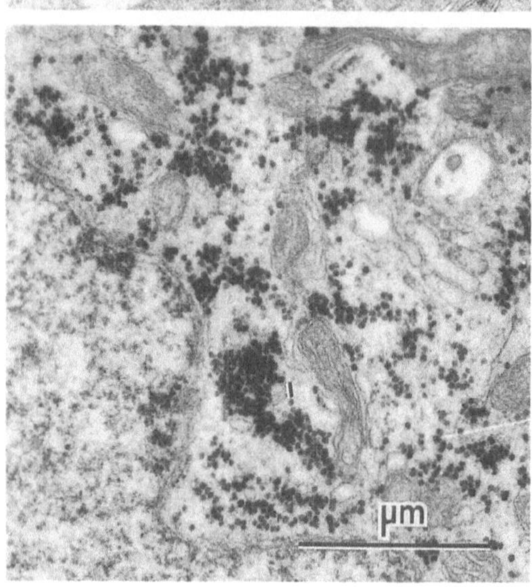

Fig. 218. (*upper*) Pinealocyte, rat. "Synaptic" ribbons in the cytoplasm

Fig. 219. (*middle*) Pinealocyte, rat. Lipid droplets (*L*) in the cytoplasm

Fig. 220. (*lower*) Pinealocyte, brush mouse. Numerous glycogen granules in the cytoplasm

dymal cells, consists of the formation of vacuoles containing flocculent material of moderate electron density by the cisternae of granular endoplasmic reticulum without apparent involvement of the Golgi apparatus; these are also believed to release their contents exocytotically from the cells. Although both these processes have been described, there is no definitive evidence that they represent true secretory mechanisms inasmuch as there is no proof that either peptides or proteins are actually released from the pineal gland. The possibility of yet other modes of pinealocyte secretion (e.g., involving clear vesicles or lipids) cannot be excluded.

Glial Cells. Although there is some inconsistency in terminology dealing with pineal glial cells, immunohistochemical data showing the presence of glial antigenic markers such as S-100 protein, GFA protein, vimentin, and S-1 antigen (Moller et al. 1978; Huang et al. 1984) provide strong support for astrocytes being typical glial components of the mammalian pineal gland. The number of glial cells varies (between 0% and 12%) in the pineal gland of mammals. Pineal astrocytes are characterized ultrastructurally by the presence of a nucleus with chromatin aggregations, by cytoplasm containing the usual variety of organelles confined mainly to the perinuclear region, and especially by the presence of numerous filaments that occur throughout the cytoplasm and processes (Fig. 221).

Nerve Cells. Nerve cells are not regular features of the mammalian pineal gland. However, the presence of intrapineal neurons has been reported at ultrastructural level in a few species (Karasek 1983; Karasek and Reiter 1992). Pineal nerve cells have a large nucleus with an electron-lucent nucleoplasm and a prominent nucleolus, large complexes of parallel-oriented cisternae of granular endoplasmic reticulum, a well-developed Golgi apparatus, numerous lysosomes, microtubules and microfilaments, and numerous granular vesicles (ca. 100 nm in diameter).

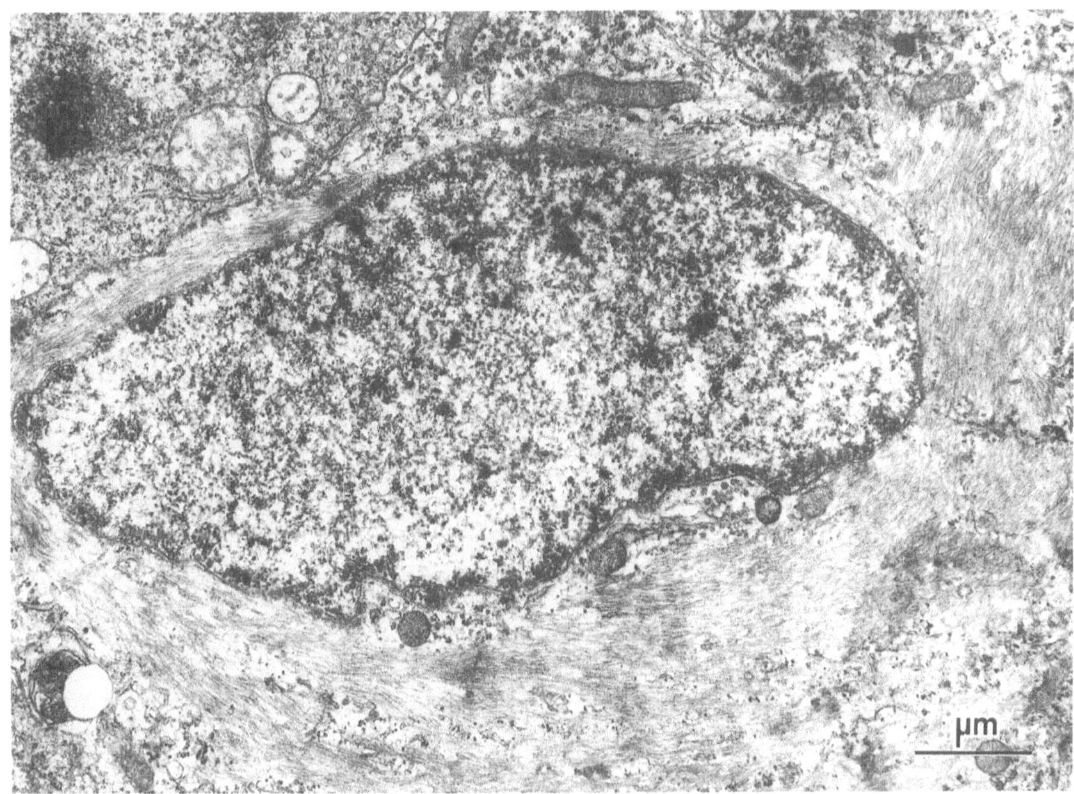

Fig. 221. Glial cell in the pineal parenchyma, fox. Note numerous microfilaments in the cytoplasm. TEM

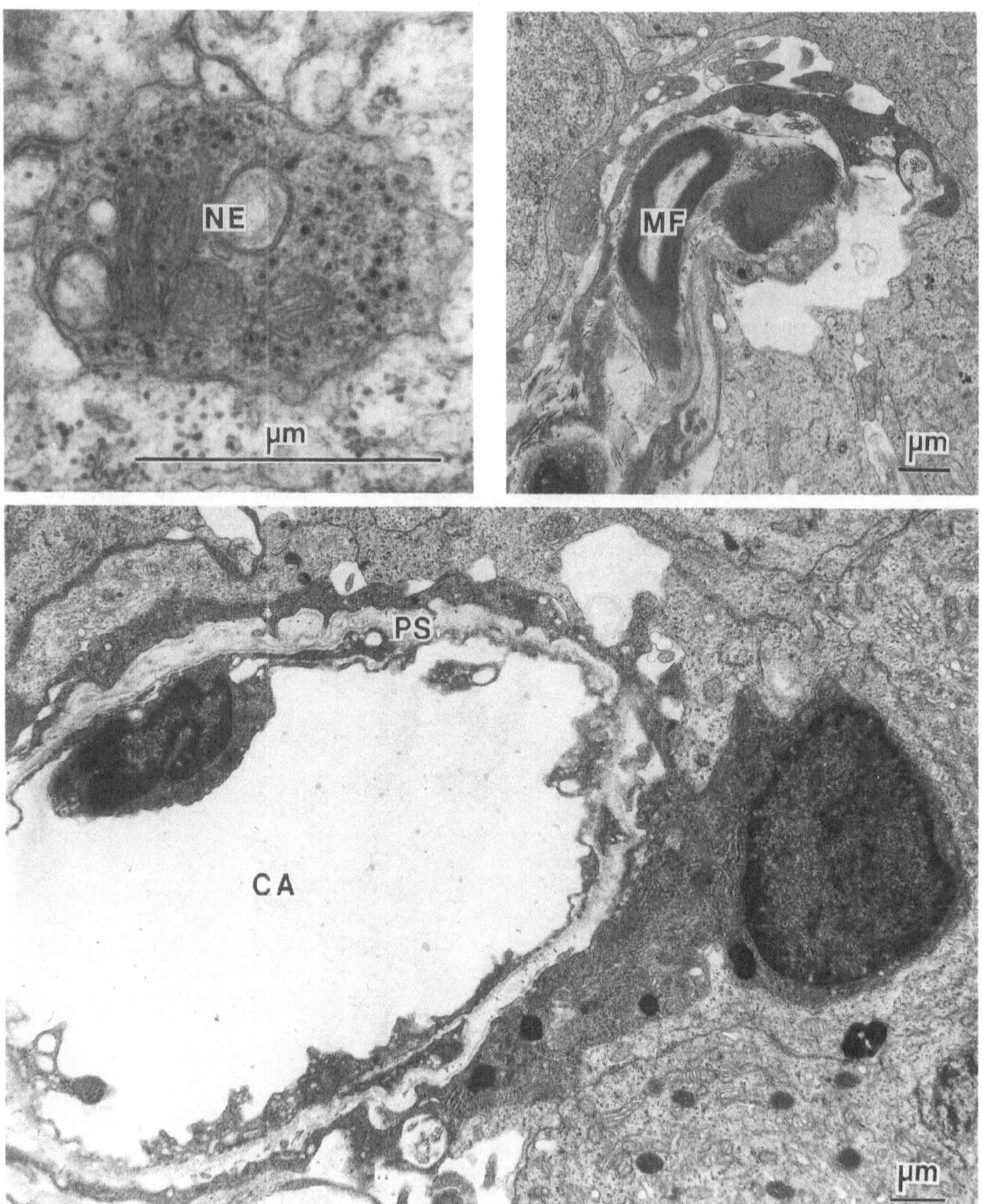

Fig. 222. (*upper left*) Pineal parenchyma, white-footed mouse. Sympathetic nerve ending (*NE*). TEM

Fig. 223. (*upper right*) Pineal parenchyma, Djungarian hamster. Myelinated nerve fiber (*MF*). TEM

Fig. 224. (*below*) Pineal parenchyma, Djungarian hamster. Capillary with fenestrated endothelium (*CA*) surrounded by perivascular space (*PS*). TEM

Nerve Fibers. The mammalian pineal gland contains mainly sympathetic nerve fibers originating in the superior cervical ganglia (Reiter 1981). Postganglionic sympathetic nerve fibers are of special importance for pineal function since the release of norepinephrine from these fibers stimulates melatonin synthesis (Ebadi and Govitrapong 1986; Reiter 1991). However, the number of sympathetic fibers varies widely among species. Most fibers and their endings are located in the perivascular areas, although they are also present within the pineal parenchyma adjacent to pinealocytes. Sympathetic nerve fibers contain numerous clear (40–80 nm in diameter) and granular vesicles (Fig. 222). Two types of granular vesicles are typically present, namely small (40–80 nm in diameter, possessing a dense core of 25 nm), and large (90–150 nm in diameter, possessing a dense core of 70–90 nm). The small vesicles outnumber the large ones by a factor of 10–20.

In addition to sympathetic nerve fibers, myelinated axons (Fig. 223) are present in the pineal of many species (Korf and Moller 1984; Moller 1992). These fibers enter the pineal gland from the posterior and habenular commissures and are located mainly in the proximal part of this organ. Relatively little is known about the functional significance of commissural nerve fibers in the mammalian pineal gland. In reference to the endocrine function of the pineal gland, the sympathetic innervation of the gland is the only one that has been shown to be functionally relevant (Kappers 1965; Reiter 1991). Recently a number of electrophysiological studies also have demonstrated the existence of central epithalamo-pineal neural connections (Korf and Moller 1984; Moller 1992).

There are also some morphological indications of a parasympathetic innervation of the mammalian pineal gland. However, the fine structure of the parasympathetic nerve terminals has never been demonstrated with certainty (Moller 1992).

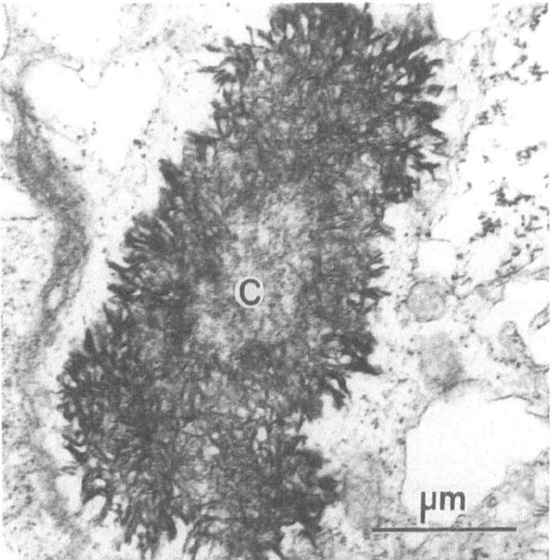

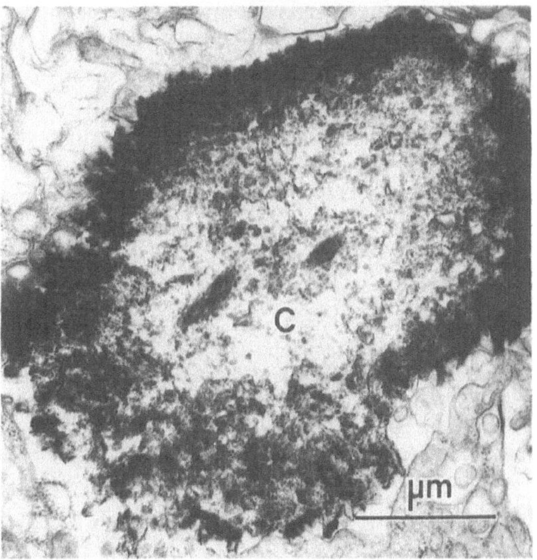

Fig. 225. (*above*). Pineal gland, gerbil. Calcareous concretion (*C*) composed of numerous needle-shaped crystals. TEM

Fig. 226. (*below*) Pineal, rat. Calcareous concretion (*C*). TEM

Capillaries and the Perivascular Spaces. The mammalian pineal gland is richly vascularized, although there are apparent species differences in the ultrastructure of the pineal capillaries (Karasek 1983; Karasek and Reiter 1992). Nonfenestrated endothelial cells are present in some species, whereas in the others a typical fenestrated endothelium is found (Fig. 224). Capillaries are surrounded in all mammals by a perivascular space which is outlined by two basal laminae, one of which faces the endothelium, and the other of which is adjacent to the parenchyma (Fig. 224). The perivascular space varies in width and contains primarily nerve fibers and their endings, terminals of pinealocyte processes, and collagen fibers. The perivascular space may be very irregular in shape, and its extensions often penetrate deeply between the pineal parenchymal cells.

Calcareous Deposits. In a limited number of species (especially in human, ungulates, and some rodents) calcareous deposits (corpora arenacea, acervuli, brain sand, pineal concretions) of unclear functional significance can be found (Karasek 1983; Welsh 1985; Krstic 1986; Karasek and Reiter 1992). They appear to be either amorphous or composed of concentric laminae. Most concretions consist of randomly and/or radially oriented needle-shaped crystals and/or filiform structures embedded in an amorphous material of moderate electron density (Figs. 225, 226).

Concluding Remarks

In general, the ultrastructural features of the mammalian pineal are unremarkable considering the high metabolic and secretory activity of the organ. Also, while the biochemical aspects of the gland display marked day-night differences (Reiter 1991), little in the morphology suggests such obvious circadian metabolic differences.

References

Collin JP (1971) Differentiation and regression of the cells of the sensory line in the epiphysis cerebri. In: Wolstenholme GEW, Knight J (eds) The pineal gland. Livingstone, Edinburgh, pp 79–120

Ebadi M, Govitrapong P (1986) Neural pathways and neurotransmitters affecting melatonin synthesis. J Neural Transm [Suppl] 21:125–155

Huang SK, Nobiling R, Schachner M, Taugner R (1984) Interstitial and parenchymal cells in the pineal gland of the golden hamster. A combined thin-section, freeze-fracture and immunofluorescence study. Cell Tissue Res 235:327–337

Kappers JA (1965) Survey of the innervation of the epiphysis cerebri and the accessory pineal organs of vertebrates. Prog Brain Res 10:87–151

Karasek M (1981) Some functional aspects of the ultrastructure of rat pinealocytes. Endocrinol Exp 15:17–34

Karasek M (1983) Ultrastructure of the mammalian pineal gland: its comparative and functional aspects. In: Reiter RJ (ed) Pineal research reviews, vol 1. Liss, New York, pp 1–48

Karasek M (1987) Functional ultrastructure of the mammalian pinealocyte. In: Reiter RJ, Fraschini F (eds) Advances in pineal research, vol 2. Libbey, London, pp 19–33

Karasek M, Reiter RJ (1992) Morphofunctional aspects of the mammalian pineal gland. Microso Res Tech 21:136–157

Korf HW, Moller M (1984) The innervation of the mammalian pineal gland with special reference to central pinealopetal projections. In: Reiter RJ (ed) Pineal research reviews, vol 2. Liss, New York, pp 41–86

Krstic R (1986) Pineal calcification: its mechanism and significance. J Neural Transm [Suppl] 21:415–432

Lerner AB, Case JD, Takahashi, Lee GH, Mori W (1958) Isolation of melatonin, the pineal factor that lightens melanocytes. J Am Chem Soc 80:2587

Moller M (1992) Fine structure of the pineopetal innervation of the mammalian pineal gland. Microso Res Tech 21:188–204

Moller M, Ingild A, Bock E (1978) Immunohistochemical demonstration of S-100 protein and GFA protein in interstitial cells of the rat pineal gland. Brain Res 140:1–13

Reiter RJ (1981) The mammalian pineal gland: structure and function. Am J Anat 162:287–313

Reiter RJ (1991) Pineal melatonin: cell biology of its synthesis and of its physiological interactions. Endocr Rev 12:151–180

Sheridan MN, Reiter RJ (1970) Observations on the pineal system of the hamster. I. Relations of the superficial and deep pineal to the epithalamus. J Morphol 131:153–162

Vollrath L (1979) Comparative morphology of the vertebrate pineal complex. Prog Brain Res 52:25–37

Vollrath L (1981) The pineal organ, Springer, Berlin Heidelberg New York

Welsh MG (1985) Pineal calcification: structural and functional aspects. In: Reiter RJ (ed) Pineal research reviews, vol 3. Liss, New York, pp 41–88

Zrenner C (1985) Theories of pineal function from classical antiquity to 1900: a history. In: Reiter RJ (ed) Pineal research reviews, vol 3. Liss, New York, pp 1–40

Tumors of the Pineal Gland, Rat

Adalbert Koestner and Henk A. Solleveld

Synonyms. Pinealoma; pineocytoma; pineoblastoma; pinealoma, benign; pinealoma, malignant WHO.*

Gross Appearance

The pineal gland in the rat can be recognized as a reddish or yellow-brown spherical elevation located just dorsal to the anterior and posterior colliculi. Its normal size is about that of the head of a pin. Unlike in the mouse, where the pineal gland often sticks to the meninges and is therefore easily lost during removal of the brain, the pineal in the rat usually remains attached to the surface of the tectum and may be plucked out without damage (Johnson 1983). Neoplasia of the pineal gland may be indicated by slight enlargements of the gland which can be confirmed only by histologic examination. This was the case in three of the five pineal gland tumors reported by Al Zubaidy and Malinowsky (1984). Pineal tumors in the rat may reach sizes exceeding 1 cm in diameter (Fig. 227) and may be further identifiable by discoloration because of hemorrhage and congestion. While these tumors are mostly well circumscribed, they may infiltrate deeply into the brain parenchyma or may spread diffusely along the meninges.

Clinical Considerations. No clinical signs have been attributed definitely to pineal gland tumors in rats. Al Zubaidy and Malinowsky (1984) suggested that some clinical signs noted in their series of five rats, such as gasping respiration, hypothermia, and weight loss may have some causal relationship to the pineal tumors. When pineal tumors become sizeable or metastasize and lead to destruction of brain parenchyma, neurologic consequences may be discernable. It has long been considered that pubertas praecox in children may be associated with germinomas of the pineal gland since the destruction of pineal tissue reduces melatonin production which exerts an inhibitory effect on sexual development (Rubinstein 1972).

* World Health Organization, International Classification of Rodent Tumors (Mohr 1994).

Microscopic Features

Since there was no general model in the past for the histologic classification of pineal tumors in the rat, all published reports referred to these tumors as pinealomas. In one report of pineal tumors in rats (Krinke et al. 1985) some pineal neoplasms were designated as pineal tumors to indicate that they carry features of both the mature pineocytoma as well as of the more primitive pineoblastoma. Al Zubaidy and Malinowski (1984) designated one of the five pineal tumors of their report as a malignant pinealoma. Based on the observations of these authors and our own experience, a spectrum of histologic features varying from poor to advanced differentiation should be expected to occur in rats as it has been established in human pineal neoplasms. Therefore it is recommended that the WHO criteria proposed for human pineal tumors be adapted to the classification of pineal parenchymal tumors of the rat.

Pineocytoma is the most differentiated neoplasm of pineal parenchymal cells. It is usually circumscribed and not invasive. The histologic pattern is reminiscent of the normal pineal gland characterized by a lobulated appearance of cell clusters separated by a delicate connective tissue stroma (Fig. 228). The rather monomorphic cell population consists of small cells with round to oval open-faced nuclei with one to three inconspicuous nucleoli (Fig. 229). The cytoplasm is pale eosinophilic, mostly polar but sometimes with poorly defined cell margins. The tumor cells have a vascular orientation and often line up around vessels (pseudo-rosettes) with processes directed toward the vascular wall (Fig. 230). Complete or incomplete rosette formation may be recognized (Fig. 231). The rate of mitosis is higher than would be expected in a neoplasm of comparable maturity.

Pineoblastoma is the more primitive form of a pineal parenchymal neoplasm. Cells are more densely and diffusely arranged, and the lobulated pattern may be discernable only occasionally. The high nucleo/cytoplasmic ratio, irregular hyperchromatic nuclei, scant cytoplasm, with poorly defined cytoplasmic borders, and the high mitotic index are all features characterizing the more primitive and anaplastic pineoblastoma cell. The

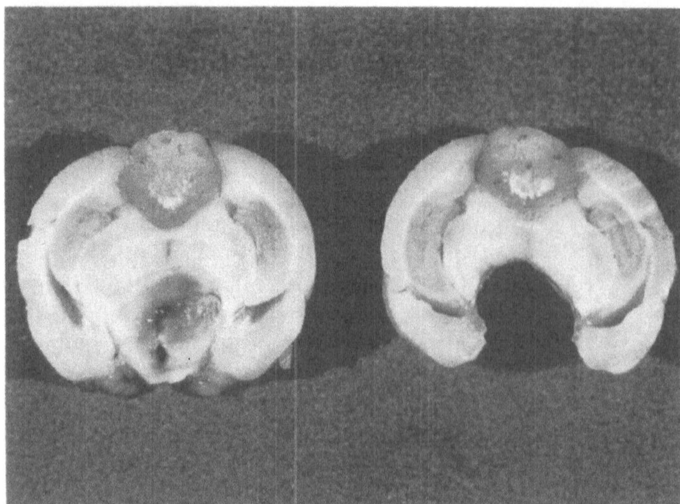

Fig. 227. Pineocytoma, rat; gross appearance. (Courtesy of Burek et al. 1983)

tendency for palisading and rosette formation can be readily recognized. Areas of necrosis are a common feature of this neoplasm (Fig. 232). Pineoblastomas often infiltrate deeply into the brain parenchyma or ventricles and may spread along the meninges or the cerebrospinal axis. Metastases of pineal tumors have not been reported in rats; however, they have been recognized in human patients.

Mixed pineocytoma-pineoblastoma represent characteristics of both types of pineal parenchymal neoplasms. In our review of seven pineal parenchymal neoplasms of rats, three fulfilled the criteria of a mixed pineocytoma-pineoblastoma. In these cases both areas of pineocytoma and pineoblastoma were recognized which usually blended into each other without a clear separating border (Fig. 233).

Tumors of the interstitial cells of the pineal gland have not been reported in rats; however, interstitial cells can be recognized in pineocytomas and also very rarely in pineoblastomas of rats. Their neoplastic transformation would be classified either as a glioma or as an astrocytoma, if astrocytic characteristics were identifiable histologically and/or by immunohistochemical demonstration of the glial fibrillary ac'dic protein (GFAP).

Special Stains and Immunohistochemistry. The histologic characteristics of pineal parenchymal cell tumors, as described above, are generally adequate to establish a diagnosis. Selected special stains and immunohistochemical biomarkers have been used successfully for further confirmation of the pineal origin of neoplastic cells. Silver impregnation (Bielschowsky's method) for identification of nerve fibers in human pineal neoplasms, demonstrated delicate tangles of fine argyrophilic processes in the centers of rosettes, reminiscent of neuroblastic rosettes. This feature may be indicative of the kinship of pineal parenchymal cells to neurons (Rubinstein 1972).

Several immunohistochemical biomarkers have been used successfully on human pineal neoplasms. Neurofilament protein, synaptophysin, and neuron-specific enolase have been used to identify specific neuronal proteins commonly present in pineal parenchymal cells. Synaptophysin has been the most consistent marker in human pineal tumors and the two pineal tumors tested from our series in rats reacted strongly positive for synaptophysin (Fig. 234). Since phylogenetically pinealocytes are derived from neurosensory photoreceptor cells, markers for photoreceptors

▶

Fig. 228. (*upper left*) Pineocytoma, rat; notice faint lobulation and clean tumor margin. H&E, ×234

Fig. 229. (*lower left*) Monomorphic cell population in a rat pineocytoma. Cytoplasm is faintly stained and nuclei are mostly open-faced with one to three nucleoli. There is a moderate rate of mitosis. H&E, ×588

Fig. 230. (*upper right*) Pseudorosette around vessel (*arrow*) in a pineocytoma, rat. H&E, ×588

Fig. 231. (*lower right*) Palisading and rosette formation (*arrow*) in a mixed pineocytoma-pineoblastoma, rat. H&E, ×234

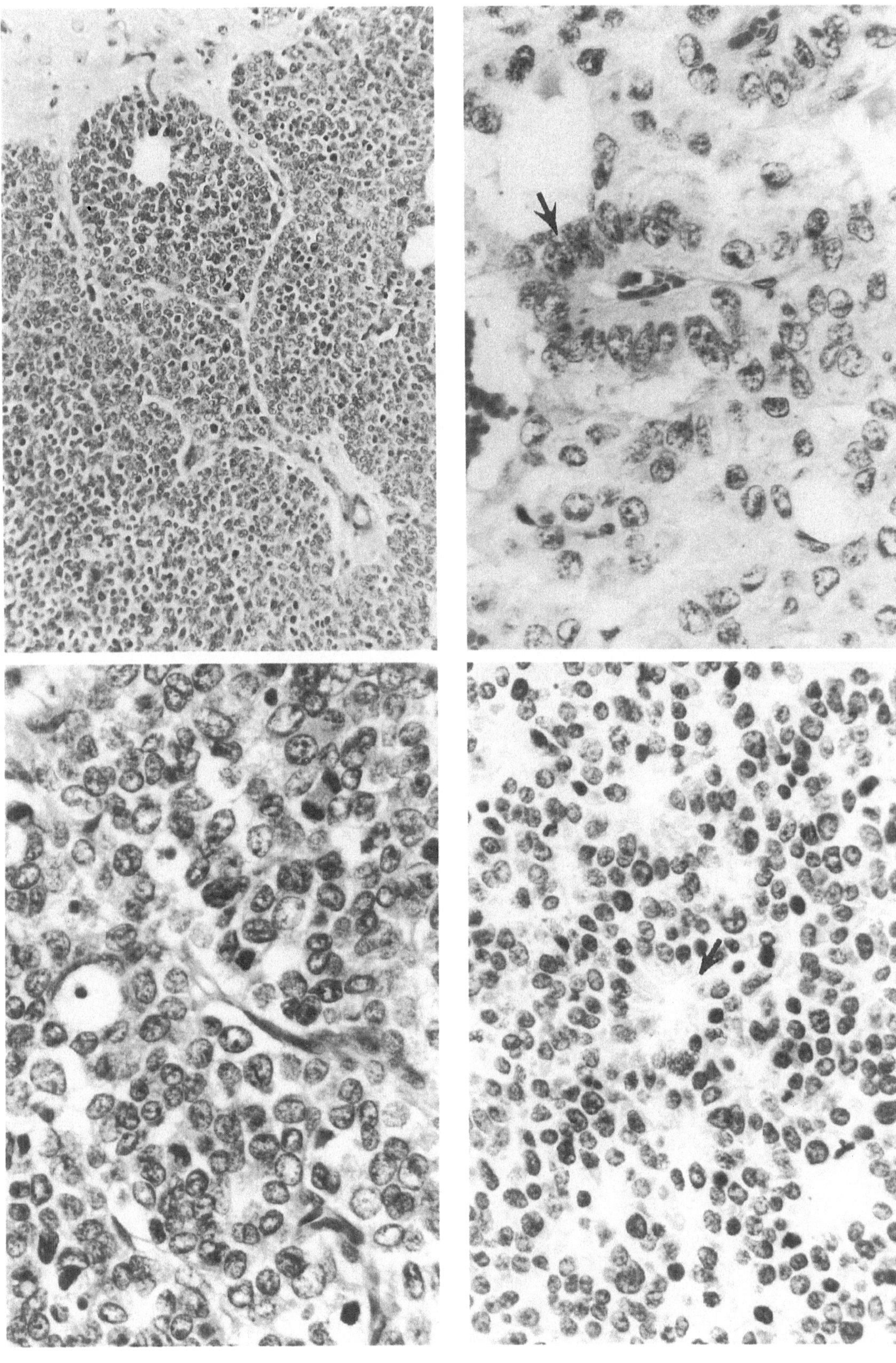

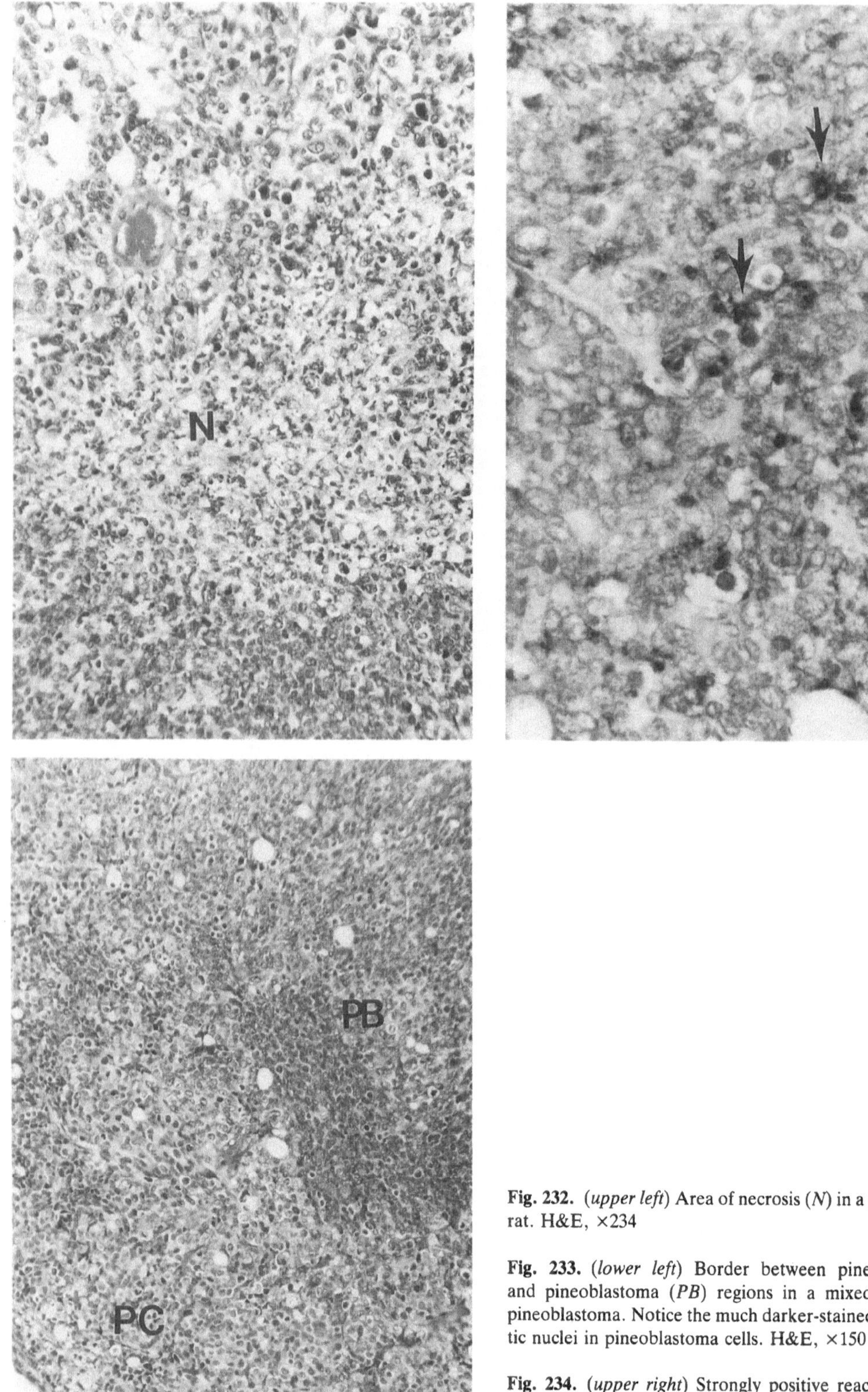

Fig. 232. (*upper left*) Area of necrosis (*N*) in a pineoblastoma, rat. H&E, ×234

Fig. 233. (*lower left*) Border between pineocytoma (*PC*) and pineoblastoma (*PB*) regions in a mixed pineocytoma-pineoblastoma. Notice the much darker-stained hyperchromatic nuclei in pineoblastoma cells. H&E, ×150

Fig. 234. (*upper right*) Strongly positive reactivity of pineal tumor cells for synaptophysin (*arrows*) indicative of the kinship of pineocytes to neurons. Mouse-derived monoclonal antibody avidin-biotin-complex method, ×588

such as retinal S-antigen (S-Ag), rhodopsin (RHO), and interphotoreceptor retinoid binding protein (IRBP) have been used. Photoreceptor cells are still present in the pineal organ of anamniotes, but they become gradually lost during evolution (Karasek and Reiter, this volume). Korf et al. (1990) reported positive S-Ag and RHO immunoreactions in midline brain neoplasms of transgenic mice, and Mena et al. (1994) detected occasional S-Ag and RHO positive cells in three human pineocytomas. Lopes et al. (1993) identified IRBP and its mRNA in a human mixed pineocytoma-pineoblastoma. IRBP is the earliest photoreceptor-associated binding protein expressed during retinal development. Its presence in pineal tumors suggests a rudimentary photosensory differentiation of a tumor with limited evidence of pineal differentiation.

A future prospective specific biomarker for pineal parenchymal cells is the hydroxyindole *O*-methyltransferase (HIOMT), a melatonin-synthesizing enzyme which converts *N*-acetylserotonin into melatonin (Kuwano et al. 1983). This marker is, to our knowledge, not yet commercially available and has not been used on pineal neoplasms of rats. Barber et al. (1978) reported a HIOMT activity in a mixed pineocytoma-pineoblastoma of a 37-year-old man to be 20% of that expected in a normal pineal gland at autopsy. The pineal gland in this case was completely replaced by neoplastic tissue. The HIOMT activity was sufficient to retain the nyctohemeral rhythmicity of melatonin concentrations in the absence of normal pineal tissue. In addition to these specific markers for pineal parenchymal cells, GFAP, and S-100 protein have been used for the identification of interstitial astrocytes. The two pineal tumors available to us for immunohistochemical examination were almost devoid of interstitial cells which was reflected in the rare presence of GFAP-positive cells within the tumors.

Ultrastructure

Electron microscopy is less specific for diagnostic purposes than immunohistochemistry since pineal tumor cells have few unique ultrastructural features (Burek et al. 1983). Neoplastic cells in the pineal tumors have been described as primitive or poorly differentiated pleomorphic cells with scant rough endoplasmic reticulum, variable amounts of free ribosomes, numerous mitochondria, and round-to-pleomorphic nuclei containing infrequent nucleoli. Cilia may be found within the cytoplasm or extending outside of the cell. When present, cilia usually are accompanied by one or more centrioles (Fig. 235). Junctional complexes resembling desmosomes are infrequently observed.

Differential Diagnosis

In the gross specimen the midline position of a mass between the cerebral hemispheres indicates the probability of a neoplasm of the pineal gland. However, on rare occasions a meningioma is found in this position. The distinctive microscopic appearance of meningioma and pineal gland tumor lead clearly to their differentiation. Teratomas and germinomas may also appear at this site in some species but can be distinguished by their histologic features.

Biologic Features

Tumors of the pineal region have been recognized in man and in several animal species and have long been called pinealomas. Because of their infrequent occurrence their histogenetic classification emerged slower than that of the more frequently encountered tumors of the central nervous system (CNS). A diversity of histologic patterns of pinealomas was first recognized in the 1940s (Russell 1944; Friedman 1947). It was observed that many pinealomas in humans resemble testicular seminomas, and that some reveal teratoid characteristics. The term germinoma was introduced at that time to separate these neoplasms from those arising from pineal parenchymal cells. Germinomas were thought to originate from primitive germ cells which migrate to widely separated areas of the embryo during early fetal life (Rubinstein 1972). Their midline location in the CNS (pineal, suprasellar, and intrasellar areas) is still unexplained. Germinomas account for over 50% of human pineal tumors.

Classification. The new World Health Organization (WHO) classification of human brain tumors (Kleihues et al. 1993) separates tumors of germ cell origin from those derived from the pineal parenchymal cells. The latter are classified as pineocytomas, pineoblastomas, and mixed pineo-

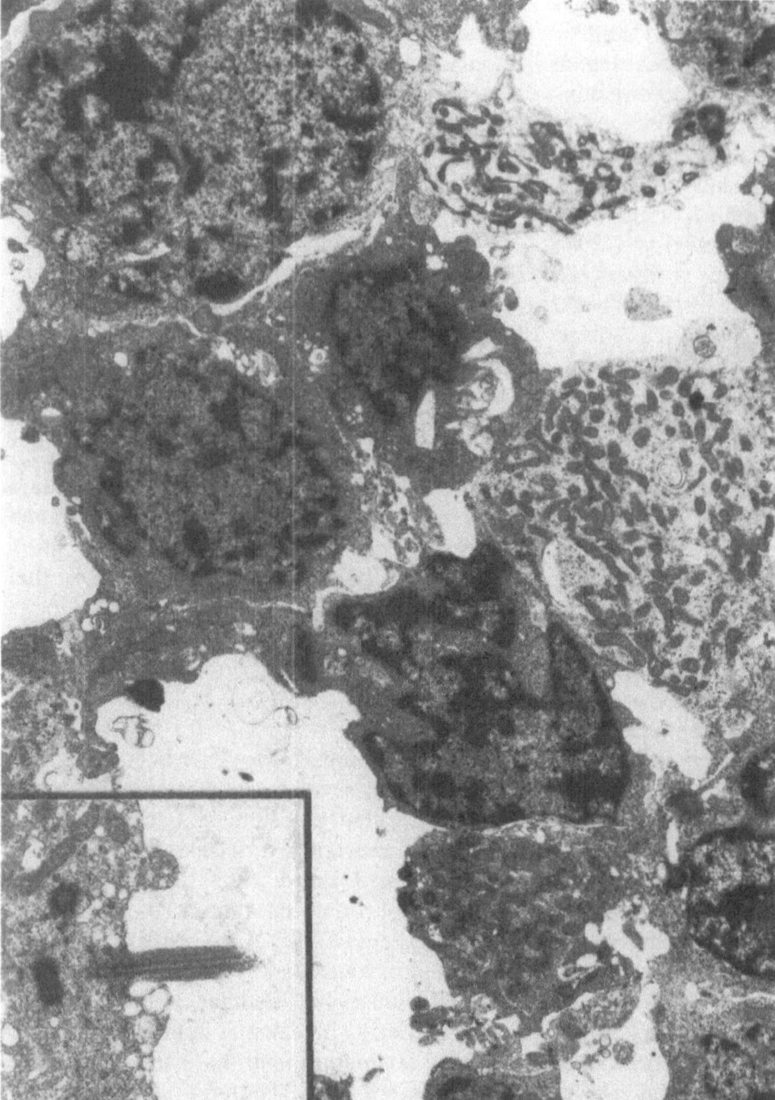

Fig. 235. Pineocytoma, rat. Ultrastructural features of cells, ×6500. Cilia and centrioles (*insert*) are frequently observed, ×20 500. (Courtesy of Burek et al. 1983)

cytoma-pineoblastomas. Tumors arising from pineal interstitial cells represent astrocytomas. Pinealoma is basically an appropriate name for pineal parenchymal cell tumors; however, its past broad use for all pineal neoplasms, including germinomas, warrants the use of a more specific nomenclature for pineal parenchymal cell tumors as reflected in the WHO classification. A WHO classification schema for animal tumors introduced after this paper was written (Mohr 1994) proposes separating neoplasms of the rat pineal into two categories: pinealoma, benign and pinealoma, malignant. Since malignancy is often based on behavior of the neoplasm (invasion, recurrence, metastasis) rather than cytologic characteristics, a cytologic classification, as proposed for human pineal tumors, will probably lead to a more specific and more discriminating diagnosis. It will also facilitate communication between veterinary and medical specialists if the same classification is used for identical neoplasms in the two species.

Incidence. The reported incidence of pineal parenchymal cell neoplasms is low in all species of animals as well as in humans. The true incidence of these tumors in the rat is difficult to assess. Only seven published reports on pineal tumors in rats are found in the literature describing a total of 15 pineal neoplasms (Table 12). Eleven of these pineal tumors were reported from countries outside the United States. It is surprising that only four pineal tumors should have been found in the hundreds of thousands of rats used in long-term toxicity studies in the United States over the past 40 years. It is of course very likely that more of these tumors have been recognized but were not reported, and that others were missed because of their very small size or were accidentally removed with the meninges during necropsy.

Based on the six publications in which both the number of pineal tumors and the total number of rats were given, 14 pineal tumors occurred in 13642 rats, for an incidence rate of 1 in 974 animals, or 0.10%. There are slight differences of pineal tumor incidences among the strains of rats used in the cited publications (Table 12); however, the number of published studies is insufficient to permit a comparison of frequencies among rat strains. Two additional pinealomas were reported from a chronic toxicity study in F344 rats; both tumors occurred in the high-dose groups together with hepatic neoplasms. A probability exists that they might have been caused by exposure to the test compound (Jackson and Blackwell 1993).

Comparison with Other Species

Germinomas of the pineal gland have, to our knowledge, not been reported in rats or in any other animal species. Only tumors believed to have originated from pineal parenchymal cells have been reported in rats. All have been detected in aged animals (average age 24 months) ranging from 10 to 34 months (Table 12). This compares well with 21 human pineocytomas, where the mean age at the time of diagnosis was 36.2 years with a range of 14–65 years (Mena et al. 1995). Human pineoblastomas and germinomas occur at younger ages, with a peak in the later half of the second decade of life (Rubenstein 1972; Fig. 236). There is a striking absence of reports of pineal neoplasms in dogs and cats, two species in which most of the intracranial neoplasms have been recognized. Textbooks of tumors for domestic animals (Moulton 1990) make no mention of pineal neoplasms. Luginbühl et al. (1968) in a review of spontaneous tumors of the nervous system in animals refer to a few publications that deal with pineal neoplasms. Affected species were a cow (Frauchiger et al. 1966), goat (Trautmann 1923), silver fox (Schlotthauer and Kernohan 1935), horse (László 1940), and zebra (Verneulen 1925). The files of the Department of Veterinary Biosciences at Ohio State University contain a pineocytoma from a 23-year old work horse (unpublished).

The rat is presently the animal species in which most of the pineal neoplasms have been reported. They are histologically very similar to pineal tumors in human beings and perfectly suitable to be classified according to the new WHO classification of brain tumors (Kleihues et al. 1993).

Acknowledgements. The authors express their appreciation to Dr. Thomas J. Bucci, National Center for Toxicological Research, for providing material from pineal tumors of two rats for this

Table 12. Pineal tumors in rats

Strain of Rat	Number in Study	Incidence of Pineal Tumors			Age (months) at Examination	Reference
		M	F	Total (%)		
Fischer F344	692		1	1 (0.11)	26.5	Maekawa et al. (1984)
Sprague-Dawley	8960	2	2	4 (0.04)	10–26	Krinke et al. (1985)
Sprague-Dawley	125	1		1 (0.80)	16	Thompson et al. (1961)
Sprague-Dawley	N.D.		1[b]	1[b]	34	Burek et al. (1983)
Wistar	1800	1	4	5 (0.28)	19–26	Al-Zubaidy et al. (1984)
* Osborne-Mendel[a]	465		2	2 (0.43)	26	Dagle et al. (1979)
Han: Wist	1600		1	1 (0.60)	13–48	Hösterey (1981)
Five strains	13642	4	10	14 (0.10)	10–48	Seven Studies

[a] Only studies listed in which pineal tumors were reported.

[b] Not be counted in incidence study since total number used in study is not known.

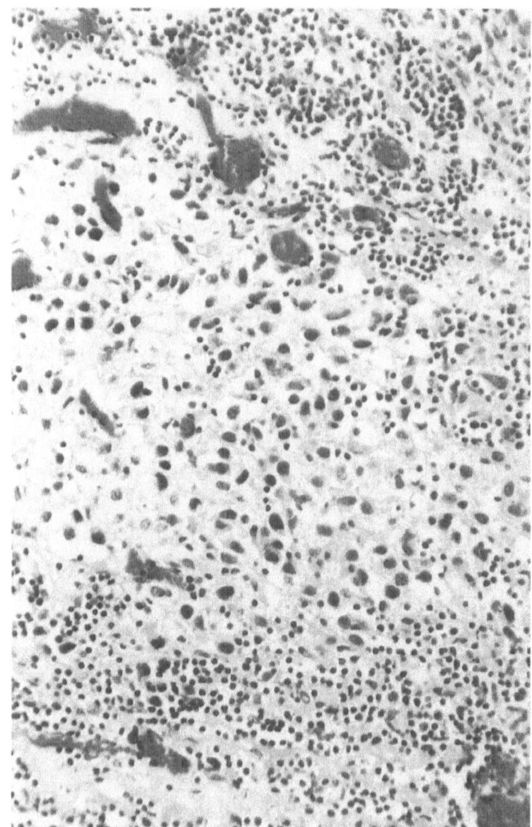

Fig. 236. Typical histologic picture of a human germinoma. Two cell types are prevalent; large spheroid cells with centrally located round to ovoid nuclei, reminiscent of testicular seminoma and lymphocytes. H&E, ×234. (Courtesy of Dr. Sandy Cottingham, Department of Pathology, Ohio State University)

study. Most illustrations (Figs. 227, 228, 231, 232, and 233) derived from this material. Thanks are also expressed to Dr. G.J. Krinke, CIBA AG, Basel, Switzerland for permitting the authors to review pineal tumor sections from five rats. Figures 229 and 230 were taken from one tumor of this collection. The authors further thank the staff of the pathology laboratory of Children's Hospital, Columbus, Ohio for performing the synaptophysin immunohistochemical test.

References

Al Zubaidy AJ, Malinowski W (1984) Spontaneous pineal body tumours (pinealomas) in Wistar rats; a histological and ultrastructural study. Lab Anim 18:224–229

Barber SG, Smith JA, Hughes RC (1978) Melatonin as a tumour marker in a patient with pineal tumour. Br Med J 2:328

Burek JD, van Zwieten MJ, Solleveld A (1983) Pinealomas, Rat. In: Jones TC, Mohr U, Hunt RD (eds). Monographs on pathology of laboratory animals, endocrine system. Springer, Berlin Heidelberg New York, pp 350–354

Dagle GE, Zwicker GM, Renne RA (1979) Morphology of spontaneous brain tumors in the rat. Vet Pathol 16:318–324

Frauchiger E, O'Hara PJ, Shortridge EH (1966) Pinealome bei Tieren. Schweiz Arch Tierheilkd 108:368–372

Friedman NB (1947) Germinoma of the pineal; its identity with germinoma ("seminoma") of the testis. Cancer Res 7:363–368

Hösterey R (1981) Histologische Klassifizierung spontaner Tumoren des Zentralen Nervensystems bei Han:Wist Ratten. Thesis, Tierärztliche Hochschule Hannover, Germany

Jackson CD, Blackwell BN (1993) Two-year toxicity study of doxylamine succinate in the Fischer 344 rat. J Am Coll Toxicol 12:1–11

Johnson JE Jr (1983) Histology, ultrastructure, pineal gland, rat. In: Jones TC, Mohr U, Hunt RD (eds) Monographs on pathology of laboratory animals; endocrine system. Springer, Berlin Heidelberg New York, pp 341–350

Kleihues P, Burger PC, Scheithauer BW (1993) The new WHO classification of brain tumors. Brain Pathol 3:255–268

Korf HW, Götz W, Herken R, Theuring F, Gruss P, Schachenmayr W (1990) S-Antigen and rod-opsin immunoreactions in midline brain neoplasms of transgenic mice: similarities to pineal cell tumors and certain medulloblastomas in man. J Neuropathol Exp Neurol 49:424–437

Krinke G, Naylor DC, Schmid S, Frölich E, Schnider K (1985) The incidence of naturally-occurring primary brain tumours in the laboratory rat. J Comp Pathol 95:175–192

Kuwano R, Iwanaga T, Nakajima T, Masuda T, Takahashi Y (1983) Immunocytochemical demonstration of hyodroxyindole O-methyltransferase (HIOMT), neuron-specific enolase (NSE) and S-100 protein in the bovine pineal gland. Brain Res 274:171–175

László P (1940) Pinaloma in der Zirbeldrüse eines Pferdes. Dtsch Tierarztl Wochenschr 47:402–403

Lopes MB, Gonzalez-Fernandez F, Scheithauer BW, VandenBerg SR (1993) Differential expression of retinal proteins in a pineal parenchymal tumor. J Neuropathol Exp Neurol 52:516–524

Luginbühl H, Fankhauser R, McGrath JT (1968) Spontaneous neoplasms of the nervous system in animals. Prog Neurol Surg 2:85–164

Maekawa A, Onodera H, Tanigawa H, Furuta K, Takahashi M, Kurokawa Y, Kokubo T, Ogiu T, Uchida O, Kobayashi K, Hayashi Y (1984) Spontaneous tumors of the nervous system and associated organs and/or tissues in rats. Gann 75:784–791

Mena H, Rushing EJ, Ribas JL, Delahunt B, McCarthy WF (1995) Tumors of pineal parenchymal cells: a correlation of histological features, including nucleolar organizer regions, with survival in 35 cases. Hum Pathol 26:20–30

Mohr U (ed) (1994) International classification of rodent tumours. I. The rat. International Agency for Research on Cancer, Lyon, pp 12–14 (IARC publication no 122)

Moulton JE (1990) Tumors in domestic animals, 3rd edn. University of California Press, Berkley, pp 279–281

Rubinstein LJ (1972) Tumors of the central nervous system. Atlas of tumor pathology, fascicle 6. Armed Forces Institute of Pathology, Washington DC

Russel DS (1944) The pinealoma: its relationship to teratoma. J Pathol Bact 56:145–150

Schlotthauer GF, Kernohan JW (1935) Glioma in a dog and pinealoma in a silver fox (*Vulpus fulvus*). Am J Cancer 24:350–356

Thompson SW, Huseby RA, Fox M, Davis CL, Hunt RD (1961). Spontaneous tumors in the Sprague Dawley rat. J Natl Cancer Inst 27:1037–1051

Trautmann A (1923) Drüsen mit innerer Sekretion. In: Joest N (ed) Anatomie der Haustiere, III. Schoetz, Berlin

Vermeulen HA (1925) Epiphyse und Epiphysen tumoren bei Tieren. Berl Munch Tierarztl Wochenschr 41:717–719

Thyroid

Hormonal Imbalances and Mechanisms of Chemical Injury of Thyroid Gland

Charles C. Capen

Introduction

Organogenesis. The thyroid gland originates as a thickened plate of epithelium in the floor of the pharynx (Fig. 237). It is intimately related to the aortic sac in its development, and this association leads to the frequent occurrence of accessory thyroid parenchyma in the mediastinum. The accessory thyroid tissue may undergo neoplastic transformation. A portion of the thyroglossal duct may persist postnatally and form a cyst due to the accumulation of proteinic material secreted by the lining epithelium. Thyroglossal duct cysts develop in the anterior cervical region. Their lining epithelium may undergo neoplastic transformation and give rise to follicular cell carcinomas. Accessory thyroid tissue is common particularly in certain animal species such as the dog and may be located anywhere from the larynx to the diaphragm. About 50% of adult dogs have accessory thyroids embedded in the fat on the intrapericardial aorta. Accessory thyroid tissue completely lacks C (parafollicular) cells, but their follicular structure and function are the same as those of the main thyroid lobes.

Histology and Ultrastructure. The thyroid gland is the largest of the organs that function exclusively as an endocrine gland. The basic structure of the thyroid is unique for endocrine glands, consisting of follicles of varying size that contain colloid produced by the follicular cells (Fig. 238). During folliculogenesis an intracytoplasmic cavity develops initially in individual cells. Follicles appear to grow during development by proliferation of component cells and coalescence of adjacent colloid-containing microfollicles in individual cells (Collins and Capen 1980; Toda and Sugihara 1990). Folliculogenesis stimulated by thyroid-stimulating hormone (TSH) in vitro appears to require integrity of both microfilaments and microtubules, since chemicals (vinblastine and colchicine) which disorganize these organelles block follicle formation (Pic et al. 1984).

The follicular cells are cuboidal to columnar and their secretory polarity is directed toward the lumen of the follicles. The luminal surfaces of follicular cells protrudes into the follicular lumen and has numerous microvillar projections that greatly increase the surface area in contact with colloid (Fig. 239). An extensive network of inter- and intrafollicular capillaries provides the follicular cells with an abundant blood supply. Follicular cells have long profiles of rough endoplasmic reticulum and a large Golgi apparatus in their cytoplasm for synthesis and packaging of substantial amounts of protein that are then transported into the follicular lumen (Fig. 239). Numerous electron-dense lysosomal bodies are present in the cytoplasm, which are important in the secretion of thyroid hormones. The interface between the luminal side of follicular cells and the colloid is modified by numerous microvilli (Fig. 239).

The biosynthesis of thyroid hormones is also unique among endocrine glands because the final assembly of the hormones occurs extracellularly within the follicular lumen. Essential raw materials, such as iodide, are trapped efficiently at the basilar aspect of follicular cells from interfollicular capillaries, transported rapidly against a concentration gradient to the lumen, and oxidized by a thyroid peroxidase in microvillar membranes to reactive iodine (I_2; Fig. 240). The assembly of thyroid hormones within the follicular lumen is made possible by a unique protein (thyroglobulin) synthesized on the rough endoplasmic reticulum and packaged in the Golgi apparatus of follicular cells.

Thyroglobulin is a high molecular weight glycoprotein synthesized in successive subunits on the

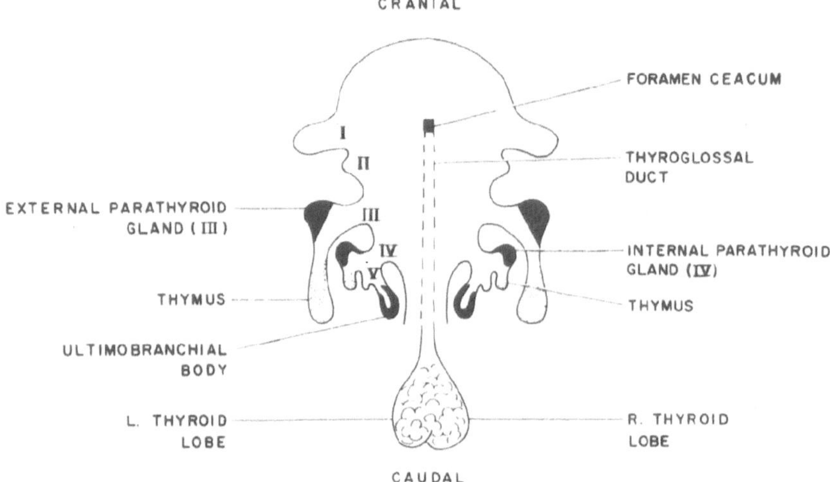

Fig. 237. Embryology of thyroid and parathyroid glands and relationship to primordia for the ultimobranchial body

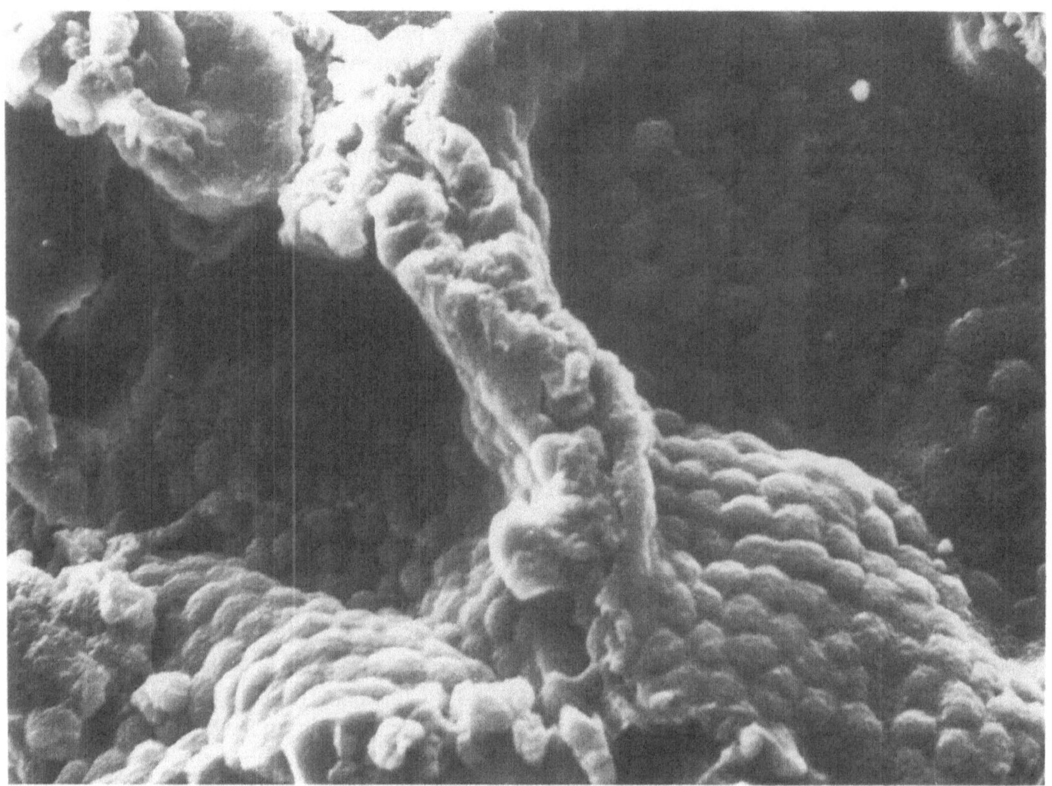

Fig. 238. Scanning electron micrograph of thyroid gland of a dog with two opened follicles (*F*). The luminal aspect of individual follicular cells protrudes into the follicular lumen (*arrowheads*). *I*, Interfollicular space with connective tissue and capillaries

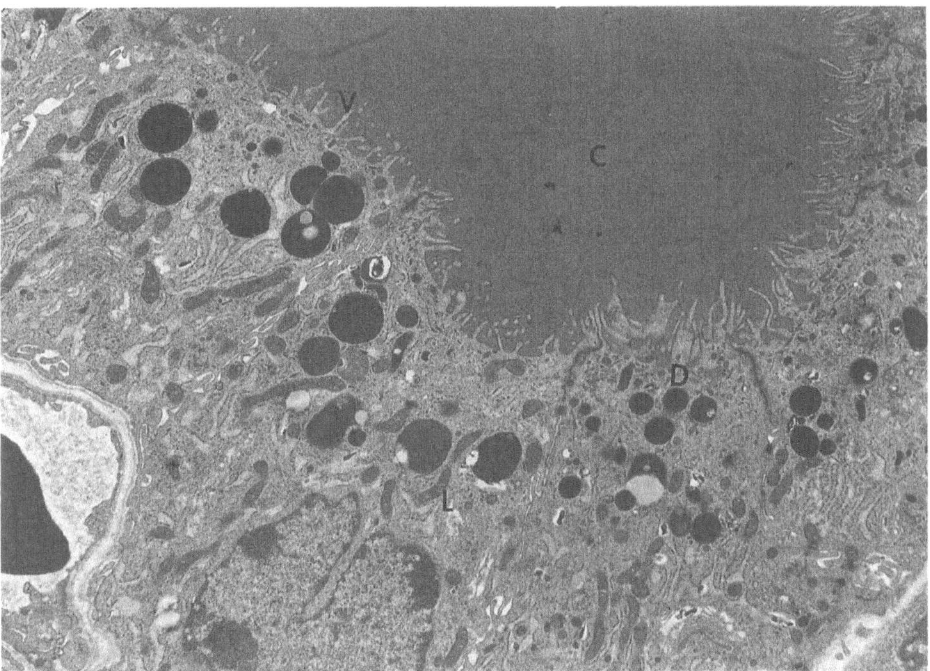

Fig. 239. Electron micrograph of normal thyroid follicular cells with long microvilli (*V*) extending into the luminal colloid (*C*). Pseudopods from the apical plasma membrane surround a portion of the colloid to form an intracellular colloid droplet (*D*). Numerous lysosomes (*L*) are present in the apical cytoplasm in close proximity to the colloid droplets. Intrafollicular capillary (*lower left*)

ribosomes in follicular cells. The constituent amino acids (tyrosine and others) and carbohydrates (i.e., mannose, fructose, galactose) come from the circulation. Recently synthesized thyroglobulin (17S) leaving the Golgi apparatus is packaged into apical vesicles and extruded into the follicular lumen. Human thyroglobulin contains complex carbohydrate units with up to four sulfate groups and units with both sulfate and sialic acid (Sakurai et al. 1990). The amino acid tyrosine is incorporated within the molecular structure of thyroglobulin. Iodine is bound to tyrosyl residues in thyroglobulin at the apical surface of follicular cells to form successively monoiodotyrosine (MIT) and diiodotyrosine (DIT). The resulting MIT and DIT combine to form the two biologically active iodothyronines (thyroxine, T_4; triiodothyronine, T_3) secreted by the thyroid gland (Fig. 241).

The majority of epithelial cells and the functionally most important cells of the thyroid are the follicular cells (Fig. 239). They vary in height depending on the intensity of stimulation by pituitary thyrotropin (TSH), between low cuboidal and tall columnar. Follicular size and shape are quite variable in the human thyroid, and there is no discernible pattern in the distribution of small and large follicles within the gland. Peripherally situated follicles in rats tend to be large and central ones are small. Uchiyama et al. (1986a,b) reported that distinct variations occur morphometrically in volume and numerical densities of follicles during a 24-h period in rats and reflect changes in subcellular organelles of follicular cells. Follicular cells in the human thyroid are relatively flat compared with those of the rat.

The histologic appearance of the thyroid is dramatically influenced by the level of circulating thyrotropin (TTH) or TSH from the adenohypophysis (Collins and Capen 1980). Thyrotropin binds to the basilar aspect of thyroid follicular cells, activates adenylate cyclase with accumulation of cyclic AMP, and increases the rate of biochemical reactions concerned with biosynthesis and secretion of thyroid hormones (Wynford-Thomas et al. 1987). One of the initial structural responses by follicular cells to TSH is the formation of numerous cytoplasmic pseudopodia, resulting in increased endocytosis of colloid and

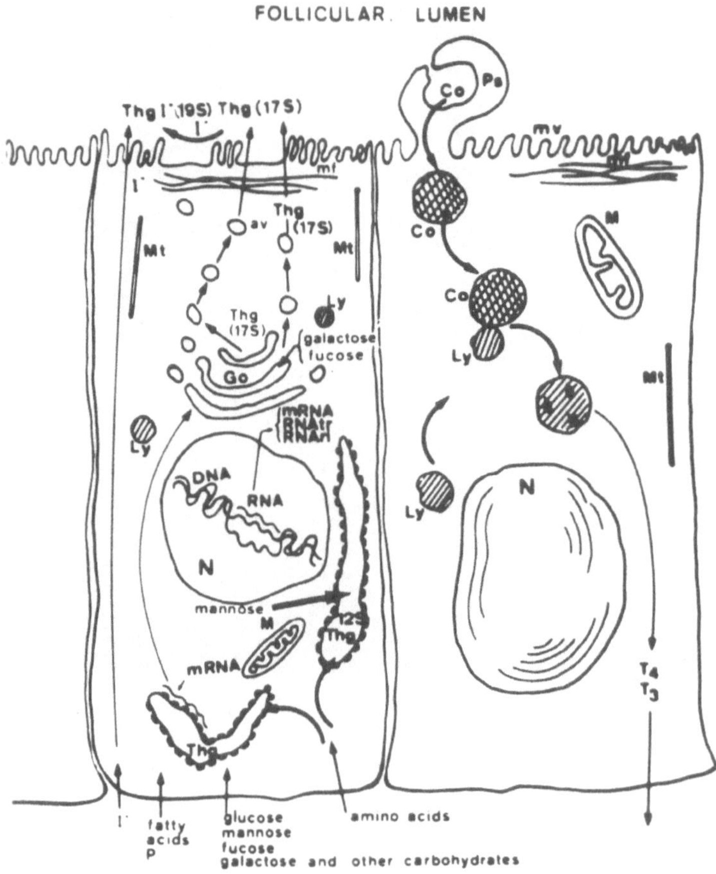

Fig. 240. Thyroid follicular cells illustrating two-way traffic of materials from capillaries into the follicular lumen. Raw materials, such as iodide ion (I^-), are concentrated by follicular cells and rapidly transported into the lumen (*left*). Amino acids (thyrosine and others) and sugars are assembled by follicular cells into thyroglobulin (*Thg*), packaged into apical vesicles (*av*), and released into the lumen. The iodination of tyrosyl residues occurs within the thyroglobulin molecule to form thyroid hormones in the follicular lumen. Elongation of microvilli and endocytosis of colloid by follicular cells occurs in response to TSH stimulation (*right*). The intracellular colloid droplets (*Co*) fuse with lysosomal bodies (*Ly*), active thyroid hormone is enzymatically cleaved from thyroglobulin, and free T_4 and T_3 released into the cytosol and eventually into the circulation. *Mt*, Microtubules, *M*, mitochondria; *mf*, microfilaments. (Courtesy of Bastenie et al. 1975)

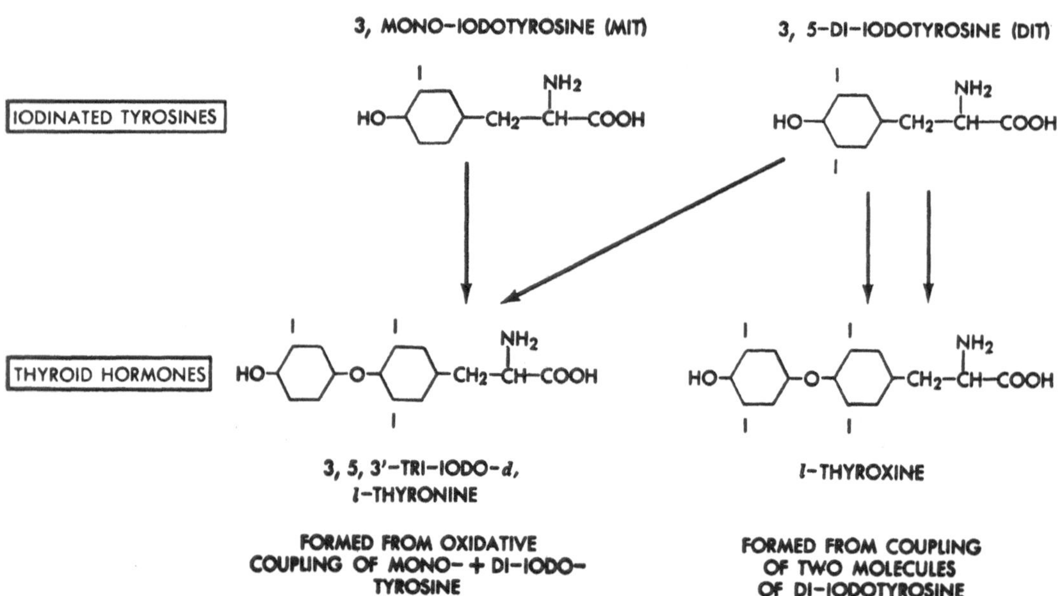

Fig. 241. Chemistry of formation of thyroid hormones from iodinated thyrosines within follicular lumen of thyroid gland. (Courtesy of R.W. Rawson and Clinical Symposia)

release of preformed thyroid hormone stored within the follicular lumen (Fig. 242). Nilsson et al. (1986) reported that follicular cells do not respond in an all-or-none mode to acute TSH stimulation but rather the response (i.e., numbers of pseudopods formed after 20 min) was graded depending upon the level of TSH.

If the secretion of TSH is sustained (hours or days), thyroid follicular cells become more columnar and follicular lumens become smaller and appear as slitlike spaces due to increased endocytosis of colloid (Fig. 243; Collins and Capen 1980; Many et al. 1985; Ericson and Engström 1978). Numerous periodic acid-Schiff (PAS) positive colloid droplets are present in the luminal aspect of the hypertrophied follicular cells. TSH stimulation not only elicits a highly individual macropinocytotic response among different follicular cells but, in addition, the fraction of TSH-responsive cells is also a function of dose (Gerber et al. 1987).

Iodine deficiency in the diet resulting in diffuse thyroid hyperplasia was common in animals and humans in many goitrogenic areas throughout the world before the widespread addition of iodized salt to the diet. Marginal iodine-deficient diets containing certain goitrogenic compounds may result in thyroid follicular cell hypertrophy and hyperplasia with clinical evidence of goiter with hypothyroidism. These goitrogenic substances include thiouracil, sulfonamides, anions of the Hofmeister series, a number of plants from the family Brassicacceae, among others.

The converse of what has been just described occurs in follicular cells as a response to an increase in circulating thyroid hormones and a corresponding decrease in circulating pituitary TTH (e.g., after exogenous T_4 therapy) or in patients with a large space-occupying pituitary lesion that markedly decreases the ability to secrete TTH (Collins and Capen 1980; Gerber et al. 1985). Thyroid follicles become greatly enlarged and distended, with densely staining colloid due to decreased TSH-mediated endocytosis of colloid. Follicular cells lining the involuted follicles are low cuboidal, and there are few endocytotic vacuoles at the interface between the colloid and follicular cells (Fig. 244). The luminal surface of follicular cells is flattened. Microvilli extending into the colloid are widely separated and short in response to a long-standing decreased secretion of TSH (Fig. 245).

The thyroid stroma is exceptionally rich in blood vessels that form extensive interfollicular capillary

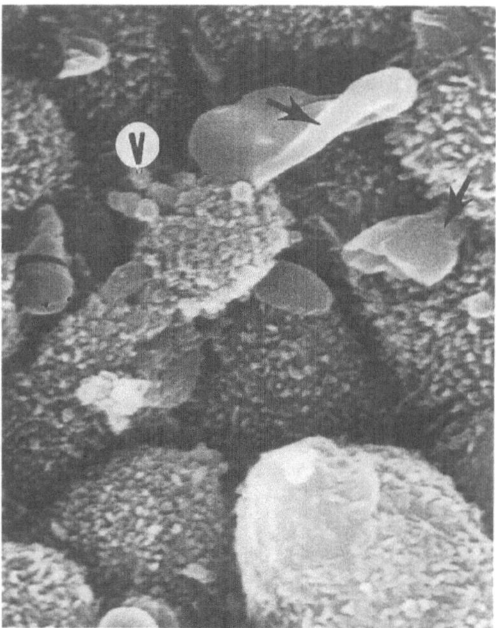

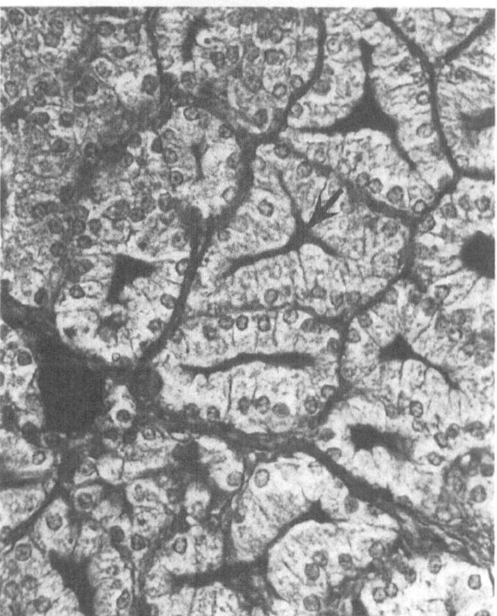

Fig. 242. (*above*) Scanning electron micrograph of apical surface of hypertrophied thyroid follicular cells 4 h after TSH stimulation. Numerous elongated microvilli (*V*) and cytoplasmic projections (*arrows*) extend into the follicular lumen to engulf colloid as part of the initial stages of thyroid hormone secretion in response to TSH. (Courtesy of Collins and Capen 1980)

Fig. 243. (*below*) Response of thyroid follicular cells 8 h after TSH stimulation. The follicular cells are hypertrophic and columnar. Many follicles are nearly depleted of colloid and partially collapsed (*arrow*)

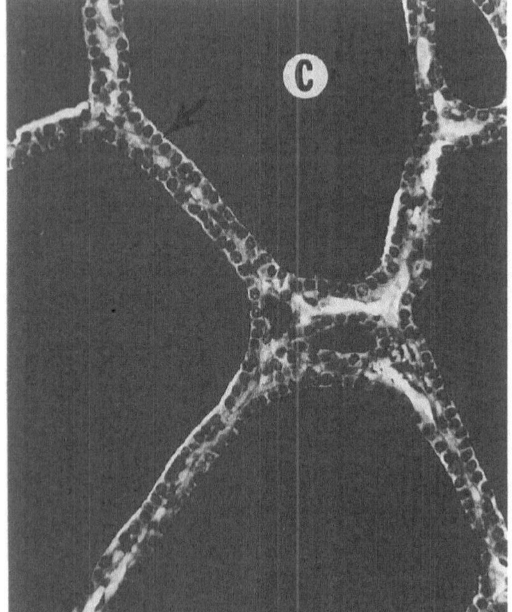

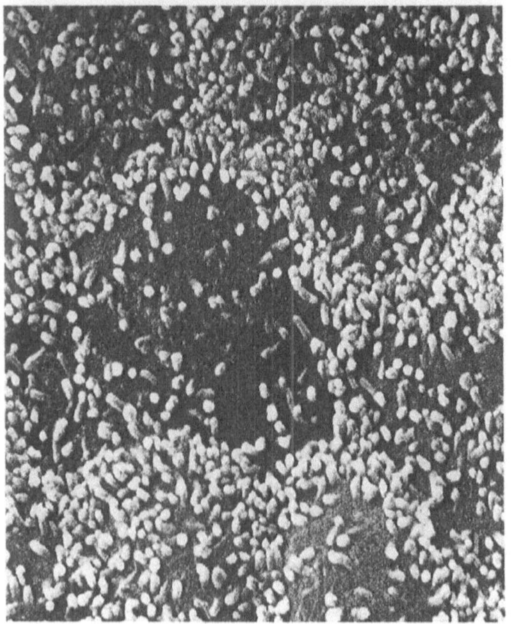

Fig. 244. (*above*) Response of thyroid follicular cells to long-term decreased levels of TSH. The follicular cells (*arrows*) are low cubiodal and thyroid follicles are distended with dense colloid (*C*) in response to decreased TSH secretion

Fig. 245. (*below*) Scanning electron micrograph of luminal surface of thyroid follicular cells from a rat administered 100 µg T_4 daily for 4 weeks. In response to decreased TSH levels microvilli are widely separated and short. There is no evidence of formation of cytoplasmic pseudopodia into the luminal colloid as in actively secreting thyroid folicles (contrast with Fig. 242). (Courtesy of Collins and Capen 1980)

plexuses lying in close proximity to the follicular basement membranes. There is also a network of lymphatics in the gland. The stroma encloses a number of nerve fibers, some of which are parasympathetic, but most are sympathetic. These nerves terminate on blood vessels or in apposition to follicular cells.

Histochemistry and Histophysiology. Follicular cells show striking polarity orientated toward the follicular lumen (Fig. 239). Varying numbers of lysosomes, histochemically stainable for enzymes such as acid phosphatase, are found in the apical portion of the cell (Wollman et al. 1964; Wetzel et al. 1965). In follicular cells soon after stimulation by TSH, intracellular droplets (phagosomes), corresponding to those demonstrated light-microscopically by the PAS reaction and representing ingested colloid, are more numerous than in the resting state (Wetzel et al. 1965). Some of these form phagolysosomes in follicular cells by fusion with lysosomes.

The apical portion of the follicular cell develop prominent elongations of microvilli shortly after stimulation by TSH which form cytoplasmic processes (pseudopods) that surround portions of the follicular colloid (Figs. 240, 242). Pseudopods appear to collect thyroglobulin located at some distance from the apical surface and may provide a mechanism of selective macropinocytosis by which newly synthesized thyroglobulin recently delivered to the follicle lumen is prevented from immediate reuptake (Ericson et al. 1983). This process, termed endocytosis, results in the formation of colloid droplets in the cytoplasm of follicular cells (Wetzel et al. 1965; Björkman et al. 1978; Ericson et al. 1980). Microtubules and microfilaments in the cytoplasm of follicular cells beneath the apical plasma membrane are important in moving colloid droplets into close proximity to lysosomal bodies (Wolff and Williams 1973). The membranes of these two organelles fuse resulting in the local release of enzymes that break down the colloid and release T_4 and T_3 into the cytosol.

The active thyroid hormones subsequently diffuse out of the cell and enter the abundant interfollicular capillaries that have a fenestrated endothelial lining. The iodinated tyrosines (MIT and DIT) released from the colloid droplets are deiodinated enzymatically, and the iodide generated either is recycled to the lumen to iodinate new tyrosyl residues or released into the circulation.

These unique structural and functional characteristics of the phylogenetically oldest endocrine gland suggest that the thyroid may have evolved toward a more "ideal" structure to perform its vital metabolic functions (Capen 1983).

The functionally most important enzyme in the thyroid hormone synthetic pathway is present in the apical plasma membrane and microvilli as well as in other structures of the follicular cells (Tice and Wollman 1974; Mizukami et al. 1985). Human thyroid peroxidase is a membrane-bound, heme-containing glycoprotein composed of 933 amino acids with a transmembrane domain (Foti and Rapoport 1990). Thyroperoxidase oxidizes iodide ion (I^-) taken up by follicular cells into reactive iodine which binds to the tyrosine residues in the thyroglobulin. Iodine is incorporated not only into newly synthesized thyroglobulin recently delivered to the follicular lumen but also into molecules already stored in the lumen (Öfverholm and Ericson 1984). Thyroperoxidase also functions as a "coupling" enzyme to combine MIT and DIT to form T_3 or 2 DIT to form T_4 (Fig. 241).

The follicular cell of the thyroid is involved concurrently in luminally directed processes of thyroglobulin synthesis and exocytosis as well as basally directed processes of colloid endocytosis with breakdown and eventual release of thyroid hormones into the interfollicular capillaries. Radioautographs prepared at increasing time intervals after pulse labeling of thyroids with a radioactive amino acid such as [^{3}H]leucine have shown that its incorporation into peptides occurs in the rough endoplasmic reticulum. Labeled material subsequently appears in the Golgi region, then over vesicles between the Golgi apparatus and the lumen, and finally in the lumen (Nadler et al. 1964). With the use of tritiated monosaccharides it can be shown that the synthesis of the carbohydrate chains of thyroglobulin starts in the endoplasmic reticulum and is completed in the Golgi apparatus (Whur et al. 1969).

The thyroid takes up iodine in the form of iodide ion. Although the active transport of iodide occurs at the base of the follicular cells near the interfollicular capillaries, iodide that has entered the thyroid cell is transported rapidly to the follicular lumen (Loewenstein and Wollman 1967). Iodide in the thyroid is oxidized to a higher valence state by the thyroperoxidase in microvilli. This oxidized form of iodine becomes rapidly attached to the tyrosyl residues in thyroglobulin in close proximity to the apical microvilli (Öfverholm et al. 1985; Wollman and Ekholm 1981).

Quantitation of Circulating Levels of TSH. In the evaluation of potential thyroid toxicity of various drugs and chemicals in laboratory rodents an accurate quantitation of circulating levels of TSH is essential in order to determine whether proliferative lesions of follicular cells are mediated by a chronic hypersecretion of TSH. The immunoassay for TSH is highly species specific with considerable interanimal and interassay variations. TSH antiserum (anti-rTSH-sp) and standard (TSH-RP-2) for use in the rat are available from the NIADDK National Hormone and Pituitary Program. When critical assessment of changes in serum or plasma TSH is required following administration of a drug or chemical, several protocol modifications are recommended: (a) increase the number of rats to 20 per interval and dose, (b) collect blood for hormone assays at sacrifice from the abdominal aorta to provide a larger sample with minimal contamination by tissue fluids, (c) freeze a separate aliquot of serum or plasma for the TSH assay and run all animals from the study in the same assay, (d) kill rats between 8 AM and noon to minimize the effects of diurnal variations on hormone levels (Ottenweller and Hedge 1982), and (e) rotate the killing of rats between all experimental groups.

Xenobiotics that disrupt either thyroid hormone synthesis, secretion, or peripheral metabolism often result in prompt increases in circulating TSH levels. It is important in the design of experiments to evaluate the effect of a xenobiotic on thyroid function to have several early collection intervals. For example, FD&C red no. 3 (a relatively mild goitrogen in rats) at a high dose (4%) resulted in a significant elevation in serum TSH at 3 days which persisted throughout a 60-day experiment (Fig. 246).

Species Differences in Thyroid Hormone Economy

Long-term perturbations of the pituitary-thyroid axis by various xenobiotics or physiologic alterations (e.g., iodine deficiency, partial thyroidectomy, and natural goitrogens in food) are more likely to predispose the laboratory rat to a higher incidence of proliferative lesions (e.g., hyperplasia and adenomas of follicular cells) in response to

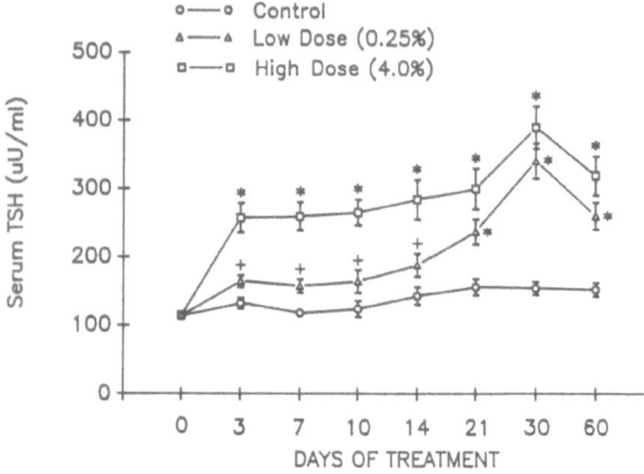

Fig. 246. Rapid significant increase in serum thyroid stimulating hormone (*TSH*) in Sprague-Dawley rats ($n = 20$ rats/group and interval) administered a mild goitrogen (FD&C red no. 3) in the feed. Blood for the TSH assay was collected terminally from the abdominal aorta. The significant increase in serum TSH persisted from days 3 to 60 of the experiment in the high dose (4%) group. (Courtesy of L.E. Braverman and W.J. DeVito, University of Massachusetts Medical School, and Certified Color Manufacturers Association, Inc)

chronic TSH stimulation than in the human thyroid (Capen and Martin 1989; Curran and DeGroot 1991). This is particularly true in the male rat, which has higher circulating levels of TSH than in females. The greater sensitivity of the rodent thyroid to derangement by drugs, chemicals, and physiologic perturbations is also related to the shorter plasma half-life of T_4 than in man due to the considerable differences between species in the transport proteins for thyroid hormones (Döhler et al. 1979).

The plasma T_4 half-life in rats is considerably shorter (12–24 h) than that in man (5–9 days). In human beings and monkeys circulating T_4 is bound primarily to thyroxine-binding globulin (TBG), but this high affinity binding protein is not present in rodents, birds, amphibians, or fish (Table 13). The binding affinity of TBG for T_4 is approximately 1000 times higher than that of prealbumin. The percent of unbound active T_4 is lower in species with high levels of TBG than in animals in which T_4 binding is limited to albumin and prealbumin. Therefore, a rat without a functional thyroid requires about ten times more T_4 (20 μg/kg body weight) for full substitution than an adult human (2.2 μg/kg body weight). T_3 is transported bound to TBG and albumin in human beings, monkey, and dog but only to albumin in mouse, rat, and chicken (Table 14). In general T_3 is bound less avidly to transport proteins than T_4 resulting in a faster turnover and shorter plasma half-life in most species. These differences in plasma half-life of thyroid hormones and binding to transport proteins between rats and humans may be one factor in the greater sensitivity of the rat thyroid to develop hyperplastic and/or neoplastic nodules in response to chronic TSH stimulation.

Goitrogenic Chemicals and Thyroid Tumors in Rodents

Numerous studies have reported that chronic treatment of rodents with goitrogenic compounds results in the development of follicular cell adenomas. Thiouracil and its derivatives have this effect in rats (Napolkov 1976) and mice (Morris 1955). This phenomenon has also been observed in rats that consumed brassica seeds (Kennedy and Purves 1941), erythrosine (FD&C red no. 3; Capen and Martin 1989; Borzelleca et al. 1987), sulfonamides (Swarm et al. 1973), and many other compounds (Hill et al. 1989; Paynter et al. 1988).

Table 13. Thyroxine (T_4) binding to serum proteins in selected vertebrate species (modified from Döhler et al. 1979)

Species	T_4-binding globulin	After albumin	Albumin	Before albumin
Human being	++		++	+
Monkey	++		++	+
Dog	+		++	
Mouse		++	++	
Rat		+	++	+
Chicken			++	

+ or ++, degree of T_4 binding to serum proteins. Empty box, absence of binding of T_4 to serum protein.

Table 14. Triiodothyronine (T_3) binding to serum proteins in selected vertebrate species (modified from Döhler et al. 1979)

Species	T_4-binding globulin	After albumin	Albumin	Before albumin
Human being	+		+	
Monkey	+		+	
Dog	+		+	
Mouse		+	+	
Rat			+	
Chicken			+	

+ or ++, degree of T_3 binding to serum proteins. Empty box, absence of binding of T_3 to serum protein.

The pathogenetic mechanism of this phenomenon has been understood for some time and is widely accepted (Furth 1968). These goitrogenic agents either directly interfere with thyroid hormone synthesis or secretion in the thyroid gland, increase thyroid hormone excretion into the bile, or disrupt the peripheral conversion of T_4 to T_3. The ensuing decrease in circulating thyroid hormone levels results in a compensatory increased secretion of pituitary TSH. The receptor-mediated TSH stimulation of the thyroid gland leads to proliferative changes of follicular cells that include hypertrophy, hyperplasia, and ultimately neoplasia in rodents. In the multistage model of carcinogenesis proliferative lesions often begin as hyperplasia, may proceed to the development of benign tumors (adenoma), and infrequently develop into a malignant tumor. Although these lesions usually are classified as discrete entities (Fig. 247), it is important to emphasize that they represent a morphologic continuum (Fig. 248), with imprecise criteria to separate borderline proliferative lesions.

Excessive secretion of TSH alone (i.e., in the absence of any chemical exposure) has also been reported to produce a high incidence of thyroid tumors in rodents. This has been observed in rats fed an iodine deficient diet (Axelrod and Leblond 1955) and in mice that received TSH-secreting pituitary tumor transplants (Furth 1968). The pathogenetic mechanism of thyroid follicular cell tumor development in rodents involves a sustained excessive stimulation of the thyroid gland by TSH. In addition, iodine deficiency is a potent promoter of the development of thyroid tumors in rodents induced by intravenous injection of *N*-methyl-*N*-nitrosourea (Table 15; Ohshima and Ward 1984).

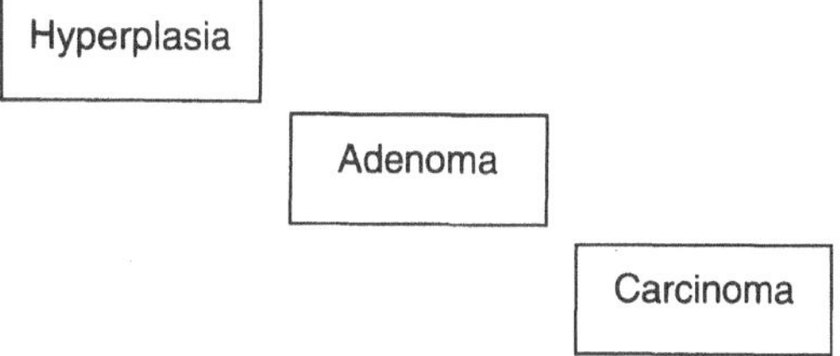

Fig. 247. Multistage model of carcinogenesis with hyperplasia, adenoma, and carcinoma as discrete stages

Morphologic Continuum

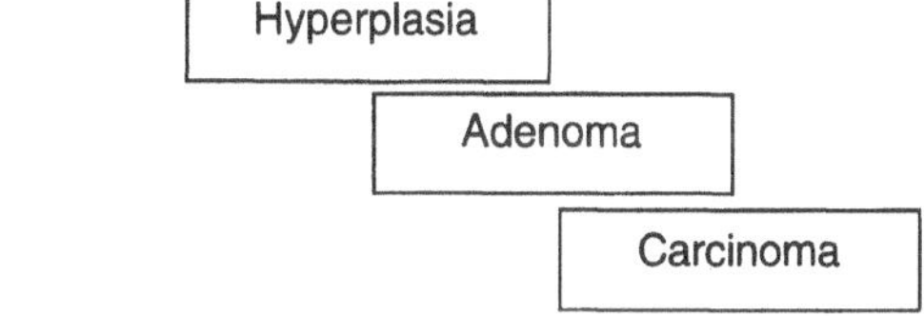

Fig. 248. Proliferative changes in the multistage model of carcinogenesis represent a morphologic continuum with an overlap in morphologic features

Chemical Inhibition of 5′-Monodeiodinase

FD&C red no. 3 (erythrosine) is an example of a well-characterized xenobiotic that results in perturbations of thyroid function in rodents and in long-term studies is associated with an increased incidence of benign thyroid tumors. Red no. 3 is a widely used color additive in foods, cosmetics, and pharmaceuticals. A chronic toxicity/carcinogenicity study revealed that male Sprague-Dawley rats fed a 4% dietary concentration of red no. 3

Table 15. Promoting effect of iodine deficiency on thyroid carcinogenesis induced by *N*-nitrosomethylurea (NMU) at 33 weeks

Group	Thyroid weight	Diffuse FC hyperplasia	Follicular cell		Total focal FC lesions (no./cm^2)
			Adenoma (%)	Carcinoma (%)	
NMU + diet	632 ± 208*	100^{5*}	100^{6*}	100^{8*}	11 ± 6
NMU + iodineadequate diet	46 ± 13**	0	70^{7*}	10	14 ± 14
NMU + control diet	29 ± 4***	0	50	0	17 ± 20
ID diet	109 ± 12^{4*}	100^{5*}	0	0	0.4 ± 0.8
Iodine-adequate diet	40 ± 16	0	0	0	0
Control diet	36 ± 4	0	0	0	0

NMU, 41 mg/kg IV at 6 weeks of age (2 weeks before diets began); control diet, sterilizable Wayne Blox diet; iodine-adequate, Remington diet plus 0.01 g/kg K iodate.
*$p < 0.01$ vs. groups 2, 3, 4, 5, or 6; **$p < 0.05$ vs. groups 3 or 4; ***$p < 0.01$ vs. group 4; $^{4*}p < 0.01$ vs. groups 5 or 6; $^{5*}p < 0.001$ vs. groups 2, 3, 5, or 6; $^{6*}p < 0.001$ vs. groups 4, 5, or 6; $^{7*}p < 0.01$ vs. groups 4, 5, or 6; $^{8*}p < 0.001$ vs. groups 2, 3, 4, 5, or 6.

Table 16. Histopathologic evaluation of thyroid follicular cells (FC) from male Sprague-Dawley rates fed FD&C red no. 3

Group	Original study					High-dose study	
	I-A	I-B	II	III	IV	I-C	V
Red no. 3 (%)	0	0	0.1	0.5	1.0	0	4.0
mg/kg per day	–	–	49	251	507	–	2464
FC adenoma (%)	0	0	0	2.9	1.5	1.5	21.8
FC carcinoma	0	0	4.5	1.5	4.4	2.9	4.4
Cystic follicular hyperplasia (%)	2.9	1.5	12	16.2	7.3	0	23.2
Diffuse or focal FC hyperplasia (%)	1.4	0	7.5	7.4	26.1	5.8	87.0
Follicular cysts (%)	10	14.5	9.0	11.8	11.6	2.9	14.5

beginning in utero and extending over their lifetime (30 months) developed a 22% incidence of well-differentiated thyroid adenomas derived from follicular cells compared to 1.5% in control rats and a historical incidence of 1.8% for this strain (Borzelleca et al. 1987; Table 16). The thyroid adenomas were well demarcated from the normal gland by a thin layer of fibrous connective tissue and adjacent follicles were slightly compressed (Fig. 249). The neoplastic cells were more hyperchromatic than the surrounding normal follicular cells and either formed variably sized colloid-containing follicles, lined large cystic spaces, or solid sheets. Some neoplastic cells formed papillary structures extending into cystic spaces. There was no evidence of vascular invasion. In addition, male rats developed a 23% incidence of follicular cystic hyperplasia (Table 16). These focal lesions were formed by the coalescence of adjacent colloid-distended follicles. The follicular wall (or remnants) was lined by one or two layers of low cuboidal epithelium with hyperchromatic nuclei that occasionally formed papillary projections (Fig. 250). There was not a significant increase in follicular cell adenomas in the lower dose groups of male rats or an increase in malignant thyroid follicular cell tumors. Female rats fed similar amounts of the color did not develop a significant increase in either benign or malignant thyroid tumors. Feeding of the color at the high dose (4%) level provided male rats with 2464 mg/kg of red no. 3 daily; by comparison human consumption in the United States is estimated to be 0.023 mg/kg per day.

The results of mechanistic studies have suggested that a primary (direct) action of FD&C red no. 3

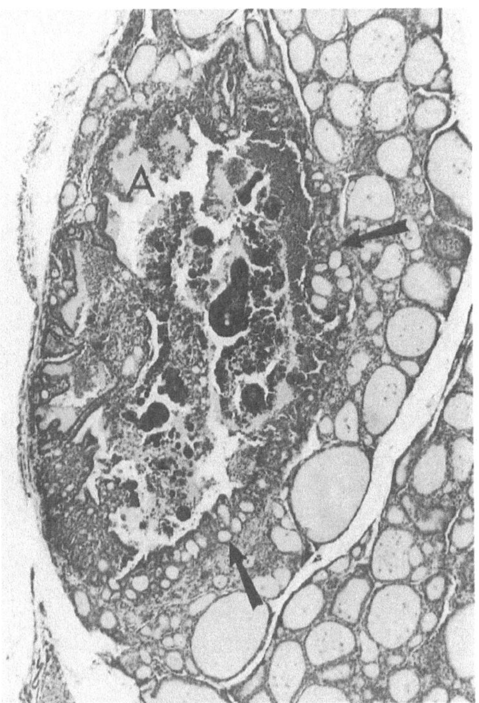

Fig. 249. Thyroid follicular cell adenoma (*A*) in a male Sprague-Dawley rat exposed to FD&C red no. 3 in utero and fed at the 4% level for a lifetime of 30 months. The adenoma is well-circumscribed (*arrows*) and adjacent follicles are slightly compressed. The hyperchromatic neoplastic cells line a cystic space and form papillary projections into the lumen. *Bar*, 100 μm (From Capen 1983)

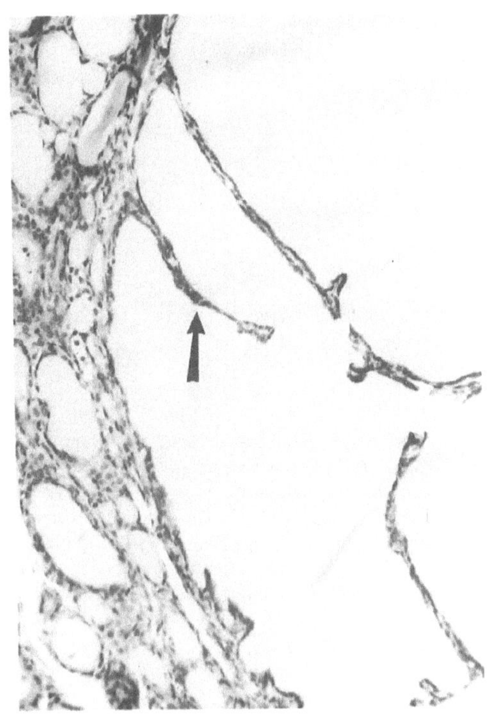

Fig. 250. Follicular cystic hyperplasia in a male Sprague-Dawley rat exposed to FD&C red no. 3 in utero and fed at the 4% level for a lifetime of 30 months. There is a coalescence of adjacent colloid-distended follicles that are lined by cuboidal epithelium with hyperchromatic nuclei and form occasional papillary projections into the cystic space (*arrow*). Adjacent thyroid follicles are only minimally compressed and there is no evidence of encapsulation. *Bar*, =100 μm. (From Capen 1983)

on the thyroid is unlikely due to: (a) failure of the color (^{14}C-labeled) to accumulate in the gland, (b) negative genotoxicity and mutagenicity assays, (c) lack of an oncogenic response in mice and gerbils, (d) a failure to result in thyroid tumor development at dietary concentrations of 1.0% or less in male and female rats (Capen and Martin 1989), and (e) a lack of increased tumor development in other organs. Investigations with radiolabeled compound have demonstrated that the color does not accumulate in the thyroid glands of rats following the feeding of either 0.5% or 4.0% FD&C red no. 3 for 1 week prior to the oral dose of ^{14}C-labeled material.

Subsequent mechanistic investigations included a 60-day study in male Sprague-Dawley rats fed either 4% (high dose) or 0.25% (low dose) of FD&C red no. 3 compared to controls in order to determine the effects of the color on thyroid hormone economy and morphometric changes in follicular cells. The experimental design of the study was to terminate groups of rats (n = 20/interval and dose) fed red no. 3 and controls after 0, 3, 7, 10, 14, 21, 30, and 60 days.

A consistent effect of red no. 3 on thyroid hormone economy was the striking increase in serum reverse T_3 (Fig. 251). In the high-dose rats reverse T_3 was increased at all intervals compared to controls and at 10, 14, and 21 days in the low dose group. The mechanisms responsible for the increased serum reverse T_3 appear to be: first, substrate (T_4) accumulation due to 5′-deiodinase inhibition with subsequent conversion to reverse T_3 rather than active T_3; and second, reverse T_3 accumulation due to 5′-deiodinase inhibition resulting in an inability to degrade reverse T_3 further to diiodothyronine (T_2). Serum T_3 was decreased significantly at all intervals in rats of the high-dose group compared to interval controls (Fig. 252). The mechanism responsible for the reduced serum

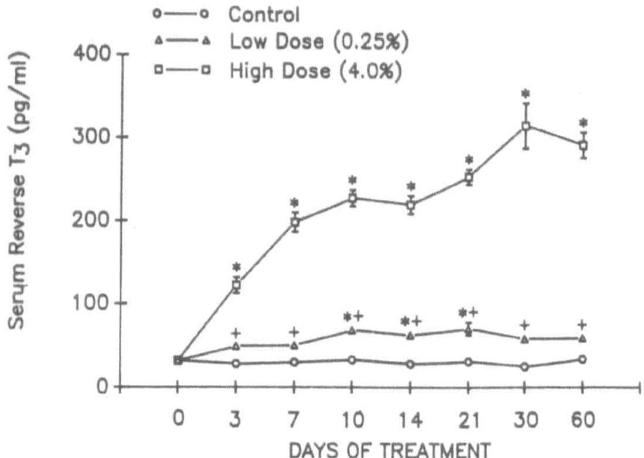

Fig. 251. Rapid and significant increase in serum reverse triiodothyronine (*rT_3*) levels in Sprague-Dawley rats (n = 20/group and interval) administered a high (4%) and low (0.25%) dose of FD&C red no. 3. The significant increase in rT_3 was detected at the initial interval of 3 days and persisted during the 60-day experiment in the high dose group. (Courtesy of the Certified Color Manfacturers Association, Inc. and Drs. L.E. Braverman and W.J. DeVito, University of Massachusetts Medical School)

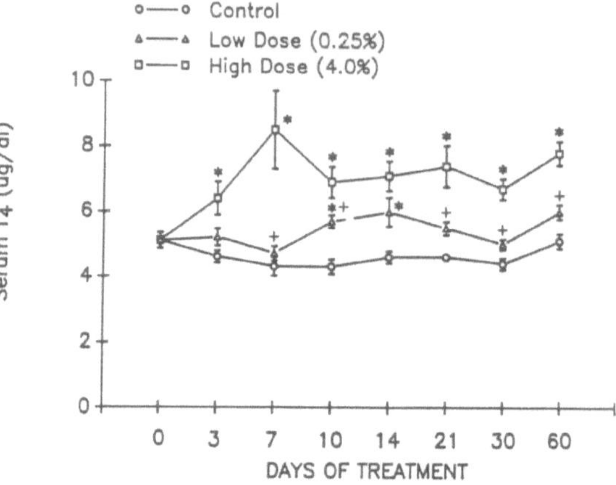

Fig. 253. Changes in serum thyroxine (*T_4*) following administration of a high (4%) and low (0.25%) dose of FD&C red no. 3 in the diet to Sprague-Dawley rats. (Courtesy of the Certified Color Manufacturers Association, Inc. and Drs. L.E. Braverman and W.J. DeVito, University of Massachusetts Medical School)

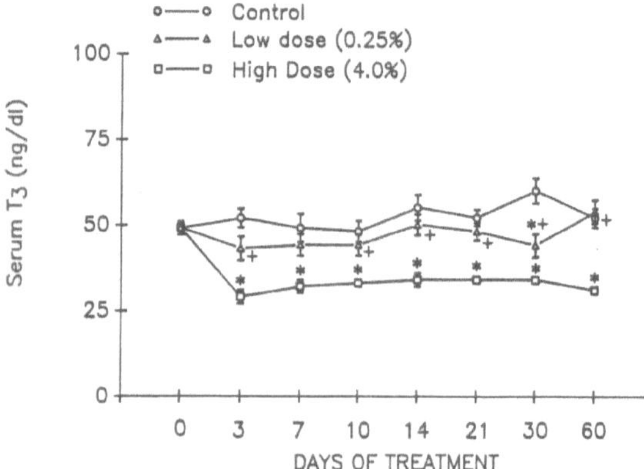

Fig. 252. Changes in serum triiodothyronine (*T_3*) following administration of a high (4%) and low (0.25%) dose of FD&C red no. 3 in the diet to Sprague-Dawley rats. (Courtesy of the Certified Color Manufacturers Association, Inc. and Drs. L.E. Braverman and W.J. DeVito, University of Massachusetts Medical School)

T_3 following feeding of red no. 3 was decreased monodeiodination of T_4 due to an inhibition of the 5′-deiodinase by the color.

Serum TSH was increased significantly at all intervals in rats of the high-dose (4%) group compared to controls. Rats fed 0.25% of red no. 3 had increased serum TSH only at days 21, 30, and 60 (Fig. 246). The mechanism responsible for the increased serum TSH following ingestion of red no. 3 was a compensatory response by the pituitary gland to the low circulating levels of T_3 that resulted from an inhibition of the 5′-deiodinase. Serum T_4 also was increased significantly at all intervals in rats fed 4% red no. 3 compared to controls (Fig. 253). The mechanism responsible for the increased serum T_4 was: first, accumulation due to an inability to monodeiodinate T_4 to T_3 in the liver and kidney from the inhibition of 5′-deiodinase by the color; and second, TSH stimulation of increased T_4 production by the thyroid gland.

^{125}I-labeled T_4 metabolism was significantly altered in liver homogenates prepared from rats fed 4% FD&C red no. 3. Degradation of labeled T_4 was decreased to approximately 40% of values in control homogenates (Fig. 254). This was associated with a 75% decrease in percent generation of ^{125}I and an approximately 80% decrease in percent generation of ^{125}I-labeled T_3 from radiolabeled T_4 substrate. These mechanistic investigations suggested that the color results in a perturbation of thyroid hormone economy in rodents by inhibiting the 5′-deiodinase in the liver (Fig. 255), resulting in long-term stimulation of follicular cells by TSH which over their lifetime predisposed to an increased incidence of thyroid tumors (Capen and Martin 1989; Borzelleca et al. 1987). The color was negative in standard genotoxic and mutagenic assays and did not increase the incidence of tumors in other organs.

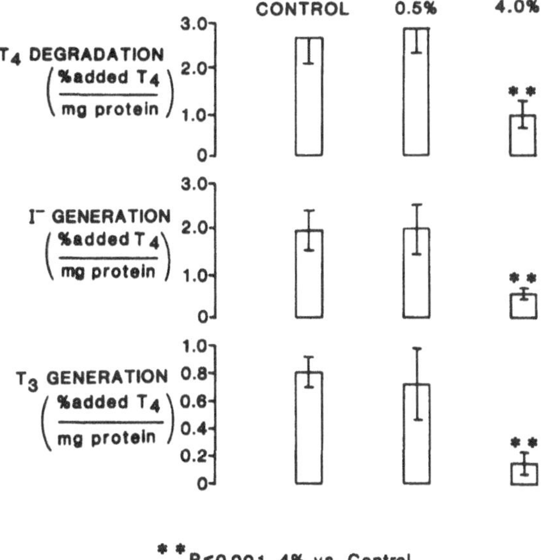

Fig. 254. Effects of dietary FD&C red no. 3 on the hepatic metabolism of ^{125}I-labeled thyroxine in male Sprague-Dawley rats. (Courtesy of the Certified Color Manufacturers Association, Inc. and the late Sidney H. Ingbar, M.D)

Morphometric evaluation was performed on thyroid glands from all rats at each interval during the 60 day study. Four levels of thyroid were evaluated with 25 measurements from each rat using a Zeiss interactive digital analysis system at a magnification ×450. The direct measurements included diameter of thyroid follicles, area of follicular colloid, and height of follicular cells. Thyroid follicular diameter was decreased significantly in both low- and high-dose groups after 3, 7, 10, and 14 days compared to interval controls. The area of follicular colloid generally reflected the decrease in thyroid follicular diameter and was decreased significantly after days 3 and 10 in high-dose rats and days 7 and 10 in the low-dose group compared to interval controls. These reductions in thyroid follicular diameter and colloid area were consistent with morphologic changes expected from an increased serum TSH concentration.

Thyroid follicular height was increased significantly only after feeding FD&C red no. 3 for 60 days in both the high- and low-dose groups compared to interval controls. The absence of morphometric evidence of follicular cell hypertrophy at the earlier intervals was consistent with the modest increase (5.8%) in thyroid gland:body weight ratio after this relatively short exposure to the color. The lack of follicular cell hypertrophy at the earlier intervals of feeding red no. 3 in rats with several-fold elevations in serum TSH levels may be related in part to the high thyroid iodine content (58% of molecular weight) interfering with the receptor-mediated response to TSH. The thyroid responsiveness to TSH is known to vary inversely with iodine content (Ingbar 1972; Lamas and Ingbar 1978). Thyroid glands of rats fed FD&C red no. 3 would be exposed to an increased iodine primarily from sodium iodide contamination of the color and, to a lesser extent, from metabolism of the compound and release of iodide.

Amiodarone. An iodinated drug used to treat tachyarrhythmias, amiodarone inhibits the in vivo 5′-monodeiodination of T_4 in rat liver. It blocks the 5′-monodeiodinase (type I enzyme) in rat liver homogenates but not the 5′-deiodinase in the rat pituitary gland (type II enzyme). Male and female Sprague-Dawley rats administered 5, 16,

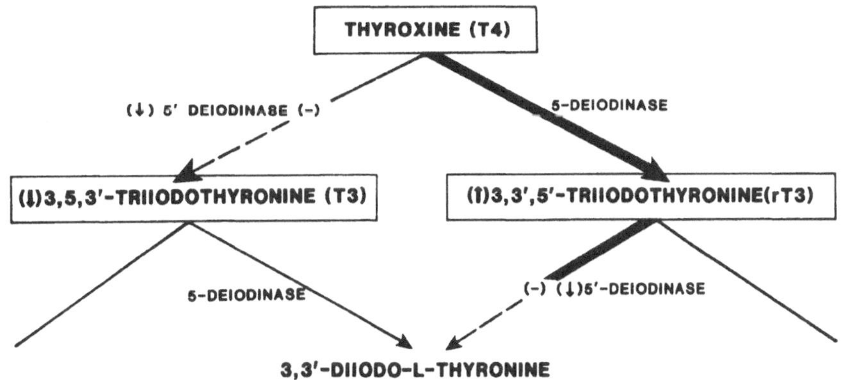

Fig. 255. Effects of FD&C red no. 3 (erythrosine) on in vivo metabolism of thyroxine. (From Capen and Martin 1989)

or 50 mg/kg per day of amiodarone by gavage in a 2-year carcinogenicity study had an increased incidence of thyroid follicular cell hyperplasia and adenomas compared to controls. There was a numerical increase in carcinomas in each treatment group when compared to controls, but there was no dose-related response. Tumors were not detected in interim sacrifices at 6 months and 1 year, and there was no increased incidence of tumors in other tissues. Male and female B6C3F1 mice that received amiodarone orally for 2 years did not develop an increased incidence of thyroid follicular cell hyperplasia or tumors. In a shorter (14-week) study male Sprague-Dawley rats that received oral amiodarone (50 mg/kg per day) had significant increases in serum TSH, T_4, and rT_3 and a significant decrease in serum T_3. These changes in thyroid hormone and TSH were similar to those observed following the administration of red no. 3. It is likely that amiodarone, as with FD&C red no. 3, produces thyroid follicular cell adenomas in rats through the TSH-mediated secondary mechanism.

The effects of amiodarone (a readily absorbed substance) on human thyroid economy are well documented and include decreased serum T_3 concentrations, increased serum T_4 and rT_3 concentrations, and initial increases in serum TSH concentrations at therapeutic doses. By comparison, FD&C red no. 3 (a poorly absorbed substance) has no effect on thyroid hormone economy in humans at doses up to 200 mg/day for 14 days except for a minimal increase in serum TSH within the normal range. This TSH increase does not appear to be caused by FD&C red no. 3 per se but rather is due to the high iodide intake associated with the large dose (200 mg/day) of the color.

Iopanoic Acid. Both type I and type II 5′-monodeiodinase in rats is inhibited by the iodinated radiographic contrast agent iopanoic acid. It shares with FD&C red no. 3 the ability to inhibit the T_4 to T_3 conversion and increase serum TSH concentrations in rats. However, iopanoic acid inhibits both type I and type II 5′-monodeiodinase whereas red no. 3 inhibits only the type I enzyme in liver and kidney and not the type II enzyme in brain, pituitary, and brown adipose tissue.

Iopanoic acid and FD&C red no. 3 differ in their ability to effect human thyroid hormone economy. Iopanoic acid in doses commonly used in clinical radiographic studies results in increased serum concentrations of T_4 and rT_3, decreased serum T_3 with a compensatory increase in basal serum TSH concentrations, and resulted in an increase in the TSH response to TRH after 5–7 days of treatment.

Hepatic Microsomal Enzyme Induction

Hepatic microsomal enzymes play an important role in thyroid hormone economy since glucuronidation is the rate limiting step in the biliary excretion of T_4 and sulfation by phenol sulfotransferase for the excretion of T_3. Long-term exposure of rats to a wide variety of different chemicals may induce these enzyme pathways and result in chronic stimulation of the thyroid by disrupting the hypothalamic-pituitary-thyroid axis (Curran and DeGroot 1991). The resulting chronic stimulation of the thyroid by increased circulating levels of TSH often results in a greater risk of developing tumors derived from follicular cells in 2-year or lifetime studies with these compounds in rats.

Xenobiotics that induce liver microsomal enzymes 'and disrupt thyroid function in rats include CNS-acting drugs (e.g., phenobarbital, benzodiazepines); calcium channel blockers (e.g., nicardipine, bepridil); steroids (spironolactone); retinoids; chlorinated hydrocarbons (e.g., chlordane; *dichlorodiphenyl-trichloroethane*, *2,3, 7,8-tetrachlorodibenzo-p-dioxin, [CE1]*), polyhalogenated biphenyls (*polychlorinated biphenyls*, PCB; *polybromated biphenyls*), among others. Most of the hepatic microsomal enzyme inducers have no apparent intrinsic carcinogenic activity and produce little or no mutagenicity or DNA damage. Their promoting effect on thyroid tumors is usually greater in rats than mice, with males more often developing a higher incidence of tumors than females. In certain strains of mice these compounds alter liver cell turnover and promote the development of hepatic tumors from spontaneously initiated hepatocytes.

Phenobarbital has been studied extensively as the prototype for hepatic microsomal inducers that increase a spectrum of cytochrome P450 isoenzymes (McClain et al. 1988). McClain et al. (1989) reported that the activity of UDP-glucuronyl transferase, the rate-limiting enzyme in T_4 metabolism, is increased in purified hepatic microsomes of male rats, expressed as picomoles per minute per milligram of microsomal protein

(1.3-fold) or as total hepatic activity (threefold). This resulted in a significantly higher cumulative (4-h) biliary excretion of ^{125}I-labeled T_4 and bile flow than in controls.

Phenobarbital-treated rats develop a characteristic pattern of changes in circulating thyroid hormone levels (McClain et al. 1988, 1989). Plasma T_3 and T_4 are markedly decreased after one week and remain decreased for 4 weeks. By 8 weeks T_3 levels return to near normal due to compensation by the hypothalamic-pituitary-thyroid axis. Serum TSH values are elevated significantly throughout the first month but often decline after a new steady state is attained. Thyroid weights increase significantly after 2–4 weeks of phenobarbital, reach a maximum increase of 40%–50% by 8 weeks, and remain elevated throughout the period of treatment.

McClain et al. (1988) in a series of experiments has shown that supplemental administration of T_4 (at doses that returned the plasma level of TSH to the normal range) blocks the thyroid tumor-promoting effects of phenobarbital, and that the promoting effects are directly proportional to the level of plasma TSH in rats. The sustained increase in circulating TSH levels results initially in hypertrophy of follicular cells, followed by hyperplasia, and ultimately places the rat thyroid at greater risk to develop an increased incidence of benign tumors.

Phenobarbital has been reported to be a thyroid gland tumor promoter in a rat initiation-promotion model. Treatment with a nitrosamine followed by phenobarbital has been shown to increase serum TSH concentrations, thyroid gland weights, and the incidence of follicular cell tumors in the thyroid gland (McClain et al. 1988, 1989). These effects could be decreased in a dose-related manner by simultaneous treatment with increasing doses of exogenous T_4. McClain et al. (1989) has demonstrated that rats treated with phenobarbital have a significantly higher cumulative biliary excretion of ^{125} I-labeled T_4 than controls. Most of the increase in biliary excretion was accounted for by an increase in T_4-glucuronide due to an increased metabolism of T_4 in phenobarbital-treated rats. This is consistent with enzymatic activity measurements which result in increased hepatic T_4-UDP-glucuronyl transferase activity in phenobarbital-treated rats. Results from these experiments are consistent with the hypothesis that the promotion of thyroid tumors in rats is not a direct effect of phenobarbital on the thyroid gland but rather an indirect effect mediated by TSH secretion from the pituitary secondary to the hepatic microsomal enzyme-induced increase of T_4 excretion in the bile.

The activation of the thyroid gland during the treatment of rodents with substances which stimulate T_4 catabolism is a well-known phenomenon and has been extensively investigated with phenobarbital and many other compounds (Curran and DeGroot 1991). It occurs particularly with rodents, first because UDP-glucuronyl transferase can easily be induced in rodent species, and second because T_4 metabolism takes place very rapidly in rats in the absence of TBG. In man a lowering of the circulating T_4 level but no change in TSH and T_3 concentrations has been observed only with high doses of very powerful enzyme-inducing compounds such as rifampicin with or without antipyrine.

There is no convincing evidence that humans treated with drugs or exposed to chemicals that induce hepatic microsomal enzymes are at increased risk for the development of thyroid cancer (Curran and DeGroot 1991). In a study of the effects of microsomal enzyme-inducing compounds on thyroid hormone metabolism in normal healthy adults, phenobarbital (100 mg daily for 14 days) did not affect the serum T_4, T_3, or TSH levels (Ohnhaus et al. 1981). A decrease in serum T_4 levels was observed after treatment with either a combination of phenobarbital plus rifampicin or a combination of phenobarbital plus antipyrine; however, these treatments had no effect on serum T_3 or TSH levels (Ohnhaus and Studer 1983). Epidemiologic studies of patients treated with therapeutic doses of phenobarbital have reported no increase in risk for the development of thyroid neoplasia (Clemmesen et al. 1974; Clemmesen and Hualgrim-Jensen 1977, 1978, 1981; White et al. 1979; Friedman 1981; Shirts et al. 1986; Olsen et al. 1989). Highly sensitive assays for thyroid and pituitary hormones are readily available clinically to monitor circulating hormone levels in patients who are exposed to chemicals that could potentially disrupt homeostasis of the pituitary-thyroid axis.

Likewise there is no substantive evidence that humans treated with drugs or exposed to chemicals that induce hepatic microsomal enzymes are at increased risk for the development of liver cancer. This is best exemplified by the extensive epidemiologic information on the clinical use of phenobarbital. Phenobarbital has been used clini-

Table 17. Serum thyroxine levels of PCB-treated and control rats determined by radioimmunoassay (from Collins et al. 1977)

Rat group	Acute effects (4 wks PCB) (μg/dl)	Chronic effects (12 wks PCB) (μg/dl)	Delayed effects (12 wks PCB; 12 wks no PCB) (μg/dl)	Long-term delayed effect (12 wks PCB; 35 wks no PCB) (μg/dl)
Controls	6.66 ± 0.3	7.18 ± 0.4	7.86 ± 0.8	6.18 ± 0.9
50 ppm PCB	4.80 ± 0.3**	1.96 ± 0.2**	4.90 ± 0.1*	5.86 ± 1.2
500/250 ppm PCB	2.10 ± 0.2***	1.78 ± 0.08***	3.01 ± 0.8**	6.02 ± 1.3

$^{*}p < 0.025$; $^{**}p < 0.05$; $^{***}p < 0.01$.
$n = 5$ rats per dose and interval.

cally as an anticonvulsant for more than eighty years. Relatively high microsomal enzyme-inducing doses have been used chronically, sometimes for lifetime exposures, to control seizure activity in human beings. A study of over 8000 patients admitted to a Danish epilepsy center from 1933 to 1962 revealed no evidence of an increased incidence of hepatic tumors in phenobarbital-treated humans when patients receiving thorotrast, a known human liver carcinogen, were excluded (Clemmesen and Hjalgrim-Jensen 1978). A more recent follow-up report on this patient population confirmed and extended this observation (Clemmesen and Hjalgrim-Jensen 1981; Olsen et al. 1989). The results of two other smaller studies (2099 epileptics and 959 epileptics) also revealed no hepatic tumors in patients treated with phenobarbital (White et al. 1979).

Another classic example of a chemical that induces hepatic microsomal enzymes and disrupts thyroid function is polychlorinated biphenyl. PCB are commonly used industrial compounds that have been released into the environment and caused widespread contamination. The disease-producing capability of these compounds includes alterations in reproduction, growth, and development. PCB cause a significant reduction in serum levels of thyroid hormones due to alterations in thyroid structure, in addition to the well-known induction of hepatic UDP-glucuronyl transferase and increased secretion of T_4-glucuronide in the bile. Feeding of PCB produced a dose-dependent significant reduction in serum T_4 levels in rats. Following withdrawal of PCB from the diet, blood T_4 levels return to the normal range at 35 weeks but not at 12 weeks (Table 17). These changes in circulating levels of T_4 were accompanied by a striking hypertrophy and hyperplasia of thyroid follicular cells compared to controls.

The most consistent lesions in follicular cells following the feeding of PCB were the accumulation of numerous large colloid droplets and irregularly shaped lysosomal bodies in the expanded cytoplasmic area. Microvilli on the luminal surface were shortened with abnormal branchings. The chronic administration (12 weeks) of PCB resulted in a striking distention of many follicular cells with large lysosomal bodies that were strongly acid phosphatase positive and colloid droplets, blunt and abnormally branched microvilli, and mitochondrial vacuolation. The principal lesion produced by PCB in follicular cells that contributed to the altered thyroid function appeared to be an interference in the interaction between the numerous colloid droplets and lysosomal bodies that is necessary for the enzymatic release of thyroid hormones.

Subsequent studies have investigated whether this direct effect on follicular cells interfering with hormone secretion contributes to the lowering of thyroid hormone levels produced by PCB. These investigations have used the Gunn rats which have an impaired ability to conjugate T_4 with glucuronic acid. The serum T_4 concentration was significantly reduced to a similar degree in both homozygous and heterozygous Gunn rats fed 500 ppm PCB daily for 6 weeks. The bile-to-plasma ratio of ^{125}I-labeled T_4 was increased more than fivefold in heterozygous Gunn rats ingesting 500 ppm PCB (Fig. 256). This was a reflection of the ability of heterozygous Gunn rats to respond to PCB with induction of hepatic UDP-glucuronyl transferase and increased conjugation and excretion of T_4-glucuronide into the bile. The bile-to-plasma ratio of homozygous control Gunn rats was only one-half that of heterozygous Gunn rats, reflecting their reduced biliary clearance of conjugated T_4. Biliary clearance of exogenous radio-

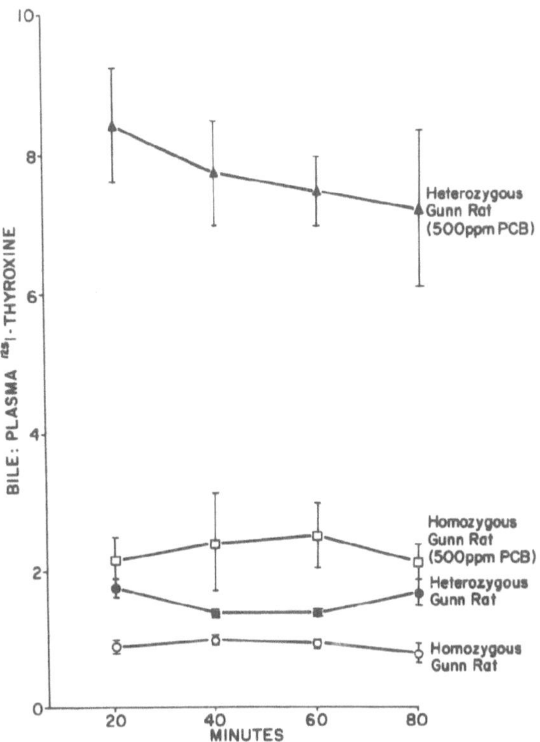

Fig. 256. Bile: plasma ^{125}I-labeled thyroxine in heterozygous and homozygous Gunn rats fed 0 or 500 ppm PCB. Rats were injected with ^{125}I-labeled T_4 18 h previously. (From Collins and Capen 1980)

labeled T_4 following the feeding of PCB was elevated only to that of control heterozygous Gunn rats.

Chemicals Directly Disrupting Thyroid Hormone Synthesis or Secretion

Inhibitors of Thyroid Hormone Synthesis. Blockage of Iodine Uptake. The initial step in the biosynthesis of thyroid hormones is the uptake of iodide from the circulation and transport against a gradient across follicular cells to the lumen of the follicle. A number of anions act as competitive inhibitors of iodide transport in the thyroid including perchlorate (ClO_4^-), thiocyanate (SCN^-), and pertechnetate (Fig. 257). Thiocyanate is a potent inhibitor of iodide transport and is a competitive substrate for the thyroid peroxidase, but it does not appear to be concentrated in the thyroid. Blockage of the iodide trapping mechanism has a similar disruptive effect on the thyroid-pituitary axis as iodine deficiency. The blood levels of T_4 and T_3 decrease resulting in a compensatory increase in the secretion of TSH by the pituitary gland. The hypertrophy and hyperplasia of follicular cells following sustained exposure results in an increased thyroid weight and the development of goiter.

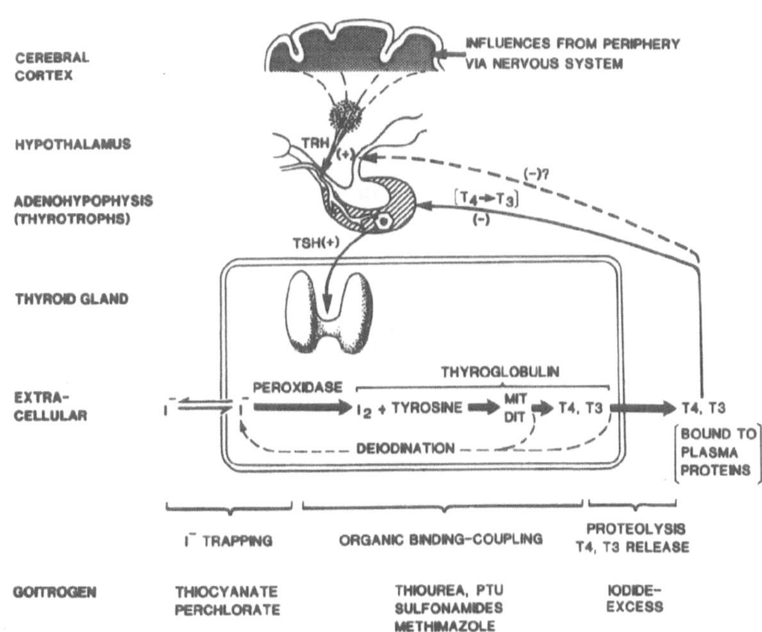

Fig. 257. Mechanism of action of goitrogens on thyroid hormone synthesis and section. (From Capen and Martin 1989)

Organification Defect: Inhibition of Thyroid Peroxidase. A wide variety of chemicals, drugs, and other xenobiotics affect the second step in thyroid hormone biosynthesis (Fig. 257). The step-wise binding of iodide to the tyrosyl residues in thyroglobulin requires oxidation of inorganic iodide (I^-) to molecular (reactive) iodine (I_2) by the thyroid peroxidase present in the luminal aspect (microvillar membranes) of follicular cells and adjacent colloid. Classes of chemicals that inhibit the organification of thyroglobulin include the (a) thionamides (such as thiourea, thiouracil, propylthiouracil, methimazole, carbimazole, and goitrin); (b) aniline derivatives and related compounds (e.g., sulfonamides, para-aminobenzoic acid, para-aminosalicylic acid, and amphenone); (c) substituted phenols (such as resorcinol, phloroglucinol, and 2,4-dihydroxybenzoic acid), and miscellaneous inhibitors (e.g., aminothiazole, tricyanoaminopropene, antipyrine and its iodinated derivative iodopyrine).

Many of these chemicals exert their action by inhibiting the thyroid peroxidase which results in a disruption both of the iodination of tyrosyl residues in thyroglobulin and also the coupling reaction of iodotyrosines (e.g., MIT and DIT) to form iodothyronines (T_3 and T_4). In rats propylthiouracil (PTU) has been shown to affect each step in thyroid hormone synthesis beyond iodide transport. The order of susceptibility to the inhibition by PTU is: the coupling reaction (most susceptible), iodination of MIT to form DIT, and iodination of tyrosyl residues to form MIT (least susceptible). Thiourea differs from PTU and other thioamides in that it does not inhibit guaiacol oxidation (standard assay for peroxidase) and does not inactivate the thyroid peroxidase in the absence of iodine. Its ability to inhibit organic iodinations is due primarily to the reversible reduction of active I_2 to $2I^-$.

The goitrogenic effects of sulfonamides have been known for approximately 50 years since the reports of the action of sulfaguanidine on the rat thyroid. Sulfamethoxazole and trimethoprim exert a potent goitrogenic effect in rats resulting in marked decreases in circulating T_3 and T_4, a substantial compensatory increase in TSH, and increased thyroid weights due to follicular cell hyperplasia. The dog also is a sensitive species to the effects of sulfonamides resulting in markedly decreased serum T_4 and T_3 levels, hyperplasia of thyrotrophic basophils, and increased thyroid weights.

By comparison, the thyroids of monkeys and human beings are resistant to the development of changes that sulfonamides produced in rodents (rats and mice) and the dog. Rhesus monkeys treated for 52 weeks with sulfamethoxazole (doses up to 300 mg/kg per day) with and without trimethoprim had no changes in thyroid weights and the thyroid histology was normal. Takayama et al. (1986) compared the effects of PTU and a goitrogenic sulfonamide (sulfamonomethoxine) on the activity of thyroid peroxidase in the rat and monkey using the guaiacol peroxidation assay. The concentration required for a 50% inhibition of the peroxidase enzyme was designated as the IC_{50}. When the IC_{50} for PTU was set at 1 for rats it took 50 times the concentration of PTU to produce a comparable inhibition in the monkey. Sulfamonomethoxine was almost as potent as PTU in inhibiting the peroxidase in rats with a factor of 2.5 times. However, it required about 500 times the concentration of sulfonamide to inhibit the peroxidase in the monkey compared to the rat.

Studies such as these with sulfonamides demonstrate distinct species differences between rodents and primates in the response of the thyroid to chemical inhibition of hormone synthesis. It is not surprising that the sensitive species (e.g., rat, mouse, and dog) are much more likely to develop follicular cell hyperplasia and thyroid nodules after long-term exposure to sulfonamides than the resistant species (e.g., subhuman primate, human beings, guinea pig, and chicken).

Inhibitors of Thyroid Hormone Secretion. Blockage of Thyroid Hormone Release by Excess Iodide and Lithium. Relatively few chemicals selectively inhibit the secretion of thyroid hormone from the thyroid gland (Fig. 257). An excess of iodine has been known for years to inhibit secretion of thyroid hormone and occasionally results in goiter and hypothyroidism in animals and human patients. High doses of iodide have been used therapeutically in the treatment of patients with Grave's disease and hyperthyroidism to lower circulating levels of thyroid hormones. Several mechanisms have been suggested for this effect of high iodide levels on the thyroid hormone secretion, including a decrease in lysosomal protease activity (human glands), inhibition of colloid droplet formation (mice and rats), and inhibition of TSH-mediated increase in cAMP (dog thyroid slices). In my laboratory rats fed an iodide-excess diet had a hypertrophy of the cytoplasmic area of follicular cells with an accumulation of numerous colloid droplets and lysosomal bodies. However, there was limited evidence ultrastructurally of fusion of the membranes of these organelles and degradation of the colloid necessary for the release of T_4 and T_3 from the thyroglobulin (Collins and Capen 1980). Circulating levels of T_4, T_3, and rT_3 all would be decreased by an iodide excess.

Lithium also has a striking inhibitory effect on thyroid hormone release (Fig. 257). The widespread use of lithium carbonate in the treatment of manic states occasionally results in the development of goiter with either euthyroidism or occasionally hypothyroidism in human patients. Lithium inhibits colloid droplet formation stimulated by cAMP in vitro and inhibits the release of thyroid hormones.

Xenobiotic (or Metabolite) Induced Thyroid Pigmentation or Changes in Colloid. The antibiotic minocycline produces a striking black discoloration of the thyroid lobes in laboratory animals and man with the formation of brown pigment granules within follicular cells. The pigment granules stain similarly to melanin and are best visualized on thyroid sections stained with the Fontana-Masson procedure. Electron-dense material first accumulates in lysosomelike granules and the rough endoplasmic reticulum. The pigment appears to be a metabolic derivative of minocycline, and the administration of the antibiotic at high dose to rats for extended periods may result in a disruption of thyroid function and the development of goiter. The release of T_4 from perfused thyroids of minocycline-treated rats was significantly decreased, but the follicular cells retained the ability to phagocytose colloid in response to TSH and had numerous colloid droplets in their cytoplasm.

Other xenobiotics [or metabolite(s)] selectively localize in the thyroid colloid of rodents resulting in abnormal clumping and increased basophilia to the colloid. Brown to black pigmented granules may be present in follicular cells, colloid, and macrophages in the interthyroidal tissues, resulting in a macroscopic darkening of both thyroid lobes. The physiochemically altered colloid in the lumen of thyroid follicles appears to be less able than normal colloid either of reacting with organic iodine in a step-wise manner to result in the orderly synthesis of iodothyronines or being phagocytized by follicular cells and enzymatically processed to release active thyroid hormones into the circulation. Serum T_4 and T_3 levels are decreased, serum TSH levels are increased by an expanded population of pituitary thyrotrophs, and thyroid follicular cells undergo hypertrophy and hyperplasia. As would be expected, the incidence of thyroid follicular cell tumors in 2-year carcinogenicity studies is significantly increased at the higher dose levels usually with a greater effect in males than females. Autoradiographic studies often demonstrate tritiated material to be preferentially localized in the colloid and not within follicular cells. Tissue distribution studies with ^{14}C-labeled compound may reveal preferential uptake and persistence in the thyroid gland compared to other tissues. However, thyroid peroxidase activity is normal, and the thyroid's ability to take up radioactive iodine is often increased compared to controls in response to the greater circulating levels of TSH. Similar thyroid changes and/or functional alterations usually do not occur in dogs, monkeys, or humans.

Secondary Mechanisms of Thyroid Oncogenesis

Understanding the mechanism of action of xenobiotics on the thyroid gland provides a more rational basis to extrapolate findings from long-term rodent studies to safety assessment of a particular compound for humans. Many chemicals and drugs disrupt one or more steps in the synthesis and secretion of thyroid hormones, resulting in subnormal levels of T_4 and T_3, associated with a compensatory increased secretion of pituitary TSH (Fig. 258). When tested in highly sensitive species, such as rats and mice, these compounds result early in follicular cell hypertrophy/hyperplasia and increased thyroid weights, and in long-term studies an increased incidence of thyroid tumors by a secondary (indirect) mechanism. In the secondary mechanism of thyroid oncogenesis in rodents the specific xenobiotic chemical or physiologic perturbation evokes another stimulus (e.g., chronic hypersecretion of TSH) that promotes the development of nodular proliferative lesions (initially hypertrophy, followed by hyperplasia, subsequently adenomas, infrequently carcinomas) derived from follicular cells. Thresholds for no effect on the thyroid gland can be established by determining the dose of xenobiotic that fails to elicit an elevation in the circulating level of TSH. Compounds acting by this indirect (second-

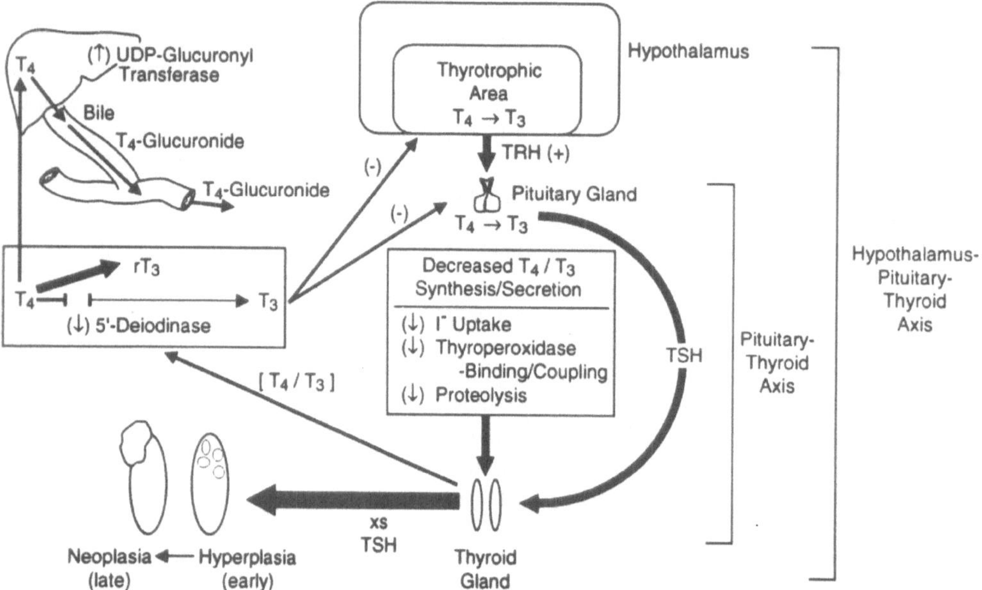

Fig. 258. Multiple sites of disruption of hypothalamic-pituitary-thyroid triad by xenobiotic chemicals. Chemicals can exert direct effects by disrupting thyroid hormone synthesis or secretion and indirectly influence the thyroid through an inhibition of 5'-deiodinase or by inducing hepatic microsomal enzymes (e.g., T_4-UDP glucuronyl transferase). All of these mechanisms can lower circulating levels of thyroid hormones (T_4 and T_3) resulting in a release from negative feedback inhibition and increased secretion of TSH by the pituitary gland. The chronic hypersecretion of TSH predisposes the sensitive rodent thyroid gland to develop an increased incidence of focal hyperplastic and neoplastic (adenomas) lesions by a secondary (epigenetic) mechanism

ary) mechanism with hormonal imbalance usually have little or no evidence for mutagenicity or for producing DNA damage.

In human patients with markedly altered changes in thyroid function and elevated TSH levels, as in areas with a high incidence of endemic goiter due to iodine deficiency, there is little if any increase in the incidence of thyroid cancer (Doniach 1970; Curran and DeGroot 1991). The relative resistance to the development of thyroid cancer in humans with elevated plasma TSH levels is in marked contrast to the response of the thyroid gland to chronic TSH stimulation in rats and mice. The human thyroid is much less sensitive to this pathogenetic phenomenon than rodents (McClain et al. 1989). Human patients with congenital defects in thyroid hormone synthesis (dyshormonogenetic goiter) and markedly increased circulating TSH levels have been reported to have an increased incidence of thyroid carcinomas (Cooper et al. 1981; McGirr et al. 1959). Likewise, thyrotoxic patients with Grave's disease where follicular cells are autonomously stimulated by an immunoglobulin (long-acting thyroid stimulator) also appear to be at greater risk to develop thyroid tumors (Pendergrast et al. 1961; Clements 1954). In summary, the literature suggests that prolonged stimulation of the human thyroid by TSH induces neoplasia only in exceptional circumstances and possibly acting together with some other metabolic or immunologic abnormality (Curran and DeGroot 1991).

Initiators of Thyroid Carcinogenesis

Specific chemicals and irradiation appear to have a direct effect on the thyroid gland resulting in genetic damage that leads to cell transformation and tumor formation. Examples of thyroid initiators include 2-acetylaminofluorine, *N*-methyl-*N*-nitrosourea (MNU), *N*-bis(2-hydroxypropyl) nitrosamine, methylcholanthrene, dichlorobenzidine, and polycyclic hydrocarbons. Chemicals in this group often increase the incidence of both benign and malignant thyroid tumors compared to controls. Iodine deficiency is a strong promoter of MNU-initiated thyroid tumors in rats (Table 15; Ohshima and Ward 1984, 1986). MNU-treated rats on an iodine-deficient diet for 52 weeks had significantly increased thyroid weights and a 90% incidence of follicular cell carcinomas compared to a 32% and 20% incidence of carcinomas in rats fed iodide-supplemented and control diets, respectively. The majority of the thyroid carcinomas were transplantable and invasive into the mammary fat pad of weanling F344/NCr rats. No other tumors induced by MNU were affected by the iodine-deficient diet.

A common component of permanent hair dye preparations (2,4-diaminoanisole sulfate, 2,4-DAAS) when fed at high doses (0.5%) to F344 rats for 107 weeks results in a 58% incidence of thyroid neoplasms in male rats and 42% in females compared to 7%-8% in controls (Ward et al. 1979). Follicular cell carcinomas are the principal type of neoplasm induced by 2,4-DAAS in thyroids without a background of diffuse hyperplasia of follicular cells. The carcinomas (papillary, cystic, and solid) were invasive but did not metastasize. 2,4-DAAS has been found to be mutagenic for *Salmonella typhimurium* but is not teratogenic. In the thyroid it results in a dose-dependent accumulation of brown granules in follicular cells that are basic fuchsin positive; PAS, acid-fast and iron negative; and ultrastructurally different than lipofuscin. The thyroid pigment may represent a reaction product of 2,4-DAAS and iodine in the cytoplasm of follicular cells.

References

Axelrod AA, Leblond CP (1955) Induction of thyroid tumors in rats by low iodine diet. Cancer 8:339-367

Bastenie PA, Ermans AM, Bonnyns M, Neve P, Delespese G (1975) Molecular pathology. Thomas, Springfield

Björkman U, Ekholm R, Ericson LE (1978) Effects of thyrotropin on thyroglobulin exocytosis and iodination in the rat thyroid gland. Endocrinology 102:460-470

Borzelleca JF, Capen CC, Hallagan JB (1987) Lifetime toxicity/carcinogenicity study of FD&C red no. 3 (erythrosine) in rats. Food Chem Toxicol 25:723-733

Capen CC (1983) Chemical injury of the thyroid: pathologic and mechanistic considerations. In: The toxicology forum, proceedings of the 1983 annual winter meeting, Arlington, VA, pp 260-268

Capen CC, Martin SL (1989) The effects of xenobiotics on the structure and function of thyroid follicular and C-cells. Toxicol Pathol 17:266-293

Clements FW (1954) Relationship of thyrotoxicosis and carcinoma of thyroid to endemic goiter. Med J Aust 2:894

Clemmesen J, Hjalgrim-Jensen S (1977) On the absence of carcinogenicity to man of phenobarbital. Statistical studies in the aetiology of malignant neoplasms. Acta Pathol Microb Scand [Suppl] 261:38

Clemmesen J, Hjalgrim-Jensen S (1978) Is phenobarbital carcinogenic? A follow-up of 8078 epileptics. Ecotoxicol Environ Safety 1:255

Clemmesen J, Hjalgrim-Jensen S (1981) Does phenobarbital cause intracranial tumors? A follow-up through 35 years. Ecotoxicol Environ Safety 5:255-260

Clemmesen J, Fuglsang-Frederiksen V, Plum CM (1974) Are anticonvulsants oncogenic? Lancet 1:705-707

Collins WT, Capen CC (1980) Ultrastructural and functional alterations of the rat thyroid gland produced by polychlorinated biphenyls compared with iodide excess and deficiency, and thyrotropin and thyroxine administration. Virchows Arch [B] 33:213-231

Collins WT Jr, Capen CC, Kasza L, Carter C, Dailey RE, et al. (1977) Effects of polychlorinated biphenyl (PCB) on the thyroid gland of rats. Ultrastructural and biochemical investigations. Am J Pathol 89:119-136

Cooper DS, Axelrod L, DeGroot LJ, et al. (1981) Congenital goiter and the development of metastatic follicular carcinoma with evidence for a leak of non-hormonal iodide: clinical, pathological, kinetic, and biochemical studies and a review of the literature. J Clin Endocrinol Metab 52:294-306

Curran PG, DeGroot LJ (1991) The effect of hepatic enzyme-inducing drugs on thyroid hormones and the thyroid gland. Endocr Rev 12:135-150

Döhler KD, Wong CC, von zur Möfchlen A (1979) The rat as model for the study of drug effects on thyroid function: consideration of methodological problems. Pharmacol Ther [B] 5:305-318

Doniach I (1970) Aetiological consideration of thyroid carcinoma. In: Smithers D (ed) Tumors of the thyroid gland. Livingstone, London, pp 55-72

Ericson LE, Engström G (1978) Quantitative electron microscopic studies on exocytosis and endocytosis in the thyroid follicle cell. Endocrinology 103:883

Ericson LE, Engstrom G, Ekholm R (1980) Effect of cycloheximide on thyrotropin-stimulated endocytosis in the rat thyroid. Endocrinology 106:1119-1126

Ericson LE, Ring KM, Öfverholm T (1983) Selective macropinocytosis of thyroglobulin in rat thyroid follicles. Endocrinology 113:1746-1753

Foti D, Rapoport B (1990) Carbohydrate moieties in recombinant human thyroid peroxidase: role in recognition by antithyroid peroxidase antibodies in Hashimoto's thyroiditis. Endocrinology 126:2983-2988

Friedman GD (1981) Barbiturates and lung cancer in humans. J Natl Cancer Inst 67:291-295

Furth J (1968) Pituitary cybernetics and neoplasia (Harvey lecture series). Academic, New York, p 47

Gerber H, Studer H, von Günigen C (1985) Paradoxical effects of thyrotropin on diffusion of thyroglobulin in the colloid of rat thyroid follicles after long term thyroxine treatment. Endocrinology 116:303-310

Gerber H, Peter HJ, Bachmeier C, Kaempf J, Studer H (1987) Progressive recruitment of follicular cells with graded secretory responsiveness during stimulation of the thyroid gland by thyrotropin. Endocrinology 120:91-96

Hill RN, Erdreich LS, Paynter O, et al. (1989) Thyroid follicular cell carcinogenesis. Fundam Appl Toxicol 12:629-697

Ingbar SH (1972) Autoregulation of the thyroid. Response to iodide excess and depletion. Mayo Clin Proc 47:814-823

Kennedy TH, Purves HD (1941) Studies on experimental goiter: effect of brassica seed diets on rats. Br J Exp Pathol 22:241

Lamas L, Ingbar SH (1978) The effect of varying iodine content on the susceptibility of thyroglobulin to hydrolysis by thyroid acid protease. Endocrinology 102:188–197

Loewenstein JE, Wollman SH (1967) Distribution of ^{125}I and ^{127}I in the rat thyroid during equilibrium labeling as determined by autoradiography. Endocrinology 81:1074

Many MC, Denef JF, Haumont S, van den Hove-Vandenbroucke MF, Cornette C, Beckers C (1985) Morphological and functional changes during thyroid hyperplasia and involution in C3H mice: effects of iodine and 3,5,3′-triiodothyronine during involution. Endocrinology 116:798–806

McClain RM, Posch RC, Bosakowski T, Armstrong JM (1988) Studies on the mode of action for thyroid gland tumor promotion in rats by phenobarbital. Toxicol Appl Pharmacol 94:254–265

McClain RM, Levin AA, Posch R, Downing JC (1989) The effects of phenobarbital on the metabolism and excretion of thyroxine in rats. Toxicol Appl Pharmacol 99:216–228

McGirr EM, Clement WE, Currie AR, Kennedy JS (1959) Impaired dehalogenase activity as a cause of goiter with malignant changes. Scott Med J 4:232

Mizukami Y, Matsubara F, Matsukawa S (1985) Cytochemical localization of peroxidase and hydrogen-peroxide-producing NAD(P)H-oxidase in thyroid follicular cells of propylthiouracil-treated rats. Histochemistry 82:263–268

Morris HP (1955) The experimental development and metabolism of thyroid gland tumors. Adv Cancer Res 3:51–115

Nadler NJ, Young BA, Leblond CP, Mitmaker B (1964) Elaboration of thyroglobulin in the thyroid follicle. Endocrinology 74:333

Napalkov NP (1976) Tumours of the thyroid gland. In: Turusov VS (ed) Pathology of tumors in laboratory animals, vol 1, part 2. International Agency for Research on Cancer, Lyon, pp 239–272 (IARC scientific publication no 6)

Nilsson M, Engström G, Ericson LE (1986) Graded response in the individual thyroid follicle cell to increasing doses of TSH. Mol Cell Endocrinol 44:165–169

Öfverholm T, Ericson LE (1984) Intraluminal iodination of thyroglobulin. Endocrinology 114:827–835

Öfverholm T, Björkman U, Ericson LE (1985) Effects of TSH on iodination in rat thyroid follicles studied by autoradiography. Mol Cell Endocrinol 40:1–7

Ohnhaus EE, Studer H (1983) A link between liver microsomal enzyme activity and thyroid hormone metabolism in man. Br J Clin Pharmacol 15:71–76

Ohnhaus EE, Burgi H, Burger A, Studer H (1981) The effect of antipyrine, phenobarbital, and rifampicin on the thyroid hormone metabolism in man. Eur J Clin Invest 11:381–387

Onshima M, Ward JM (1984) Promotion of N-methyl-N-nitrosurea-induced thyroid tumors by iodine deficiency in F344/NCr rats. J Natl Cancer Inst 73:289–296

Ohshima M, Ward JM (1986) Dietary iodine deficiency as a tumor promoter and carcinogen in male F344/NCr rats. Cancer Res 46:877–883

Olsen JH, Boice JD Jr, et al. (1989) Cancer among epileptic patients exposed to anticonvulsant drugs. J Natl Cancer Inst 81:803–808

Ottenweller JE, Hedge GA (1982) Diurnal variations of plasma thyrotropin, thyroxine, and triiodothyronine in female rats are phase shifted after inversion of the photoperiod. Endocrinology 111:509–514

Paynter SH, Burin GJ, Jaeger RB, Gregorio CA (1988) Goitrogens and thyroid follicular cell neoplasmia: evidence for a threshold process. Regul Toxicol Pharmacol 8:102

Pendergrast WJ, Milmore BK, Marcus SC (1961) Thyroid cancer and toxicosis in the United States: their relation to endemic goiter. J Chronic Dis 13:22

Pic P, Remy L, Athouel-Haon AM, Mazzella E (1984) Evidence for a role of the cytoskeleton in the in vitro folliculogenesis of the thyroid gland of the fetal rat. Cell Tissue Res 237:499–508

Sakurai S, Fogelfeld L, Ries A, Schneider AB (1990) Anionic complex-carbohydrate units of human thyroglobulin. Endocrinology 127:2056–2063

Shirts SB, Annegers JF, Hauser WA, Kurland LT (1986) Cancer incidence in a cohort of patients with seizure disorders. J Natl Cancer Inst 77:83–87

Swarm RL, Roberts GKS, Levy AC, Hines LR (1973) Observations on the thyroid gland in rats following the administration of sulfamethoxazole and trimethoprim. Toxicol Appl Pharmacol 24:351–363

Takayama S, Aihara K, Onodera T, Akimoto T (1986) Antithyroid effects of propylthiouracil and sulfamonomethoxine in rats and monkeys. Toxicol Appl Pharmacol 82:191–199

Tice LW, Wollman SH (1974) Ultrastructural localization of peroxidase on pseudopods and other structures of the typical thyroid epithelial cell. Endocrinology 94:1555–1567

Toda S, Sugihara H (1990) Reconstruction of thyroid follicles from isolated porcine follicle cells in three-dimensional collagen gel culture. Endocrinology 126:2027–2034

Uchiyama Y, Oomiya A, Murakami G (1986a) Fluctuations in follicular structures of rat thyroid glands during 24 hours: fine structural and morphometric studies. Am J Anat 175: 23–33

Uchiyama Y, Murakami G, Igarashi M (1986b) Changes in colloid droplets and dense bodies in rat thyroid follicular cells during 24 hours: fine structural and morphometric studies. Am J Anat 175:15–22

Ward JM, Stinson SF, Hardisty JF, Cockrell BY, Hayden DW (1979) Neoplasms and pigmentation of thyroid glands in F344 rats exposed to 2,4-diaminoanisole sulfate, a hair dye component. J Natl Cancer Inst 62:1067–1073

Wetzel BK, Spicer SS, Wollman SH (1965) Changes in fine structure and acid phosphatase localization in rat thyroid cells following thyrotropin administration. J Cell Biol 25:593

White SJ, McLean AE, Howland C (1979) Anticonvulsant drugs and cancer. A cohort study in patients with severe epilepsy. Lancet 2:458–461

Whur P, Herscovics A, Leblond CP (1969) Radioautographic visualization of the incorporation of galactose-^{3}H and mannose-^{3}H by rat thyroids in vitro in relation to the stages of thyroglobulin synthesis. J Cell Biol 43:289–311

Wolff J, Williams JA (1973) The role of microtubules and microfilaments in thyroid secretion. Recent Prog Horm Res 29:229–285

Wollman SH, Ekholm R (1981) Site of iodination in hyperplastic thyroid glands deduced from autoradiographs. Endocrinology 108:2082–2085

Wollman SH, Spicer SS, Burstone MS (1964) Localization of esterase and acid phosphatase in granules and colloid droplets in rat thyroid epithelium. J Cell Biol 21:191

Wynford-Thomas D, Smith P, Williams ED (1987) Proliferative response to cyclic AMP elevation of thyroid epithelium in suspension culture. Mol Cell Endocrinol 51:163–166

Ectopic Thyroid, Mouse

Charles H. Frith

Synonym. Aberrant thyroid tissue.

Gross Appearance

Ectopic thyroid tissue in the mouse is not visible grossly.

Microscopic Features

Ectopic thyroid tissue in the mouse may be found at the base of the heart in multilocular fat. The tissue consists of a group of isolated thyroid follicles similar in appearance to normal thyroid tissue. The follicles are lined by a single layer of low cuboidal epithelium and filled with eosinophilic colloid (Fig. 259).

Ultrastructure

The ultrastructural characteristics of ectopic thyroid tissue in the mouse have not been studied. It may be assumed that these structures have the same features observed with the electron microscope in thyroid glands in the usual anatomic location. This point needs to be established, however, by appropriate studies.

Differential Diagnosis

The presence of typical thyroid follicular cells, with acini containing colloid, at an aberrant site in histologic sections is adequate for the diagnosis.

Biologic Features

Ectopic thyroid tissue results from the failure of all or part of the thyroid anlage to descend from the floor of the pharynx to its normal cervical location (Ficarra 1958).
Ectopic thyroid tissue is of practical importance in experimental thyroidectomies since persistent normal thyroid function can result from its presence. Complete removal of the thyroid gland in the mouse does not ensure removal of all functional thyroid tissue because of the occurrence of ectopic thyroid tissue.

Comparison with Other Species

Hunt (1963) reported the presence of ectopic thyroid tissue in seven of 2634 (0.27%) BALB/c mice. Such tissue was not seen in any of 1033 Strong A mice. Ectopic thyroid has also been described in the rat (Van Dyke 1953), guinea pig

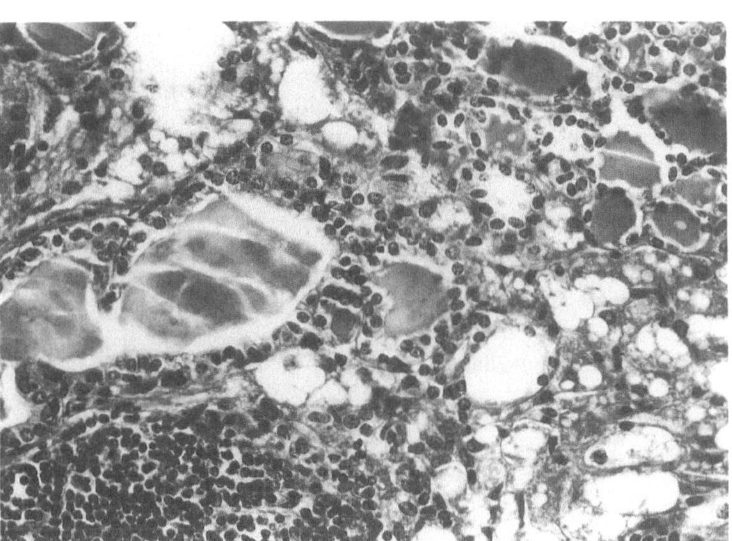

Fig. 259. Ectopic thyroid tissue in the mouse, demonstrating follicles with colloid. H&E, ×300

(Kochakian and Cockrell 1958), dog (Geil 1961), and humans (Ficarra 1958).

References

Ficarra BJ (1958) Diseases of the thyroid and parathyroid glands. Intercontinental Medical Book, New York, pp 211–222

Geil RG (1961) Intrathoracic thyroid gland in a dog-case report. J Am Vet Med Assoc 138:539–540

Hunt RD (1963) Aberrant thyroid tissue in the mouse. Science 141:1054–1055

Kochakian CD, Cockrell D (1958) Presence of aberrant thyroid tissue in the guinea pig. Endocrinology 63:385–388

Van Dyke JH (1953) Experimental aberrant mediastinal goiters (thymic) in the rat. Arch Pathol 55:412–422

Ectopic Thyroid, Rat

George A. Parker and Marion G. Valerio

Synonym. Thyroid rests.

Gross Appearance

Thyroid rests are rarely large enough to be seen grossly. The identity of those few grossly visible nodules must be confirmed microscopically; thus, gross diagnosis is virtually impossible.

Microscopic Features

Ectopic thyroid consists of small aggregates of thyroid follicles near the midline of the body in the neck and thoracic cavity, particularly near the thymus and aorta (Anderson and Capen 1978; McCarrison 1917). The ectopic follicles are histologically identical to the normal thyroid, but the calcitonin-secreting C cells are not present (Anderson and Capen 1978; Hardisty and Boorman 1990).

Ultrastructure

No information is available.

Differential Diagnosis

None.

Biologic Features

Thyroid rests that are cranial to the primary thyroid gland are thought to arise from remnants of the thyroglossal duct or stalk, while whose caudal to the thyroid are believed to arise from detached fragments of the thyroid primordia that are carried with the heart into the thoracic cavity (Arey 1965). Ectopic thyroid tissue often is functional and responds to the same stimuli as the primary gland; it may thus give rise to aberrant goiters or neoplasms (Nieberle and Cohrs 1967). No data are available on the frequency of occurrence of ectopic thyroid in the rat. As with many other ectopias in rodents, detection of ectopic thyroid usually results from the fortuitous inclusion of small islands of thyroid tissue in sections of another organ. Reliable estimation of the frequency would probably require serial sectioning of the head, neck, and thorax of a number of rats in each strain.

Comparison with Other Species

Ectopic thyroid tissue is not infrequently found near the thyroid, in the tongue, near the hyoid bones, along the entire length of the trachea, on the aortic arch, and in or on the pericardium of many species (Snell 1965). Thyroid rests are found within the pericardium or in the periaortic fat in about 50% of dogs (Snell 1965). (See also Ectopic Thyroid, Mouse, this volume.)

References

Anderson MP, Capen CC (1978) The endocrine system. In: Benirschke K, Garner FM, Jones TC (eds) Pathology of laboratory animals, vol 1. Springer, Berlin Heidelberg New York, pp 423–499

Arey LB (1965) Developmental anatomy, 7th edn. Saunders, Philadelphia, p 243

Hardisty JF, Boorman GA (1990) Thyroid Gland. In: Boorman GA, Eustis SL, Elwell MR, Montgomery CA, MacKenzie WF (eds) Pathology of the Fischer Rat, Academic, New York, p 523

McCarrison R (1917) The thyroid gland in health and disease. Tindall and Cox, London Bailliere, p 7

Nieberle K, Cohrs C (1967) Textbook of the special pathological anatomy of domestic animals. Pergamon, New York, p 916

Snell KC (1965) Spontaneous lesions of the rat. In: Ribelin WE, McCoy JR (eds) Pathology of laboratory animals, Thomas, Springfield, chap 10

Ectopic Thymus, Thyroid, Rat

George A. Parker and Marion G. Valerio

Synonym. Thymic rests.

Gross Appearance

Thymic rests are rarely large enough to be seen grossly. The identity of those few grossly visible nodules must be confirmed microscopically; thus, gross diagnosis is virtually impossible.

Microscopic Features

Ectopic thymus consists of small nests of thymic tissue in the region between the thyroid and heart. In standard sections from laboratory rats the nests are most commonly seen adjacent to or within the thyroid or parathyroid (Stefanski et al. 1990). The nests have distinct cortical and medullary regions, which may not be apparent in tangential sections through the cortical region. Ectopic thymus is characterized by a mixture of thymic epithelium and mature thymic lymphocytes and has occasionally Hassall's corpuscles (Figs. 260–262); Arey 1965; Hardisty and Boorman 1990).

Ultrastructure

No information is available.

Differential Diagnosis

Ectopic thymus must be distinguished from lymph nodules. The presence of corticomedullary microarchitecture and thymic epithelium is essential to identifying ectopic thymus. Presence of Hassall's corpuscles is a definitive identifying feature, but may not be present in all rests.

Biologic Features

The thymic primordia arise from the third pharyngeal pouches early in embryonic life. The lower end becomes attached to the pericardium and migrates with the heart into the thoracic cavity. During the migration the upper ends become drawn out and eventually disappear. Small secondary thymic masses are frequently encountered in embryos. The slender upper ends sometimes persist, thus continuing the thymus to the level of the thyroid. Isolated nests of accessory thymic tissue result from discontinuities in this slender thymic projection (Arey 1965).

The frequency of ectopic thymus in the rat is not documented in the literature. Detection of ectopic thymus usually results from fortuitous inclusion of the rests in sections of other organs, particularly the thyroids. Some of the small lymphoid nodules seen in the neck region of the rat may in fact be tangential sections through the cortical part of thymic rests. Serial sectioning of such nodules reveals whether a medullary region exists, thus identifying the nodule as ectopic thymus.

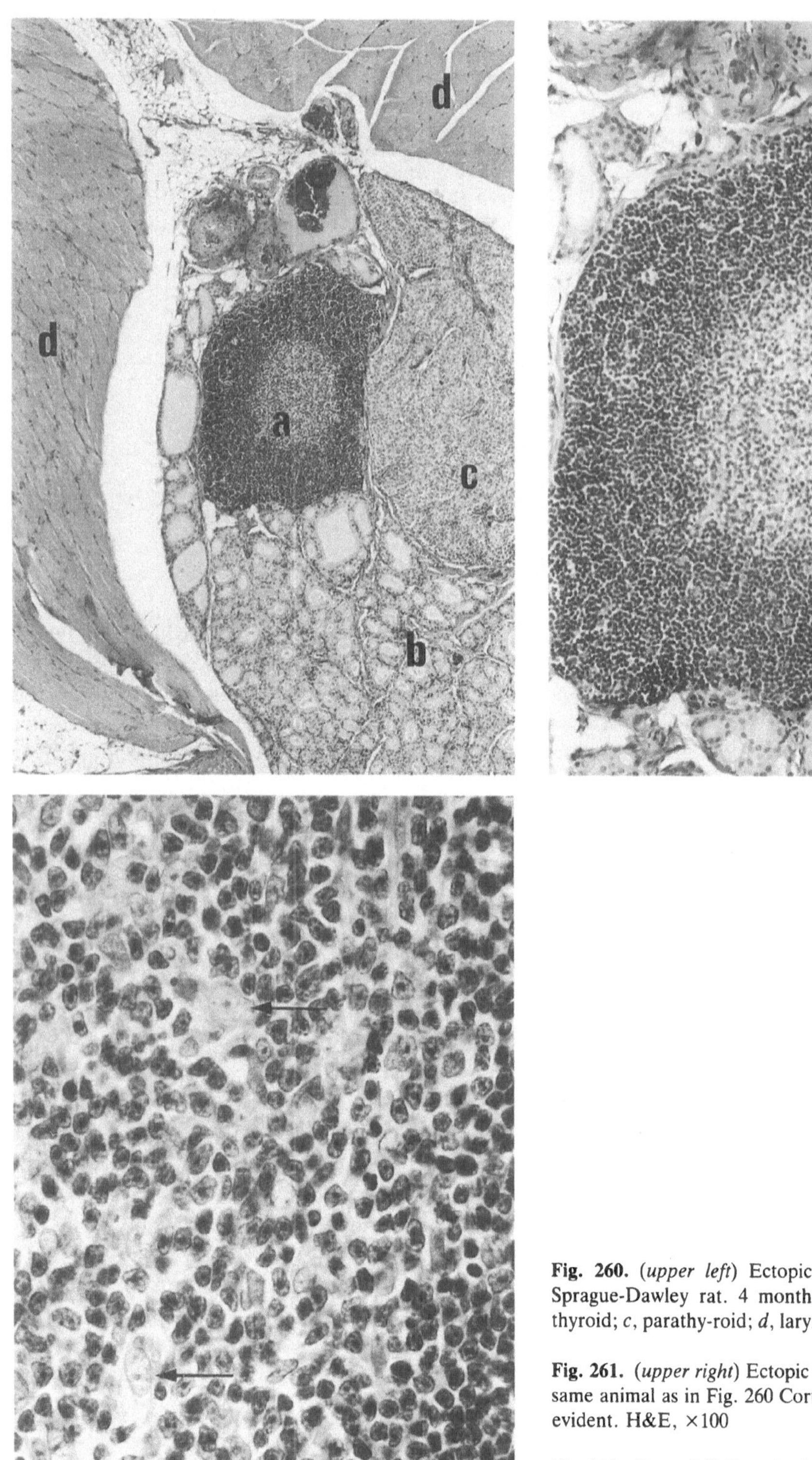

Fig. 260. (*upper left*) Ectopic thymus in the thyroid of a Sprague-Dawley rat. 4 months old. *a*, Ectopic thymus; *b*, thyroid; *c*, parathy-roid; *d*, laryngeal musculature. H&E; ×32

Fig. 261. (*upper right*) Ectopic thymus in the thyroid of a rat: same animal as in Fig. 260 Cortex and medulla of thymus are evident. H&E, ×100

Fig. 262. (*lower left*) Ectopic thymus in the thyroid of a rat: same animal as in Fig. 260. Mixed population of darkly stained lymphocytes and thymic epithelial cells (*arrows*). H&E, ×300

Comparison with Other Species

No significant information is available on this subject at present.

References

Arey LB (1965) Developmental anatomy: a textbook and laboratory manual of embryology, 7th edn. Saunders, Philadelphia

Hardisty JF, Boorman GA (1990) Thyroid gland. In: Boorman GA, Eustis SL, Elwell MR, Montgomery CA, MacKenzie WF (eds) Pathology of the Fischer rat. Academic, San Diego, p 523

Stefanski SA, Elwell MR, Stromberg PC (1990) Spleen, lymph nodes and thymus. In: Boorman GA, Eustis SL, Elwell MR, Montgomery CA, MacKenzie WF (eds) Pathology of the Fischer rat. Academic, San Diego, p 389

Follicular Cell Hyperplasia, Adenoma, and Carcinoma, Thyroid, Rat

Gary A. Boorman and Michael R. Elwell

Synonyms. Follicular cell hyperplasia: follicular cystic hyperplasia, diffuse or nodular hyperplasia; follicular cell adenoma: follicular adenoma, trabecular adenoma, microfollicular cell adenoma, papillary adenoma, adenoma, cystadenoma; follicular cell carcinoma: follicular carcinoma, trabecular carcinoma, microfollicular carcinoma, papillary carcinoma, carcinoma, adenocarcinoma, cystadenocarcinoma.

Gross Appearance

Diffuse hyperplasia, which may occur in prechronic toxicity studies, has been grossly described as goiter (Latin *gutter*, throat). This is characterized by diffuse, uniform, bilateral enlargement of the thyroid gland; the weight of a hyperplastic gland may be ten times that of the normal thyroid gland. The diffusely hyperplastic thyroid gland is generally a darker red-brown color than the glands of control rats. This color difference has been attributed to increased vascularity and decreased follicular colloid in the hyperplastic gland. In short-term studies the capsular surface of the gland may be smooth but may become lobulated in studies of longer duration. The lobulated appearance has been attributed to the capsular fibrosis that may occur in more severe cases of hyperplasia.

Milder cases of diffuse or focal hyperplasia as well as small adenomas are often not detected grossly. Large adenomas and carcinoma of the thyroid gland may cause unilateral or bilateral, asymmetrical enlargement or occur as nodular masses.

Microscopic Features

Follicular cell hyperplasia occurs as a treatment-related proliferative lesion in short-term toxicity studies and as a spontaneous or treatment-related effect in chronic toxicity and carcinogenicity studies. With iodine deficiency or with short-term (2- to 13-week) administration of goitrogenic compounds (Gopinath et al. 1987; Hayden et al. 1978; Kanno et al. 1992) the hyperplasia typically involves the entire thyroid gland (Fig. 263). In diffuse hyperplasia thyroid follicles appear smaller, contain little or no colloid, and are lined by a cuboidal to columnar hyperchromatic epithelium (Fig. 264). In more severe lesions the vascularity of the thyroid gland may be increased. Short or blunt papillary projections may extend into the follicle lumen. In cases of marked diffuse hyperplasia the capsule may be thickened by proliferation of fibrous tissue that extends into the lobes of the thyroid gland (Fig. 265). In studies of longer duration the hyperplastic changes in thyroid follicles are less uniform. Frequently there are large portions which appear normal but may represent areas with regression of previously diffuse hyperplasia. These thyroid glands can have focal follicular cell (cystic) hyperplasia characterized by one or several cystic or dilated, colloid-filled follicles lined by low cuboidal or flattened epithelium. Larger cystic follicles may slightly compress the adjacent surrounding tissue (Fig. 266). Such follicles are lined by a single layer of cuboidal, hyperchromatic epithelial cells that frequently form simple or blunt papillary structures which project into the follicular lumen (Fig. 267). Whereas a morphologic continuum from the focal hyperplasia to adenoma or carcinoma may be identified, the complexity of structure and degree of cellular atypia are helpful morphologic features for distinguishing these proliferative lesions (Hardisty and Boorman 1990).

Follicular cell adenoma often compresses adjacent thyroid follicles but usually lacks a well-defined capsule or are partially encapsulated. The tumor cells are typically more hyperchromatic than those

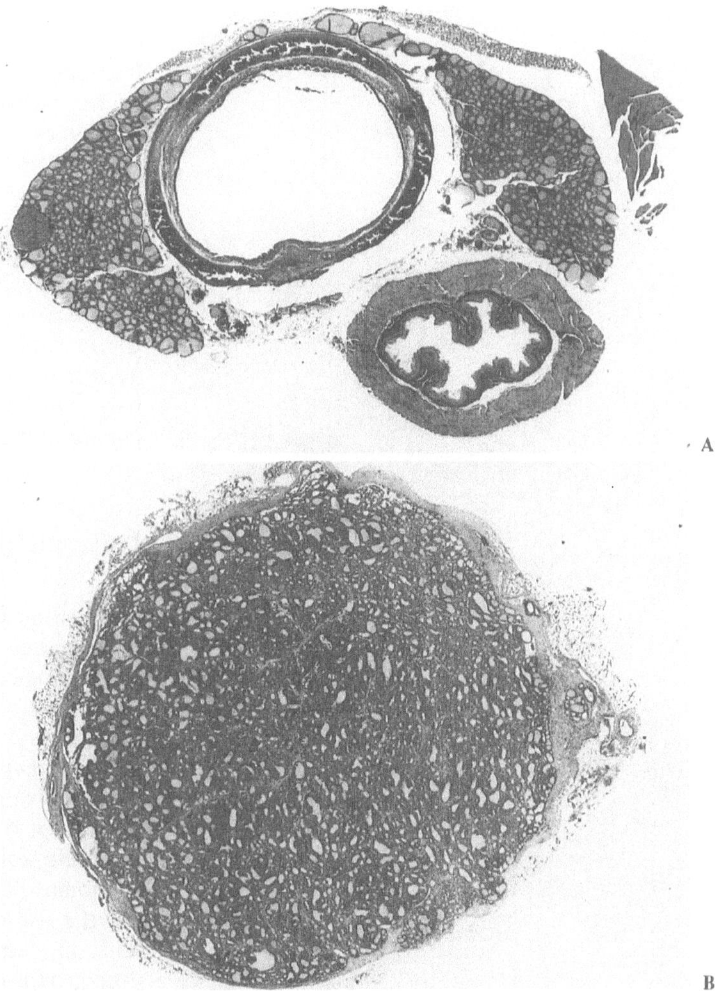

Fig. 263A,B. Thyroid, rat. **A** Control male rat. **B** Diffuse follicular cell hyperplasia in male rat exposed to a concentration of 50 mg/m^3 2-mercaptobenzimidazole for 13 weeks. Note the thickened fibrous capsule and increased size of this transverse section of one lobe compared to the entire thyroid gland of the control. H&E, ×15

of surrounding thyroid follicular epithelium (Fig. 268). They form variable-sized follicles (Fig. 269) or line large cystic spaces, frequently forming irregular papillary structures (Fig. 270). These papillary structures may be more complex than those seen in hyperplastic lesions and often show a greater degree of nuclear crowding and cellular atypia (Figs. 271, 272).

Follicular cell carcinoma may have a follicular (Fig. 273), papillary (Fig. 274), or solid growth pattern or may have a combination of these patterns. While follicular cell carcinoma is often a well-differentiated neoplasm, the presence of disorganized or heterogeneous growth patterns, cellular pleomorphism, and a scirrhous reaction are criteria for malignancy. Follicular cells in carcinomas may be highly pleomorphic and form small follicles with a scirrhous reaction (Fig. 275), and both follicular (acinar) and solid areas may be present in the same neoplasm (Figs. 276, 277). Extension through the thyroid capsule into adjacent tissues, vascular invasion, or metastatic foci are the unequivocal features of malignancy.

Ultrastructure

Features of diffuse hyperplasia include increased size of follicle cells and accumulation of colloid material in dilated endoplasmic reticulum (Gopinath et al. 1987). The ultrastructural features of rat follicular cell adenoma and carcinoma have also been studied (Christov 1981). The principal changes seen in adenomatous cells include elongated microvilli, pseudopodia, and protrusions of plasma membrane from the apex of tumor

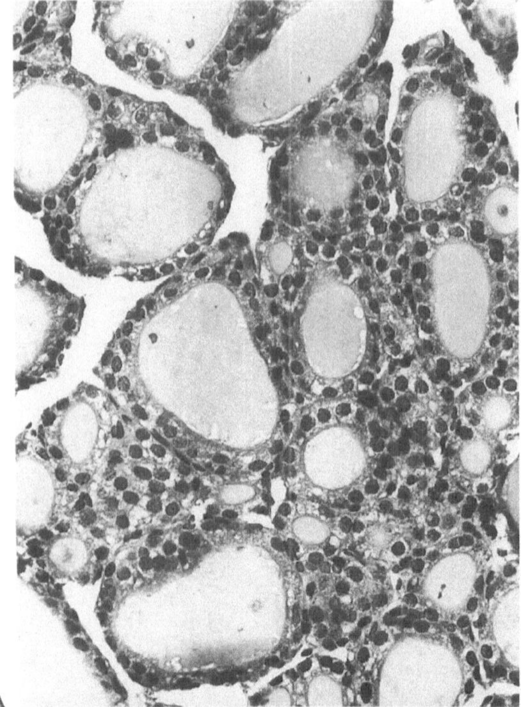

A

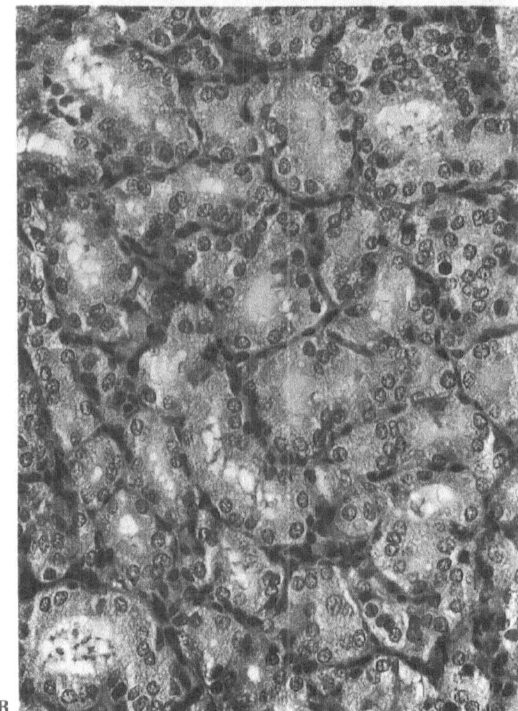

B

Fig. 264A,B. Thyroid, rat. **A** Control male rat. **B** Diffuse follicular cell hyperplasia in male rat administered 5000 ppm 2,6-toluenediamine dihydrochloride in the feed for 13 weeks. Gland is comprised of hyperchromatic follicular epithelial cells forming small follicles that contain little or no colloid compared to the thyroid gland of the control. H&E, ×250

cells. Near the apical border a heterogeneous population of colloid droplets, small vesicles, and lysosomes are present. In the intermediate region of the tumor cells, enlarged Golgi apparatus, lysosomes, mitochondria, and filamentous structures predominate. Membranes of the rough endoplastic reticulum are often arranged in parallel arrays and sometimes form vacuoles and cisternae differing in size and optical density. Follicular cell carcinomas have more conspicuous dilated cisternae and pseudopodia in the lumen of acini. Tumor cells may be linked together by desmosomes, pseudodesmosomes, and terminal bars. The basal lamina is well defined and rarely disrupted by tumor cells, even in carcinomas.

Differential Diagnosis

Progression from focal follicular cell hyperplasia to adenoma and carcinoma in rats is evident morphologically (Hardisty and Boorman 1990). Clear distinction between these categories is sometimes difficult. Morphologic criteria are not often predictive of biologic behavior and removal of thyroid-stimulating hormone stimulation causes reversal of some but not all proliferative lesions, including some lesions that may appear to be adenomas (Todd 1986). In spite of these difficulties the use of standardized criteria applied in a uniform fashion allows comparisons between dose groups and between different studies. Follicular cell hyperplasia can be distinguished from follicular cyst and from follicular cell adenoma. Follicular cyst is lined by flattened epithelium and often occurs near the periphery of the gland. Follicular cell adenoma has a more complex pattern than hyperplasia. An important feature is the occurrence of multiple layers of follicular cells on the basement membrane. Follicular cell adenoma is more solid than hyperplasia and often has a papillary or follicular pattern. Follicular cell adenoma must be distinguished from follicular cell carcinoma. Adenoma often consists of a single morphological pattern, but carcinoma may have a heterogeneous growth pattern and some cellular pleomorphism. Follicular cell carcinoma is often distinguished by a scirrhous response forming a capsule. Invasion of the capsule or adjacent musculature is a hallmark of malignancy. Some chemically induced carcinomas may be quite anaplastic.

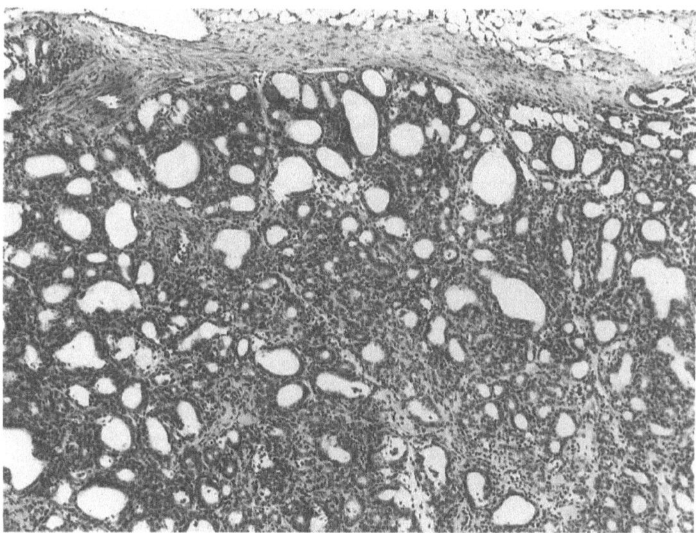

Fig. 265. Thyroid, rat. Diffuse hyperplasia from thyroid gland in Fig. 263B. Note the small compact follicles and larger irregular shaped follicles with small amount of faintly staining colloid material. Note also the interfollicular fibrosis. H&E, ×125

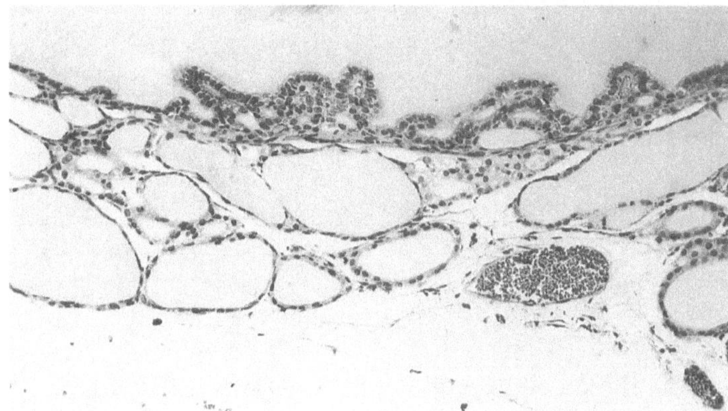

Fig. 266. Thyroid, rat. Follicular cell hyperplasia. Enlarged follicle lined by a single layer of follicular cells that project into the lumen. H&E, ×60

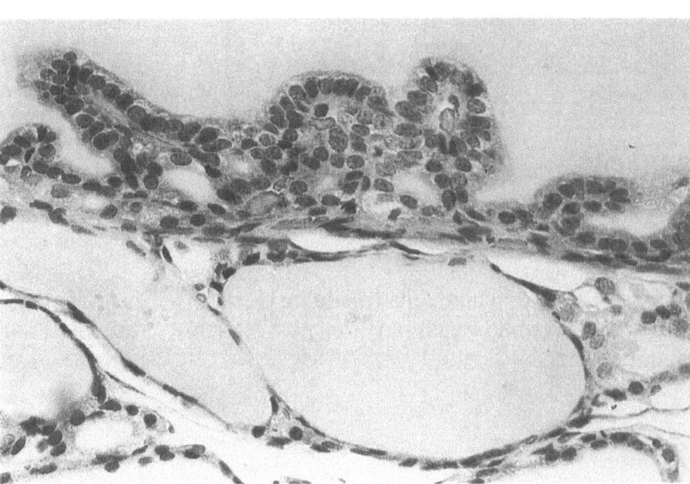

Fig. 267. Thyroid, rat. Follicular cell hyperplasia. Higher magnification of Fig. 266. H&E, ×384

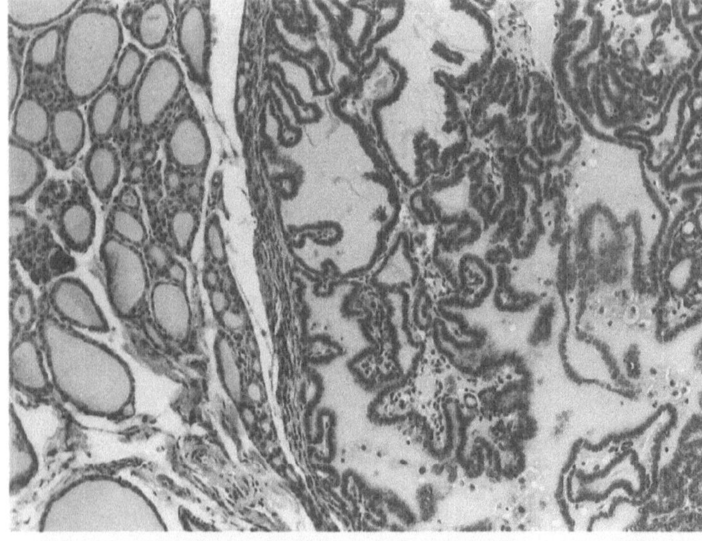

Fig. 268. Thyroid, rat; follicular cell adenoma with hyperchromasia of tumor cells. Irregular and varying-sized follicles are formed by the tumor cells. H&E, ×40

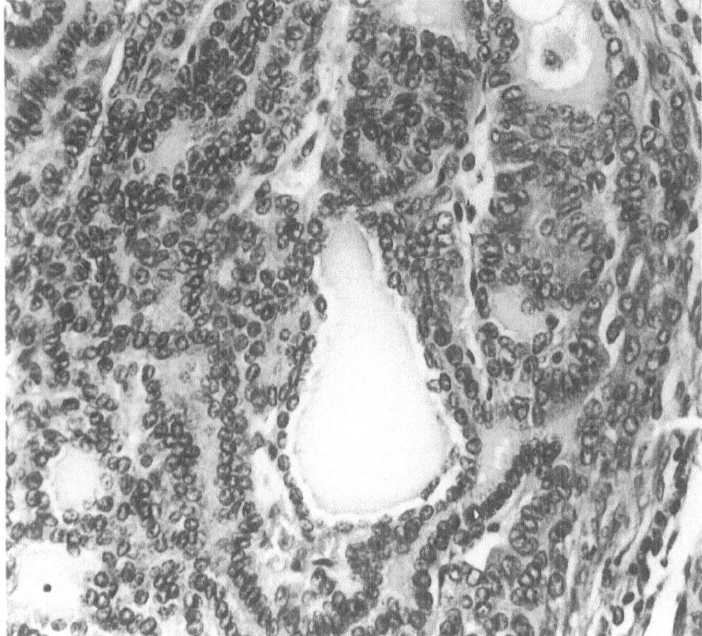

Fig. 269. Thyroid, rat; follicular adenoma. Note nuclear crowding, irregular acini, and expansive growth. H&E, ×200. (Tissue section courtesy of Dr. C.H. Frith)

Lesions of parafollicular cells (medullary cells, C cells) are described separately on p. 262 (this volume).

Biologic Features

Follicular cell hyperplasia is uncommon as a spontaneous lesion in aging studies; however, it occurs frequently in studies where follicular cell adenomas and carcinomas are induced by a variety of goitrogenic substances (Hayden et al. 1978, Murthy 1980, Ward et al. 1979). Spontaneous follicular cell adenomas are also uncommon in rats. They are reported to occur in 4% of male and 2% of female Osborne-Mendel rats (Goodman et al. 1980) but in only 0.7% of male and 0.6% of female F344 rats from 2-year studies (Hardisty and Boorman 1990; Haseman et al. 1990). Numerous studies have shown that follicular cell adenomas and carcinomas can be induced by goitrogenic substances such as thiourea or

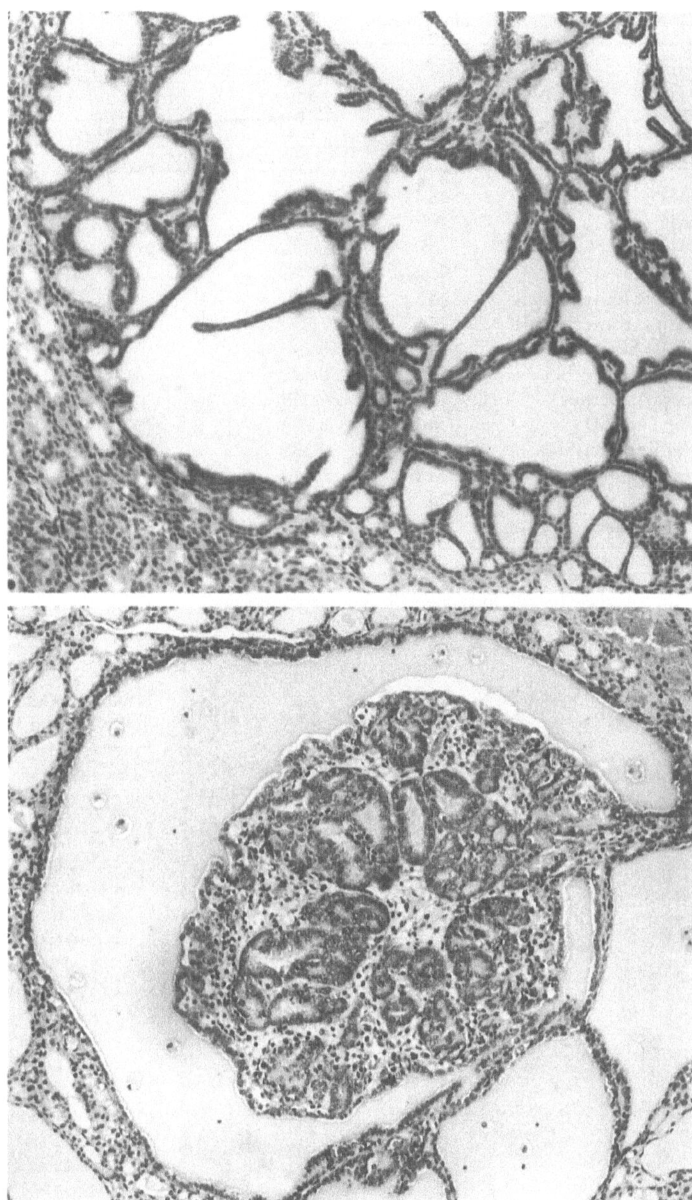

Fig. 270. Thyroid, rat; follicular adenoma with tendency to form cystic follicles. H&E, ×40

Fig. 271. Thyroid, rat; follicular adenoma projecting into a cystic follicle. H&E, ×40

thiouracil (Napalkov 1990). Iodine-restricted diets over prolonged periods will induce follicular cell adenomas or carcinomas. Exposure to either ^{131}I (Doniach 1957) or ^{125}I (deRuiter et al. 1976) induces both follicular cell adenomas and carcinomas. Partial destruction of the thyroid with concomitant decreased thyroxine production results in prolonged thyroid-stimulating hormone secretion and subsequent thyroid tumorigenesis (Axelrad and Leblond 1955). Follicular cell carcinomas are not as frequent in rats as carcinomas of C cell origin but a low incidence has been reported in a variety of rat strains (Table 18). It is interesting to note that although a variety of spontaneous tumors in F344 rats have been increasing in frequency over the past 15 years (Haseman 1992), the rate of thyroid follicular cell adenomas and carcinomas has remained constant (Table 18). Induced thyroid tumorigenesis (Table 19) has been the subject of numerous reviews (Biels-

Table 18. Follicular cell tumors in rats

Strain	Sex	Follicular cell adenoma		Follicular cell carcinoma		Reference
		n	%	*n*	%	
F344	M	11/1794	0.6[a]	19/1794	1[b]	Goodman et al. 1979
F344	F	5/1754	0.3[a]	12/1754	0.7[b]	Goodman et al. 1979
F344	M	13/1904	0.7	10/1904	0.5	Haseman et al. 1990
F344	F	12/1938	0.6	7/1938	0.4	Haseman et al. 1990
Wistar (conventional)	M	0/83	–	1/83	1	Kroes et al. 1981
Wistar (conventional)	F	1/83	1	0/83	–	Kroes et al. 1981
Wistar SPF	M	0/192	–	0/192	–	Kroes et al. 1981
Wistar SPF	F	0/192	–	0/192	–	Kroes et al. 1981
Sprague/Dawley	M/F	0/258	–	0/258	–	MacKenzie and Garner 1973
Holtzman-SD	M/F	0/268	–	0/268	–	MacKenzie and Garner 1973
Charles River-SD	M/F	0/535	–	2/535	0.4	MacKenzie and Garner 1973
Osborne-Mendel	M/F	0/673	–	0/673	–	MacKenzie and Garner 1973
Osborne-Mendel	M	42/975	4	27/975	3	Goodman et al. 1980
Osborne-Mendel	F	18/970	2	15/970	1.5	Goodman et al. 1980

[a] Adenoma and follicular cell adenoma combined.
[b] Adenocarcinoma and follicular cell carcinoma combined.

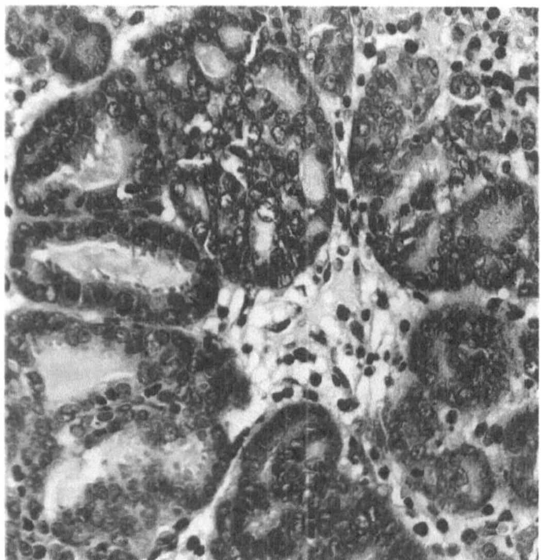

Fig. 272. Thyroid, rat; follicular adenoma. Same lesion as in Fig. 269. H&E, ×300

chowsky 1955; Burek 1978; Goodman et al. 1979; Hill et al. 1989; Kroes et al. 1981; MacKenzie and Garner 1973).

Comparison with Other Species

Spontaneous thyroid tumors in rats are infrequent and have not been studied extensively. The growth

Table 19. Chemicals in the NCI/NTP bioassay program causing evidence of thyroid follicular cell neoplasia (from Hardisty and Boorman 1990)

Thionamides
- *N*,*N'*-Dicyclohexylthiourea (M)
- *N*,*N'*-Diethylthiourea (M,F)
- Trimethylthiourea (F)

Aromatic amines
- Single ring
  - *O*-Anisidine hydrochloride (M)
  - 2,4-Diaminoanisole sulfate (M,F)
- Bridged double rings
  - 4,4'-Methylenebis(*N*,*N*-dimethyl)benzenamine (M,F)
  - 4,4'-Methylenedianiline dihydrochloride (M,F)
  - 4,4'-Oxydianiline (M,F)
  - 4,4'-Thiodianiline (M,F)
- Miscellaneous
  - C.I. Basic Red 9 monochloride (M,F)

Complex halogenated hydrocarbons
- Aldrin (M,F)
- Chlordane (M,F)
- Chlorinated paraffins (C_{12}, 60% chlorine) (F)
- 2,3,7,8-Tetrachlorodibenzo-*p*-dioxin (M,F)
- Tetrachlorodiphenylethane (*p*,*p'*-DDD) (M)
- Toxaphene (M,F)

Organophosphorous compounds
- Azinphosmethyl (M)
- Tetrachlorvinphos[a] (M)

M, Male rats; F, female rats.
[a] Response primarily limited to follicular cell hyperplasia.

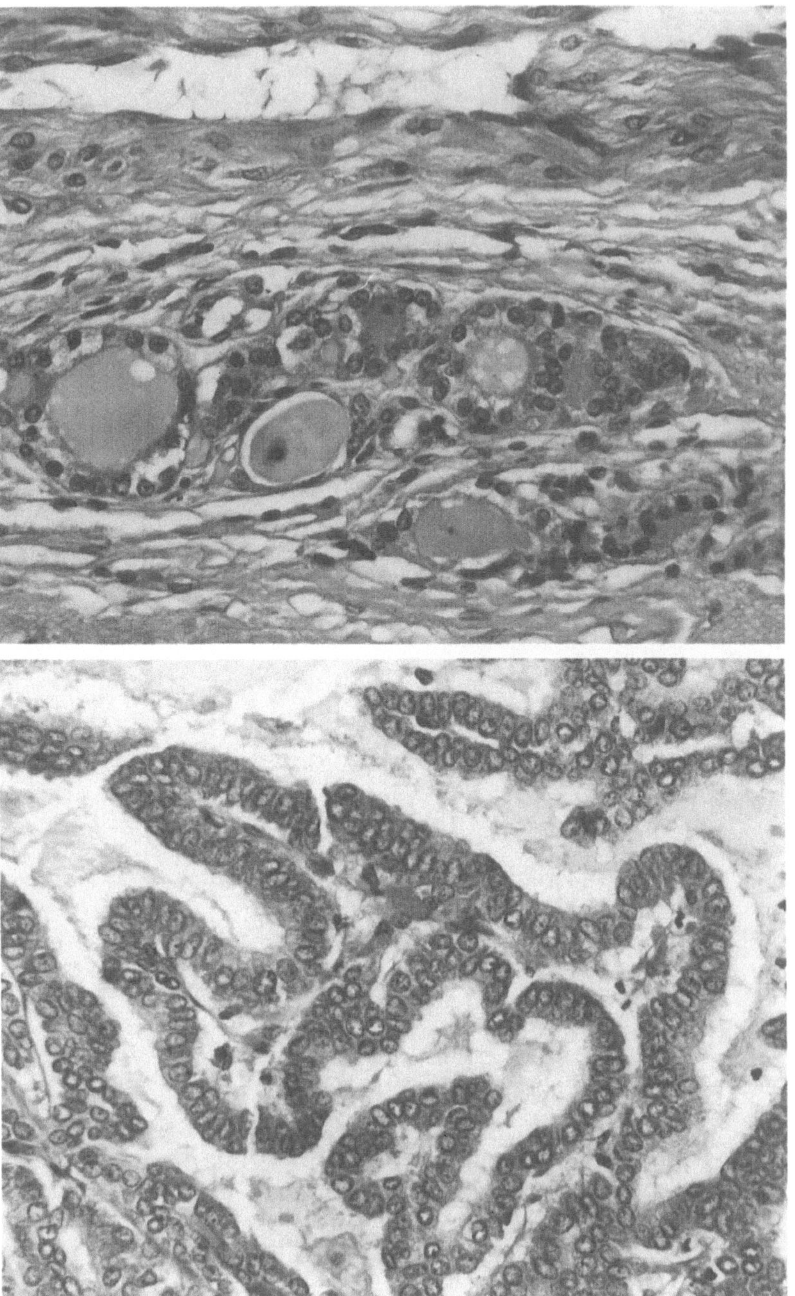

Fig. 273. (*above*) Follicular cell carcinoma in the thyroid of a female Wistar rat, 574 days old, control. Tumor cells forming acini and colloid in capsule of thyroid adjacent to an artery. H&E, ×240. (Courtesy of Dr. Charles H. Frith)

Fig. 274. (*below*) Follicular cell carcinoma in the thyroid of a female Wistar rat, 574 days old, control. Papillary pattern formed by cells in some parts of the tumor. H&E, ×240. (Courtesy of Dr. Charles H. Frith)

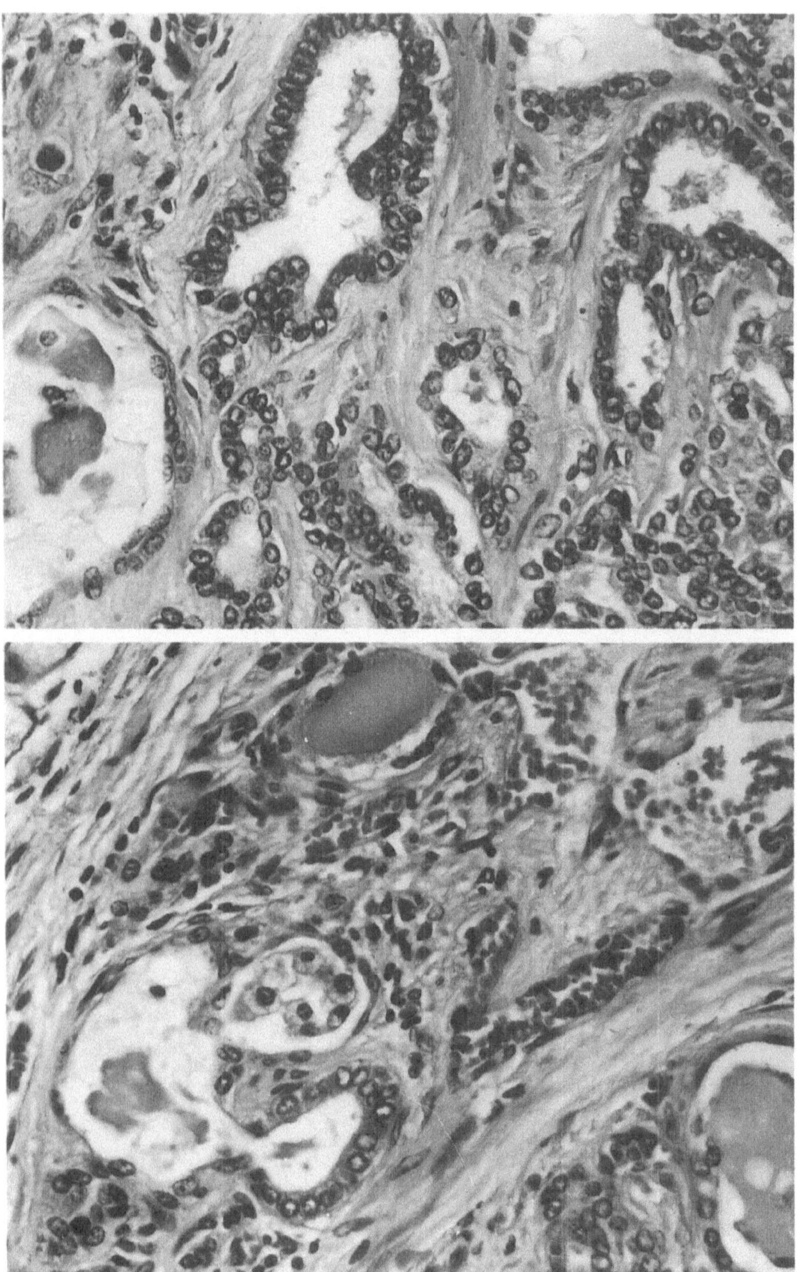

Fig. 275. (*above*) Follicular cell carcinoma, thyroid, female Wistar rat; same section as Fig. 273. Pleomorphism and scirrhous reaction. H&E, ×240. (Courtesy of Dr. Charles H. Firth)

Fig. 276. (*below*) Follicular cell carcinoma, thyroid, rat; same section as Fig. 273. Acini containing colloid and plemorphic tumor cells. H&E, ×240. (Courtesy of Dr. Charles H. Frith)

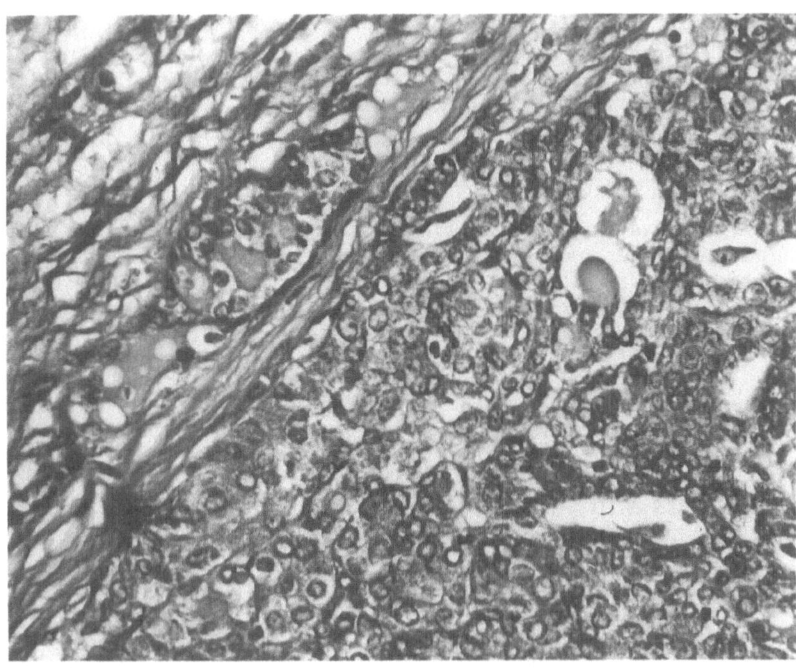

Fig. 277. Follicular cell carcinoma in the thyroid of a male Wistar rat, 702 days old, given 2-naphtylamine. Acini and colloid (*A*) are present, as well as solid areas (*S*). Tumor has invaded lymphatic in capsule (*C*). H&E, ×240. (Courtesy of Dr. Charles H. Frith)

patterns and cellular morphology of spontaneously occurring proliferative lesions of the thyroid gland are similar to those reported for mice and other species. Malignant tumors of the thyroid gland are more common in the rat than in the mouse. Follicular cell carcinomas in man have been subclassified, but this has not proven to be particularly useful for predicting biologic behavior (Meissner and Warren 1969).

References

Axelrad AA, Leblond CP (1955) Induction of thyroid tumors in rats by a low iodine diet. Cancer 8:339–367

Bielschowsky F (1955) Neoplasia and internal environment. Br J Cancer 9:80–116

Burek JD (1978) Pathology of aging rats. CRC, Boca Raton

Christov K (1981) Ultrastructure of thyroid tumors. I. Follicular adenomas and carcinomas in rats and hamsters. Pathol Res Pract 173:30–44

deRuiter J, Hollander CF, Boorman GA, Hennemann G, Docter R, van Putten LM (1976) Comparison of carcinogenicity of ^{131}I and ^{125}I in thyroid gland of the rat. In: Biological and environmental effects of low-level radiation: proceedings of a symposium on biological effects of low-level radiation pertinent to the protection of man and his enviroment. International Atomic Energy Agency, Vienna, pp 21–33

Doniach I (1957) Comparison of the carcinogenic effect of xirradiation with radioactive iodine on rat's thyroid. Br J Cancer 11:67–76

Goodman DG, Ward JM, Squire RA, Chu KC, Linhart MS (1979) Neoplastic and nonneoplastic lesions in aging F344 rats. Toxicol Appl Pharmacol 48:237–248

Goodman DG, Ward JM, Squire RA, Paxton MB, Reichardt WD, Chu KC, Linhart MS (1980) Neoplastic and nonneoplastic lesions in aging Osborne-Mendel rats. Toxicol Appl Pharmacol 55:433–447

Gopinath C, Prentice DE, Lewis DJ (1987) Atlas of experimental toxicological pathology. MTP, Lancaster

Hardisty JF, Boorman GA (1990) Thyroid gland. In: Boorman GA, Eustis SL, Elwell MR, Montgomery CAJ, MacKenzie WF (eds) Pathology of the Fischer rat. Academic, San Diego, pp 519–536

Haseman JK (1992) Value of historical controls in the interpretation of rodent tumor data. Drug Inform J 26:191–200

Haseman JK, Arnold J, Eustis SL (1990) Tumor incidences in Fischer 344 rats: NTP historical data. In: Boorman GA, Eustis SL, Elwell MR, Montgomery CAJ, MacKenzie WF (eds) Pathology of the Fischer rat. Academic, San Diego, pp 555–564

Hayden DW, Wade GG, Handler AH (1978) The goitrogenic effect of 4,4′-oxydianiline in rats and mice. Vet Pathol 15:649–662

Hill RN, Erdreich LS, Paynter OE, Roberts PA, Rosenthal SL, Wilkinson CF (1989) Review. Thyroid follicular cell carcinogenesis. Fund Appl Toxicol 12:629–697

Kanno J, Onodera H, Furuta K, Maekawa A, Kasuga T, Hayashi Y (1992) Tumor-promoting effects of both iodine deficiency and iodine excess in the rat thyroid. Toxicol Pathol 20:226–235

Kroes R, Garbis-Berkvens JM, deVries T, van Nesselrooy HJ (1981) Histopathological profile of a Wistar rat stock including a survey of the literature. J Gerontol 36:259–279

MacKenzie WF, Garner FM (1973) Comparison of neoplasms in six sources of rats. J Natl Cancer Inst 50:1243–1257

Meissner WA, Warren S (1969) Tumors of the thyroid gland. In: Armed Forces Institute of Pathology (ed) Atlas of tumor pathology, 2nd edn. Armed Forces Institute of Pathology, Bethesda, p 135

Murthy AS (1980) Morphology of the neoplasms of the thyroid gland in Fischer 344 rats treated with 4,4′-methylene-bis-(N, N-dimethyl)-benzenamine. Toxicol Lett 6:391–397

Napalkov NP (1990) Tumours of the thyroid gland. In: Turusov VS, Mohr U (eds) Pathology of tumours in laboratory animals. International Agency for Research on Cancer, Lyon, pp 539–572

Todd GC (1986) Induction and reversibility of thyroid proliferative changes in rats given an antithyroid compound. Vet Pathol 23:110–117

Ward JM, Stinson SF, Hardisty JF, Cockrell BY, Hayden DW (1979) Neoplasms and pigmentation of thyroid glands in F344 rats exposed to 2,4-diaminoanisole sulfate, a hair dye component. J Natl Cancer Inst 62:1067–1074

Adenoma and Carcinoma, Thyroid Follicular Cell, Mouse

James E. Heath

Synonyms. Thyroid adenoma, thyroid carcinoma, thyroid adenocarcinoma.

Gross Appearance

Thyroid follicular cell adenomas are usually not visible grossly although they occasionally occur as a mildly enlarged thyroid gland or a flesh-colored to brownish nodule up to 3–4 mm in diameter. Follicular cell carcinomas may be undetectable at necropsy, but they often appear as tan to dark brown spherical or lobulated nodules up to 10 mm or more in diameter. They are most often unilateral, and the larger tumors may displace or encompass the trachea, larynx or esophagus.

Microscopic Features

Follicular cell adenomas usually occur as a single, well-circumscribed proliferation of follicular cells which form atypical follicles or papillary structures (Figs. 278–281). Individual cells are cuboidal to columnar in shape. They may be normal in size but are usually slightly enlarged and are often hyperchromatic. Mitotic activity is usually low. The cellular arrangement may vary from solid areas of closely packed cells to follicular or papillary formations and cystic structures filled with colloid. The papillary formations consist of a single layer of cells relative to the basement membrane. Any of the cellular arrangements may predominate in such a way that the tumor can be classified as solid, follicular or papillary. Some adenomas, however, contain varying combinations of two or all three cellular configurations which may make classification using these criteria difficult. The adjacent nonneoplastic follicles are often compressed, and although the larger adenomas may protrude beyond the normal contours of the thyroid, there is no evidence of infiltration or extension beyond the gland.

Follicular cell carcinomas vary considerably in their appearance. They often consist of follicular or glandular structures composed of pleomorphic cells with a high nuclear to cytoplasmic ratio. The cells frequently coalesce to form cords several cell

▶

Fig. 278. *(upper left)* Thyroid gland: follicular cell adenoma, mouse, with a combination of papillary and follicular structures. Note the typical, well-circumscribed growth pattern. H&E, ×63

Fig. 279. *(lower left)* Follicular cell adenoma, thyroid, mouse, with papillary morphology. H&E, ×100

Fig. 280. *(upper right)* Higher magnification of Fig. 279. Note papillary structures composed of a single layer of columnar cells. H&E, ×250

Fig. 281. *(lower right)* Follicular cell adenoma, thyroid, mouse, with solid to follicular architecture compressing nonneoplastic thyroid follicles. H&E, ×100

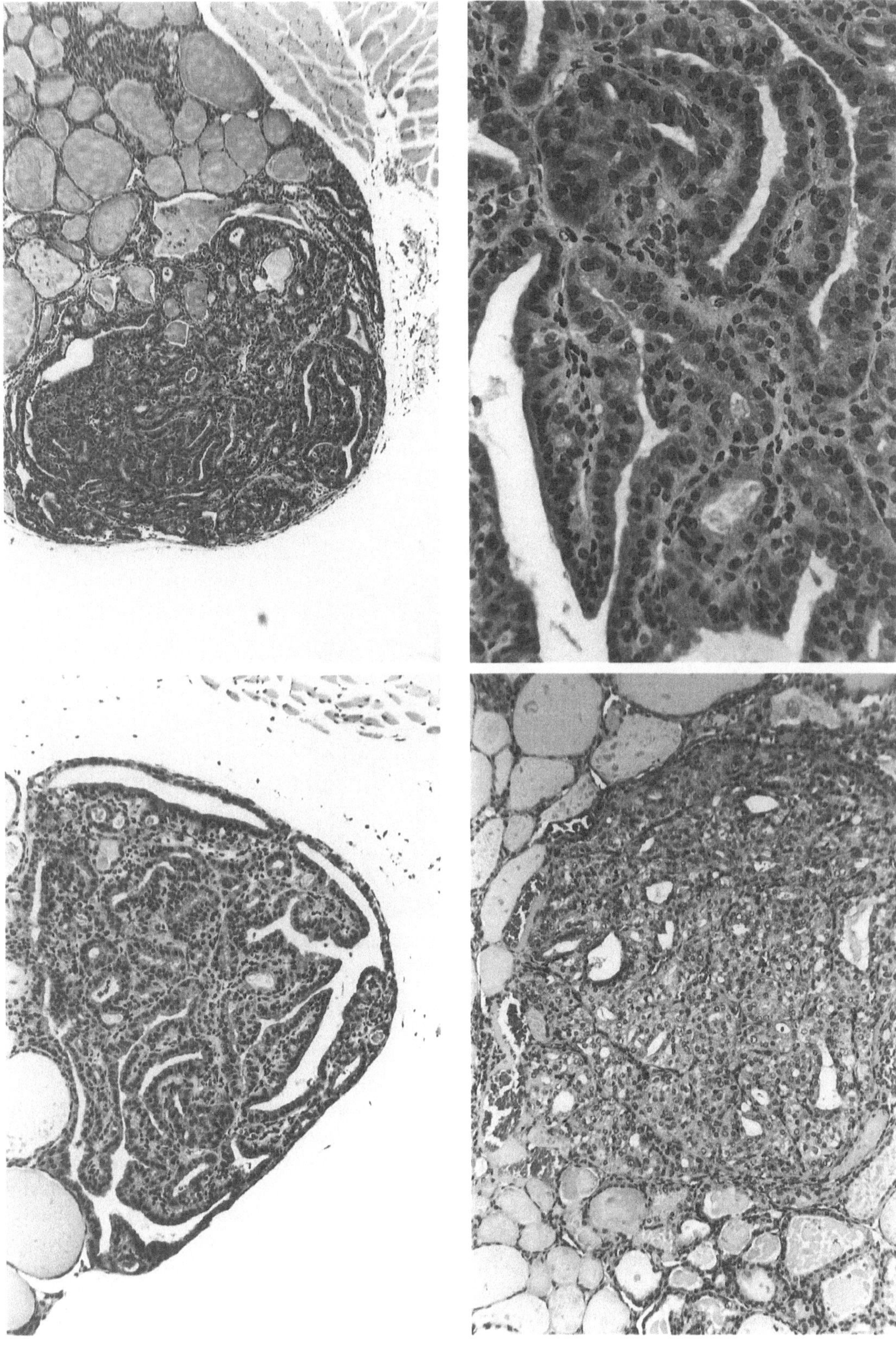

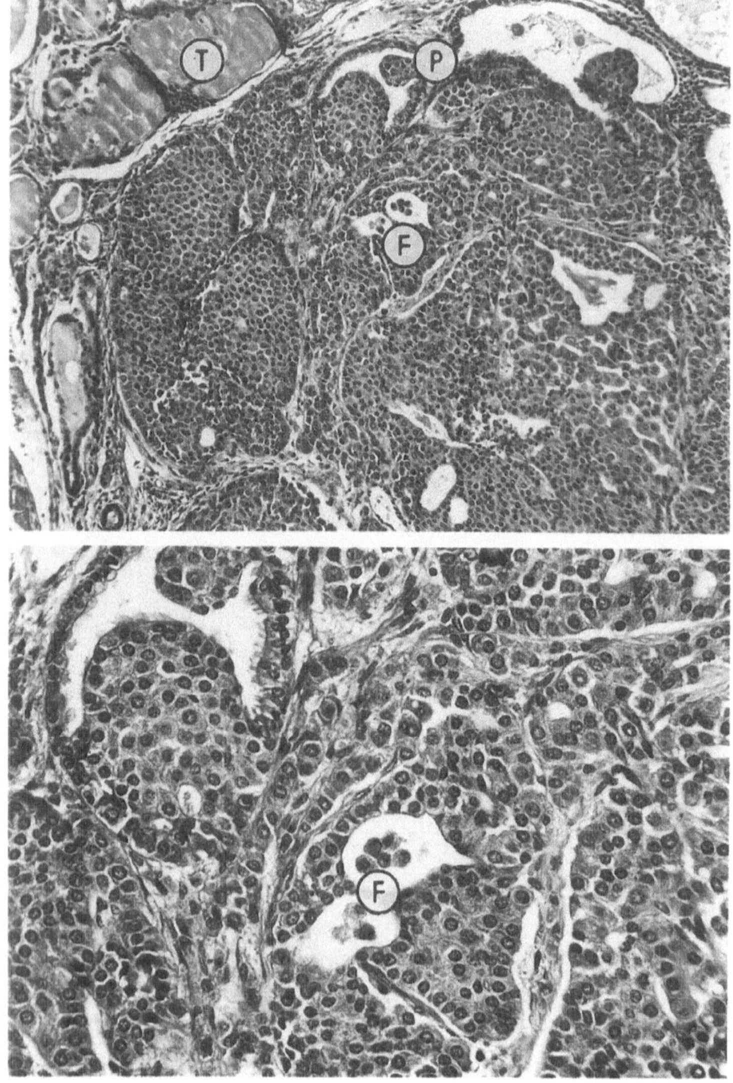

Fig. 282. (*above*) Follicular cell carcinoma, thyroid, mouse, wtih papillary (*P*) and follicular (*F*) structures encroaching on nonneoplastic thyroid (*T*). H&E, ×100

Fig. 283. (*below*) Higher magnification of Fig. 282, with cords of neoplastic cells and follicular structures (*F*). H&E, ×250

layers thick with no intervening basement membrane, and cystic spaces filled with colloid are less common than is seen in adenomas. The cellular architecture can range from follicular or papillary structures and cysts to solid sheets of relatively monomorphic cells (Figs. 282, 283). The number of mitotic figures varies but is often high. The more anaplastic carcinomas may have a mesenchymal pattern composed of fusiform cells with or without a scirrhous response. Residual follicles occurring singularly or in groups may be seen among the neoplastic components and occasionally tumor cells are observed in direct continuity with these isolated follicles (Fig. 284). Frequently no remaining nonneoplastic thyroid gland is visible, and invasion of adjacent tissues such as trachea, esophagus, and salivary gland may occur. Metastasis occurs occasionally and most often involves the regional lymph nodes.

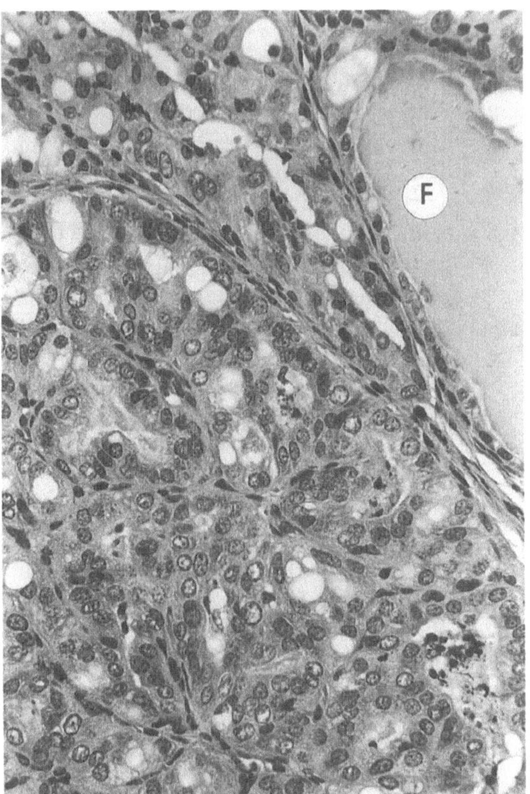

Fig. 284. Follicular cell carcinoma, thyroid, mouse, with cellular pleomorphism and a nonneoplastic follicle (*F*). H&E, ×250

Ultrastructure

Ultrastructural studies of mouse thyroid follicular cell neoplasms are limited. Transmission electron microscopy was performed on follicular cell adenocarcinomas from transgenic mice (Ledent et al. 1991). The classical follicular structure was absent, and follicular cells had lost their normal abundant rough endoplasmic reticulum although free ribosomes were abundant. The tumor cells could still be recognized as epithelial; cell polarity was evident, and microfollicles containing microvilli were discernible between the densely packed neoplastic cells.

Differential Diagnosis

Follicular cell adenomas must be distinguished from follicular cysts, follicular cell hyperplasia, colloid goiter, parathyroid gland adenomas, C cell tumors, and follicular cell carcinomas. Follicular cysts usually consist of cystic spaces that exceed the size of the larger follicles normally found at the gland periphery. They are filled with eosinophilic colloid material and are bounded by low cuboidal or flattened follicular cells. The cysts occasionally have multilocular patterns and could be confused with cystic adenomas. They are distinguished from adenomas by the absence of increased cell size, hyperchromasia, and well-developed papillary formations.

Follicular cell hyperplasia, either focal or diffuse, is relatively common in some strains of old mice and frequently occurs in conjunction with follicular cysts. Follicular cell hyperplasias are less circumscribed than adenomas and merge imperceptibly with the normal follicles rather than causing compression, as do adenomas. The increase in cell numbers in the hyperplastic areas may result in contortions and infoldings of the follicular epithelium, but the overt papillary formations seen with adenomas are not present. It is believed that focal follicular cell hyperplasia can progress to adenoma and the distinction between the two may be vague.

Colloid goiter, which is seen occasionally in experimental mice administered iodinated compounds, consists of universally enlarged, spherical follicles distended with colloid and bordered by flattened epithelium.

Parathyroid gland adenomas, which are extremely rare in mice, usually can be seen emanating from the affected parathyroid gland and are composed of small basophilic cells similar to the chief cells that comprise the parathyroid gland.

Follicular cell carcinomas must be differentiated from follicular cell adenomas, diffuse hyperplastic goiter, and C cell tumors. Features that distinguish follicular cell adenoma from follicular cell carcinoma were described in a previous section. Diffuse hyperplastic goiter is observed in animals administered goitrogenic agents or in animals with dietary imbalances (either excess or deficiency) of iodine (Capen and Martin 1989). The change is manifested by marked hyperplasia and hypertrophy of follicular cells, often with formation of papillary projections, which may mimic neoplasia. In contrast to follicular cell carcinoma, hyperplastic goiter is usually bilaterally symmetrical and lacks the anaplastic cellular features and invasive nature of carcinomas. Thyroid gland C cell neoplasms (parafollicular cell tumor, medullary carcinoma) have been reported in mice but are rare (Van Zwieten et al. 1983). These tumors consist of large solid nests of polyhedral or slightly fusiform cells that are separated by delicate connective tissue septa (Figs. 285, 286). Diagnosis can be aided with the use of electron microscopy or immunocytochemistry to demonstrate the cytoplasmic secretory granules of C cells (Fig. 287).

Biologic Features

Natural History and Pathogenesis. Follicular cell carcinoma in mice represents a series of cellular responses which are first recognizable microscopically as focal follicular cell hyperplasia. Foci of hyperplasia may evolve to adenomas and adenomas may progress to carcinomas. This concept is supported by the occasional occurrence of follicular cell neoplasms that appear ostensibly as adenomas, but which may contain focal areas of apparent carcinomatous transformation. Spontaneous follicular cell neoplasms occur most often in old mice. In a recent evaluation involving 400 untreated $B6C3F_1$ mice (200 male, 200 female) at Southern Research Institute, follicular cell tumors were observed in 25 animals (12 male, 13 female). Of these 25 the tumors in all except three mice were seen at the terminal killing (approximately 105 weeks), and the mean period of time on study for the remaining three animals with tumors was 99 weeks.

Etiology. Follicular cell neoplasms have been induced in mice by administration of several agents including sulfonamides (Littlefield et al. 1989), estrogen (Greenman et al. 1990), dyestuffs (Ito et al. 1986), and cancer chemotherapeutic agents (Weisburger et al. 1975), as well chemicals used in the manufacture of such materials as epoxy resins, flame retardants, plasticizers, and polyurethane foams (Bucher et al. 1987; Lamb et al. 1986; Weisburger et al. 1984). The feeding of goitrogenic agents such as methyl thiouracil has been shown to promote thyroid tumors in mice fed iodine-deficient diets (Jemec 1977). This finding correlates with the increased frequency of thyroid follicular cell neoplasia arising from hyperplastic goiter, which has been historically observed in human beings and animals living in iodine-deficient areas (Meissner and Warren 1969). Dietary deficiency of iodine has been shown to promote the thyroid follicular cell carcinogenicity of *N*-methyl-*N*-nitrosourea in rats (Ohshima and Ward 1984).

Frequency. Spontaneous thyroid follicular cell tumors in mice occur rarely (Table 20). Data from studies for which the incidence of tumors in both sexes is available indicate the frequency to be slightly greater for females than for males in most strains of mice. Thyroid tumors in mice are much more likely to be benign than malignant; of 83 follicular cell neoplasms observed in 5204 untreated mice from nine strains at the National Center for Toxicological Research only seven were considered to be carcinomas (Heath and Frith 1983). Because of the relative infrequency of spontaneous follicular cell tumors in mice this species is considered a good model for use in thyroid gland carcinogenicity assays.

Comparison with Other Species

As in mice, the incidence of spontaneous thyroid follicular cell tumors in rats is low. However, the incidence of carcinomas relative to adenomas is considered higher for rats than for mice, the

Table 20. Incidence of spontaneous thyroid cell neoplasms in various mouse strains

Strain	Sex	Experimental Period (Weeks)	Incidence (%)		Reference
			Adenoma	Carcinoma	
CD-1	Male	0–104	8/891 (0.9)	0/891 (0.0)	Maita et al. 1988
	Female	0–104	6/890 (0.7)	0/890 (0.0)	
$B6C3F_1$	Male	0–110	16/2543 (0.6)	7/2543 (0.3)	Ward et al. 1979
	Female	0–110	30/2522 (1.2)	6/2522 (0.2)	
C57BL/6	Male	>30	2/294 (0.7)	0/294 (0.0)	Frith and Heath 1984
	Female	>30	16/369 (4.3)	0/369 (0.0)	
BALB/c	Male	>30	0/431 (0.0)	0/431 (0.0)	Frith and Heath 1984
	Female	>30	3/2226 (0.1)	0/2226 (0.0)	

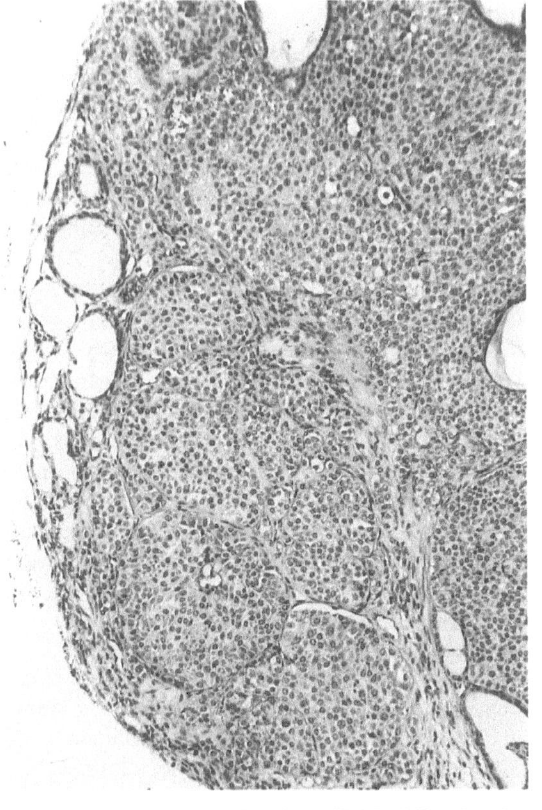

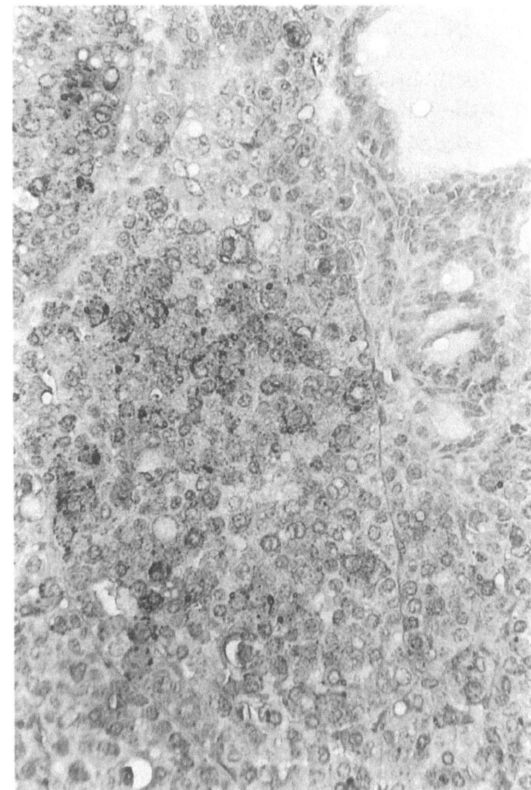

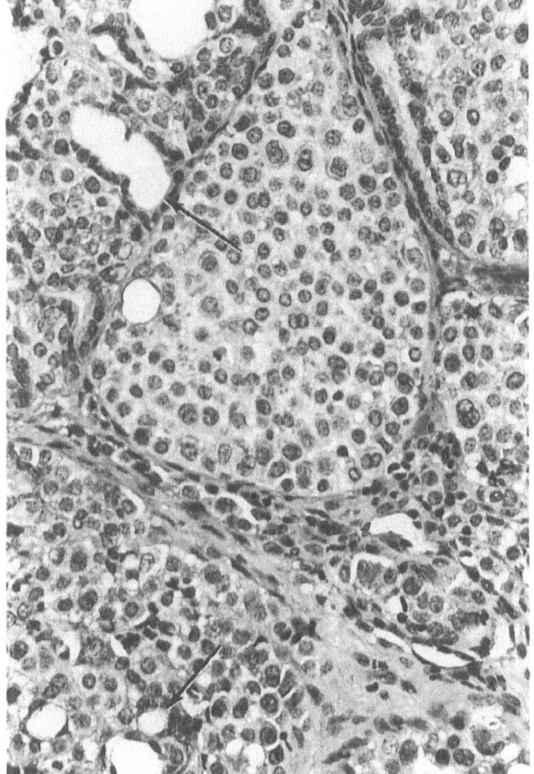

Fig. 285. (*upper left*) Thyroid gland, mouse. C-cell tumor with thick cords and masses of pale staining cells encroaching on thyroid follicles. H&E, ×100 (Specimen provided by Dr. Winslow Sheldon, National Center for Toxicological Research, Jefferson, Arkansas)

Fig. 286. (*lower left*) Higher magnification of Fig. 285, with solid nests of monomorphic C-cells with pale staining cytoplasm encompassing thyroid follicles (*arrows*). H&E, ×250

Fig. 287. (*upper right*) Tumor in Figs. 285 and 286, with positive staining for calcitonin. Immunoperoxidase, ×250

ratio for Fischer 344 rats being approximately 60% adenomas to 40% carcinomas (Haseman et al. 1990). In contrast to mice, in which virtually all neoplasms involve the follicular epithelium, thyroid gland tumors in rats much more commonly arise from the parafollicular cells (C cells). Thyroid gland tumors are relatively rare in hamsters. Thirty-eight thyroid tumors, six of which were considered malignant, were observed in an evaluation of 1500 Syrian hamsters, an incidence of 2.5% (Kirkman and Algard 1968). Thyroid neoplasms are very rare in rabbits and guinea pigs (Weisbroth 1974; Blumenthal and Rogers 1965). In the domestic animals thyroid follicular cell tumors occur most frequently in older dogs and cats, are relatively common in horses, and are rarely reported in cattle, sheep, and swine (Capen 1993). The reported low incidence in the latter three species may be attributed at least in part to the generally early age at slaughter seen with these animals. In dogs follicular cell carcinomas, which are often poorly differentiated, occur more frequently than do adenomas while the reverse is true for cats (Brodey 1970; Leav et al. 1976). Malignant mixed thyroid gland tumors, which contain a mixture of malignant thyroid follicular cells and mesenchymal elements, have been reported in dogs (Johnson and Patterson 1981; Buergelt 1968). A syndrome characterized clinically by signs of hyperthyroidism and morphologically by multinodular goiter, adenoma, and occasionally carcinoma of follicular cells has been reported in older cats (Jones and Johnstone 1981; O'Brien et al. 1980). Reported cases of follicular cell tumors in nonhuman primates are limited; one was an adenocarcinoma from an adult marmoset (Williamson and Hunt 1970), and two other reports involved adenomas from baboons (Fox 1936; Weber and Greet 1973).

In humans proliferative lesions of the thyroid gland include nodular hyperplasia, adenoma, and carcinoma of the follicular cells, and clearcut distinctions are often difficult to determine. Follicular cell carcinomas in man are classified as papillary, follicular, and undifferentiated (anaplastic) types (Franssila 1985). About 95% of all thyroid neoplasms in man derive from the follicular epithelium, with the remaining 5% arising from the parafollicular cells (C cells). Epidemiological studies indicate an incidence rate of approximately two or three cases of thyroid carcinoma per 100 000 in the general population (Meissner and Warren 1969). The tumors are more common in older individuals and occur two to three times more frequently in women than in men. Most follicular cell cancers are considered spontaneous although cases resulting from radiation therapy have occurred (Noltenius 1988). Unlike the malignant tumors of mice, which are believed to evolve from adenomas, most follicular cell carcinomas in man are believed to arise de novo from nonproliferating epithelium (Meissner and Warren 1969). Another species difference is that of the papillary type carcinomas seen in human beings; occurrence in children and young adults is relatively high (Franssila 1985) whereas follicular cell carcinomas in young mice have not been reported. Of interest is the reported increase in frequency of thyroid neoplasms, most often "papillary carcinomas," among children under 15 years of age, living in the Republic of Belarus at the time of the nuclear accident in 1986 at the Chernobyl Atomic Power Station, in what was then the Soviet Union (Furmanchuk et al. 1992)

Acknowledgement. The author wishes to thank Dr. Thomas S. Winokur, University of Alabama at Birmingham, Birmingham, Alabama, for immunocytochemical staining procedures.

References

Blumenthal HT, Rogers JB (1965) Spontaneous and induced tumors in the guinea pig. In: Ribelin WE, McCoy JR (eds) The pathology of laboratory animals. Thomas, Springfield, pp 183–209

Brodey RS (1970) Canine and feline neoplasia. Adv Vet Sci Com Med 14:309–354

Bucher JR, Alison RH, Montgomery CA, Huff J, Haseman JK et al (1987) Comparative toxicity and carcinogenicity of two chlorinated paraffins in F344/N rats and B6C3F$_1$ mice. Fundam Appl Toxicol 9:454–468

Buergelt CD (1968) Mixed thyroid tumors in two dogs. J Am Vet Med Assoc 152:1658–1663

Capen CC (1993) The endocrine glands. In: Jubb KV, Kennedy PC, Palmer N (eds) Pathology of domestic animals, vol III. Academic, San Diego, pp 267–347

Capen CC, Martin SL (1989) The effects of xenobiotics on the structure and function of thyroid follicular and C-cells. Toxicol Pathol 17:266–293

Fox, H (1936) Mortality and matters of pathologic interest. Penrose Research Laboratory, Philadelphia, pp 14–19

Franssila KO (1985) Thyroid gland. In: Kissane JM, Anderson WA (eds) Anderson's pathology. Mosby, St Louis, pp 1399–1419

Frith CH, Heath JE (1984) Morphological classification and incidence of thyroid tumors in untreated aged mice. J Gerontol 39(1):7–10

Furmanchuk AW, Averkin JI, Egloff B, Ruchti et al. (1992) Pathomorphological findings in thyroid cancer of children from the Republic of Belarus: a study of 86 cases occurring between 1986 ("post-Chernobyl") and 1991. Histopathology 21(5):401-408

Greenman DL, Highman B, Chen J, Sheldon W, Gass G (1990) Estrogen-induced thyroid follicular cell adenomas in C57BL/6 mice. J Toxicol Environ Health 29(3):269-278

Haseman JK, Arnold J, Eustis SL (1990) Tumor incidences in Fischer 344 rats: NTP historical data. In: Boorman GA, Eustis EL, Elwell MR, Montgomery CA, McKenzie WF (eds) Pathology of the Fischer rat: reference and atlas. Academic, San Diego, pp 555-564

Heath JE, Frith CH (1983) Carcinoma, thyroid mouse. In: Jones TC, Mohr U, Hunt RD (eds) Monographs on pathology of laboratory animals - endocrine system. Springer, Berlin Heidelberg New York, pp 188-191

Ito A, Watanabe H, Naito M, Aoyama H, Nakagawa Y et al (1986) Induction of thyroid tumors in (C57BL/6N × C3H/N)F_1 mice by oral administration of 9-3', 4', 5', 6'-tetrachloro-o-carboxy phenyl6-hydroxy-2,4,5,7-tetraiodo-3-isoxanthone sodium (Food Red 105, Rose Bengal B). J Natl Cancer Inst 77(1):277-281

Jemec B (1977) Studies of the tumorigenic effect of two goitrogens. Cancer 40:2188-2202

Johnson JA, Patterson JM (1981) Multifocal myxedema and mixed thyroid neoplasm in a dog. Vet Pathol 18:13-20

Jones BR, Johnstone AC (1981) Hyperthyroidism in an aged cat. NZ Vet J 29:70-72

Kirkman H, Algard FT (1968) Spontaneous and nonviral-induced neoplasms. In: Hoffman RA, Robinson PF, Magalhaes H (eds) The golden hamster: its biology and use in medical research. Iowa State University Press, Ames, pp 227-240

Lamb JC, Huff JE, Haseman JK, Murthy AS, Lilja H (1986) Carcinogenesis studies of 4',4-methylenedianiline dihydrochloride given in drinking water to F344/N rats and B6C3FI mice. J Toxicol Environ Health 18(3):325-337

Leav I, Schiller AL, Rijnberk A, Legg MA, der Kinderen PJ (1976) Adenomas and carcinomas of the canine and feline thyroid. Am J Pathol 83:61-122

Ledent C, Dumont J, Vassart G, Parmentier M (1991) Thyroid adenocarcinomas secondary to tissue-specific expression of simian virus-40 large T-antigen in transgenic mice. Endocrinology 129(3):1391-1401

Littlefield NA, Gaylor DW, Blackwell BN, Allen RR (1989) Chronic toxicity/carcinogenicity studies of sulfamethazine in B6C3F_1 mice. Food Chem Toxicol 27(7):455-463

Maita K, Hirano M, Harada T, Mitsumori K, Yoshida A, et al. (1988) Mortality, major cause of moribundity and spontaneous tumors in CD-1 mice. Toxicol Pathol 16(3):340-349

Meissner WA, Warren S (1969) Tumors of the thyroid gland. In: Armed Forces Institute of Pathology (ed) Atlas of tumor pathology. Armed Forces Institute of Pathology, Washington, pp 55-70

Noltenius H (1988) Tumors of the thyroid and parathyroid gland. In: Noltenius H (ed) Human oncology. Pathology and clinical characteristics, vol II. Urban and Schwarzenburg, Baltimore, pp 599-638

O'Brien SE, Riley JH, Hagemoser WA (1980) Unilateral thyroid neoplasm in a cat. Vet Rec 107:199-200

Ohshima M, Ward JM (1984) Promotion of N-methyl-N-nitrosourea-induced thyroid tumors by iodine deficiency in F344/NCr rats. J Natl Cancer Inst 73:289-296

Van Zwieten MJ, Frith CH, Nooteboom AL, Wolfe HJ, DeLellis RA (1983) Medullary thyroid carcinoma in female BALB/c mice. Am J Pathol 110:219-229

Ward JM, Goodman DG, Squire RA, Chu KC, Linhart MS (1979) Neoplastic and nonneoplastic lesions in aging (C57BL/6N × C3H/HeN)F_1 (B6C3F_1) mice. J Natl Cancer Inst 63:849-854

Weber HW, Greet MJ (1973) Observations on spontaneous pathological lesions in chacma baboons (*Papio ursinus*). Am J Phys Anthropol 38:407-413

Weisbroth SH (1974) Neoplastic diseases. In: Weisbroth SH, Flatt RE, Kraus AL (eds) The biology of the laboratory rabbit. Academic, New York, pp 331-375

Weisburger EK, Griswold DP, Prejean JD, Casey AE, Wood HB (1975) The carcinogenic properties of some of the principal drugs used in clinical cancer chemotherapy. In: Rentchnick P, Herfarth C, Senn HJ (eds) Recent results in cancer research, vol 52. Springer, Berlin Heidelberg New York, pp 1-17

Weisburger EK, Murthy AS, Lilja HS, Lamb JC (1984) Neoplastic response of F344 rats and B6C3F_1 mice to the polymer and dyestuff intermediates 4,4'-methylenebis(N,N-dimethyl)-benzenamine, 4,4'-oxydianiline, and 4,4'-methylenedianiline. J Natl Cancer Inst 72(6):1457-1463

Williamson ME, Hunt RD (1970) Adenocarcinoma of the thyroid in a marmoset (*Sanguinus nigricollis*). Lab Anim Care 20:1139-1141

C-Cell Hyperplasia, C-Cell Adenoma, and C-Cell Carcinoma*, Thyroid, Rat

Gary A. Boorman, Ronald A. DeLellis, and Michael R. Elwell

Synonyms. C-cell hyperplasia: parafollicular cell hyperplasia; light cell hyperplasia; clear cell hyperplasia.
C-Cell Adenoma: parafollicular cell adenoma; light cell adenoma; clear cell adenoma; nodular hyperplasia of C cells; early C-cell carcinoma; carcinoma in situ.
C-Cell Carcinoma: medullary carcinoma; parafollicular cell carcinoma; light cell carcinoma; clear cell carcinoma.

Gross Appearance

C-cell hyperplasia and adenoma are usually not visible grossly. C-cell carcinoma may appear as a unilateral or bilateral nodule or irregularly shaped enlargement of the thyroid. When incised, C-cell carcinoma is a moderately firm, uniform, white to tan mass that contrasts sharply with the red-brown color of the normal thyroid parenchyma.

Microscopic Appearance

The C cells are named for their main secretory product, calcitonin, and are located within the thyroid follicles, principally at the base of the follicular cells. In young rats (12 months old), especially of the Long-Evans strain, the C cells are more numerous in the center of the lateral lobes of the thyroid, each follicle containing four to eight C cells. These cells are readily identified by the immunoperoxidase method for calcitonin (Figs. 288, 289). In addition to calcitonin, C cells may also contain somatostatin (O'Briain et al. 1979), neurotensin (Bidard et al. 1993), neuromedin (Bidard et al. 1993), and calcitonin gene-related peptide (CGRP; Denijn et al. 1992; Haller-Brem et al. 1987).
Hyperplasia of C cells is a common change in many strains of older rats and may be either a diffuse or focal lesion. Some degree of diffuse hyperplasia is generally present in aging rats in addition to an increasing incidence of focal C-cell hyperplasia. For example, between 12 and 24 months of age rats of the Long-Evans strain develop a diffuse, uniform increase in the number of C cells between the basement membrane and the follicular epithelium of the thyroid follicles (Figs. 290, 291). In diffuse hyperplasia many of the follicles have one or two layers of C cells peripheral to the follicular epithelium (Fig. 292). These hyperplastic cells have a pale-staining cytoplasm and indistinct cell boundaries. The cells have a uniformly round to slightly oval nucleus

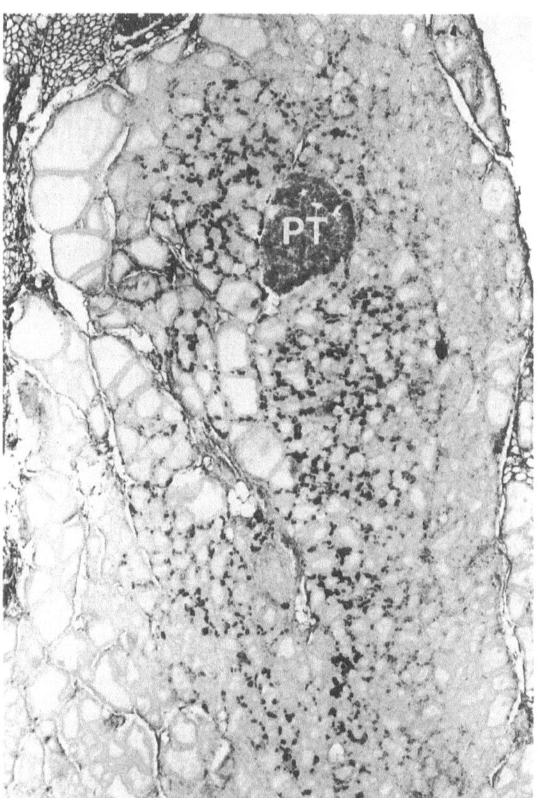

Fig. 288. C cells in the central portion of lateral lobe of the thyroid of a young rat. The parathyroid is nonspecifically stained (*PT*). Immunoperoxidase method for calcitonin, ×100. (DeLellis et al. 1979)

* World Health Organization, International Classification of Rodent Tumors (Mohr 1994).

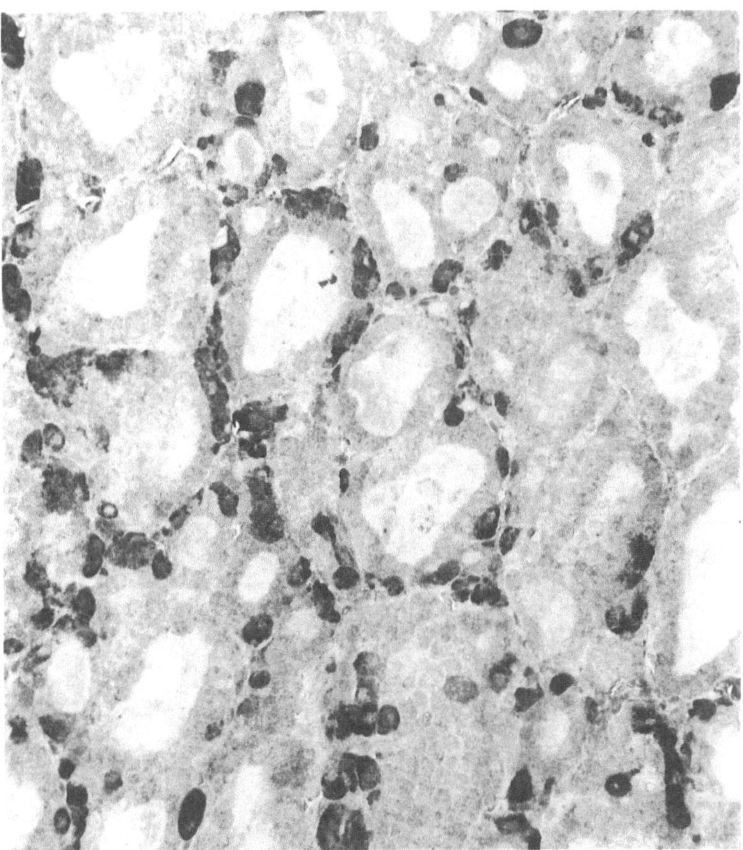

Fig. 289. Higher magnification of Fig. 288, showing the calcitonin-bearing C cells within the thyroid follicles, predominately at the base of the follicular cells. Immunoperoxidase method for calcitonin, ×250. (DeLellis et al. 1979)

with a finely stippled chromatin pattern. With continued proliferation of C cells there may be compression of thyroid follicles resulting in a small lumen lined by flattened follicular cell epithelium (Fig. 293). As this lesion progresses, follicles may become filled with C cells (Fig. 294). While diffuse C-cell hyperplasia is easily recognized, with progression focal, distinct C-cell lesions may develop which must be distinguished from adenoma.

C-cell adenoma is a common lesion in older rats that varies in incidence in different strains (Table 21). It is characterized by one or multiple small masses of C cells in one or both lobes of the thyroid (Fig. 295). The lesion is usually well-circumscribed and may cause compression of the adjacent parenchyma but rarely has a well-defined capsule. The cytologic features are similar to C-cell hyperplasia although there may be some minimal cellular atypia consisting of enlarged or more fusiform-shaped cells with more intensely staining cytoplasm and hyperchromatic or enlarged nuclei (Fig. 296).

C-cell carcinoma, less common than adenoma also varies considerably in incidence with different strains (Table 21). C-cell carcinoma consists of solid sheets to irregular clusters of tumor cells that fill contiguous follicles. The more solid areas often contain focal areas of hemorrhage. Vascular invasion (Fig. 297), extension into adjacent musculature, or distant metastases are seen in advanced lesions. There is usually evidence of capsular invasion in cases where a fibrous capsule is present. The deep cervical lymph nodes are often the first site of metastases. In some rats metastatic foci occur in the lungs. The cytologic features are usually similar to benign lesions consisting primarily of a uniform population of cells, with round to oval nuclei that have finely stippled chromatin (Fig. 298). In some malignant tumors mitotic figures are common, and there is more pleomorphism including spindle-shaped cells. Amyloid deposits, which are a common feature in human tumors, are rare in the rat but have been reported (Boorman et al. 1972).

Table 21. C cell tumors in rats

Strain	Sex	C-cell adenoma	C-cell carcinoma	Reference
F344	M	68/1794 4%	31/1794 2%	Goodman et al. 1979
F344	F	70/1754 4%	30/1754 2%	Goodman et al. 1979
F344	M	147/1904 8%	73/1904 4%	Haseman et al. 1990
F344	F	156/1938 8%	66/1938 3%	Haseman et al. 1990
Osborne-Mendel	M	18/975 4%	5/975 0.5%	Goodman et al. 1980
Osborne-Mendel	F	32/970 3%	16/970 2%	Goodman et al. 1980
Sprague-Dawley	M/F[a]	15/223 7%	–	MacKenzie and Garner 1973
Holtzman-Sprague-Dawley	W/F	9/200 4%	–	MacKenzie and Garner 1973
Charles River–Sprague-Dawley	M/F	12/466 3%	–	MacKenzie and Garner 1973
Diablo Sprague-Dawley	M/F	8/196 4%	–	MacKenzie and Garner 1973
Oregon	M/F	3/647 0.5%	–	MacKenzie and Garner 1973
WAG/Rij	M	–	41/124 33%[b]	Boorman et al. 1974
WAG/Rij	F	–	47/101 47%	Boorman et al. 1974
BN/BI	M	–	7/74 9%	Burek 1978
	F		6/236 6%	Burek 1978
Long-Evans	M	8/33 25%	7/33 21.5%	DeLellis et al. 1979

[a] Males and females combined (approximately equal numbers). All tumors were classified as light-cell adenomas even though one had distant metastases.

[b] Tumors were classified as carcinomas when more than one contiguous follicle was involved.

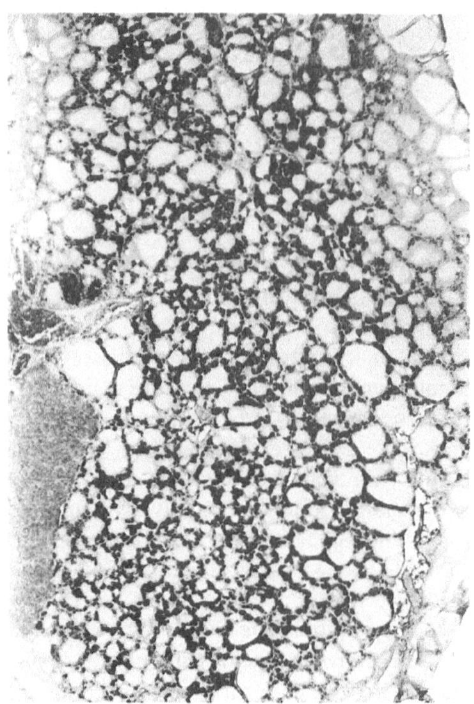

Fig. 290. Hyperplasia of C cells in thyroid of a 24-month-old Long-Evans rat, stained by immunoperoxidase method for calcitonin. Increase in numbers of C cells throughout the gland. ×100. (DeLellis et al. 1979)

Ultrastructure

The C cells are located at the base of the follicular cells within the basal lamina of the thyroid follicle (Fig. 299). The follicular cells are thus interposed between the C cells and the colloid in the lumen of the follicle. The cytoplasm of the C cells contains a variable number of membrane-bound secretory granules. While C cells in the storage phase of the secretory cycle contain large numbers of granules, cells in the early synthetic phase are sparsely granulated (Fig. 299; DeLellis et al. 1977; Ekholm and Ericson 1968) Calcitonin-containing secretory granules are of two morphologic types, although each contains immunoreactive calcitonin. Type I granules have a mean diameter of 190 nm and are characterized by moderately electron-dense, finely granular contents which are close to the limiting membrane. Type II granules have a mean diameter of 125 nm and are characterized by more electron-dense contents which are separated from the limiting membranes by a small but distinct electron-lucent space (DeLellis 1994; DeLellis et al. 1979). While the diagnosis of hyperplasia, adenoma, or carcinoma is based upon the morphologic features evident by light microscopy, the characteristic features of C cells can be identified ultrastructurally in adenoma (Fig. 300) or carcinoma. In one C-cell carcinoma extracellular fibrils with a periodicity characteristic of

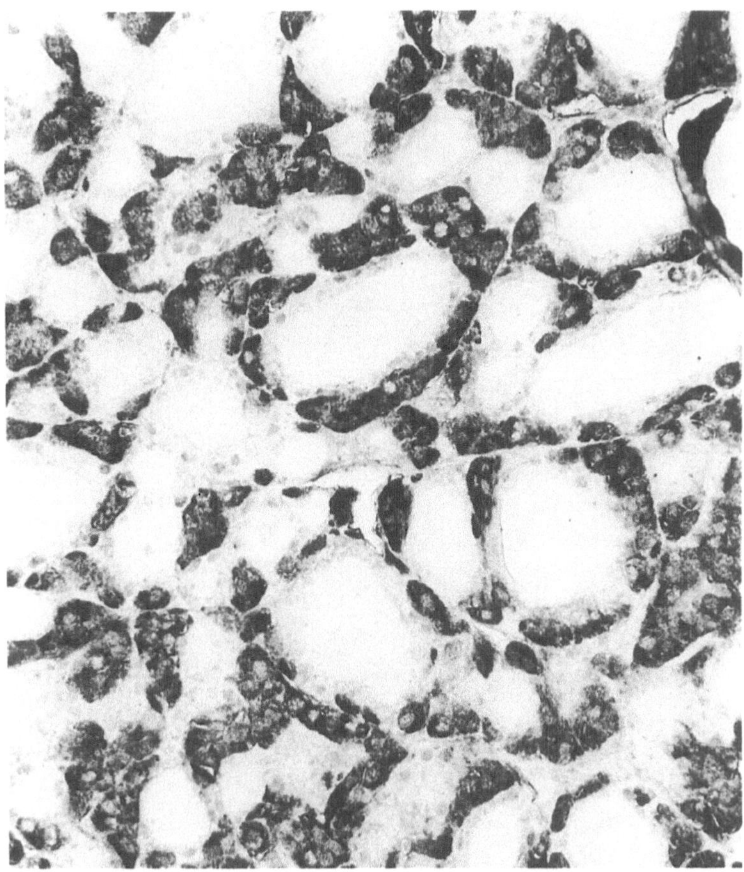

Fig. 291. Higher magnification of Fig. 290, showing C cells at base of follicular cells, usually surrounding each follicle. ×250. (DeLellis et al. 1979)

amyloid fibrils (Boorman et al. 1972) were demonstrated (Fig. 301).

Differential Diagnosis

C-cell hyperplasia may be difficult to distinguish from C-cell adenoma or C-cell carcinoma because proliferative lesions of the C cell appear to progress gradually from diffuse hyperplasia and focal hyperplasia to adenoma, and then to obvious carcinoma with distant metastases (Fig. 302). The difficulty in establishing definitive diagnostic criteria is heightened by the lack of cytologic alteration with malignancy.

In diffuse C-cell hyperplasia the cells are increased and diffusely distributed within the thyroid follicles (DeLellis 1994) versus focal C-cell hyperplasia. The hyperplastic C cells in diffuse and focal lesions are not essentially different in appearance from normal C cells (Figs. 289, 291). Diffuse hyperplasia (Fig. 292) is easily distinguished from focal hyperplasia (Fig. 293), as supported by the ultrastructural studies of DeLellis et al. (1977, 1979). Focal hyperplasia may represent early neoplasia. In humans C-cell nodules (similar to the rat lesion shown in Fig. 294) were shown ultrastructurally to represent thyroid follicles that had become completely filled with C cells rather than stromal expansion or intrathyroid metastases, as has been suggested by light microscopic studies (Fig. 295).

The diagnostic criteria for adenoma is defined for consistency within and between studies. We consider a focal nodule of C cells greater in diameter than five contiguous follicles with no invasion of capsule or adjacent structures to be a C-cell adenoma (Hardisty and Boorman 1990). These contiguous follicles (Fig. 295) compress adjacent or surrounding thyroid tissue. There may be atypia

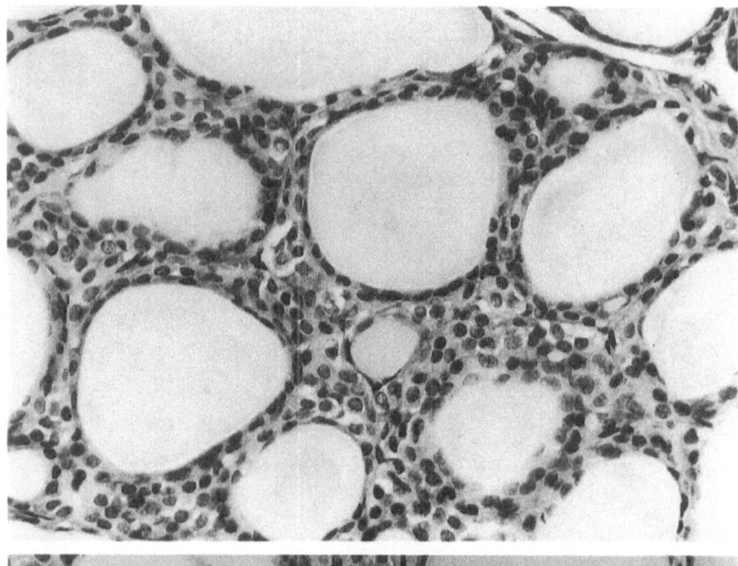

Fig. 292. Diffuse C-cell hyperplasia, thyroid, rat. H&E, ×168

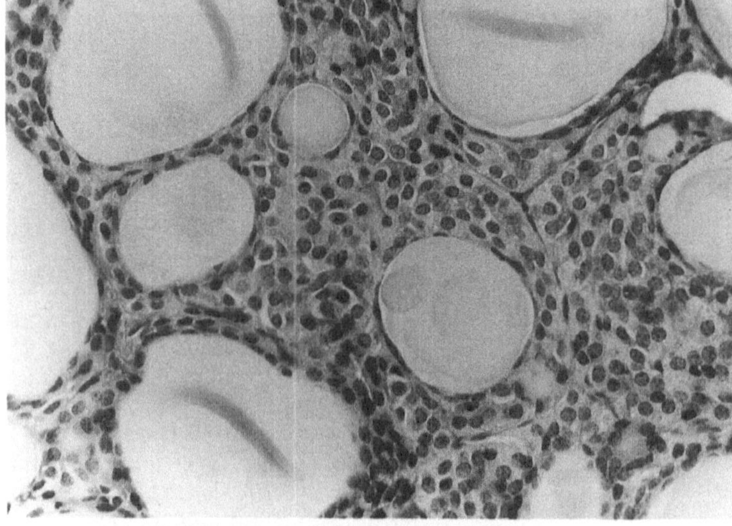

Fig. 293. Focal C-cell hyperplasia, thyroid, rat. C cells with clear cytoplasm are beginning to fill some thyroid follicles, resulting in compression of some follicular epithelial cells. H&E, ×168

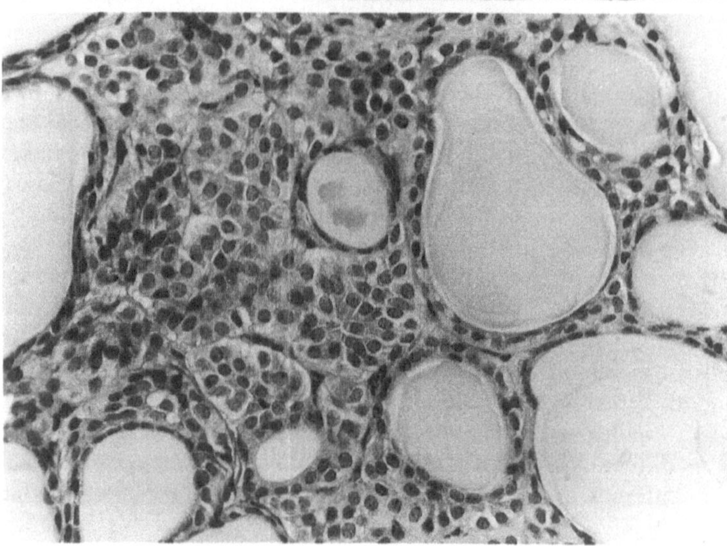

Fig. 294. Focal C-cell hyperplasia. Several thyroid follicles are filled with C cells. H&E, ×168

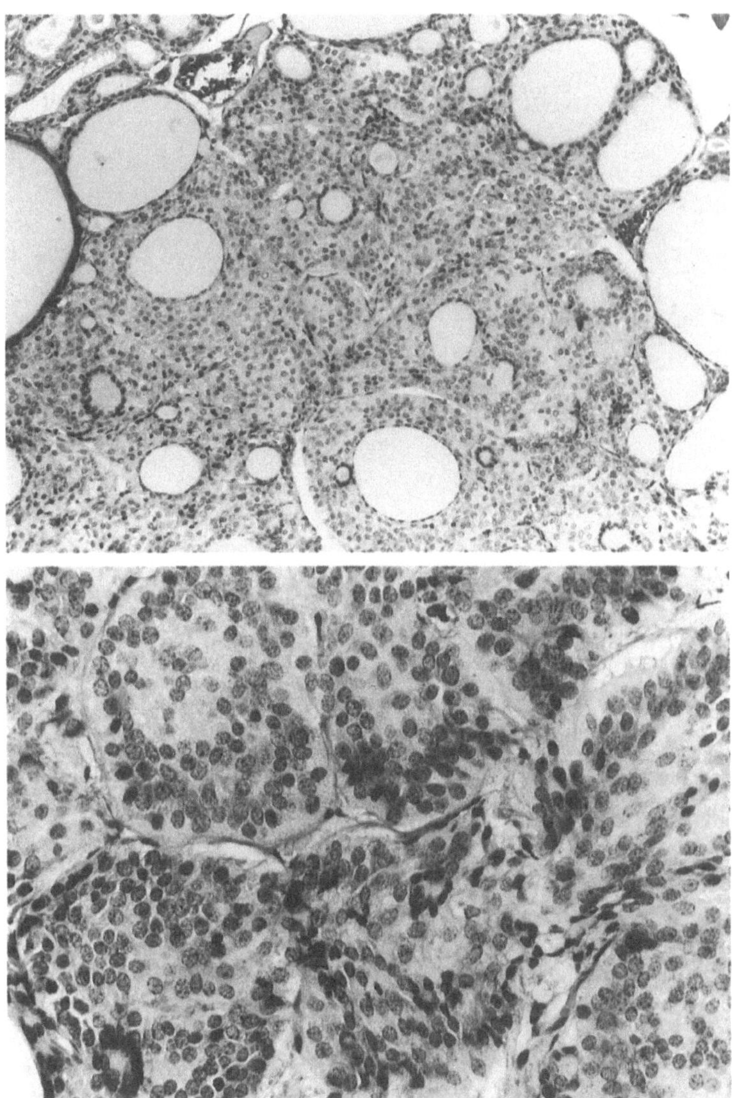

Fig. 295. C-cell thyroid adenoma, rat. A circumscribed collection of C cells found filling contiguous follicles, H&E, ×80

Fig. 296. C-cell thyroid adenoma, rat. Contiguous follicles are filled with uniform C cells. H&E, ×380

of some of the cells in the adenoma. However, even in the metastatic foci of C cells seen in C-cell carcinoma mitotic figures may be rare, and the cellular morphology may be similar to that in hyperplasia. In C-cell carcinoma the lesion often fills almost the entire thyroid lobe or has histologic features of invasion or metastases (Goodman et al. 1979, 1980; Hardisty and Boorman 1990). In early malignancy invasion of the capsule and blood vessels may be seen. Generally, a lesion involving the entire lobe of the thyroid is considered C-cell carcinoma even if invasion cannot be demonstrated. In these advanced cases metastases can frequently be found in the deep cervical lymph nodes (Boorman and Hollander 1976; Boorman et al. 1972; DeLellis 1994). Rarely a smaller lesion showing marked atypia may be also be diagnosed as C-cell carcinoma.

Occasionally a C-cell carcinoma is more pleomorphic and must be distinguished from solid follicular cell carcinoma or oxyphilic follicular cell carcinoma. Cells in solid follicular cell carcinoma have more hyperchromatic cytoplasm, better defined cell boundaries, and more coarse chromatin than cells of the C-cell carcinoma. Oxyphilic follicular cell carcinomas often show some tendency to form small follicles, are uncommon in humans, and have not been reported in the rat. A specific diagnosis of C-cell (medullary) thyroid carcinoma may be made by the demonstration of

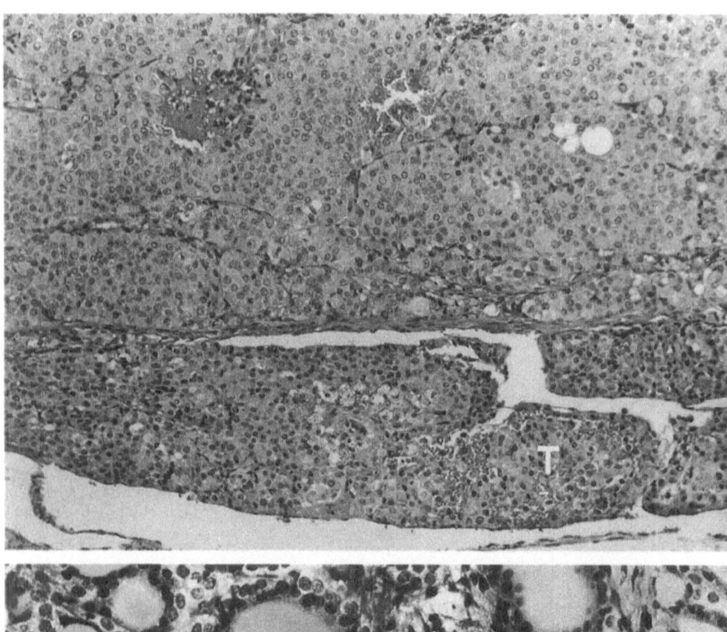

Fig. 297. Medullary thyroid carcinoma, rat. Solid tumor (*T*) invading a vessel adjacent to the thyroid. H&E, ×160

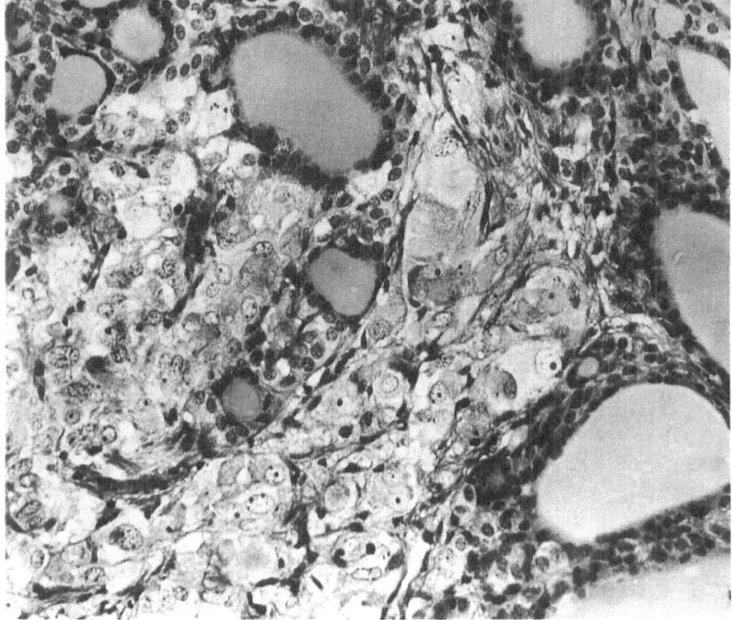

Fig. 298. Medullary thyroid carcinoma, rat. Infiltrating nests and cords of tumor cells between isolated thyroid follicles. H&E, ×250. (DeLellis et al. 1979)

calcitonin with the tumor cells using the immunoperoxidase technique (Boorman et al. 1974; DeLellis et al. 1979; Emmertsen 1985; Le Guellec et al. 1993; Milhaud 1985) and/or by demonstration of CGRP (Carter et al. 1991; DeLellis 1994; Henninger et al. 1988; Poston et al. 1987).

Biologic Features

In the young rat C cells are few in number and are found in the central part of the lateral lobe, but by 2 years of age C-cell hyperplasia is very common (Figs. 290, 291). The gradual increase in the number of C cells in the thyroid of rat with increasing age has been observed in Fischer 344

▶

Fig. 299. Control thyroid gland, young rat. C cells (*C*) are located at the bases of the follicular cells, separated from the colloid (*CO*) by the follicular cells (*F*). Portions of two cells *at bottom* are heavily granulated; the C cells *at top* is sparsely granulated. *Cap*, Capillary; *BL*, basal lamina. TEM, ×5200 (DeLellis et al. 1979)

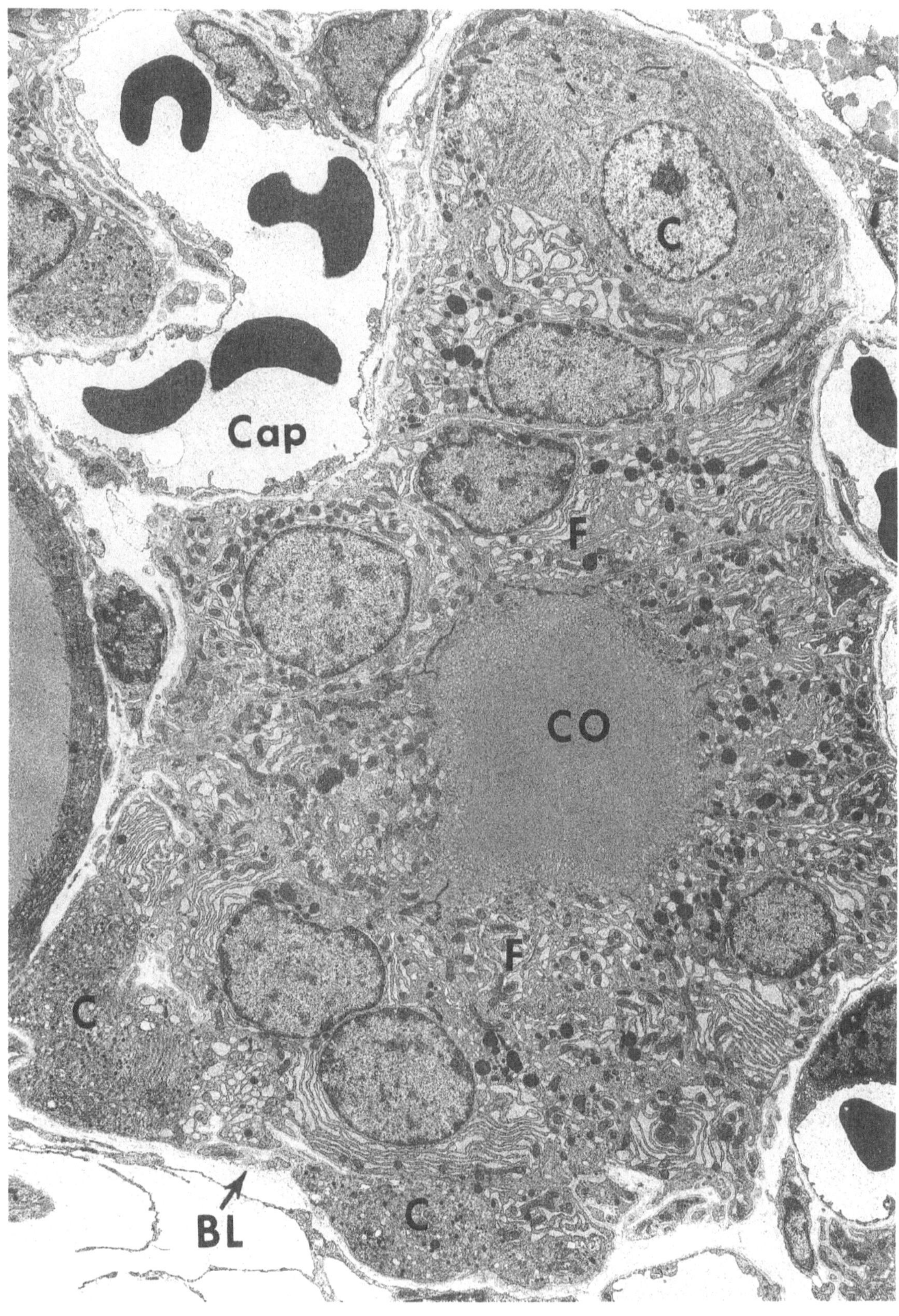
C
Cap
F
CO
F
C
C
BL

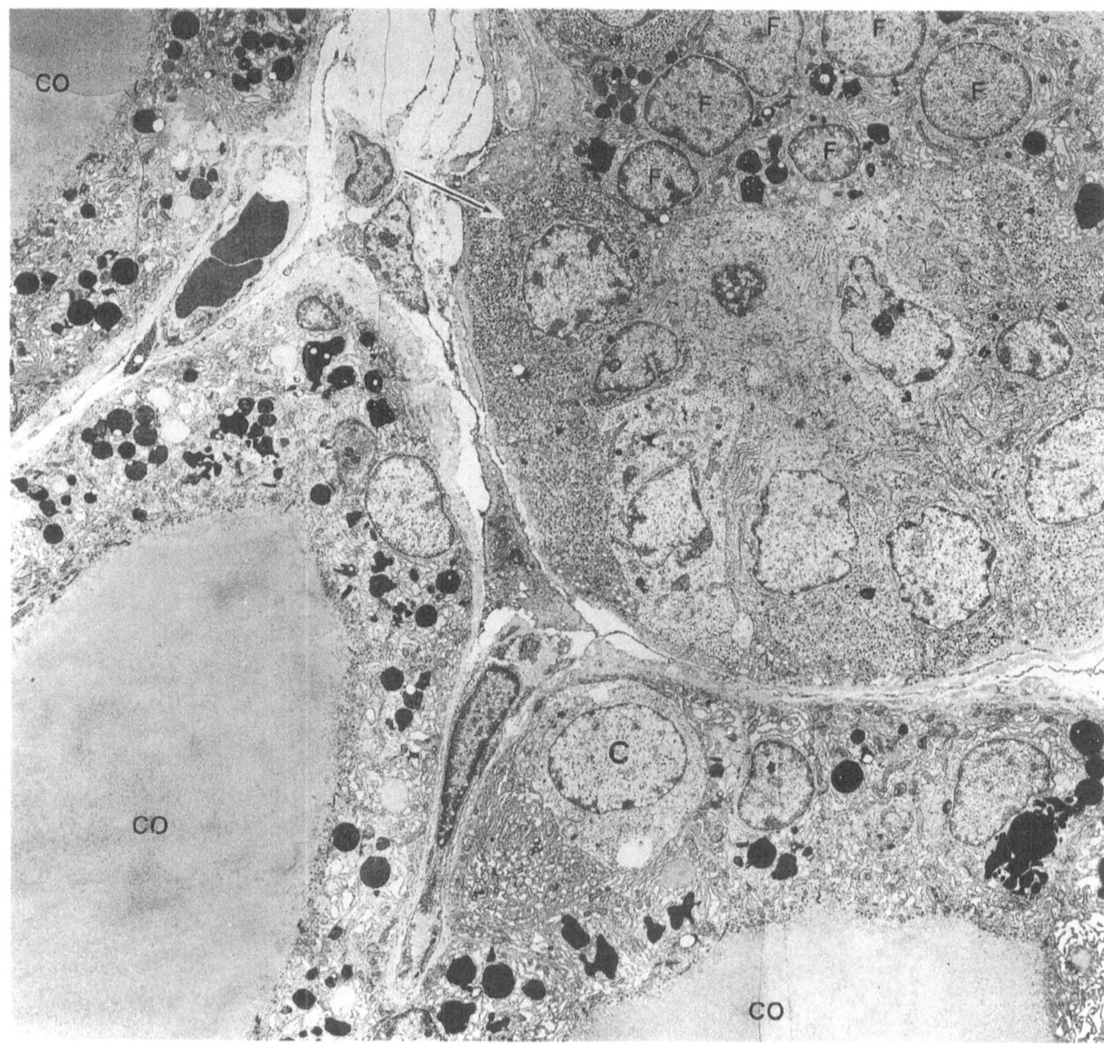

Fig. 300. C-cell adenoma, or nodular hyperplasia, thyroid, rat. Thyroid follicle in upper right is largely replaced by C cells. Follicular cells (*F*) are compressed and contain cytoplasmic accumulation of lipofuscin. Heavily granulated C cells (*arrow*) are present in the periphery of a follicle. One sparsely granulated C cell is present at lower center (*C*). *CO*, Colloid. TEM, ×3300 (DeLellis et al. 1979)

and WAG/Rij strains (Boorman and Hollander 1973, 1976; Boorman et al. 1972; Burek 1978; Hardisty and Boorman 1990). The progression of C-cell lesions from mild to severe diffuse hyperplasia, nodular hyperplasia, adenoma, and then to medullary thyroid carcinoma (C-cell carcinoma) has been demonstrated in the Long-Evans strain of rat by DeLellis et al. (1979) and is depicted in Fig. 303. The frequency of C-cell adenomas and C-cell carcinomas in various rat strains is shown in Table 21. C-cell adenomas occur in approximately 8% of male and female Fischer 344 rats (Haseman et al. 1990), nearly double the rate of 15 years ago (Goodman et al. 1979) while the incidence is 2% in male and 3% in female Osborne-Mendel rats (Goodman et al. 1980).

Serum calcitonin abnormalities have been demonstrated in Long-Evans rats with C-cell hyperplasia (DeLellis et al. 1979) and in young WAG/Rij rats before the appearance of tumors (Delehaye et al. 1989) or in WAG/Rij rats with either spontaneous or transplanted C-cell neoplasms (Delehaye et al. 1989; Denijn et al. 1992). Long-Evans rats with severe diffuse C-cell hyper-

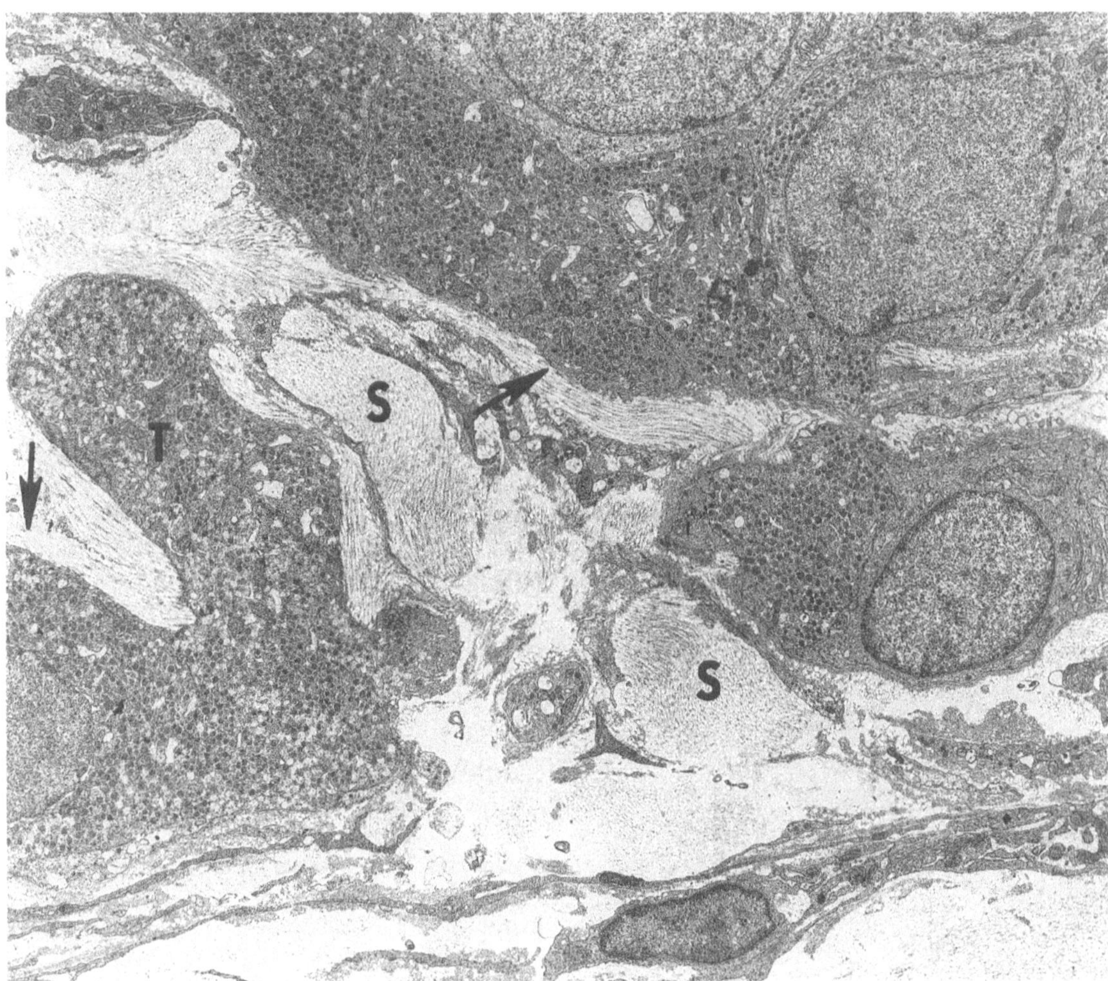

Fig. 301. Medullary thyroid carcinoma, rat. Stromal invasion by tumor cells (*T*). Focally deficient basal lamina (*arrows*). Increased amount of collagen in the stroma (*S*). TEM, ×6000 (DeLellis et al. 1979)

plasia have mean serum calcitonin levels of 0.5 ± 0.1 ng/ml (normal, <0.10 ng/ml). Plasma calcitonin levels appear to be the preferable assay for C-cell (medullary) carcinoma in humans, but CGRP may help predict metastatic lesions (Carter et al. 1991; Henninger et al. 1988). Calcitonin and CGRP are encoded by a single gene, the CALC-1 gene (Denijn et al. 1992), and both calcitonin and CGRP (serum levels and mRNA levels) are useful tools in detecting C-cell carcinomas in WAG/Rij rats (Delehaye et al. 1989; Denijn et al. 1992; Poston et al. 1987). In the Long-Evans rat strain, tumor-bearing animals have serum calcitonin levels of 0.40 ± 0.1 ng/ml (DeLellis et al. 1979). The etiology of C-cell carcinogenesis is not established, but it is known that C cells secrete calcitonin as part of a feed-back mechanism to maintain blood calcium within precise limits (Deftos et al. 1976). High dietary calcium may play a role in the development of C-cell carcinomas in bulls of dairy cattle breeds (Black et al. 1973). More than 450 chemicals have been evaluated for carcinogenicity in the National Toxicology Program, and only five chemicals (phosphamidon, picloram, 4,4′-methylenedianiline dihydrochloride in female rats; ziram and stannous chloride in male rats) showed evidence of increased C-cell neoplasia with chemical exposure (Hardisty and Boorman 1990). The C-cell carcinoma in the rat has been shown to be transplantable and to secrete calcitonin (Boorman et al. 1974; Delehaye et al. 1989; DeLellis 1994). Rats bearing transplantable C-

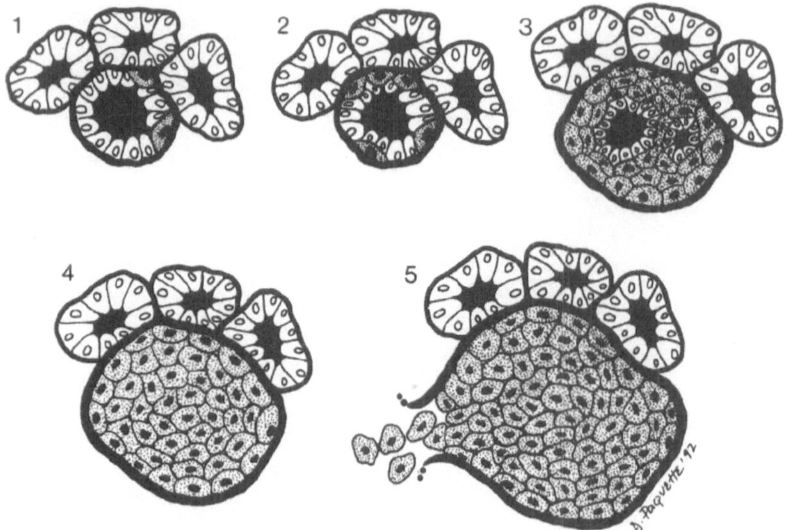

Fig. 302. Stages in the development of medullary thyroid carcinoma. C cells are depicted with closed nuclei and stippled cytoplasm, while follicular cells are shown with opened nuclei and cytoplasm. *1*, Normal C-cell distribution in young rat; *2*, C-cell hyperplasia, diffuse; *3*, C-cell hyperplasia, nodular (focal); *4*, C-cell adenoma; *5*, C-cell carcinoma. *Heavy black line*, follicular basal lamina surrounding the follicle. (Courtesy of R.A. DeLellis and ILSI Press)

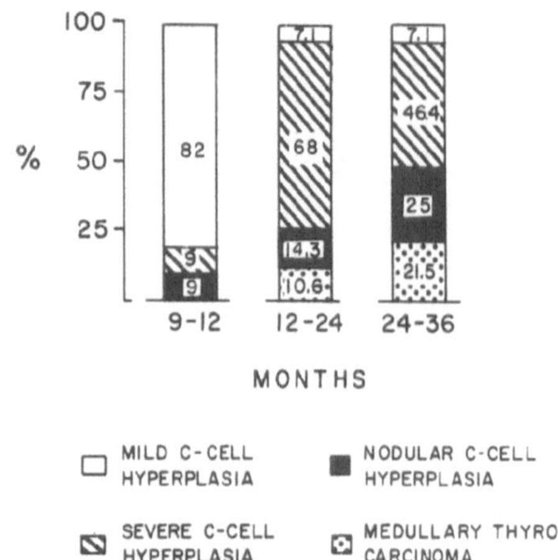

Fig. 303. C-cell lesions in Long-Evans rats (from DeLellis et al. 1979)

cell carcinomas responded to infusions of calcium, pentagastrin, and prostaglandin E_2 by a two- to sevenfold increase in plasma calcitonin (Deftos et al. 1976) while human and rat C-cell carcinoma cell lines respond to an elevation in extracellular calcium with increased calcitonin and CGRP synthesis (Haller-Brem et al. 1987). C-cell neoplasms may also synthesize and secrete somatostatin (Birnbaum et al. 1980) and neurotensin (Zeytinoglu et al. 1980).

Comparison with Other Species

In the mouse C-cell tumors are very rare; only four tumors (one adenoma and three carcinomas) have been recognized in B6C3F1 mice from the NTP chronic toxicity and carcinogenicity studies (Jokinen and Botts 1994). In humans C-cell adenoma and carcinoma occurs as a sporadic entity and also as a genetic disorder with an autosomal dominant mode of inheritance (Emmertsen 1985; Milhaud 1985). In these familial cases the tumors are almost always bilateral and frequently multicentric. The thyroid neoplasms may be accompanied by bilateral and multicentric pheochromocytomas and parathyroid hyperplasia (type IIa multiple endocrine neoplasia). Medullary thyroid carcinomas in humans are often accompanied by bilateral C-cell hyperplasia, which is one antecedent to the malignant tumor (DeLellis et al. 1979; Meissner and Warren 1969). In humans, C-cell carcinomas typically contain amyloid, unlike the rat where amyloid is uncommon (Napalkov 1990). However, the C-cell neoplasms in the Long-Evans rat have similarities to the familial disorder in man. Diffuse and nodular hyperplasia of C cells may be observed in this strain starting at 9 months of age and increasing in severity as the animals become older. The focal hyperplasia becomes increasing nodular, or adenomatous, and as rats reach 12–24 months C-cell adenoma and medullary (C-cell) carcinomas are very prevalent (Table 21). This has made the rat an excellent model to study not only C-cell neoplasia but C cells in general and the endocrinologic intricacies of the regulation of calcium levels (Bidard et al. 1993; Delehaye et al. 1989; Denijn et al. 1992; Haller-Brem et al. 1987; Le Guellec et al. 1993; Milhaud 1985; Okimura et al. 1989; Oskam et al. 1985; Poston et al. 1987).

References

Bidard JN, de Nadai F, Rovere C, Moinier D, Laur J, Martinez J, Cuber JC, Kitabgi P (1993) Immunological and biochemical characterization of processing products from the neurotensin/neuromedin N precursor in the rat medullary thyroid carcinoma 6–23 cell line. J Biochem 291:225–233

Birnbaum RS, Muszynski M, Roos BA (1980) Tumor and plasma somatostatin-like immunoreactivity in transplantable rat medullary thyroid carcinoma. Cancer Res 40:4192–4196

Black HE, Capen CC, Young DM (1973) Ultimobranchial thyroid neoplasms in bulls. A syndrome resembling medullary thyroid carcinoma in man. Cancer 32:865–878

Boorman GA, Hollander CF (1973) Spontaneous lesions in the female WAG/Rij rat. J Gerontol 28:152–159

Boorman GA, Hollander CF (1976) Animal model of human disease: medullary carcinoma of the thyroid. Am J Pathol 83:237–240

Boorman GA, van Noord MJ, Hollander CF (1972) Naturally occurring medullary thyroid carcinoma in the rat. Arch Pathol 94:35–41

Boorman GA, Heersche JNM, Hollander CF (1974) Transplantable calcitonin-secreting medullary carcinomas of the thyroid in the WAG/Rij rat. J Natl Cancer Inst 53:1011–1015

Burek JD (1978) Pathology of aging rats. CRC, West Palm Beach

Carter WB, Taylor RL, Kao PC, Heath H III, Heath H (1991) Determination of plasma calcitonin gene-related peptide concentrations by a new immunochemiluminometric assay in normal persons and patients with medullary thyroid carcinoma and other neuroendocrine tumors. J Clin Endocrinol Metab 72:327–335

Deftos LJ, Boorman GA, Roos BA (1976) Immunoassay of calcitonin in rat medullary thyroid carcinoma. Horm Metab Res 8:83–84

Delehaye MC, Cohen R, Segond N, Pidoux E, Treilhou-Lahille F, Milhaud G, Moukhtar MP (1989) Elevated levels of calcitonin mRNA: a marker for the spontaneous development of medullary thyroid carcinoma in rats. Biochem Bioshys Res Commun 159:528–535

DeLellis RA (1994) Changes in structure and function of thyroid C cells. In: Mohr U, Dungworth DL, Capen CC (eds) Pathobiology of the aging rat. ILSI, Washington DC, pp 285–299

DeLellis RA, Nunnemacher G, Wolfe HJ (1977) C-cell hyperplasia. An ultrastructural analysis. Lab Invest 36:237–248

DeLellis RA, Nunnemacher G, Bitman WR, Gagel RF, Tashjian AH Jr, Blount M, Wolfe HJ (1979) C-cell hyperplasia and medullary thyroid carcinoma in the rat. An immunohistochemical and ultrastructural analysis. Lab Invest 40:140–154

Denijn M, de Weger RA, den Otter W, van Unnik JA, Lips CJ (1992) Expression of the first calcitonin/CGRP gene in spontaneous and transplanted rat medullary thyroid carcinoma: a comparison of dot-blot analysis, in situ hybridization, and immunohistochemistry. J Histochem Cytochem 40:1761–1767

Ekholm R, Ericson LE (1968) The ultrastructure of the parafollicular cells of the thyroid gland in the rat. J Ultrastruct Res 23:378–402

Emmertsen K (1985) Medullary thyroid carcinoma and calcitonin. Dan Med Bull 32:1–28

Goodman DG, Ward JM, Squire RA, Chu KC, Linhart MS (1979) Neoplastic and nonneoplastic lesions in aging F344 rats. Toxicol Appl Pharmacol 48:237–248

Goodman DG, Ward JM, Squire RA, Paxton MB, Reichardt WD, Chu KC, Linhart MS (1980) Neoplastic and nonneoplastic lesions in aging Osborne-Mendel rats. Toxicol Appl Pharmacol 55:433–447

Haller-Brem S, Muff R, Petermann JB, Born W, Roos BA, Fischer JA (1987) Role of cytosolic free calcium concentration in the secretion of calcitonin gene-related peptide and calcitonin from medullary thyroid carcinoma cells. Endocrinology 121:1272–1277

Hardisty JF, Boorman GA (1990) Thyroid gland. In: Boorman GA, Eustis SL, Elwell MR, Montgomery CA Jr, MacKenzie WF (eds) Pathology of the Fischer rat. Academic, San Diego, pp 519–536

Haseman JK, Arnold J, Eustis SL (1990) Tumor incidences in Fischer 344 rats: NTP historical data. In: Boorman GA, Eustis SL, Elwell MR, Montgomery CA Jr, MacKenzie WF (eds) Pathology of the Fischer rat. Academic, San Diego, pp 555–564

Henninger S, Schatz H, Stracke H, Wagner U, Kracht J (1988) Immunohistochemical hormone content in medullary and undifferentiated thyroid carcinoma and prognosis after surgery. Acta Histochem 83:51–56

Jokinen MP, Botts S (1994) Tumours of the thyroid gland. In: Turusov V, Mohr U (eds) Pathology of tumours in laboratory animals. International Agency for Research on Cancer, Lyon, pp 565–594

Le Guellec P, Dumas S, Volle GE, Pidoux E, Moukhtar MS, Treilhou-Lahille F (1993) An efficient method to detect calcitonin mRNA in normal and neoplastic rat C-cells (medullary thyroid carcinoma) by in situ hybridization using a digoxigenin-labeled synthetic oligodeoxyribonucleotide probe. J Histochem Cytochem 41:389–395

Meissner WA, Warren S (eds) (1969)Tumors of the thyroid gland. In: Firminger HI (ed) Atlas of tumor pathology, vol 4, 2nd edn. Armed Forces Institute of Pathology, Bethesda, p 135

Milhaud G (1985) Current progress in medullary carcinoma of the thyroid. Int Congr Ser 684:55–58

Mohr U (1994) International classification of rodent tumours, part 1. World Health Organization, IARC Science Publication no 122

Napalkov NP (1990) Tumours of the thyroid gland. In: Turusov VS, Mohr U (eds) Pathology of tumours in laboratory animals. International Agency for Research on Cancer, Lyon, pp 539–572

O'Briain DS, DeLellis RA, Wolfe HJ, Reichlin S, Bollinger J, Tashjian AH Jr (1979) Somatostatin immunoreactive cells in C cell hyperplasia and medullary thyroid carcinoma. Lab Invest 40:275–276

Okimura Y, Kitajima N, Uchiyama T, Yagi H, Abe H, Shakutsui S, Chihara K (1989) Insulin-like growth factor I (IGF-I) production and the presence of IGF-I receptors in rat medullary thyroid carcinoma cell line 6–23 (clone 6). Biochem Bioshys Res Commun 161:589–595

Oskam R, Rijksen G, Lips CJ, Staal GE (1985) Enolase isozymes in differentiated and undifferentiated medullary thyroid carcinomas. Cancer 55:394–399

Poston GJ, Seitz PK, Townsend CM Jr, Alexander RW, Rajaraman S, Cooper CW, Thompson JC (1987) Calcitonin gene-related peptide: possible tumor marker for medullary thyroid cancer. Surgery 102:1049–1054

Zeytinoglu FN, Gagel RF, Tashjian AH Jr, Hammer RA, Leeman SE (1980) Characterization of neurotensin production by a line of rat medullary thyroid carcinoma cells. Proc Natl Acad Sci USA 77:3741–3745

Goiter, Nodular Hyperplasia, Adenoma, and Carcinoma of the Thyroid Induced by Amitrole and Ethylenethiourea, Rat

Hiroyuki Tsuda

Synonyms. Goiter: diffuse hyperplastic goiter, hyperplasia, thyroid; carcinoma: follicular carcinoma; adenoma: papillary adenoma.

Gross Appearance

The greatly enlarged thyroid lobes of surviving rats that have received amitrole (0.25% in drinking water) have a combined weight of as much as 1.0–2.5 g. The affected thyroids usually appear whitish in color because of their thickened fibrous capsule. Their surface is usually smooth, but the capsule may adhere to the adjacent fatty or muscular tissue. Occasionally the enlarged thyroid is surrounded by a mass of coagulated blood due to the rupture of subcapsular blood vessels in hypertrophied thyroid tissue (Fig. 304).

In rats given amitrole after partial thyroidectomy, goiters of various sizes develop from the residual tissue and often have fibrous adhesions to adjacent tissue. In rats subjected to partial thyroidectomy only, the thyroid regenerates to almost the same size and weight as the controls. Rats given ethy-

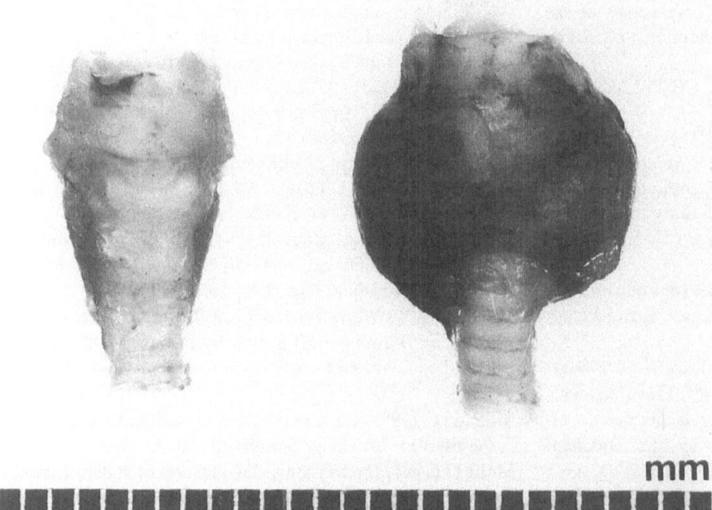

Fig. 304. Normal thyroid (*left*) and enormously enlarged amitrole-treated thyroid (*right*)

Table 22. Effects of amitrole (AT; 0.25% in drinking water) and partial thyroidectomy (PTx) on the induction of goiter and neoplasms in rat thyroid

Group	Treatment	total no. of rats	Effective[a]	Lesions of the thyroid (%)					
				Goiter	Follicular carcinoma				Nodules of papillary adenoma
					With invasion of			Total no.	
					Capsule	Adjacent fatty tissue	Blood vessels		
1	AT	40	26	26 (100)*	16 (61.5)	4 (15.4)	5 (19.2)	19 (73.1)*	3 (11.5)
2	AT + PTx	30	14	14 (100)*	11 (78.6)	10 (71.4)	3 (21.4)	14 (100)*	1 (7.1)
3	PTx	10	7	0	0	0	0	0	0
4	–	10	7	0	0	0	0	0	0

* Significantly different from values in groups 3 and 4.
[a] No. of rats that survived longer than 30 weeks.

Table 23. Effects of ethylenethiourea (ETU; 0.025% in drinking water) and amitrole (AT; 0.25% in drinking water) on the induction of goiter and neoplasms in rat thyroid

Group	Treatment	Total no. of rats	Effective[a]	Lesions of the thyroid (%)						
				Goiter	Follicular carcinoma				Nodules of papillary adenoma	Total
					With invasion of					
					Capsule	Adjacent fatty tissue	Blood vessels	Metastasis to Lung		
1	ETU	30	17	17 (100)*	17 (100)	12 (70.6)	2 (11.8)	2 (11.8)	14 (82.4)*,**	17 (100)*
2	ETU + AT	30	17	17 (100)*	17 (100)	7 (41.2)	3 (17.6)	0	5 (29.4)*	17 (100)*
3	AT	20	13	13 (100)*	8 (61.5)	2 (15.4)	2 (15.4)	0	2 (15.4)	10 (76.9)*
4	–	20	16	0	0	0	0	0	0	

* Significantly different from the value for group 4; ** significantly different from the values for groups 2 and 3.
[a] No. of rats that survived longer than 30 weeks.

lenethiourea alone or in combination with amitrole develop goiters weighing 1.5–2.0 g, slightly smaller but in gross appearance quite similar to those induced by amitrole alone (Tables 22, 23).

Microscopic Features

Four lesions are encountered in the thyroid of rats treated with amitrole or ethylenethiourea under specific experimental conditions: goiter, nodular hyperplasia, follicular adenocarcinoma, and papillary adenoma.

Goiter. The enlarged thyroid induced by amitrole and/or ethylenethiourea consists of small, diffusely proliferated follicles lined by cuboidal to columnar epithelium in which the cytoplasm stains clearly with routine hematoxylin and eosin. The nuclei of these follicular cells are located toward the base of the cell. The lumina of these small follicles contain little or no colloid (Fig. 305). Abundant dilated vascular spaces lie between the follicles, which is also responsible for enlargement of the thyroid tissue (Rognoni et al. 1987). Stromal tissue separating small proliferated follicles may be partially hyalinized. Capsules of the goitrous thyroid are usually thick. Papillary projections of the follicular epithelium into the follicular lumen may be a characteristic feature of goiter in rats given amitrole and/or ethylenethiourea for a long period. However, mitoses are rarely found.

Recent investigation indicated that the goiter tissue contains a subpopulation of TSH-responsive follicular cells which respond to further TSH stimulation (Groch and Clifton 1992).

Nodular Hyperplasia. Although at low incidence, hypertrophic nodular lesions arising from diffuse goiters may be found. These consist of hypertrophied follicular tissue, closely resembling goiters themselves, and exhibit compression of the surrounding thyroid to a variable degree. The lesion does not have any obvious fibrous capsule and nuclear irregularities and basophilia are absent.

Follicular Adenocarcinoma. This malignant neoplasm resembles the hyperplasic goiter histologically but is distinguished by cellular irregularity and structural and nuclear atypia, invasion of the capsule, adjacent adipose or muscular tissue, and blood vessels (Figs. 306–309). This lesion is often seen in advanced hyperplastic, goitrous thyroid (Table 22).

Papillary Adenoma. Nodules of neoplastic thyroid tissue are a frequent finding, and they consist of small basophilic follicular cells with a conspicuous papillary growth into somewhat enlarged follicular spaces (Fig. 310). These are usually encapsulated by a thin fibrovascular stroma, and their nodular and papillary features readily distinguish them from surrounding hyperplastic follicular (goitrous) tissue.

Ultrastructure

The appearance of the thyroid under the electron microscope is similar in rats treated with amitrole and ethylenethiourea and in those treated with ethylenethiourea alone. During the early stage of treatment (4 weeks) the low columnar or cuboidal epithelium contains widely dilated endoplasmic reticulum and slightly elongated microvilli, which project into the lumen. At 10–20 weeks, when the thyroid gland is enlarged severalfold, the size and shape of follicles are varied. Most of them contain no colloid. Intrafollicular papillary growth of the follicular epithelium is a prominent feature. The follicular epithelium is tall and columnar and possesses a basal nucleus and long microvilli projecting into the follicular lumen. The endoplasmic reticulum is greatly distended, and the cisternae do not stain for peroxidase activity (Figs. 311, 312). Perinuclear cisternae are also negative to the peroxidase stain. After prolonged treatment with amitrole, when variety in follicular size and papillary growth of follicular epithelium become more prominent, the cisternae of the endoplasmic reticulum and greatly dilated and filled with amorphous flocculent material. Peroxidase activity is greatly diminished throughout the cell, as indicated by histochemical stains (Tsuda et al. 1973). No fundamental difference is found in the ultrastructural feature of lesions showing invasive and noninvasive growth.

Differential Diagnosis

Since amitrole and ethylenethiourea act as antithyroid agents (Alexander 1959; Doniach 1953; International Agency for Research on Cancer 1974; Jukes and Shaffer 1960), they indirectly stimulated increased secretion of thyroid-stimulating hormone (TSH) which induces hyperplasia in the thyroid, i.e., goiter. Therefore the histopathologic features of amitrole- and ethylenethiourea-induced goiters are indistinguishable from those induced by other antithyroid agents such as thiouracil, methylthiouracil, and propylthiouracil or by a low iodine diet (Matovinovic et al. 1965). However, invasive lesions of proliferating follicular tissue are more frequent in animals treated with amitrole or ethylenethiourea (Tables 22, 23).

The essential differentiating feature of goiter is the diffuse enlargement of the thyroid by increased numbers of small follicles containing little or no colloid and lined with cuboidal to columnar epithelium. The papillary adenoma is made up of nodules of small basophilic follicular cells which project into the lumen owing to papillary growth. The cells of the follicular carcinoma resemble

▶

Fig. 305. (*upper left*) Hyperplastic follicular tissue in amitrole-induced goiter. Follicles are small and contain no colloid; the epithelium is cuboidal to columnar. H&E, ×240

Fig. 306. (*lower left*) Thyroid, rat invasion of capsule (*C*) by follicular carcinoma. H&E, ×33, ×120

Fig. 307. (*upper right*) Thyroid, rat; invasive growth into connective tissue outside the capsule. H&E, ×100

Fig. 308. (*lower right*) Thyroid, rat; intravascular invasion by follicular carcinoma (*arrows*). H&E, ×100

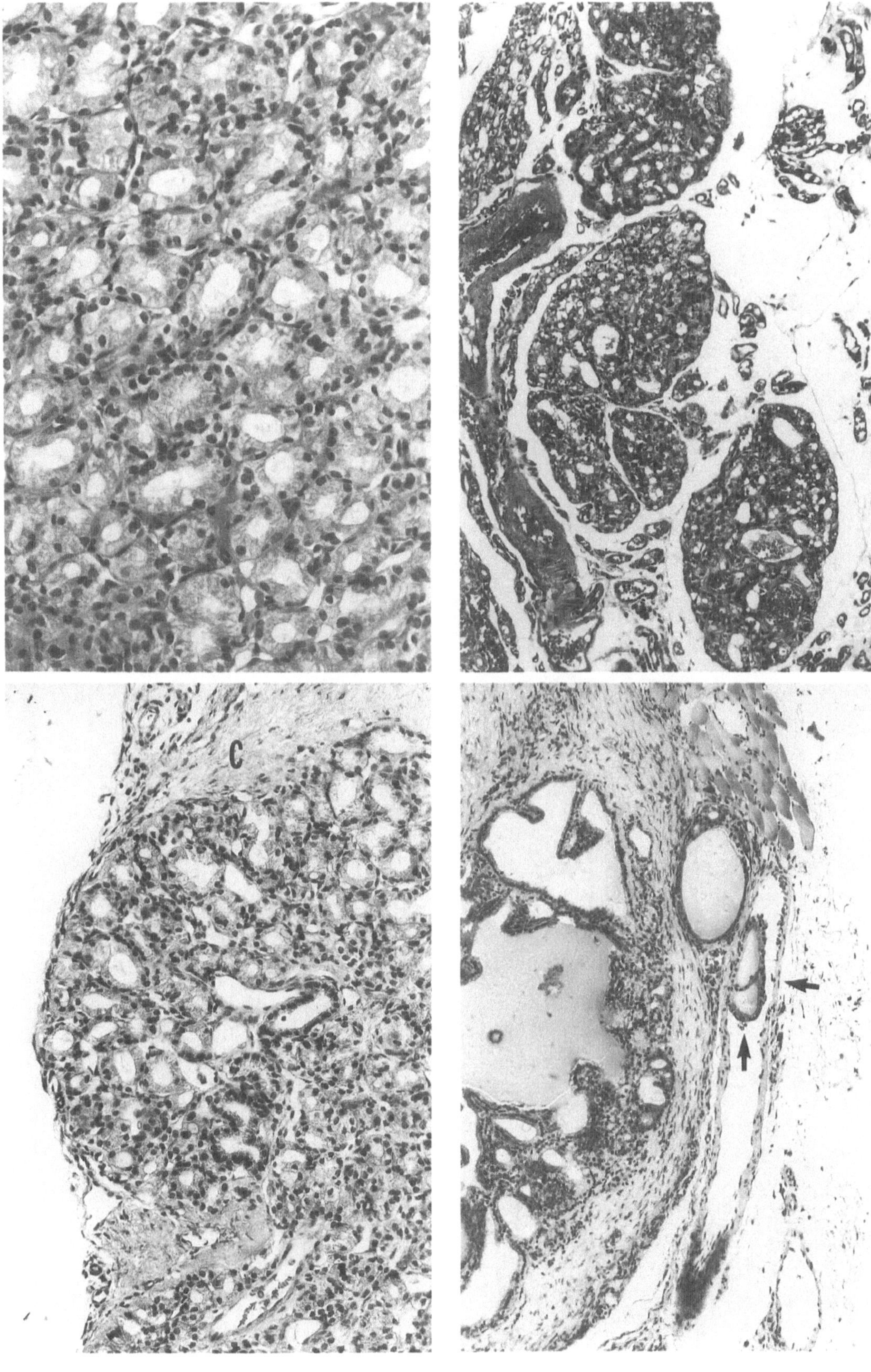
C

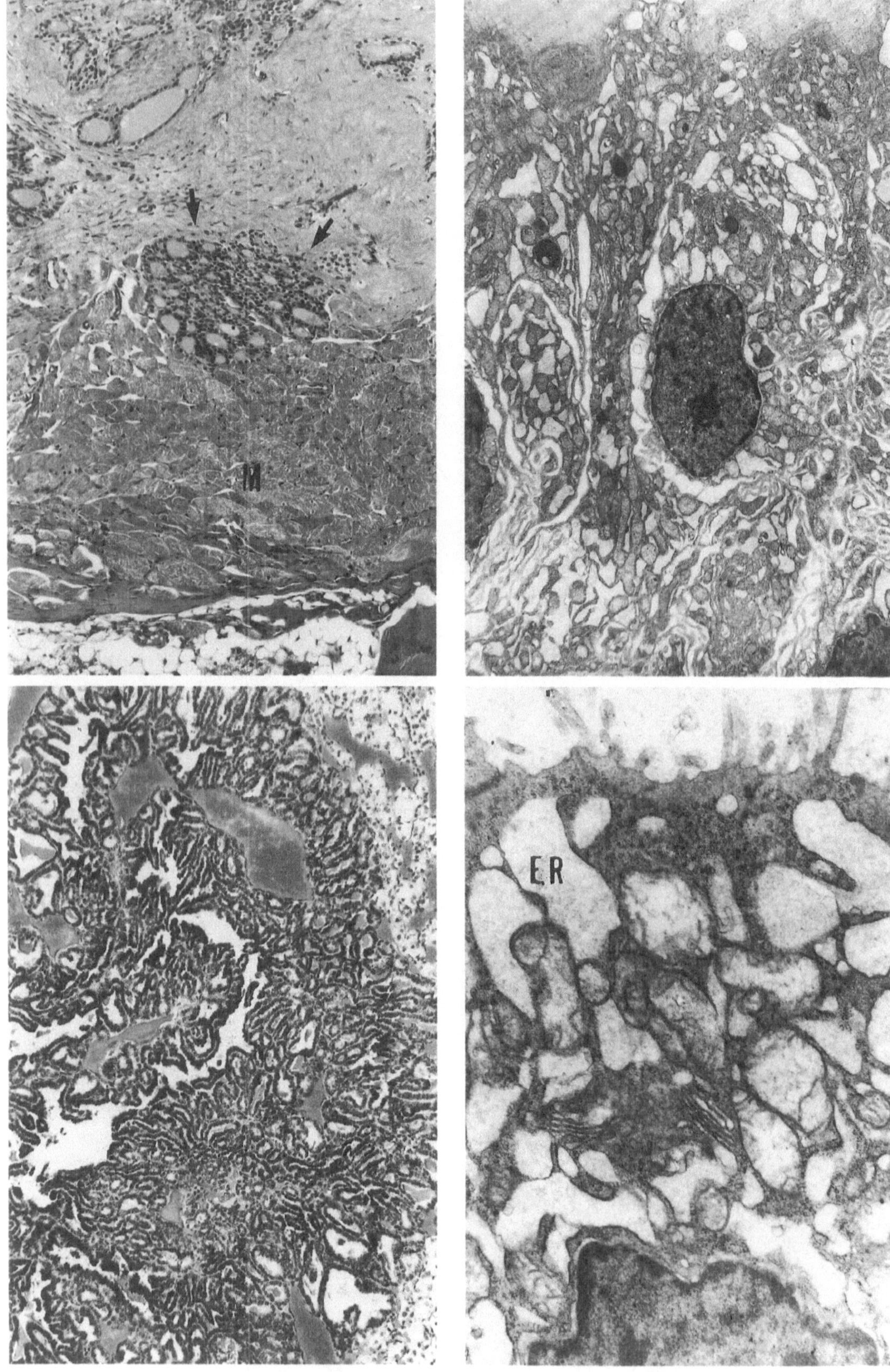
M
ER

hyperplastic follicular cells but invade the capsule, adjacent tissue, and blood vessels and may metastasize.

Biologic Features

Pathogenesis of Induced Tumors. Amitrole is known to inhibit peroxidase activity and is goitrogenic in experimental animals due to its indirect effect on release of excess pituitary thyrotropic hormone (Alexander 1959; Jukes and Shaffer 1960; Strum and Karnovsky 1971). The antithyroid drugs propylthiouracil and methylthiouracil, when administered alone or in combination with injected ^{131}I, have a tumorigenic effect on rat thyroid (Graham and Hansen 1972; Lindsay et al. 1966; Money and Rawson 1950). Amitrole alone induces carcinoma of the thyroid under certain experimental conditions. Ethylenethiourea, which also has antithyroid activity, induces goiters and invasive carcinomas (Graham et al. 1973, 1975; Ulland et al. 1972). These tumors may develop because the continuous stimulation of goiter tissue by TSH, released indirectly by amitrole, provides an opportunity for amitrole to cause some alteration in DNA of the epithelial cells. Antithyroid agents have an effect to promote thyroid carcinogenesis, possibly due to increase in TSH level similar to low iodine condition (Kanno et al. 1990; Ohshima and Ward 1984).

Malignancy of Tumors. Invasion of follicular tissue through the capsule into adjacent stromal tissue and into blood vessels represents a malignant condition. Metastases of this follicular tissue have been reported in animals maintained on antithyroid drugs such as thiouracil (Doniach 1950; Goldberg et al. 1964; Lindsay et al. 1966; Money and Rawson 1950). In the tissue of animals given amitrole, examination of serial sections revealed no remote metastasis to other organs, but such metastasis was certainly possible. Similar lesions were also induced by ethylenethiourea, and their malignant potential was demonstrated by the finding of pulmonary metastases. Nodules of papillary adenomas with cellular and structural atypia were found within follicular tissues. It is not clear why this type of lesion which shows more atypia was not invasive, but this type may correspond to microfollicular adenomas in humans.

◀
Fig. 309. (*upper left*) Thyroid, rat; follicular carcinoma (*arrows*). Invasion of muscular tissue (*M*) in a rat treated with ethylenethiourea. H&E, ×100

Fig. 310. (*lower left*) Thyroid, rat; papillary adenoma following amitrole treatment. The cytoplasm and nuclei are more basophilic than surrounding follicular tissue. H&E, ×40

Fig. 311. (*upper right*) Thyroid, amitrole-treated rat; follicular epithelial cell is tall and columnar; cisternae of endoplasmic reticulum are extremely dilated. EM, ×6000

Fig. 312. (*lower right*) Thyroid, amitrole-treated rat; goitrous follicular cell with enormously dilated cisternae of endoplasmic reticulum (*ER*). EM, ×18000

Modifying Factors. Partial Thyroidectomy. Invasive lesions are significantly more frequent in groups subjected to partial thyroidectomy followed by treatment with amitrole than in those given amitrole alone. This is probably due to an increase in the level of TSH, which stimulates the regeneration of thyroid tissue and may thus provide more opportunity for malignant change in the follicular cells.

Combined Effect of Amitrole and Ethylenethiourea. Amitrole has a mild inhibitory effect on ethylenethiourea carcinogenesis. The mechanism of this inhibitory effect is unclear; possibly detoxification or excretion of ethylenethiourea is accelerated by amitrole owing to activation of some enzymatic process. A similar phenomenon has been observed following combined treatment with 3-methylcholanthrene or α-benzene hexachloride and hepatocarcinogens (Doniach 1950; Marugami et al. 1967; Thamavit et al. 1974). It is also possible that TSH is a cocarcinogen, but that ethylenethiourea reacts directly with the thyroid to produce carcinoma.

Low-Iodine Diet. It is known that thyroid tumors can be induced by a low-iodine diet. However, a low-iodine diet does not increase the incidence of carcinoma on administration of ethylenethiourea (Tsuda et al. 1978). A possible explanation is that animals given a low iodine diet take less water containing ethylenethiourea than animals on a control diet.

References

Alexander NM (1959) Antithyroid action of 3-amino-1,2,4-triazole. J Biol Chem 234:148–150

Doniach I (1950) The effect of radioactive iodine alone and in combination with methylthiouracil and acetylaminofluorene upon tumor production in the rat's thyroid gland. Br J Cancer 4:223–234

Doniach I (1953) The effect of radioactive iodine alone and in combination with methylthiouracil upon tumour production in the rat's thyroid gland. Br J Cancer 7:181–202

Goldberg RC, Lindsay S, Nichols CW Jr, Chaikoff IL (1964) Induction of neoplasms in thyroid glands of rats by subtotal thyroidectomy and by the injection of one microcurie of I^{131}. Cancer Res 24:35–43

Graham SL, Hansen WH (1972) Effects of short-term administration of ethylenethiourea upon thyroid function of the rat. Bull Environ Contam Toxicol 7:19–25

Graham SL, Hansen WH, Davis KJ, Perry CH (1973) Effects of one year administration of ethylenethiourea upon the thyroid of the rat. J Agric Food Chem 21:324–329

Graham SL, Davis KJ, Hansen WH, Graham CH (1975) Effects of prolonged ethylenethiourea ingestion on the thyroid of the rat. Food Cosmet Toxicol 13:493–499

Groch KM, Clifton KH (1992) The plateau phase of rat goiter contains a sub-population of TSH-responsive follicular cells capable of proliferation following transplantation. Acta Endocrinol (Copenh) 126:85–96

International Agency for Research on Cancer (1974) IARC monographs on the evaluation of carcinogenic risk of chemicals to man, no 7. Some antithyroid and related substances, nitrosofurans and industrial chemicals. IARC, Lyon

Jukes TH, Shaffer CB (1960) Antithyroid effects of aminotriazole. Science 132:296–297

Kanno J, Matsuoka C, Furuta K, Onodera H, Miyajima H. Maekawa A, Hayashi Y (1990) Tumor promoting effect of goitrogens on the rat thyroid. Toxicol Pathol 18:239–246

Lindsay S, Nichols CW Jr, Chaikoff IL (1966) Induction of benign and malignant thyroid neoplasms in the rat. Arch Pathol 81:308–316

Marugami M, Ito N, Konishi Y, Hiasa Y, Farber E (1967) Influence of 3-methylcholanthrene on liver carcinogenesis in rats ingesting DL-ethionine, 3′-methyl-4-dimethylaminoazobenzene, and N-2fluorenylacetamide. Cancer Res 27: 2011–2019

Matovinovic J, Hilbert RD, Armstrong WF, Helgensen RT (1965) Thyroid tumor and thyroid transplant tumor in iodine-deficient rat. In: Cassano C, Andreoli M (eds) Current topics in thyroid research. Academic, New York, pp 920–932

Money WL, Rawson RW (1950) The experimental production of thyroid tumors in the rat exposed to prolonged treatment with thiouracil. Cancer 3:321–335

Ohshima M, Ward JM (1984) Promotion of N-methyl-N-nitrosourea-induced thyroid tumors by iodine deficiency in F344/NCr rats. JNCI 73:289–296

Rognoni JB, Penel C, Bastiani P (1987) Involution of hyperplastic goiter in the adult male rat. Tissue compartment process with early iodine effect: a stereological and biochemical study. Virchows Arch [B] 53:166–175

Strum JM, Karnovsky MJ (1971) Aminotriazole goiter. Fine structure and localization of thyroid peroxidase activity. Lab Invest 24:1–12

Thamavit W, Hiasa Y, Ito N, Bhamarapravati N (1974) The inhibitory effects of alpha-benzene hexachloride on 3′-methyl-4-dimethylaminoazobenzene and DL-ethionine carcinogenesis in rats. Cancer Res 34:337–340

Tsuda H, Takahashi M, Fukushima S, Endo Y (1973) Fine structure and localization of peroxidase activity in aminotriazole goiter. Nagoya Med J 18:183–197

Tsuda H, Hananouchi M, Tatematsu M, Hirose M, Hirao K, Takahashi M, Ito N (1976) Tumorigenic effect of 3-amino-1H-1,2,4-triazole on rat thyroid. JNCI 57:861–864

Tsuda H, Takahashi M, Murasaki G, Ogiso T, Tatematsu M (1978) Effect of 3-amino-1H-1,2,4-triazole or low iodine diet on rat thyroid carcinogenesis induced by ethylenethiourea. Nagoya Med J 23:83–92

Ulland BM, Weisburger JH, Weisburger EK, Rice JM, Cypher R (1972) Thyroid cancer in rats from ethylene thiourea intake. JNCI 49:583–584

Ganglioneuroma, Thyroid Gland, Rat

James W. Crissman

Gross Appearance

Ganglioneuromas of the thyroid gland have not been identified at necropsy because of their small size, 1.5 mm or less, and frequent association with larger C cell tumors.

Microscopic Features

Ganglioneuromas of the thyroid are generally easily identifiable in standard hematoxylin and eosin sections because of their characteristically large ganglion cells and abundant eosinophilic matrix with Schwann's cells (Figs. 313–315). The tumors are unencapsulated and grow by infiltration and expansion, frequently trapping thyroid follicles. One small ganglioneuroma has been observed to have infiltrated the parathyroid gland, but the tumors have been benign in all other respects. Ganglion cells are seen singly or in clusters embedded in moderate to broad bands of eosinophilic matrix (Fig. 316). These clusters are sometimes cystic, with ballooned and degenerating ganglion cells at their center (Fig. 317). The ganglion cells are large, pale staining, and angular, with large, eccentric, pale nuclei and prominent, usually single, nucleoli. The degree of ganglion cell differentiation and cell size is variable within individual tumors. Smaller cells clustered with large ganglion cells generally bear adequate resemblance to the ganglion cells to be considered to be of the same lineage (Fig. 318). Uncommonly, smaller cells form rosettes suggestive of neuroblastoma (Fig. 317). In many tumors the smaller cells within the ganglioneuromas may appear to be extensions of C cell proliferations (Figs. 314, 315). The eosinophilic matrix has many small, spindle-shaped Schwann's cells, cross sections of neurites (axons and dendrites), and a scant fibrovascular component. Bielschowsky's silver impregnation technique provides excellent morphologic definition of the tumors; it demonstrates clearly the many neuritic processes extending from ganglion cells and the many neuritic processes embedded in the matrix (Fig. 319).

Immunohistochemical staining for calcitonin may be carried out to exclude the diagnosis of "pleomorphic C cell tumor." The technique clearly identifies C cells at the periphery of thyroid follicles entrapped in ganglioneuromas (Fig. 320) as well as C cell tumors adjoining ganglioneuromas. Large ganglion cells of the tumors may stain weakly for calcitonin – similarly to neurons in CNS tissues used as positive controls. Cells on intermediate morphology have reacted with intermediate intensity to calcitonin antibodies.

Ultrastructure

Electron microscopy provides confirmation of the light-microscopic diagnosis (Fig. 321). The ganglion cells have large eccentric nuclei with dispersed chromatin and prominent nucleoli. The cytoplasm is abundant, with a homogeneous distribution of organelles including mitochondria, numerous free ribosomes, occasional neurosecretory granules and multivesicular bodies. Stacks of rough endoplasmic reticulum in the perikaryon (Nissl's bodies) are small but occasionally observed near the nucleus. The areas seen as broad band of eosinophilic matrix by light microscopy consist primarily of many neuritic processes with a scant matrix of collagen, small vessels, basement membrane, and Schwann's cells. Schwann's cell processes partially envelope ganglion cells and their neurites, resembling the morphology of normal nonmyelinated nerve tissue (Jones and Cowan 1983). The ultrastructural morphologic appearance is very distinct from normal or neoplastic C cells, which are smaller, have marginated nuclear chromatin, have many secretory granules, and lack cell processes.

Differential Diagnosis

Pleomorphic C cell tumor, and ganglioneuroblastoma, should be considered in the differential diagnosis. These are described, respectively, on pp. 262 and 280, this volume.

Biologic Features

Natural History. In the two studies in which these tumors were observed (Crissman et al. 1991), the earliest identified occurrence was in a 16-monoth-old female rat; the great majority were seen in rats surviving to the scheduled termination at 26 mo. of age. They had no discernable effect on the health of the rats. It should be noted that rarely, solitary, apparently normal ganglion cells have been observed in the thyroid gland of young rats of similar lineage used in subacute studies in the laboratory where these tumors were described.

Pathogenesis. It is generally agreed that the C cells of the thyroid gland originate from the neural crest (LiVolsi 1980; Pearse 1986). Ganglion cells of the autonomic system also arise from neural crest and invest the gland (Jones and Cowan 1983). These cells then comingle with the thyroid follicular tissue which has arisen from entodermal downgrowth of the base of the tongue (Tice 1983). C cells and the cells of the autonomic ganglia are of neural crest origin, which may explain the close association observed between C cell tumors and ganglioneuromas. Ganglioneuromas of the adrenal gland usually occur in association with

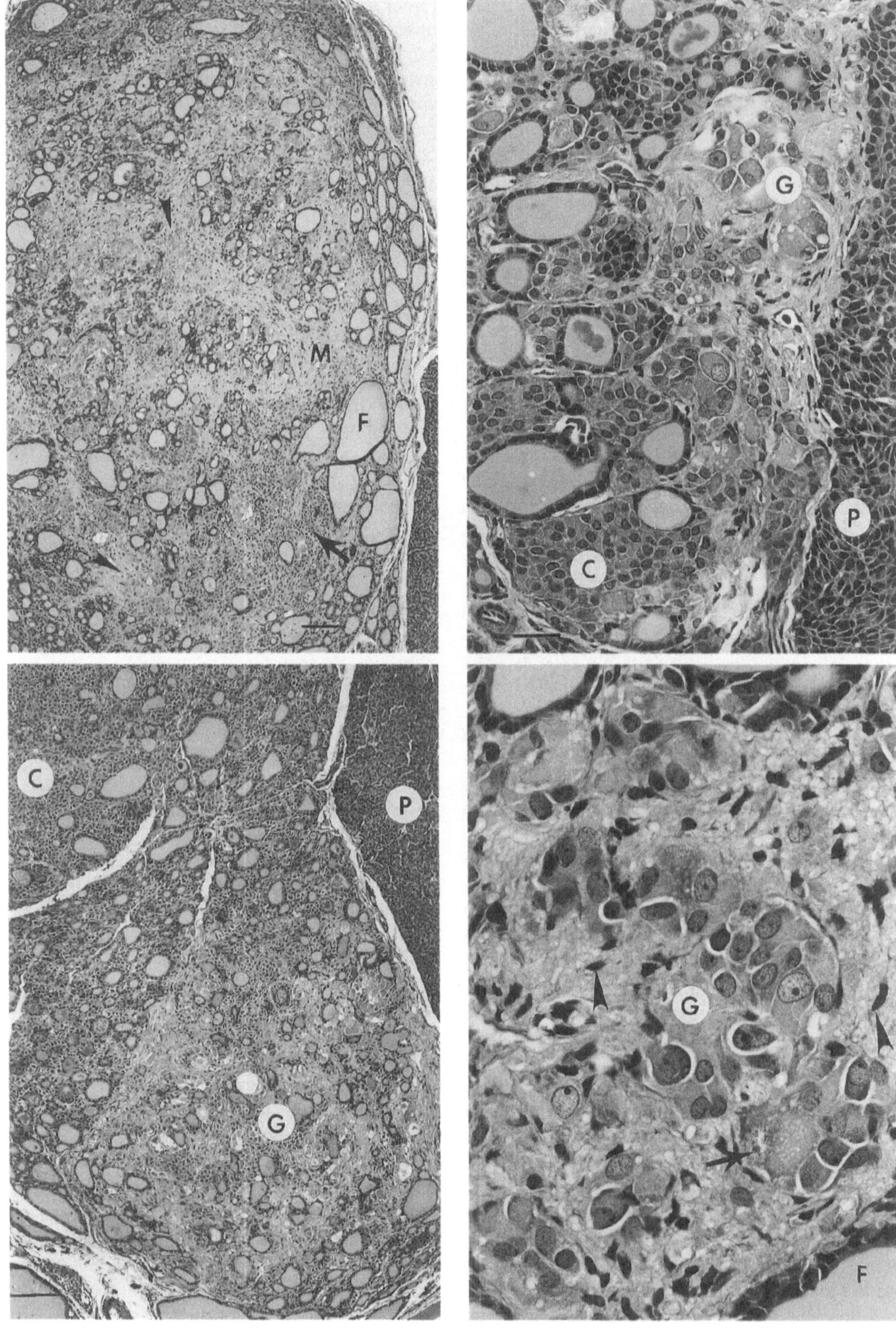
M
F
G
C
P
C
P
G
G
F

◄

Fig. 313. (*upper left*) Ganglioneuroma of the thyroid gland; 26-month-old female rat. Note isolated thyroid follicles (*F*), matrix (*M*), clusters of large ganglion cells (*arrowheads*), and area of smaller, primitive neuronal cells (*arrow*). *Bar*, 100 μm. H&E

Fig. 314. (*lower left*) Ganglioneuroma of the thyroid gland; 25-month-old male rat. A ganglioneuroma (*G*) of the thyroid gland adjacent to, and blending with, a C cell tumor (*C*). *P*, Parathyroid. *Bar*, 100 μm. H&E

Fig. 315. (*upper right*) Ganglioneuroma of the thyroid gland; 26-month-old female rat. Small ganglioneuroma (*G*) is adjacent to a focus of C cell hyperplasia (*C*) and parathyroid gland (*P*). *Bar*, 50 μm. H&E

Fig. 316. (*lower right*) Higher magnification of Fig. 313. A cluster of ganglion cells (*G*) is in the matrix with many Schwann cells (*arrowheads*). Degenerating ganglion cell (*arrow*) with cytoplasmic vacuolation and karyorrhexis. Thyroid follicle (*F*). *Bar*, 20 μm. H&E

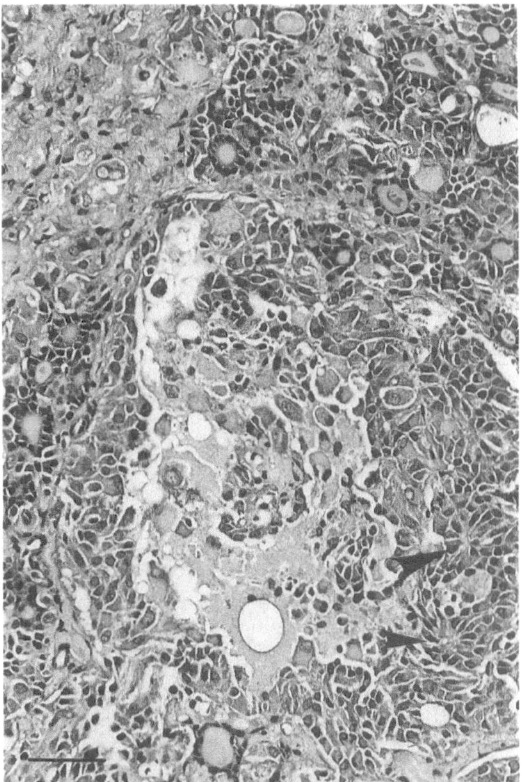

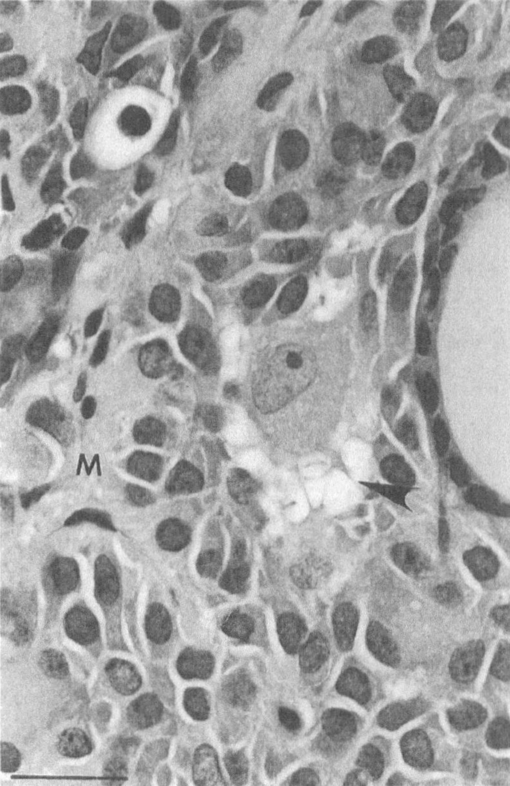

►

Fig. 317. (*above*) Ganglioneuroma of the thyroid gland; 24-month-old male rat. Ganglioneuroma with area of cystic degeneration. Adjacent smaller cells form rosettes (*arrowheads*). *Bar*, 50 μm. H&E

Fig. 318. (*below*) Higher magnification of Fig. 313 from the area of smaller cells. A large ganglion cell adjacent to a thyroid follicle is surrounded by smaller, more primitive neuronal cells. Note the long cell process (*arrowhead*). The matrix (*M*) is similar to the more differentiated areas of the neoplasm. *Bar*, 20 μm. H&E

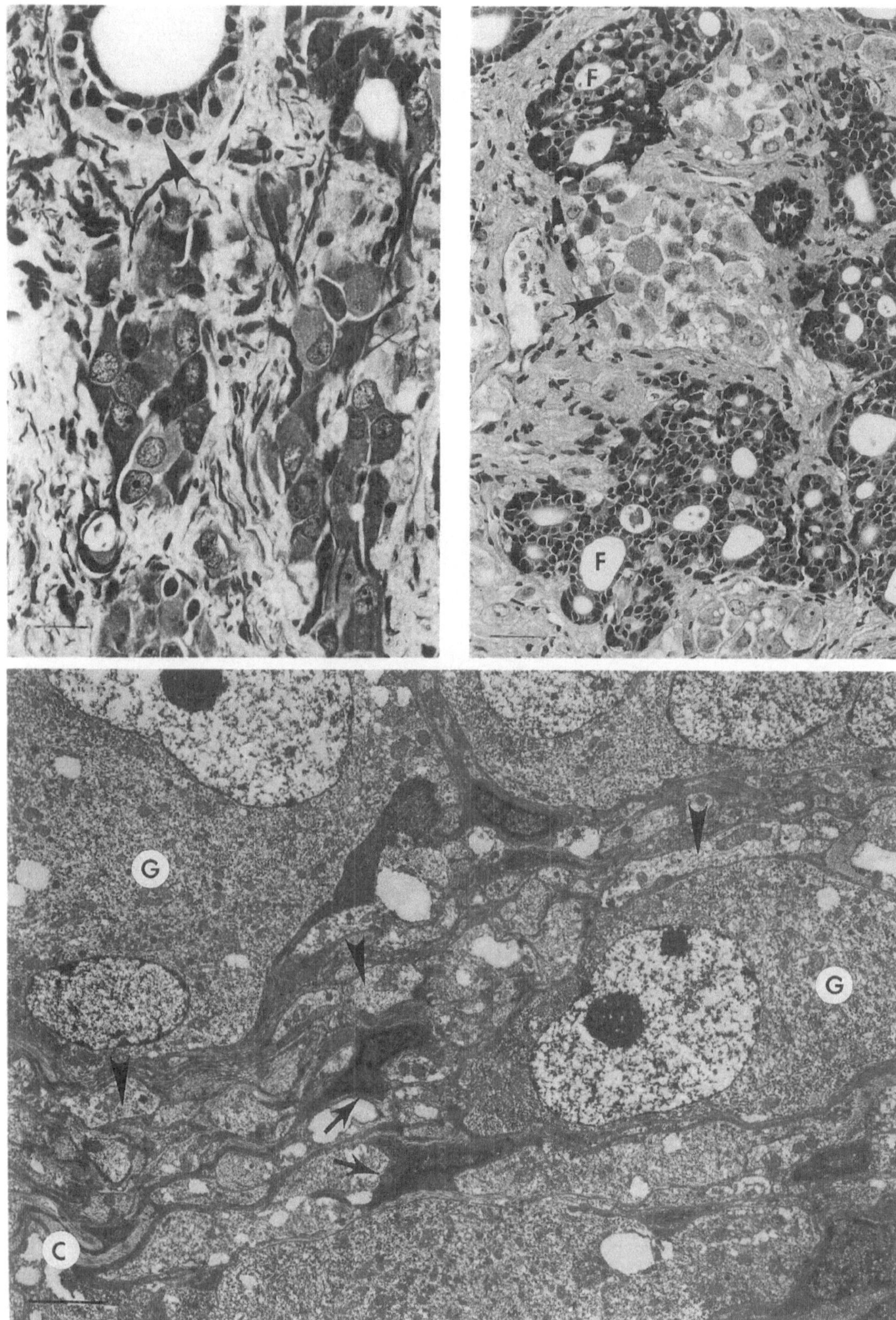
F
F
G
G
C

pheochromocytomas in F344 rats (Reznik et al. 1980) and may also be coincident in man (Alba et al. 1988). Some areas of such mixed tumors are of intermediate morphology, suggesting a common stem cell for the dimorphic components (Reznik et al. 1980). Ganglioneuromas and C cell proliferations of the thyroid may have a parallel relationship – and similar questions of cellular identity and lineage result.

Etiology. The high incidence that occurred in the two studies where these tumors were observed is unexplained. The incidence was unrelated to the presence of test compounds in the diet.

Frequency. Ganglioneuromas of the thyroid gland have not been reported except for the two studies performed at ICI Pharmaceuticals in the middle 1980s, described below, in which they were observed as common findings. This may be because Sprague-Dawley rats are an outbred stock; both genetic diversity and colony isolation contribute to genetic drift and divergence over many generations. The affected rats were from Hilltop Lab Animals' colony 23 (Scottdale, PA), this stock was derived from NIH Sprague-Dawley rats in 1982. Examination by the author of the thyroids of 127 Sprague-Dawley rats used as controls in 2-year studies conducted at the Dow Chemical Company (Midland, MI) during the middle to late 1970s revealed no ganglioneuromas – but these rats were only distantly related to the affected colony. In the two unrelated 2-year studies in which they occurred, a total of 52 ganglioneuromas were identified in the thyroid glands of 698 rats. Fifty rats (7.1%) were affected; of these, two rats, both control females, had bilateral ganglioneuromas. Of the 50 affected rats 58% were females and 42% males (not significant, χ^2 test, 95% confidence interval). An association with C cell proliferations (focal hyperplasias, adenomas, or carcinomas) was evident; 63.5% of the 52 ganglioneuromas were contiguous or mixed with a C cell proliferation. Another 17.3% had one or more noncontiguous C cell proliferations in the same or contralateral lobe. The total incidence of C cell proliferations in the 50 rats with ganglioneuroma was 80%, significantly greater (χ^2 test, 99% confidence level), than the overall incidence of 52.4% of rats with one or more C cell proliferations.

◄

Fig. 319. (*upper left*) Same ganglioneuroma as Fig. 313. Ganglion cell bodies are dark gray to black. Black fibers are neurites seen extending from ganglion cells and in the matrix. C cells (*arrowhead*) surround a thyroid follicle. *Bar*, 20 µm. Bielschowky's silver stain

Fig. 320. (*upper right*) Same ganglioneuroma as Fig. 316. C cells around trapped follicles (*F*) stain deeply for calcitonin. Ganglion cells (*arrowhead*) are negative. *Bar*, 50 µm. Immunohistochemical stain for calcitonin

Fig. 321. (*below*) Ganglioneuroma, thyroid, rat. Same case as Fig. 313. Several ganglion cells (*G*) with eccentric nuclei and dispersed neuclear chromatin. Numerous neuritic processes (*arrowheads*), Schwann's cells (*arrows*), and collagen (*C*) are present in the stromal band bisecting the figure. *Bar*, 3 µm. TEM

Comparison with Other Species

Ganglioneuromas of the thyroid gland have not been reported in any other species. However, they have been reported at other sites in several species including rats (Maekawa et al. 1984; Reznik et al. 1980; Reznik and Ward 1983a), cattle (Cimprich and Ardington 1975; Sokale and Ladds 1983), water buffalo (Gupta and Singh 1978), a puppy (Hawkins and Summers 1987), a kitten (Patnaik et al. 1978), and man (Hale et al. 1987; Russel and Rubinstein 1977; Triche 1989). Neuroblastomas are malignant tumors of similar histogenesis and have been diagnosed in cattle (Anderson and Cordy 1981), cats (Cox and Powers 1989), dog (Helman et al. 1980), rat adrenal gland (Reznik and Ward 1983b), and man (Triche 1989). Neuroblastomas of the adrenal gland are the most common tumors that cause abdominal masses in young children (Cotran et al. 1989), and in some cases in very young children they may spontaneously differentiate to ganglioneuromas without persistent blastic elements (Bolande 1979; Triche 1989).

References

Anderson BC, Cordy DR (1981) Olfactory neuroblastoma in a heifer. Vet Pathol 18:536–540

Alba M, Hirayama A, Ito Y, Fujimoto Y, Nakagami Y, Demura H, Shizume K (1988) A compound adrenal medullary tumor (pheochromocytoma and ganglioneuroma) and a cortical adenoma in the ipsilateral adrenal gland. Am J Surg Pathol 12:559–566

Bolande RP (1979) Developmental pathology. Am J Pathol 94:627–683

Cimprich R, Ardington P (1975) Spinal ganglioneuroma in a steer. Vet Pathol 12:59–60

Cotran RS, Kumar V, Robbins SL (1989) The pathologic basis of disease, 4th edn. Saunders, Philadelphia, pp 1262–1268
Cox NR, Powers RD (1989) Olfactory neuroblastomas in two cats. Vet Pathol 26:341–343
Crissman JW, Valerio MG, Asiedu SA, Evangelista-Sobel I (1991) Ganglioneuromas of the thyroid gland in a colony of Sprague-Dawley rats. Vet Pathol 28:354–362
Gupta PP, Singh B (1978) Ocular ganglioneuroma in Indian water buffaloes (Bubalus bubalis). Vet Pathol 15:138–139
Hale PJ, Suarez V, Williams A, Baddeley RM, Nattrass M (1987) Insulinoma and ganlioneuroma. Br J Surg 74:1183
Hawkins KL, Summers BA (1987) Mediastinal ganglioneuroma in a puppy. Vet Pathol 24:283–285
Helman RG, Adams LG, Hall CL, Read WK (1980) Metastatic neuroblastoma in a dog. Vet Pathol 17:769–773
Jones EG, Cowan WM (1983) The nervous tissue. In: Weiss L (ed) Histology: cell and tissue biology, 5th edn. Elsevier, New York, pp 282–370
LiVolsi VA (1980) Calcitonin: the hormone and its significance. In: Fenoglio CM, Wolff M (eds) Progress in surgical pathology, vol 1. Masson, New York, pp 71–103
Maekawa A, Onodera H, Tanigawa H, Furuta K, Takahashi M, Kurokawa Y, Kokubo T, Ogiu T, Uchida O, Kobayashi K, Hayashi Y (1984) Spontaneous tumors of the nervous system and associated organs and/or tissues in rats. Gann 75:784–791
Patnaik AK, Lieberman PH, Johnson GF (1978) Intestinal ganglioneuroma in a kitten – a case report and review of the literature. J Small Anim Pract 19:735–742
Pearse AGE (1986) The diffuse neuroendocrine system: peptides, amines, placodes and the APUD theory. In: Hokfelt T, Fuxe, K, Pernow B (eds) Progress in brain research, vol 68. Elsevier, New York, pp 25–31
Reznik G, Ward JM (1983a) Ganglioneuroma, adrenal, rat. In: Jones TC, Mohr U, Hunt RD (eds) ILSI monographs on pathology of laboratory animals. Endocrine system. Springer, Berlin Heidelberg New York, pp 30–34
Reznik G, Ward JM (1983b) Neuroblastoma, adrenal, rat. In: Jones TC, Mohr U, Hunt RD (eds) ILSI Monographs on pathology of laboratory animals. Endocrine system. Springer, Berlin Heidelberg New York, pp 35–37
Reznik G, Ward JM, Reznik-Schuller (1980) Ganglioneuromas in the adrenal medulla of F344 rats. Vet Pathol 17: 614–621
Russel DS, Rubinsein LJ (1977) Ganglioneuromas. In: Russell DS, Rubinstein LJ (eds) Pathology of tumours of the nervous system, 4th edn. Williams and Wilkins, Baltimore, pp 417–424
Sokale EO, Ladds PW (1983) Multicentric ganglioneuroma in a steer. Vet Pathol 20:767–770
Tice LW (1983) The thyroid gland. In: Weiss L (ed) Histology, cell and tissue biology, 5th edn. Elsevier, New York, pp 1090–1101
Triche TJ (1989) Tumors of the neuroendocrine (APUD) system. In: Schuller HM (ed) Comparative ultrastructural pathology of selected tumors in man and animals. CRC Press, Boca Raton, pp 133–196

Lymphocytic Thyroiditis, Rat

George E. Sandusky and Glen C. Todd

Synonyms. Autoimmune thyroiditis, immune complex thyroiditis, Hashimoto's thyroiditis, lymphadenoid goiter.

Gross Appearance

The gross appearance varies with the stage of the disease. The thyroid glands may not appear abnormal when only minimally involved. However, if there is considerable lymphocytic infiltration, the glands are symmetrically enlarged and the cut surfaces are pale. The thyroids may weigh up to ten times their normal weight. The capsule is intact and usually smooth, but can be lobulated.

Microscopic Features

The thyroid glands have a multifocal to diffuse infiltration of lymphocytes, plasma cells, and macrophages (Fig. 322). The degree of cellular infiltration varies, but eventually becomes diffuse with secondary lymphoid follicle formation. The thyroid follicles become compressed, with reduced size and depletion of colloid. The epithelial cells are large and appear hyperplastic. Some follicles may be atrophic, while others may have degenerative changes and infiltration of the epithelium with lymphocytes (Fig. 323). Fibrosis in uncommon.

Ultrastructure

Ultrastructural investigations confirm the findings described under microscopic features. Moderate electron-dense deposits in the basement membrane region, assumed to represent immune complexes, have been identified by immunofluorescence (Bigazzi and Rose 1975; Clagett et al. 1974; Kalderon et al. 1977; Kitchen et al. 1979). Plasma cells are present in the regions of these deposits.

Differential Diagnosis

The histopathologic diagnosis of lymphocytic thyroiditis is not difficult because of the characteristic infiltration of lymphoid cells. The morphologic appearance of spontaneous or experimentally induced lymphocytic thyroiditis is similar. The demonstration of circulating thyroid antibodies is confirmatory evidence. Autoantibodies to thyroglobulin are present, and immune complexes can be identified in the affected glands by immunofluorescence and immunocytochemistry. These studies strongly indicate that the disease process is autoimmune (Allison 1976; Gosselin et al. 1980; Kalderon and Bogaars 1977; Kitchen et al. 1979).

Biologic Features

Natural History. Most rats with spontaneous or experimentally induced lymphocytic thyroiditis have no clinical evidence of thyroid disease. However, thyroid function decreases slowly, and the decrease is often not recognized until the thyroiditis has been present for a considerable time. It is a slowly progressive disease with minimal effect on survival.

Pathogenesis and Etiology. Lymphocytic thyroiditis has been produced experimentally in guinea pigs, rats, hamsters, rabbits, monkeys, dogs, and baboons by immunization with thyroid antigens, usually thyroglobulin mixed with adjuvants (Volpe 1978). This disease has been produced in

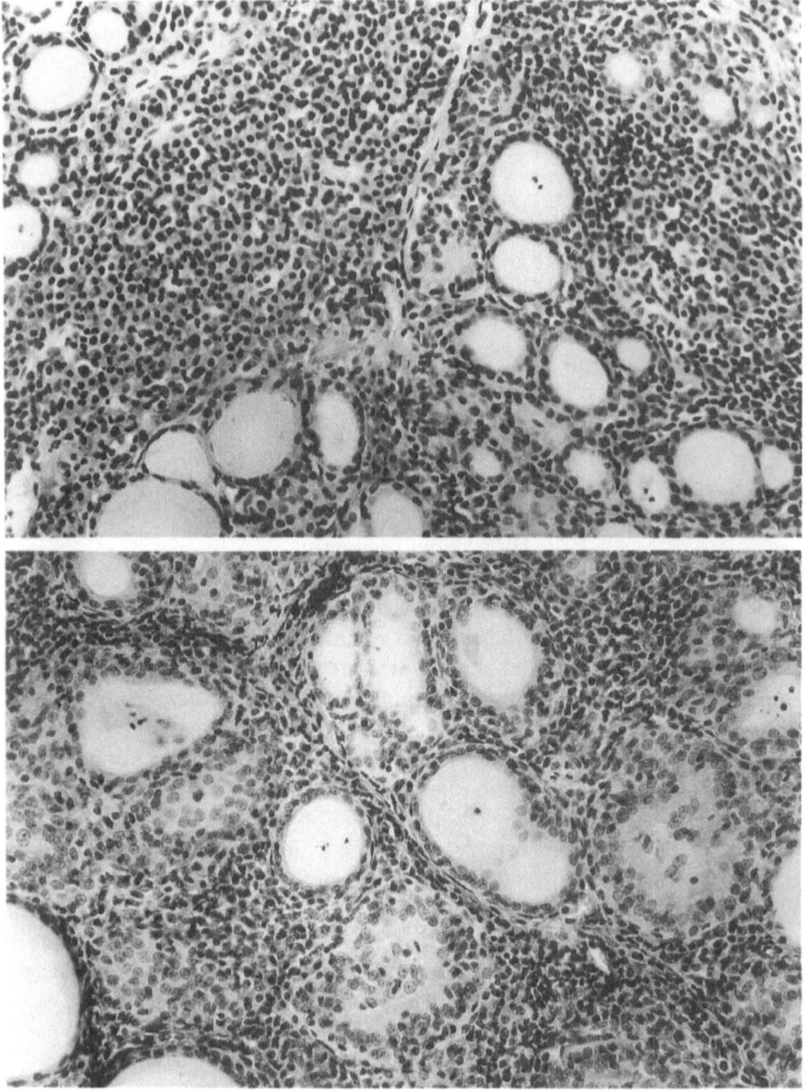

Fig. 322. (*above*) Lymphocytic thyroiditis, rat, with extensive infiltration of the interstitium and follicles by lymphocytes, plasma cells, and macrophages. The follicular epithelial cells are hyperplastic. ×125. H&E

Fig. 323. (*below*) Lymphocytic thyroiditis, rat. Loss of colloid and variation in the size of thyroid follicles; follicular cells hyperplastic in some follicles. ×125. H&E

rats by administration of chemicals (Kitchen et al. 1979; Reuber and Glover 1976; Silverman and Rose 1971, 1975) and by thymectomy and irradiation (Penhale and Ahmed 1982). Spontaneous lymphocytic thyroiditis has been reported in chickens, rats, beagle dogs, monkeys, *Mastomys*, and man (Bigazzi and Rose 1975; Gosselin et al. 1981; Solleveld 1981).

Considerable evidence has been accumulated which indicates that lymphocytic thyroiditis is the prototype of autoimmune disease. However, there are several factors which can influence the development of the disease, such as heredity, active thymus, age, and sex. The role of genetic factors has been identified in chickens (Rose et al. 1973), rats (Bigazzi and Rose 1975), mice (Kojima et al. 1976; Wick et al. 1978), and man (Volpe 1978). The incidence of spontaneous lymphocytic thyroiditis can be greatly increased by selective inbreeding in animals. The best example of this is the establishment of the Obese strain of White Leghorn chickens, which originally had an incidence of 1% in females but now has greater than a 90% incidence in both sexes (Bigazzi and Rose 1975). Neonatal thymectomy increases the incidence and severity of lymphocytic thyroiditis in rats, mice, an chickens (Kojima et al. 1976; Penhale and Ahmed 1982; Rose 1975). Young rats given an immunosuppressive compound developed a 50% incidence of lymphocytic thyroiditis (Kitchen et al. 1979). Cyclosporin A completely inhibited the development of lymphocytic thyroiditis in the BB/W or rat (Jaworski et al. 1986).

Thyroglobulin or microsomal antibodies have been present in the blood of nearly all human and animal cases. Cellular destruction has been thought to be related to a dysfunction of suppressor T lymphocytes allowing helper T lymphocytes to stimulate production of cytotoxic autoantibodies against thyroid tissue (Rallison 1987). Recent data in the BB/W or rat, Obese strain chicken, hamster, and man has shown that the level of iodine intake is the one predisposing factor which leads to the development of lymphocytic thyroiditis (Allen et al. 1986a; Allen and Bravennan 1990; Bagchi et al. 1985). In the BB/W or rat the level of iodine intake in the diet influences the rate of development of lymphocytic thyroiditis (Allen et al. 1986a). It has been demonstrated that excess iodine ingestion for 2 months increased the incidence of lymphocytic thyroiditis in young BB/W or rats while low iodine ingestion decreased the incidence (Allen et al. 1986a). Further research has shown that methimazole and L-thyroxine decreased the incidence of lymphocytic thyroiditis in control BB/W rats, but did not effect the progression of iodine induced disease (Allen et al. 1986a; Reinhardt et al. 1988; Braverman et al. 1987; Banovac et al. 1988). Daily doses of interleukin-1β accelerated the onset of lymphocytic thyroiditis in genetically prone BB/Wor rats (Vertrees et al. 1991).

Recent studies in the BB/Wor rat indicated that iodine increased the number of dendritic cells in the early stages of the disease process. This was followed by the appearance of activated T lymphocytes, many of which were T helper cells. Ia antigen positivity was a late finding in the disease and associated with thyrocytes adjacent to large lymphocytic aggregations (Li et al. 1993). Dendritic cells have also been seen in increased numbers in Hashimoto's thyroiditis in man (Kabel et al. 1988). It is likely that dendritic cells may transport autoantigens to the draining lymph node of the thyroid to initiate the immune response (Knight et al. 1988). It is still uncertain whether the effects of iodine on antigen presenting cells is a direct effect on dendritic cells and T helper lymphocytes, or whether iodine is directly toxic to organelles in the thyroid follicular cells.

Frequency. Common strains of rats usually have less than a 1% incidence of spontaneous lymphocytic thyroiditis. However, the Buffalo strain has a 48% incidence at 30 months of age (Bigazzi and Rose 1975).

Comparison with Other Species

Spontaneous or experimental lymphocytic thyroiditis in rats and other experimental species mimics the clinical, immunologic, and pathophysiologic features of lymphocytic (Hashimoto's) thyroiditis in human beings.

References

Allen EM, Bravennan LE (1990) The effect of iodine on lymphocytic thyroiditis in the thymectomized buffalo rat. Endocrinology 127:1613-1616

Allen EM, Appel MC, Braverman LE (1986a) The effect of iodine ingestion on the development of spontaneous lymphocytic thyroiditis in the diabetes-prone BB/W rat Endocrinology 118:1977-1981

Allen EM, Rajatanavin R, Nogimori T, Cushing G, Ingbar SH, Braverman, LE (1986b) The effect of methimazole on the development of spontaneous lymphocytic thyroiditis in the diabetes-prone BB/W rat. Am J Med Sci 292:267-271

Allison AC (1976) Self-tolerance and autoimmunity in the thyroid. N Engl J Med 295:821-827

Bagchi N, Brown TR, Urdanivia E (1985) Induction of autoimmune thyroiditis in chickens by dietary iodine. Science 230:325-327

Banovac K, Ghandur-Mnaymneh L, Zakarija M, Rabinovitch A, McKenzie JM (1988) The effect of thyroxine on spontaneous thyroiditis in BB/W rats. Int Arch Allergy Appl Immunol 87:301-305

Bigazzi PR, Rose NR (1975) Spontaneous autoimmune thyroiditis in animals as a model of human disease. Prog Allergy 19:245-274

Braverman LE, Paul T, Reinhardt W, Appel MC, Allen EM (1987) Effect of iodine intake and methimazole on lymphocytic thyroiditis in the BB/W rat. Acta Endocrinol (Copenh) [Suppl] 281:70-76

Clagett JA, Wilson CB, Weigle WO (1974) Interstitial immune complex thyroiditis in mice. The role of antibody to thyroglobulin. J Exp Med 140:1439–1456

Gosselin SJ, Capen CC, Martin SL, Targowski SP (1980) Biochemical and immunological investigations on hypothyroidism in dogs. Can J Comp Med 44:158–168

Gosselin SJ, Capen CC, Martin SL (1981) Histologic and ultrastructural evaluation of thyroid lesions associated with hypothyroidism in dogs. Vet Pathol 18:299–309

Jaworski MA, Honore L, Jewell LD, Mehta JG, McGuire-Clark P, Schouls JJ, Yap WY (1986) Cyclosporin prophylaxis induces long-term prevention of diabetes, and inhibits lymphocytic infiltration in multiple target tissues in the high-risk BB rat. Diabetes Res 3:1–6

Kabel PJ, Voorbij HA, de Hann M, van der Gaag RD, Drexhage HA (1988) Intrathyroidal dendritic cells. J Clin Endocrinol Metab 65:199–207

Kalderon AE, Bogaars HA (1977) Immune complex deposits in Graves-disease and Hashimoto's thyroiditis. Am J Med 63:729–734

Kalderon AE, Bogaars HA, Jolly G, Diamond I (1977) Electron-dense deposits in the follicular basal lamina of obese strain chickens with spontaneous hereditary autoimmune thyroiditis. Lab Invest 37:487–496

Kitchen DN, Todd GC, Meyers DB, Paget C (1979) Rat lymphocytic thyroiditis associated with ingestion of an immunosuppressive compound. Vet Pathol 16:722–729

Knight SC, Farrant J, Chan J, Bryant A, Bedford PA Bateman C (1988) Induction of autoimmunity with dendritic cells: studies on thyroiditis mice. Clin Immunol Immunopathol 48:277–289

Kojima A, Tanaka-Kojima Y, Sakakura T, Nishizuka Y (1976) Spontaneous development of autoimmune thyroiditis in neonatally thymectomized mice. Lab Invest 34:550–557

Li M, Eastman CJ, Boyages SC (1993) Iodine induced lymphocytic thyroiditis in the BB/W rat: early and late immune phenomena. Autoimmunity 14:181–187

Penhale WJ, Ahmed SA (1982) Animal model of human disease. Lymphocytic thyroiditis. Autoimmune thyroiditis in rats induced by thymectomy and irradiation. Am J Pathol 106:300–302

Rallison L (1987) Chronic lymphocytic (autoimmune) thyroiditis in children. Wien Klin Wochenschr 99:289–294

Reinhardt W, Paul TL, Allen EM, Alex S, Yang YN, Appel MC, Braverman LE (1988) Effect of L-thyroxine on the incidence of iodine induced and spontaneous lymphocytic thyroiditis in the BB/Wor rat. Endocrinology 122:1179–1181

Reuber MD, Glover EL (1976) Role of age and sex in chronic thyroiditis in rats fed 3-methyl-4-dimethylaminoazobenzene. Vet Pathol 13:295–302

Rose NR (1975) The role of the thymus in spontaneous autoimmune thyroiditis. Ann NY Acad Sci 249:116–124

Rose NR, Kite JH Jr, Vladutiu AO, Tomazic V, Bacon LD (1973) Genetic aspects of autoimmune thyroiditis. Int Arch Allergy Appl Immunol 45:138–149

Silverman DA, Rose NR (1971) Autoimmunity in methylcholanthrene-induced and spontaneous thyroiditis in Buffalo strain rats. Proc Soc Exp Biol Med 138:579–584

Silverman DA, Rose NR (1975) Spontaneous and methylcholanthrene-enhanced thyroiditis in BUF rats. J Immunol 114:148–150

Solleveld HA (1981) Praomys (Mastomys) natalensis in aging research with emphasis on autoimmune phenomena. Public Institute for Experimental Gerontology, TNO, Rijswijk

Vertrees S, Wilson CA, Ubungen R, Wilson D, Baskin DG, Toivola B, Jacobs C, Boiani N, Baker P, Lemmark A (1991) Interleukin-1 beta regulation of islet and thyroid autoimmunity in the BB rat. J Autoimmun 4:717–732

Volpe R (1978) Lymphocytic (Hashimoto's) thyroiditis. In: Wemer SC, Ingbar SH (eds) The thyroid. Harper and Row, New York, pp 996–1008

Wick G, Schwarz S, Muller PU (1978) No development of experimental autoimmune thyroiditis in nude mice. Z Immunitatsforsch Immunobiol 154:162–168

Parathyroids

Pathobiology of Parathyroid Gland Structure and Function in Animals

Charles C. Capen

Introduction

Calcium plays a key role in many fundamental biologic processes and is also an essential structural component of the skeleton. These processes include neuromuscular excitability, membrane permeability, muscle contraction, enzyme activity, hormone release, blood coagulation. The precise control of calcium in extracellular fluids is vital to health. To maintain a constant concentration of calcium, despite marked variations in intake and excretion, endocrine control mechanisms have evolved that consist primarily of the interactions of three major hormones: parathyroid hormone (PTH), calcitonin (CT), and cholecalciferol (vitamin D). This chapter summarizes recent advances in the pathobiology of parathyroid glands and selected disease problems in animals associated with perturbation of parathyroid structure and function in animals.

Functional Cytology of Parathyroid Gland

Parathyroid glands are composed of a single cell type concerned with the biosynthesis of one hormone (Fig. 324). Chief cells have a normal secretory cycle, with the majority being in the inactive stage under steady-state conditions. In response to a low calcium ion signal, chief cells enter the active phase with synthesis and packaging of a "batch" of hormone. After secretion of PTH the chief cell involutes back to the resting (inactive) phase. In response to long-term stimulation chief cells undergo a sequence of morphologic changes culminating in the formation of water-clear cells. Conversely, long-term suppression by elevated blood calcium ion results in parathyroids with predominantly inactive and atrophic chief cells. Mitochondrion-rich oxyphil cells form in parathyroids of humans and certain animal species with advancing age. Synthetic and secretory organelles are largely crowded out by the proliferation of mitochondria in the cytoplasm, suggesting that oxyphil cells are not actively involved in the biosynthesis of PTH.

Chief cells that are interpreted to be in an inactive (resting or involuted) stage predominate in the parathyroid glands under normal conditions. Inactive chief cells are cuboidal and have uncomplicated interdigitations between contiguous cells. The relatively electron-transparent cytoplasm contains poorly developed organelles and infrequent secretory granules. The cytoplasm often has either numerous lipid bodies and lipofuscin granules or aggregations of glycogen particles. Chief cells in the active stage occur less frequently in the parathyroid glands of most species. The cytoplasm of active chief cells has an increased electron density due to the close proximity of organelles and secretory granules, increased density of the cytoplasmic matrix, and loss of glycogen particles and lipid bodies.

The second cell type in the parathyroid glands of certain animal species and human beings is the oxyphil cell (Fig. 324). They are absent in parathyroids of the rat, chicken, and many species of lower animals. Oxyphil cells are observed either singly or in small groups interspersed between chief cells. They are larger than chief cells and their abundant cytoplasmic area is filled with numerous large, often bizarrely shaped mitochondria. Glycogen particles and free ribosomes are interspersed between the mitochondria. Granular endoplasmic reticulum, Golgi apparatuses, and secretory granules are poorly developed in oxyphil cells of normal parathyroid glands, suggesting that oxyphil cells do not have an active function in the biosynthesis of PTH. Oxyphil cells have been shown histochemically to have a higher oxidative and hydrolytic enzyme activity than chief cells, associated with the marked increase in mitochondria.

Cells are observed with cytoplasmic characteristics intermediate between those of chief and oxyphil cells. These transitional oxyphil cells have numerous mitochondria, but other organelles are present including rough endoplasmic reticulum, Golgi apparatuses, and secretory granules. The significance of oxyphil cells in the pathophysiology of the parathyroid glands has not been elucidated completely. They are not altered in response to either short-term hypocalcemia or hypercalcemia in animals, but both oxyphil cells and transitional forms may be increased in response to long-term stimulation of human parathyroid glands. There-

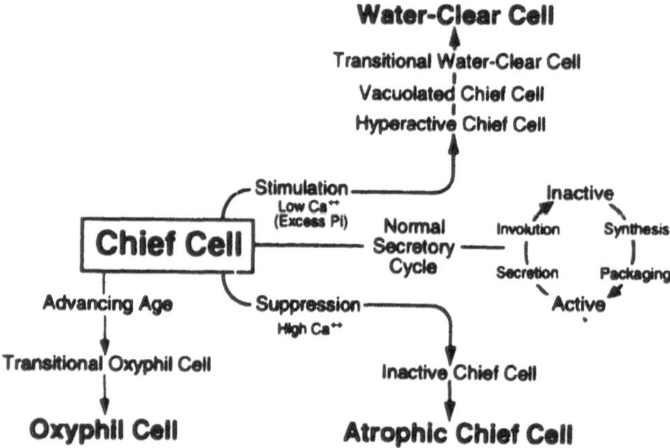

Fig. 324. Functional cytology of parathyroid gland under normal and pathologic conditions

fore oxyphil cells do not appear to be degenerate chief cells, as previously suggested, but rather are derived from chief cells as the result of aging or some other metabolic derangement.

Biosynthesis of Parathyroid Hormone by Chief Cells

Parathyroid chief cells in humans and many animal species store relatively small amounts of preformed hormone but respond quickly to variations in need for hormone by changing the rate of synthesis. PTH, as with many peptide hormones is first synthesized as a larger biosynthetic precursor molecule that undergoes post-translational processing in chief cells. PreproPTH is the initial translation product synthesized on ribosomes of the rough endoplasmic reticulum in chief cells. It is composed of 115 amino acids and contains a hydrophobic signal or leader sequence of 25 amino acid residues that facilitates the penetration and subsequent vectorial discharge of the nascent peptide into the cisternal space of the rough endoplasmic reticulum (Kronenberg et al. 1986). PreproPTH is rapidly converted within 1 min or less of its synthesis to proPTH by the proteolytic cleavage of 25 amino acids from the NH_2-terminal end of the molecule (Habener 1981). The intermediate precursor, proPTH, is composed of 90 amino acids and moves within membranous channels of the rough endoplasmic reticulum to the Golgi apparatus (Fig. 325). Enzymes within membranes of the Golgi apparatus cleave a hexapeptide from the NH_2-terminal (biologically active) end of the molecule forming active PTH (Fig. 325). Active PTH is packaged into membrane-limited, macromolecular aggregates in the Golgi apparatus for subsequent storage in chief cells. Under certain conditions of increased demand (i.e., low calcium ion concentration in extracellular fluid com-

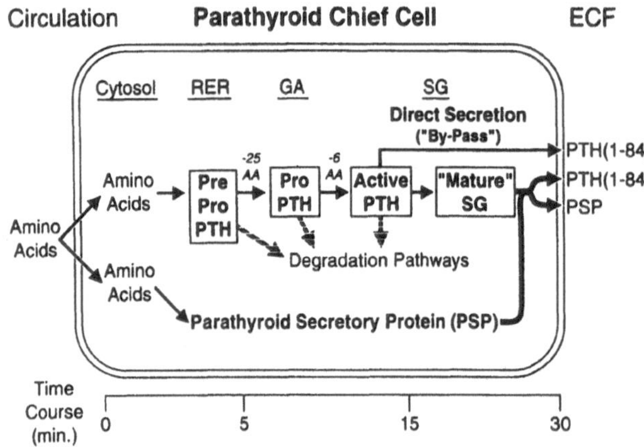

Fig. 325. Biosynthesis of parathyroid hormone (*PTH*) and parathyroid secretory protein (*PSP*) by chief cells. Preproparathyroid hormone (*preproPTH*) is the initial translation product from ribosomes of the rough endoplamic reticulum, which is rapidly converted to proparathyroid hormone (*ProPTH*). Active PTH either is stored in the cytosol as mature secretory granules (*SG*) or may be secreted directly from chief cells (*"By-pass"*). Chief cells also synthesize another protein designated parathyroid secretory protein, which is incorporated into secretory granules along with active PTH. PSP is released in parallel with PTH by a low calcium ion concentration in extracellular fluids

partment), PTH may be released directly from chief cells without being packaged into secretion granules by a process termed "bypass secretion." Although the principal form of active PTH secreted from chief cells is a straight chain peptide of 84 amino acids (molecular weight 9500), the molecule is rapidly cleaved into amino- and carboxy-terminal fragments in the peripheral circulation and especially in the liver. The purpose of this fragmentation is uncertain since the biologically active amino-terminal fragment is no more active than the entire PTH molecule (1-84). The plasma half-life of the N-terminal fragment is considerably shorter than that of the biologically inactive carboxy-terminal fragment of PTH. The C-terminal and other portions of the PTH molecule are degraded primarily in the kidney and tend to accumulate with chronic renal disease. The immunoheterogeneity caused by the multiple circulating fragments of PTH created significant problems in the development and application of highly specific radioimmunoassays to diagnostic problems in human patients and experimental animals (Goltzman et al. 1986).

Control of Parathyroid Hormone Secretion

Secretory cells in the parathyroid gland store small amounts of preformed hormone but are capable of responding to minor fluctuations in calcium concentration by rapidly altering the rate of hormonal secretion and more slowly by altering the rate of hormonal synthesis (Roth and Raisz 1964). In contrast to most endocrine organs that are under complex controls involving both long and short feedback loops, the parathyroids have a unique feedback controlled by the concentration of calcium (and to a lesser extent magnesium) ion in serum. If the blood calcium is elevated by the intravenous infusion of calcium, there is a rapid and pronounced reduction in circulating levels of immunoreactive PTH (iPTH). Conversely, if the blood calcium is lowered by ethylenediaminetetraacetic acid (EDTA), there is a brisk and substantial increase in iPTH levels.

The concentration of blood phosphorus has no direct regulatory influence on the synthesis and secretion of PTH; however, several disease conditions with hyperphosphatemia in both animals and man are associated clinically with secondary hyperparathyroidism. An elevated blood phosphorus level may lead indirectly to parathyroid stimulation by virtue of its ability to lower blood calcium. If the blood phosphorus is elevated significantly by an infusion of phosphate and calcium administered simultaneously in amounts to prevent the accompanying reduction of blood calcium, plasma iPTH levels remain within the normal range. Magnesium ion has an effect on parathyroid secretion ratmilar to that of calcium, but its effect is not equipotent to that of calcium (Mayer and Hurst 1978). The more potent effects of calcium ion in the control of PTH secretion, together with its preponderance over magnesium in the extracellular fluid, suggests a secondary role for magnesium ion in parathyroid control.

Calcium ion not only controls the rate of biosynthesis and secretion of PTH, but also other metabolic and intracellular degradative processes within chief cells (Chu et al. 1973). An increase in calcium ions in extracellular fluids rapidly inhibits the uptake of amino acids by chief cells, synthesis of proPTH and conversion to PTH, and secretion of stored PTH. A shift in the percentage of flow of proPTH from the degradative pathway to the secretory route represents a key adaptive response of the parathyroid gland to a low-calcium diet. Parathyroids from rats fed a low-calcium (0.02%) diet convert approximately 40% of proPTH to PTH, compared to a 20% conversion in rats fed a control diet (normal calcium; Chu et al. 1973). During periods of long-term calcium restriction the enhanced synthesis and secretion of PTH would be accomplished by an increased capacity of the entire pathway in individual hypertrophied chief cells and through hyperplasia of active chief cells. Degradation of "mature PTH" by lysosomal enzymes increases after prolonged exposure to a high calcium environment.

Recently synthesized and processed active PTH may be released directly after passing through the Golgi complex, most likely in small vesicles, in response to increased demand and bypass the storage pool of mature secretory granules in the cytoplasm of chief cells. Bypass secretion of PTH can be stimulated only by a low circulating concentration of calcium ion whereas beta agonists as well as low calcium can mobilize PTH stored in secretory granules (Fig. 326).

Parathyroid chief cells have several adaptive responses to hypocalcemia, which otherwise would be life-threatening. The first is bypass

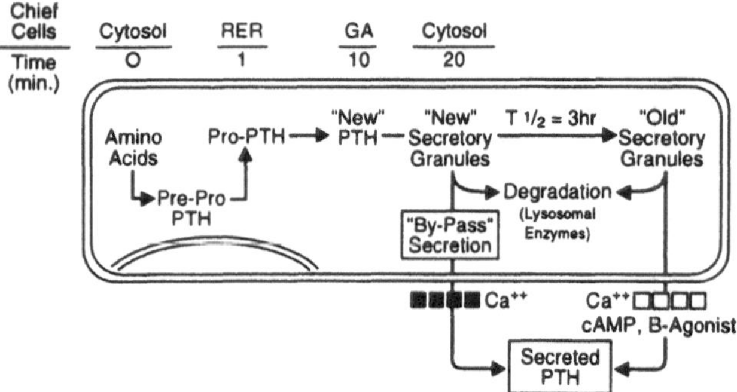

Fig. 326. Bypass secretion of parathyroid hormone in response to increased demand signaled by decreased blood calcium ion concentration. Recently synthesized and progressed active PTH (1-84) may be released directly and not enter the storage pool of mature (*"old"*) secretory granules in the cytoplasm of chief cells. PTH from the storage pool can be mobilized by cyclic adenosine monophosphate (*cAMP*) and β (*B*) agonists (such as epinephrine, norepinephrine, and isoproterenol) as well as by lowered blood calcium ion, whereas secretion from the pool of recently synthesized PTH can be stimulated only by a decreased calcium ion concentration. *RER*, Rough endoplasmic reticulum; *GA*, Golgi apparatus. (Redrawn from Cohn and MacGregor 1981)

secretion of PTH in response to a low calcium ion signal. The second is to increase the efficiency of conversion of inactive proPTH into active PTH and its subsequent release from chief cells. This process under normal conditions is quite inefficient and therefore provides a point of regulation in response to increased demand for hormone. Longer term adaptive responses to hypocalcemia are the result of hypertrophy and hyperplasia of parathyroid chief cells.

Chief cells synthesize and secrete another major protein termed "parathyroid secretory protein (I)" or chromogranin A. It is a higher molecular weight molecule (70 kDa) composed of 430–448 amino acids that is costored and secreted with PTH. A similar molecule has been found in secretory granules of a wide variety of hormone peptide-secreting cells and in neurotransmitter secretory vesicles. An internal region of the parathyroid secretory protein or chromogranin A molecule is identical in sequence to pancreastatin, a C-terminal amidated peptide that inhibits glucose-stimulated insulin secretion. This 49 amino acid proteolytic cleavage product (amino acids 240–280) of parathyroid secretory protein has been reported recently to inhibit low calcium stimulated secretion of PTH and chromogranin A from parathyroid cells. These findings suggest that chromogranin A derived peptides may act locally in an autocrine manner to inhibit the secretion of active hormone by endocrine cells, such as those of the parathyroid gland (Barbosa et al. 1991; Fasciotto et al. 1990).

Biologic Actions of Parathyroid Hormone

PTH is the principal hormone involved in the minute-to-minute fine regulation of blood calcium in mammals. It exerts its biologic actions by directly influencing the function of target cells primarily in bone and kidney, and indirectly in the intestine to maintain plasma calcium at a level sufficient to ensure the optimal functioning of a wide variety of body cells. The action of PTH on bone is to mobilize calcium from skeletal reserves into extracellular fluids (Raisz and Kream 1983). The administration of PTH causes an initial decline followed by a sustained increase in circulating levels of calcium. This transitory decrease in blood calcium is considered to be the result of a sequestration of calcium-phosphate in bone and soft tissues. The subsequent increase in blood calcium results from an interaction of PTH with osteoblasts and osteoclasts in bone and increased tubular reabsorption of calcium in the kidney (High et al. 1981; Sutton and Dirks 1978).

Interaction of PTH with Target Cells in Bone. Osteoclasts appear to be primarily responsible for the catabolic action of PTH on bone by increasing bone resorption (Chambers 1980; Chambers et al. 1984; Wong 1986). PTH has been known for some time to stimulate an increased activity of preformed osteoclasts. This is interesting in light of recent findings which have failed to demonstrate specific receptors for PTH on osteoclasts; however, receptors were present on

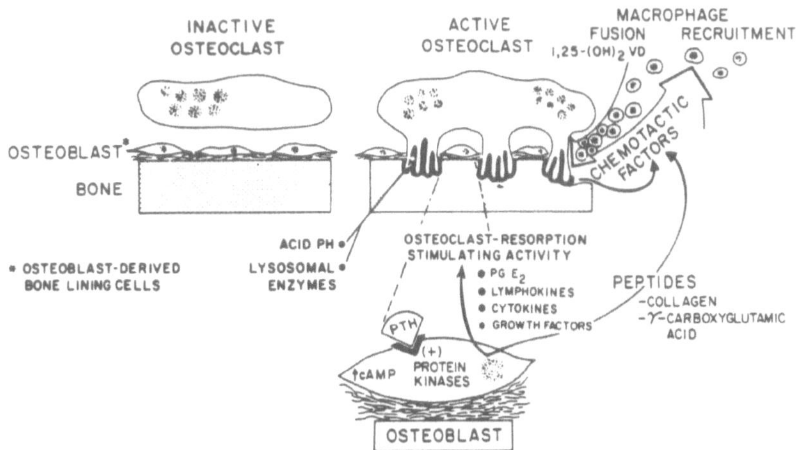

Fig. 327. Paracrine control of bone resorption. Specific receptors for parathyroid hormone are present on osteoblasts but not osteoclasts

osteoblasts (Pliam et al. 1982; Silve et al. 1982). Isolated osteoclasts do not respond to PTH without the concurrent presence of osteoblasts (McSheehy and Chambers 1986).

The mechanisms by which binding of PTH to osteoblasts results in stimulation of osteoblastic secretory products which are capable of stimulating osteoclastic bone resorption is not known but may include direct effects on the osteoblast and/or stimulation of osteoclastic secretory products capable of stimulating osteoblastic bone resorption (Fig. 327; Vaes 1988). If the increase in PTH is sustained, the size of the active osteoclast pool in bone is increased by activation of osteoprogenitor cells in the endosteal bone cell envelope.

The initial binding of PTH to osteoblasts lining bone surfaces appears to cause the cells to contract thereby exposing the underlying mineral to osteoclasts (Fig. 327; Rodan and Martin 1981). The change in shape of osteoblasts associated with PTH may be critical to mediation of osteoclastic bone resorption stimulated by the hormone. Osteoblastic contraction is associated with microfilament disaggregation (Wong 1986). The alteration in osteoblast shape exposes osteoid-covered bone matrix to osteoclasts; however, osteoclasts attach preferentially to mineralized bone matrix.

Osteoblasts secrete a latent collagenase and neutral proteases (such as plasminogen activator that can activate latent collagenase) which result in degradation of the osteoid matrix and exposes the underlying calcified matrix for osteoclastic bone resorption (Eeckhout et al. 1988). Bone-resorbing hormones such as PTH, prostaglandin E_2 (PGE_2), and 1,25-dihydroxyvitamin D stimulate plasminogen activator activity in osteoblasts. A collagenase inhibitor (Cl-1, an analogue of collagen α-chain sequence) can inhibit PTH-induced bone resorption (Delaisse et al. 1985). Bone-resorption products, particularly osteocalcin, can attract osteoclast precursors and enhance the resorption process.

Osteoblasts also may elaborate unidentified paracrine chemical mediators of osteoclastic bone resorption. None of the known bone-resorbing factors (PTH, PGE_2, lymphokines, growth factors) have been shown to directly stimulate osteoclasts without the presence of osteoblasts (de Vernejoul et al. 1988). The only substance that was found to stimulate bone resorption by isolated chicken osteoclasts in one investigation was murine splenic conditioned medium (de Vernejoul et al. 1988). Bone resorption by isolated osteoclasts is inhibited by calcitonin and PGE_2 which induce cAMP production in osteoclasts.

PTH stimulation of osteoblasts results in induction of bone resorption due to osteoclast activation and increased osteoclast numbers. The plasma membrane of osteoclasts in intimate contact with the resorbing surfaces is modified to form a series of membranous projections referred to as the brush ("ruffled") border. The brush border of activated osteoclasts is isolated from the extracellular fluids by adjacent transitional ("sealing") zones, thereby localizing the lysosomal enzymes and acidic environment to the immediate area undergoing dissolution. PTH and other bone-resorbing agents increase proteolytic, lysosomal, and acid-producing enzymes in osteoclasts which include acid phosphatase, β-glucuronidase, and carbonic anhydrase (Wong 1986). Carbonic anhydrase is localized to the brush border and induces acidification of the brush border area.

Binding of PTH to specific receptors on bone cells results in the activation of adenylate cyclase in the plasma membrane (Fig. 327). The adenylate cyclase catalyzes the conversion of ATP to cAMP in target cells. The accumulation of cAMP in target cells functions as an intracellular messenger of PTH action in osteoblasts. PTH also induces an increase in cytoplasmic calcium and stimulates phosphatidyl inositol turnover in osteoblasts; however, it has not been determined which intracellular messenger is required for induction of bone resorption by PTH stimulation of osteoblasts (Donahue et al. 1988; Farndale et al. 1988; Herrmann-Erlee et al. 1988). The increase in cytosolic calcium is partially dependent on cAMP accumulation. Calcium concentration in the osteoblast also may be increased by the activation of protein kinase C resulting in the production of inositol triphosphate and subsequent release of calcium from the endoplasmic reticulum (Yamaguchi et al. 1987).

Interaction of PTH with Target Cells in Kidney. PTH has a rapid (within 5–10 min) and direct effect on renal tubular function leading to decreased reabsorption of phosphate and phosphaturia (Knox and Haramati 1985). The site of PTH on blocking tubular reabsorption of phosphate has been localized by micropuncture methods to the proximal tubule of the nephron. Parathyroidectomy decreases renal phosphate excretion. PTH binds to a receptor on the basolateral aspect of renal epithelial cells. The hormone stimulates adenylate cyclase, increases intracellular cAMP, and inhibits phosphate reabsorption across the brush border through the actions of protein kinases. PTH also increases the transport of calcium across the basolateral renal cell membrane and increases intracellular calcium which inhibits the formation of cAMP, thus decreasing the phosphaturic effects of PTH (Beck et al. 1974; Knox and Haramati 1985). PTH is capable of stimulating inositol triphosphate and diacylglycerol production in renal tubular cells (Hruska et al. 1987). Therefore, regulation of phosphate transport by PTH may be mediated by two classes of receptors and transmembrane-signaling systems, one which activates adenylate cyclase and one which activates protein kinase C and increases intracellular calcium (Cole et al. 1987).

Although the effects of PTH on the tubular reabsorption of phosphate have been considered to be of major importance, evidence has accumulated indicating that the ability of PTH to enhance the reabsorption of calcium plays a considerable role in the maintenance of calcium homeostasis. This effect of PTH upon tubular reabsorption of calcium appears to be due to a direct action on the distal convoluted tubule (Sutton and Dirks 1978). The biochemical mechanism by which PTH enhances calcium reabsorption is unknown, but it is coupled to increases in intracellular cAMP (Hanai et al. 1986). There are two calcium active transport systems in the basolateral membrane of renal cells, a high-affinity calcium ATPase and a Na^+/Ca^{2+} exchanger.

The other important effect of PTH on the kidney is on the regulation of the conversion of 25-hydroxycholecalciferol to 1,25-dihydroxycholecalciferol and other metabolites of vitamin D. PTH has been shown to promote the absorption of calcium from the gastrointestinal tract in animals under a variety of experimental conditions (Norman 1986). This effect is not as rapid as the action on the kidney and is not observed in vitamin D deficient animals. The increase in intestinal calcium transport appears to be an indirect effect of PTH on absorptive cells by its action on stimulating synthesis of the biologically active metabolite of vitamin D by mitochondria in renal tubular epithelial cells (de Vernejoul et al. 1988). The effects of PTH on the metabolism of 25-hydroxycholecalciferol appear to be mediated by cAMP and not dependent on calcium ion concentration (Henry 1985). The active metabolites of vitamin D make bone cells more sensitive to the direct effects of PTH ("permissive effect") as well as greatly enhancing the gastrointestinal absorption of calcium, thereby amplifying the effect of PTH upon plasma calcium concentration. In addition, vitamin D metabolites exert negative feedback control on parathyroid chief cells at the level of transcription to decrease mRNA for preproPTH (Fig. 329). As blood levels of 1,25-dihydroxycholecalciferol are increased, and its action to increase intestinal calcium absorption the animal requires less PTH synthesis and

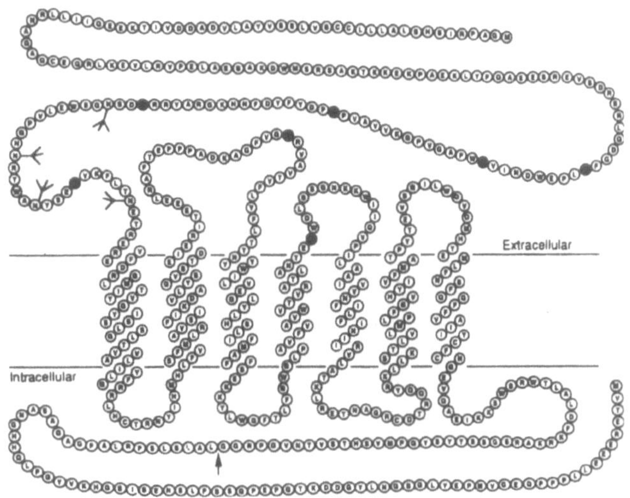

Fig. 328. PTH-PTHrP receptor (*at top*, NH_2 terminus) cloned and sequenced from cDNA isolated from kidney cells. *Y*, Potential N-glycosylation sites; •, cysteine residues conserved in the calcitonin receptor. (From Jüppner et al. 1991)

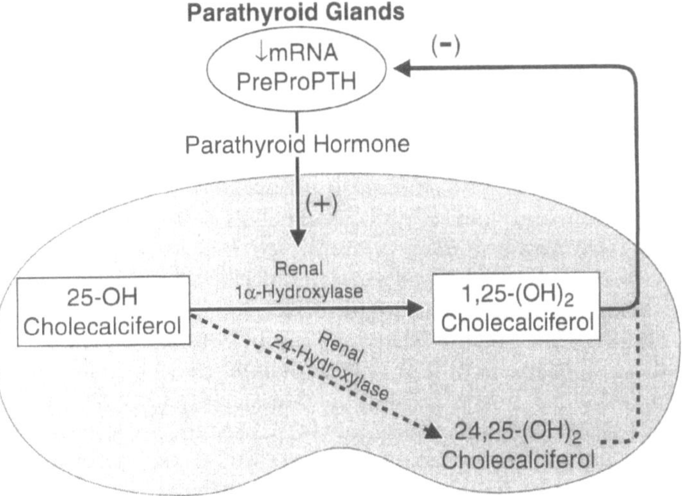

Fig. 329. Circulating levels of 1,25-dihydroxycholecalciferol exert negative feedback control on parathyroid chief cells at the level of transcription to decrease mRNA for preproPTH and the synthesis of parathyroid hormone. Conversely, parathyroid hormone is one major factor for the renal x-hydroxylase that synthesizes 1,25-$(OH)_2$-cholecalciferol from 25-OH-cholecalciferol

release from the parathyroid gland to maintain calcium homeostasis.

The kidney also is a major organ for the degradation of PTH. Biologically active PTH from the peritubular capillaries is degraded by specific proteases on the surface of renal tubular cells. In addition, both biologically active (NH_2 1–34) and inactive (34–84 COOH) fragments are degraded intracellularly by lysosomal enzymes within renal tubular cells (Hruska et al. 1987).

The PTH receptor has been recently cloned and sequenced from cDNA isolated from kidney cells (Jüppner et al. 1991; Fig. 328). It belongs to a class of receptors that has seven potential transmembrane domains and is linked to a specific G protein in the target cells. The expressed receptor binds PTH and PTH-related protein (PTHrP) with equal affinity, resulting in the activation of adenylate cyclase and phospholipase C. The PTH/PTHrP receptor has a striking degree of sequence homology (approximately 56%) with the calcitonin receptor but lacks similarity with other G protein-linked receptors other than secretin (Loveridge et al. 1991). The receptors for these calcium regulating hormones appear to belong to a new family of G protein-linked receptors with seven transmembrane spanning domains that activate adenylate cyclase and phospholipase C.

Special Methods for Study of Parathyroids

Assay Methods for Parathyroid Hormone. PTH in the circulation of animals can be measured by sensitive radioimmunoassays or immunoradiometric assays. Although the hormone is secreted from chief cells primarily as a straight chain (1–84 amino acids) peptide, molecular fragments (amino and carboxy terminal) are formed in the periphery (primarily by Kupffer's cells in the liver). The immunoheterogenicity created by the multiple circulating fragments of PTH has caused significant problems in the development of sensitive assays in both human patients and experimental animals. Since the amino (N-) terminal end of the molecule (that portion which interacts with the receptor in target cells) is highly conserved in man and all other mammalian species thus far tested, assays directed against this end of PTH are the most sensitive and accurate in assessing parathyroid function. The amino-terminal assay is particularly useful in measuring ongoing or recent functional changes in the parathyroid following exposure to various xenobiotics or physiologic perturbations.
The intact N-terminal PTH assay (Nichols Institute, Los Angeles, CA) is useful for toxicity testing since the antibody is generated in chickens to the highly conserved end of the molecule (1–34 PTH synthetic human). The assay can be run on either serum (preferred) or plasma that has been separated and frozen (−70°C in either glass or plastic tubes) as soon as possible after collection. In contrast to some peptide hormones PTH as quantitated by radioimmunoassays is relatively stable in serum at ice or refrigerator temperatures so that it is possible to collect representative specimens from large numbers of experimental rats such as at the end of a chronic study. Circulating levels of PTH using N-terminal assays in most animals are near 20 pg/ml (e.g., rat 29 ± 7 pg/ml; mouse 19 ± 3 pg/ml; dog 20 ± 5 pg/ml; cat 17 ± 2 pg/ml) with levels in nonhuman primates being slightly lower.
PTH assays utilizing antibody generated against the carboxy (C-) terminal end of the human PTH molecule usually give less consistent results in animals than in human patients. The amino acid sequence of the C-terminal portion of PTH is less well conserved between animal species and man than the N-terminal region, thereby rendering the antibody less specific and the assay less sensitive. It is important to emphasize that the C-terminal fragment in the circulation is biologically inactive and has a longer plasma half-life than the N-terminal end of the PTH molecule. Therefore C-terminal assays for PTH in species where a specific antibody is available tend to give a more integrated evaluation of parathyroid function over time due to the slower turnover rate of this portion of the molecule in the circulation.

Morphologic Evaluation by Light and Electron Microscopy. The parathyroid gland is infrequently injured directly in rats by the acute or chronic administration of xenobiotics. However, parathyroid function may be altered by a wide variety of chemicals that either elevate or lower the blood concentration of calcium (particularly calcium ion). In response to hypocalcemia chief cells undergo hypertrophy and eventually hyperplasia. On formalin or Bouin's fixed tissue sections the expanded cytoplasmic area is lightly eosinophilic and vacuolated compared with chief cells in normal animals. Perivascular spaces are narrow in a hyperplastic parathyroid, and there are few fat cells in the interstitium. In response to hypercalcemia the cytoplasmic area of chief cells is decreased and more densely eosinophilic, often with a widening of intercellular and pericapillary spaces. If the hypercalcemia is prolonged, there is an overall reduction in glandular parenchyma with increased fibrous or adipose connective tissue in the interstitium. Subtle differences between treated and control groups can be best evaluated by morphometric evaluation of parenchyma-to-interstitium ratio, cell and nuclear areas, numbers of mitochondria, and numbers of secretory and prosecretory granules in chief cells (Gröne et al. 1992).
Ultrastructural evaluation of chief cells is a sensitive means of morphologically assessing whether a particular drug or chemical affects the parathyroid gland. Perfusion of the thyroid-parathyroid area with glutaraldehyde-based fixatives followed by postfixation with osmium tetroxide results in the best retention of structural detail in parathyroids of animals. Morphometric studies at the ultrastructural level can be used to quantitate total cytoplasmic area and area occupied by a particular organelle (e.g., secretory granules).
In response to an acute lowering of blood calcium a larger percentage of chief cells ultrastructurally are in the active stage of synthesis and secretion than under steady-state conditions. This is

indicated by a peripheral migration of secretory granules and alignment along the plasma membrane, aggregation of the endoplasmic reticulum into lamellar arrays, and enlargement of the Golgi apparatus associated with many small dense granules in the process of formation. It should be pointed out that chief cells of rats have few mature secretory granules compared to most animal species and human beings. Conversely, chief cells in response to hypercalcemia are predominantly in the inactive stage as evaluated by electron microscopy with dispersed profiles of endoplasmic reticulum, small Golgi complexes with few granules, and often accumulations of either glycogen or lipid in the cytoplasm. Atrophic chief cells develop in response to sustained and/or more severe hypercalcemia. Their cytoplasm is more electron dense and irregularly shrunken with widened intercellular spaces. Cytoplasmic organelles are poorly developed and may have early degenerative changes suggested by mitochondrial vacuolation with disruption of cristae and distention of endoplasmic reticulum with loss of ribosomes (Capen 1971).

Embryonic Development and Parathyroid Cysts

Parathyroid (Kürsteiner's) Cyst. Embryologically, parathyroids are of entodermal origin, being derived from the III or IV pharyngeal pouches in close association with primordia of the thymus (Fig. 330). Rats have a single pair of parathyroids in contrast to other laboratory animals and human beings, which have two pairs of parathyroids. Parathyroid (Kürsteiner's) cysts develop from a persistence and dilatation of remnants of the duct that connects the parathyroid (anterior portion) and thymic (caudal portion) primordia during embryonic development. The cyst fluid has been reported to contain higher levels of iPTH (1–84 intact molecule and 39–84 COOH fragments) than serum (Ayer et al. 1989). The lining cells stain for PTH by immunohistochemistry. Similar cysts may be present in the anterior mediastinum when remnants of the embryonic duct are displaced with the caudal migration of the thymus.

Small cysts are frequently observed within the parenchyma of the parathyroid or in the immediate vicinity of the glands in rats (Capen 1983; Fig. 331). Parathyroid cysts usually are multiloculated, lined by a cuboidal to columnar (often partially ciliated) epithelium, and contain a densely eosinophilic proteinic material. The lining epithelial cells have an electron-dense cytoplasm and numerous microvilli projecting into the lumen of the cyst, but they have poorly developed synthetic and secretory organelles (Fig. 332).

Parathyroid cysts are distinct from midline cysts derived from remnants of the thyroglossal duct. The latter are lined by multilayered thyroidogenic

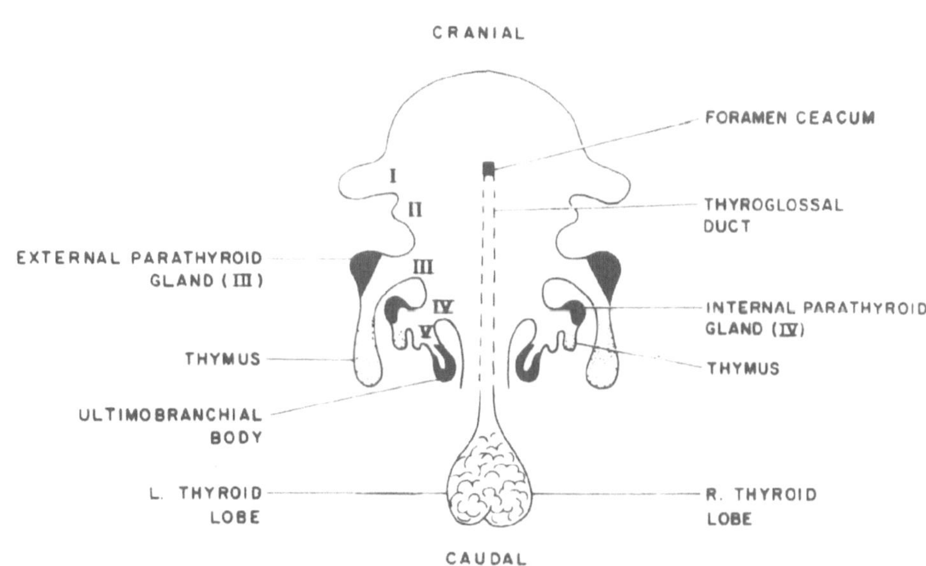

Fig. 330. Embryology of parathyroid glands and relationship to primordia of thyroid gland and ultimobranchial body

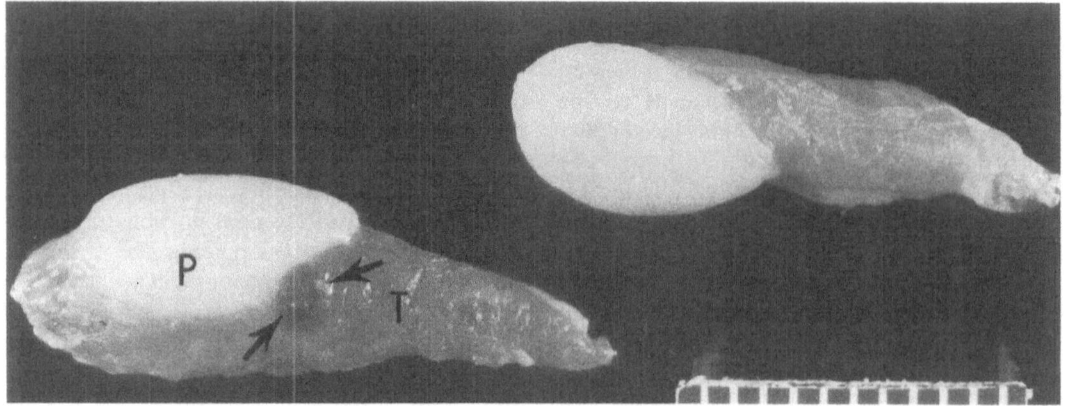

Fig. 331. Parathyroid cyst (*arrows*) derived from persistence and distension of embryonic duct that connects parathyroid thymic primordia in the third and fourth pharyngeal pouches (Kürsteiner's cyst). *T*, Thyroid gland. Hyperplastic parathyroids (*P*) from dog with chronic renal failure. *Scale* (*bottom*), 1 cm

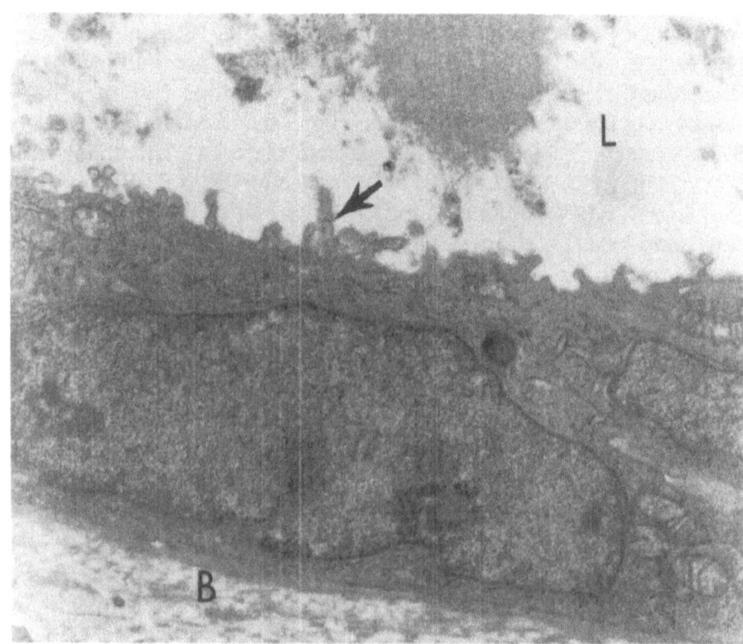

Fig. 332. Epithelial cell, lining parathyroid cyst (see Fig. 331) derived from embryonic duct connecting parathyroid and thymic primordia in third and fourth pharyngeal pouches. Cuboidal cells have microvilli (*arrow*) projecting into lumen (*L*) that contains proteinic material; small cytoplasmic area has poorly developed synthetic and secretory organelles. *B*, Basement membrane of cyst wall. ×9000

epithelium that often has colloid-containing follicles. They usually are located near the midline from the base of the tongue caudally into the mediastinum.

Age-Related Changes in Parathyroid Function

Serum iPTH [as well as calcitonin (iCT)] have been reported to be different in young compared to aged Fischer 344 (F344) rats; however, the serum calcium concentration does not change with age (Wongsurawat and Armbrecht 1987). This suggests that the regulation of iPTH (and iCT) secretion may be affected by the process of aging. Parathyroid glands from F344 rats of different ages (2–3 months = young; 12–13 months = adult; 24–27 months = old) have been removed and incubated in vitro with media containing either low (1.0 m*M*) or high (2.5 m*M*) calcium for 3 h. The iPTH secretion per pair of glands was significantly higher from older rats regardless of the medium concentration of calcium. The decrease in iPTH secretion in response to high (2.5 mM) calcium was smaller in old than in young rats.

The decreased responsiveness of chief cells to calcium may be due to age-related changes in the regulation of the secretory pathway. This could include age-related changes in the effect of calcium on release of stored PTH, intracellular degradation of PTH, or modification of adenylate cyclase activity as observed in other tissues that utilize calcium as an intermediary signal (Brown 1982). Therefore the sensitivity of parathyroid chief cells to calcium appears not to be fixed but rather may change during development and aging and in response to certain disease processes.

The increased secretion of iPTH with advancing age in rats could be due to several factors; first, an increased number of parathyroid secretory cells with age, and second, an altered regulation of chief cells in response to calcium ion associated with the process of aging (Wongsurawat and Armbrecht 1987). For example, a decreased sensitivity of chief cells to negative feedback by calcium ion could result in the higher blood levels of iPTH in aged F344 rats. Wada et al. (1992) reported that the early age-related rise in plasma PTH in F344 rats was neither a consequence of low plasma calcium nor of renal insufficiency. Age-related changes in the responsiveness of chief cells to circulating levels of other factors which modulate iPTH secretion, particularly 1,25-dihydroxycholecalciferol and α-and β-adrenergic catecholamines, also could contribute to the variations in blood levels of iPTH in rats of different ages. In addition, target cell responsiveness to PTH also decreases with advancing age in rats. PTH does not increase the renal production of 1,25-dihydroxyvitamin D in adult (13-month-old) male F344 rats compared to young (2-month-old) rats, where its production was increased 61% (Armbrecht et al. 1982). Older rats have a decreased calcemic response and decreased renal production of 1,25-dihydroxycholecalciferol compared to young rats (Armbrecht et al. 1982; Kalu et al. 1982).

The set-point for PTH release has been investigated in male F344 rats at 3, 6, 12, 18, 24, and 28 months (Uden et al. 1992). The basal maximally stimulated and suppressed levels of iPTH were determined as well as the concentration of ionized calcium sufficient to produce half-maximal suppression of the plasma iPTH ("set point for PTH release"). Basal iPTH levels increased 2.3-fold from 3 to 28 months of age, whereas basal blood ionized calcium remained unchanged. The set-point for PTH release increased steadily from 1.19 ± 0.09 mM at 3 months to 1.37 ± 0.13 mM at 24 months; basal serum iPTH levels correlated significantly with set point. Neither maximally stimulated nor suppressed iPTH levels showed any significant change with advancing age. These results suggest that the age-related increase in basal iPTH in the rat was related in part to the increased set-point for PTH release from parathyroid chief cells (Uden et al. 1992).

Studies in male Sprague-Dawley rats revealed that basal iPTH (NH_2-terminal assay) were 68% higher in aged (24–26-month) than in adult (6-month-old) rats. The initial (5–10 min) secretory response to acute constant hypocalcemic stimulus (0.32 mM decrease in ionized Ca^{2+} for 2 h by EDTA) was reduced in aged compared to adult rats (1.9 vs. 3.1-fold increase), suggesting reduced PTH stores. However, higher sustained iPTH levels (30 min–2 h) were maintained in aged rats, indicating increased synthesis and secretion. The EDTA infusion rate necessary to maintain a constant hypocalcemia was less in aged rats, suggesting a possible skeletal resistance to PTH. Slow EDTA and calcium infusions were used to determine iPTH secretion at plasma CA^{2+} levels from 0.7 to 1.5 mM. In aged rats iPTH levels were higher at all Ca^{2+} concentrations, but the set-point for iPTH release by Ca^{2+} was the same as in adult rats. Therefore the elevated iPTH secretion in aged Sprague-Dawley rats was not caused by a change in the set-point for iPTH release but did result in decreased PTH stores in the gland (Fox 1991).

Renal cortical cells in senescent (24-month-old) rats are known to have a blunted or inhibited response of PTH-stimulated Na^+-Ca^{2+} activity compared to young adults (6-month-old; Hanai et al. 1986). PTH is known to regulate renal Na^+-Ca^{2+} exchange via both cAMP-dependent and independent pathways. The findings of decreased G_S and G_i in renal membranes are consistent with the hypothesis that prolonged exposure to elevated circulating iPTH levels in aged rats results in a heterologous desensitization of the adenylate cyclase complex (Hanai et al. 1989). The number of binding sites for PTH in basolateral renal membranes prepared from adult (6-month-old) and old (24-month-old) male Wistar rats has been quantitated by the binding of synthetic analogue ^{125}I-labeled [Nle$^{8, 18}$, Tyr]bPTH-(1–34) amide to the renal membranes (Hanai et al. 1990). The maximum number of specific PTH binding sites was 92.7 ± 9.3 and 36.7 ± 6.1 fmol/mg protein, respectively, in membranes prepared from adult and old rats. The affinity of the PTH receptor was unaffected with age. The level of PTH binding components, estimated by ligand affinity blot technique using biotinylated bPTH-(1–34), was similarly reduced in renal membranes isolated from senescent rats. The decreased number of PTH binding sites and binding components were partially or completely reversed by parathyroidectomy. These findings suggested that the blunting of PTH-stimulated Na^+-Ca^{2+} exchange and adenylate cyclase activities in the kidney of aged rats are due in part to the loss of PTH receptors in the basolateral membranes, and that the defect was reversible (Hanai et al. 1990). The results of this study were consistent with the development of homologous desensitization to PTH in aging rats. Desensitization of PTH responses at the receptor site also has been reported in a variety of model systems including PTH pretreatment of cultured renal cells (Henry et al. 1983) and bone cells (Goldring et al. 1984; Teitelbaum et al. 1986), prolonged infusion of exogenous PTH (Mahoney and Nissenson 1983), and feeding animals a vitamin D deficient or low-calcium diet (Forte et al. 1982).

Lee et al. (1984) reported an increase in urinary phosphorus excretion in old (28- to 29-month-old) F344 rats compared to younger (12- to 15-month-old) adult rats fed equal amounts of dietary phosphorus. The increase in renal phosphorus excretion in old F344 rats was PTH-independent since the phosphaturia was not reversed by thyroparathyroidectomy and the renal cortical generation of cAMP in response to PTH did not differ between the two age groups of rats. However, there was a clear decrease in phosphorus uptake by renal brush border membrane vesicles prepared from old (28- to 29-month-old) rats in response to PTH compared to those from younger (12- to 15-month-old) rats. Alkaline phosphatase activity in the renal cortical vesicles did not differ between the two age groups of rats.

Kiebzak and Sacktor (1986) demonstrated a significant age-related phosphaturia (i.e., elevated urinary phosphorus excretion and fractional excretion) in Wistar-derived male rats fed a normal (0.5%) phosphorus diet. Studies compared young, rapidly growing (2- to 3-month-old), young adults (6-month-old), and mature adults (12-month-old), transition rats from adults to senescence (18-month-old) and senescent (24-month-old) rats. Plasma phosphorus decreased significantly and progressively with advancing age. There was an age-related decrease in the transport of phosphorus by renal brush border membrane vesicles but the Na^+ gradient-dependent uptake of glucose and proline was unaffected, demonstrating the specificity of the phosphorus transport decrement. An elevation in serum PTH did not appear to be related to the renal phosphorus conservation since urinary cAMP was not elevated in the intact senescent rat and phosphorus excretion was not normalized in the senescent rats 3 days after parathyroidectomy. However, the senescent and young adult Wistar rats adapted to a low (0.1%) phosphorus diet by a marked (>100%) increase in phosphorus intake by renal brush border membrane vesicles compared to those prepared from rats fed a normal phosphorus diet. Therefore, the kidney of senescent Wistar rats retained the ability to respond appropriately to a low intake of dietary phosphorus.

Inflammation of Parathyroid: Immune-Mediated Parathyroiditis

Isoimmune hypoparathyroidism has been induced experimentally by repeated injections of parathyroid emulsions with Freund's adjuvant for 4 months (Lupulescu et al. 1968). The parathyroids had lymphocytic infiltration, disorganization in the pattern of arrangement and atrophy of chief cells, and progressive fibrosis (Fig. 333). Mitochondria in chief cells were irregularly swollen, and cristae were disrupted, giving a vacuolated appearance. The granular endoplasmic reticulum was poorly developed, and secretory granules were reduced in number.

Hypoparathyroidism results when subnormal amounts of PTH are secreted by pathologic parathyroids, or the hormone secreted is unable to interact normally with target cells (Capen 1985b). Hypoparathyroidism is often associated with a diffuse lymphocytic parathyroiditis resulting in extensive degeneration of chief cells and replacement by fibrous connective tissue (Fig. 332). In the early stages of lymphocytic parathyroiditis there is infiltration of the gland with

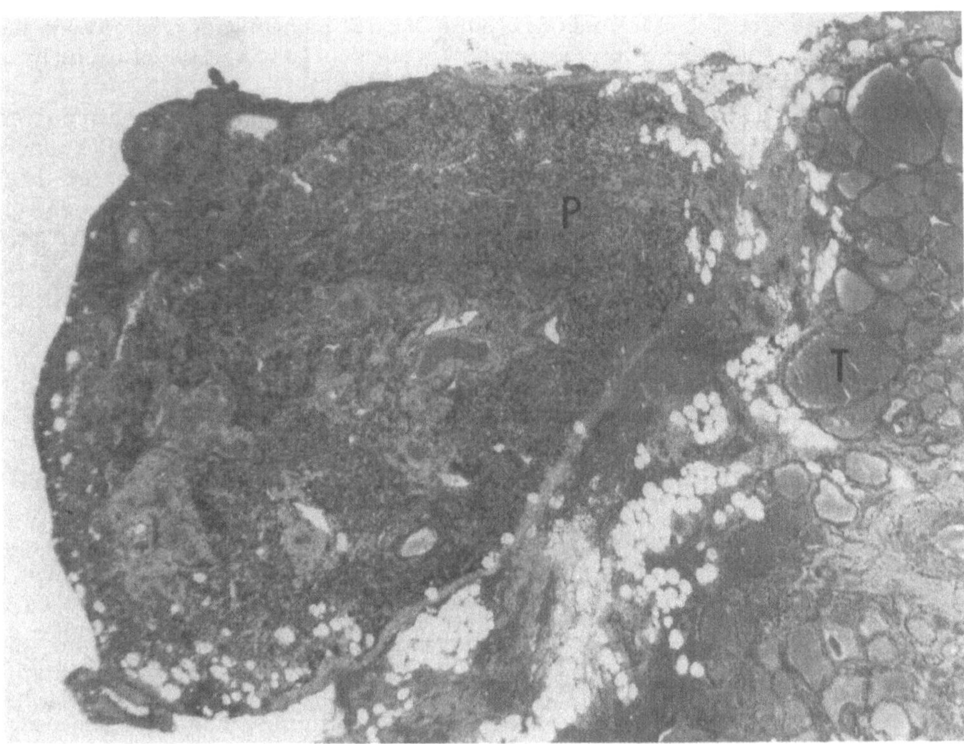

Fig. 333. Diffuse lymphocytic parathyroiditis (*P*), dog with hypoparathyroidism and hypocalcemia. Complete replacement of external parathyroid gland by lymphocytes, plasma cells, fibroblasts, and neocapillaries. *T*, Thyroid gland. ×16

lymphocytes and plasma cells with nodular regenerative hyperplasia of the remaining chief cells. The lymphocytic parathyroiditis appears to develop by an immune-mediated mechanism since a similar destruction of secretory parenchyma and lymphocytic infiltration has been produced experimentally by repeated injections of parathyroid tissue immulsions. Bone resorption is decreased because of a lack of PTH and blood calcium levels diminish progressively.

Xenobiotic-Induced Toxic Injury of Parathyroids

Ozone. Inhalation of a single dose of ozone (0.75 ppm) for 4–8 h has been reported to produce light- and electron-microscopic changes in parathyroid glands (Atwal and Wilson 1974). Subsequent studies have used longer (48-h) exposure to ozone to define the pathogenesis of the parathyroid lesions (Atwal 1979; Atwal et al. 1975). Initially (1–5 days postozone exposure) many chief cells undergo compensatory hypertrophy and hyperplasia, with areas of capillary endothelial cell proliferation, interstitial edema, degeneration of vascular endothelium, formation of platelet thrombi, leukocyte infiltration of the walls of larger vessels in the gland, and disruption of basement membranes. Chief cells had prominent Golgi complexes and endoplasmic reticulum, aggregations of free ribosomes, and swelling of mitochondria (Atwal and Pemsingh 1981).

Inactive chief cells with few secretory granules predominate in the parathyroids in the later stages of exposure to ozone. There was evidence of parathyroid atrophy from 12 to 20 days after ozone exposure with mononuclear cell infiltration and necrosis of chief cells. The reduced cytoplasmic area contained vacuolated endoplasmic reticulum, a small Golgi apparatus, and numerous lysosomal bodies. Plasma membranes of adjacent chief cells were disrupted, resulting in coalescence of the cytoplasmic area. Fibroblasts with associated collagen bundles were prominent in the interstitium and the basal lamina of the numerous capillaries often was duplicated.

The parathyroid lesions in ozone-exposed animals are similar to isoimmune parathyroiditis in other species (Lupulescu et al. 1968). Antibody against parathyroid tissue was localized near the periphery of chief cells by indirect immunofluorescence, especially 14 days following ozone injury (Atwal et al. 1975).

Aluminum. Evidence for a direct effect of aluminum on the parathyroid is suggested from studies of patients with chronic renal failure treated by hemodialysis with aluminum-containing fluids or orally administered drugs containing aluminum. These patients often had normal or minimal elevations of iPTH, little histologic evidence of osteitis fibrosa in bone, and a depressed response parathyroid to acute hypocalcemia (Bourdeau et al. 1987). Morrissey et al. (1983) reported that an increase in aluminum concentration in vitro over a range of 0.5–2.0 m*M* in a low-calcium medium (0.5 m*M*) progressively inhibited the secretion of iPTH. At 2.0 m*M* aluminum iPTH secretion was inhibited by 68% while high medium calcium (2.0 m*M*) without aluminum maximally inhibited iPTH secretion only 39%. The inhibition of PTH secretion by aluminum does not appear to be due to an irreversible toxic effect since normal secretion was restored when parathyroid cells were returned to 0.5 m*M* calcium medium without aluminum. The incorporation of [^{3}H]leucine into total cell protein, parathyroid secretory protein, proPTH, or PTH was not affected by aluminum; however, the secretion of radiolabeled protein by dispersed parathyroid cells was inhibited by aluminum (Morrissey et al. 1983).

The molecular mechanism by which aluminum inhibits PTH secretion appears to be similar to that of calcium ion by reducing diglyceride levels in chief cells (Morrissey and Slatopolsky 1986). Aluminum appears to decrease diglyceride synthesis, which is reflected in a corresponding decrease in synthesis of phosphatidylcholine and possible triglyceride; however, phosphatidylinositol synthesis was not affected by aluminum. The mechanism whereby aluminum decreases diglycerides and maintains phosphatidylinositol synthesis in parathyroid cells is not known.

L_l-Asparaginase. Tettenborn et al. (1970) and Chisari et al. (1972) reported that rabbits administered L-asparaginase develop severe hypocalcemia and tetany characterized by muscle tremors, opisthotonos, carpopedal spasms, paralysis, and coma. This drug was of interest in cancer chemotherapy because of the beneficial effects of guinea pig serum against lymphosarcoma in mice.

Parathyroid chief cells appeared to be selectively destroyed by L-asparaginase (Young et al. 1973). Chief cells were predominately in the inactive stage of the secretory cycle; degranulated and large autophagic vacuoles were present in the cytoplasm of degenerating cells. Cytoplasmic organelles concerned with synthesis and packaging of secretory products were poorly developed in chief cells. The rabbits developed hyperphosphatemia, hypomagnesemia, hyperkalemia, and azotemia in addition to the acute hypocalcemia. Rabbits with clinical hypocalcemic tetany did not recover spontaneously; however, administration of parathyroid extract prior to or during treatment with L-asparaginase decreased the incidence of hypocalcemic tetany.

The development of hypocalcemia and tentany have not been observed in other experimental animals administered L-asparaginase (Oettgen et al. 1970). However, this response may not be limited to the rabbit since some human patients receiving the drug also have developed hypocalcemia (Jaffe et al. 1972). The L-asparaginase induced hypoparathyroidism in rabbits is a valuable model to investigate drug-endocrine cell interactions, somewhat analogous to the selective destruction of pancreatic beta cells by alloxan with production of experimental diabetes mellitus.

Parathyroid Changes Associated with Metabolic Disorders

Renal Hyperparathyroidism. As a complication of chronic renal failure, secondary hyperparathyroidism is a metabolic state characterized by an excessive, but not autonomous, rate of PTH secretion (Capen and Rosol 1989). The secretion of hormone by the hyperplastic parathyroid gland usually remains responsive to fluctuations in blood calcium. The primary etiologic mechanism in this disorder is long-standing progressive renal disease resulting in severely impaired function. When the renal disease progresses to the point at which there is significant reduction in glomerular filtration rate, phosphorus is retained and progressive hyperphosphatemia develops (Fig. 334). Although the concentration of blood phosphorus has no direct regulatory influence on the synthesis and secretion of PTH, when elevated, it con-

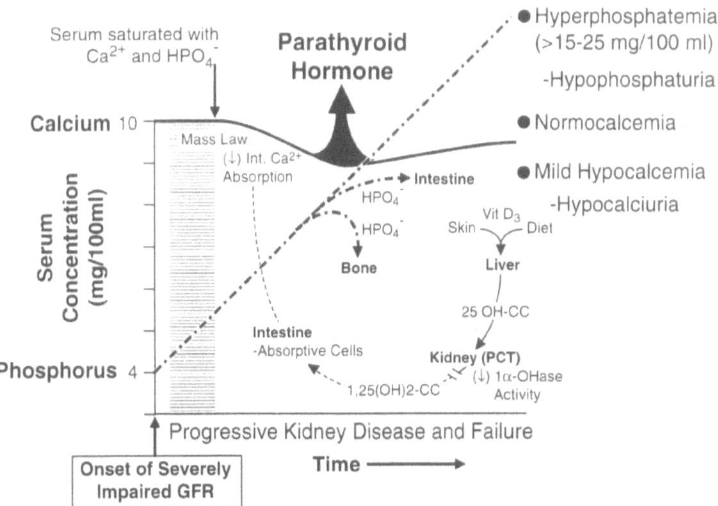

Fig. 334. Alterations in serum calcium and phosphorus during the pathogenesis of secondary hyperparathyroidism associated with progressive renal disease and failure

tributes to parathyroid stimulation by virtue of its ability to lower blood calcium levels.

Parathyroid stimulation associated with chronic renal disease can be attributed directly to the hypocalcemia. An impaired intestinal absorption of calcium due to an acquired defect in vitamin D metabolism plays an important role in the development of hypocalcemia associated with renal insufficiency. Chronic renal disease interferes with the production of 1,25-dihydroxycholecalciferol by the kidney, thereby diminishing intestinal calcium transport. All parathyroids are considerably enlarged as a result initially of hypertrophy of chief cells and subsequently by hyperplasia as compensatory mechanisms to increase hormonal synthesis and secretion in response to the hypocalcemic stimulus.

Chronic renal insufficiency occurs frequently as a result of several acquired, induced, or congenital kidney lesions (Capen and Martin 1974). All four parathyroid glands undergo marked chief-cell hyperplasia and the bones have varying degrees of generalized osteitis fibrosa. Ultrastructurally, chief cells in the parathyroid glands of dogs with chronic renal disease are primarily in the actively synthesizing stage (Fig. 335). These chronically stimulated chief cells have extensive lamellar aggregations of endoplasmic reticulum, numerous ribosomes, large mitochondria, and prominent Golgi apparatuses with many prosecretory granules. The numbers of mature storage granules are less than in chief cells from normal dogs, and they are situated in the peripheral parts of the cell. Plasma membranes of adjacent cells are frequently interdigitated. Aggregations of glycogen particles are observed in many chief cells, but droplets of neutral lipid and lysosomelike bodies are infrequent.

Nutritional Hyperparathyroidism. The increased secretion of PTH in this disorder is a compensatory mechanism directed against a disturbance in mineral homeostasis induced by nutritional imbalances (Capen 1985a). The disease occurs in dogs, cats, monkeys, laboratory rodents, among other animals, fed improper diets. Dietary mineral imbalances of etiologic importance in the pathogenesis are a low content of calcium, excessive phosphorus with normal or low calcium, and inadequate amounts of cholecalciferol (vitamin D_3) in New World nonhuman primates housed indoors without exposure to sunlight. The significant end result is hypocalcemia, which results in parathyroid stimulation (Fig. 336).

A diet low in calcium fails to supply the daily requirement, even though a greater proportion of ingested calcium is absorbed, and hypocalcemia develops (Fig. 336). Ingestion of excessive phosphorus results in increased intestinal absorption and elevation in blood phosphorus levels. Hyperphosphatemia does not stimulate the parathyroid gland directly but does so indirectly by virtue of its ability to lower blood calcium levels and suppress the synthesis of 1,25-$(OH)_2$-cholecalciferol by the kidney. In response to the nutritionally induced hypocalcemia all parathyroid glands undergo cellular hypertrophy and hyperplasia.

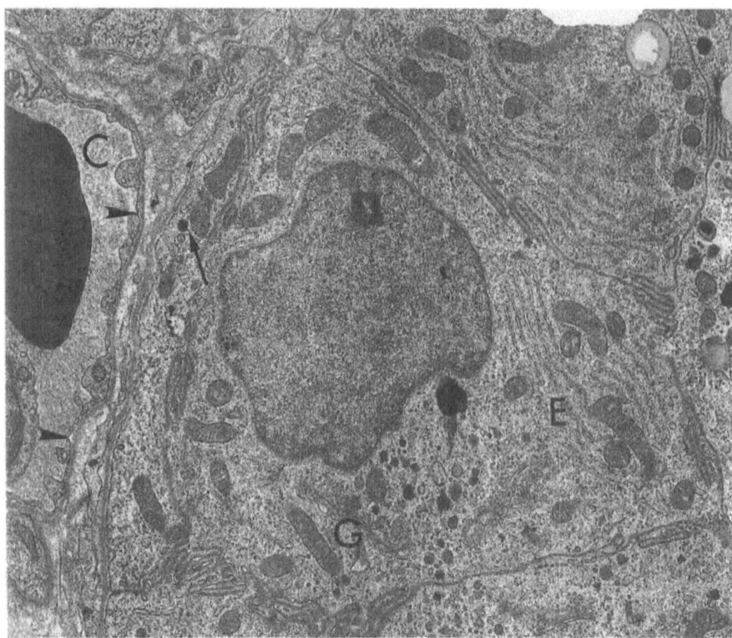

Fig. 335. Chronically stimulated parathyroid chief cells from a dog with chronic renal failure and generalized osteitis fibrosa. Note extensive aggregations of endoplasmic reticulum (*E*), clusters of free ribosomes, large Golgi apparatus (*G*) with prosecretory granules, and large mitochondria. Mature storage granules (*arrow*) are infrequent and situated in parts of chief cells near capillaries (*C*) with fenestrae (*arrowheads*). Plasma membranes of adjacent hyperactive chief cells are interdigitated. ×10 300

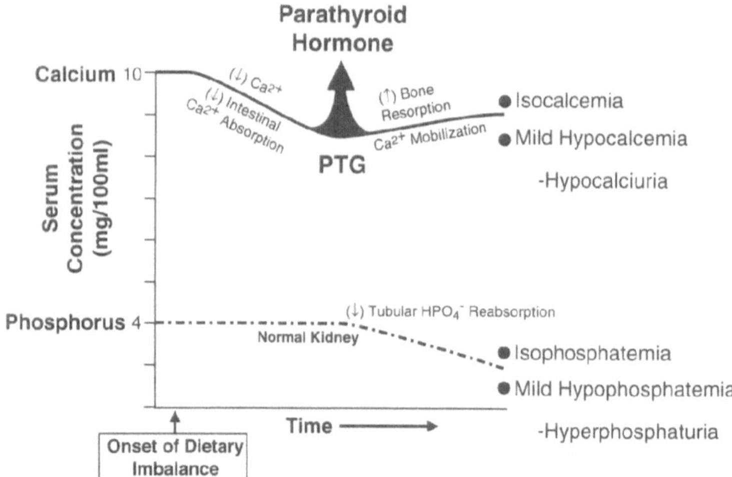

Fig. 336. Alterations in serum calcium and phosphorus in the pathogenesis of nutritional secondary hyperparathyroidism caused by feeding a diet low in calcium or deficient in cholecalciferol but with normal amounts of phosphorus

In response to the diet-induced hypocalcemia, chief cells undergo hypertrophy and eventually hyperplasia. The expanded cytoplasmic area is lightly eosinophilic and vacuolated (Fig. 337) compared with chief cells in control animals (Fig. 338). Perivascular spaces are narrow, and there are few fat cells in the interstitium. Ultrastructurally the cytoplasmic area of chief cells is increased, and organelles concerned with protein synthesis and packaging of secretory products are well developed after low-calcium feeding for 1 week. An increased number of chief cells have the endoplasmic reticulum aggregated into lamellar arrays and an enlarged Golgi apparatus

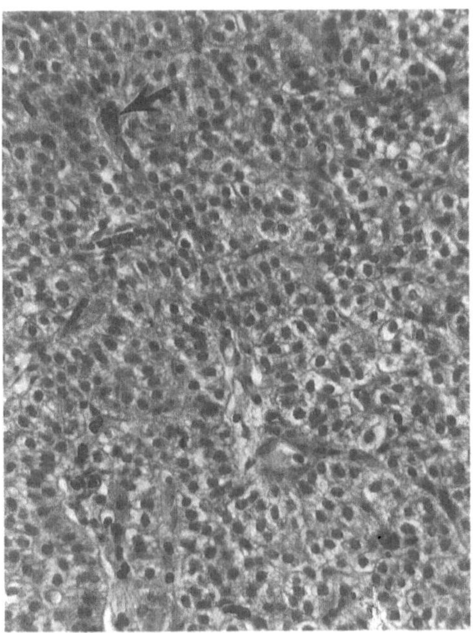

Fig. 337. Diet-induced parathyroid chief cell hyperplasia. Kitten with nutritional secondary hyperparathyroidism induced by being fed low calcium diet for 9 weeks. Hyperactive chief cells are enlarged, lightly eosinophilic, vacuolated, and packed closely together with narrow perivascular spaces (*arrow*). H&E, ×315

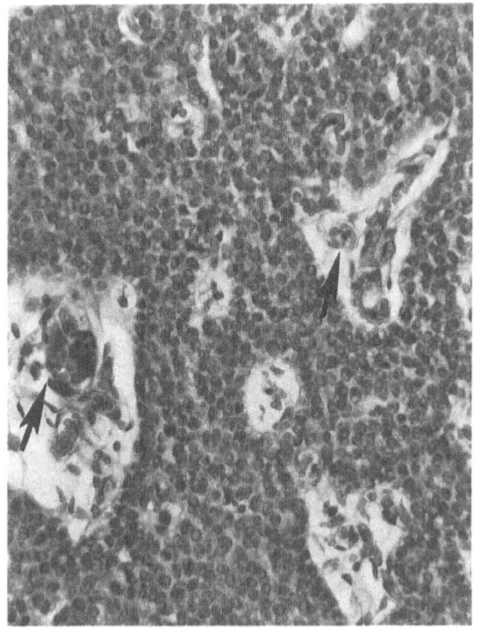

Fig. 338. Chief cells in parathyroid gland of control kitten fed balanced control diet that supplied daily requirements for calcium and phosphorus. Chief cells are smaller (especially cytoplasmic area) and more loosely arranged, and perivascular spaces (*arrows*) are more prominent than in gland with chief cell hyperplasia (compare Fig. 337). H&E, ×315

associated with many prosecretory granules. Secretory granules are present in numbers similar to those in control kittens, but are situated more peripherally (Capen and Rowland 1968).

Hypoparathyroidism. The metabolic disorder of hypoparathyroidism is one in which either subnormal amounts of PTH are secreted by pathologic parathyroids or the hormone secreted is unable to interact normally with target cells (Capen 1985b). Hypoparathyroidism is often associated with a diffuse lymphocytic parathyroiditis (Fig. 333), resulting in extensive degeneration of chief cells and replacement by fibrous connective tissue. In the early stages of lymphocytic parathyroiditis there is infiltration of the gland with lymphocytes and plasma cells with nodular regenerative hyperplasia of the remaining chief cells. The lymphocytic parathyroiditis appears to develop by an immune-mediated mechanism since a similar destruction of secretory parenchyma and lymphocytic infiltration has been produced experimentally by repeated injections of parathyroid tissue immulsions. The functional disturbances of hypoparathyroidism are the result primarily of increased neuromuscular excitability and tetany. Bone resorption is decreased because of a lack of PTH and blood calcium levels diminish progressively (Fig. 339).

The functional disturbances and clinical manifestations of hypoparathyroidism are primarily the result of increased neuromuscular excitability and tetany. Because of the lack of PTH bone resorption is decreased, and blood calcium levels diminish progressively (4–6 mg/100 ml). Affected animals are restless, nervous, and ataxic, with weakness and intermittent tremors of individual muscle groups that progress to generalized tetany and convulsive seizures. Concurrently, blood phosphorus levels are substantially elevated owing to increased renal tubular reabsorption (Fig. 339).

Primary Hyperparathyroidism. In primary hyperparathyroidism PTH is produced in excess by a functional tumor in the gland. The normal control of PTH secretion by the concentration of blood calcium is lost in primary hyperpara-

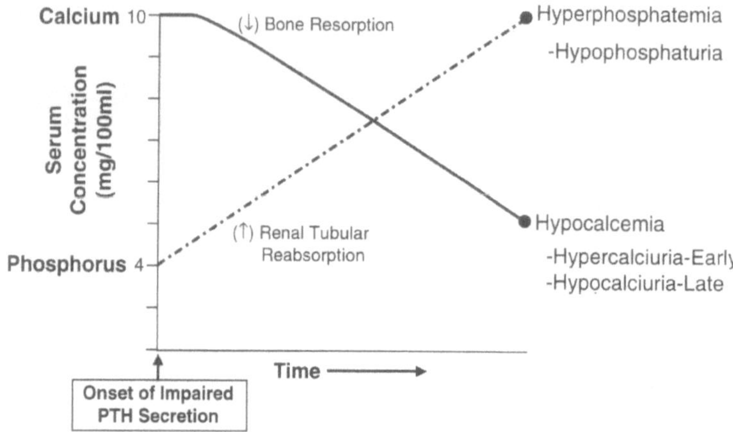

Fig. 339. Alterations in serum calcium and phosphorus in response to an inadequate secretion of parathyroid hormone. There is a progressive increase in serum phosphorus and a marked decline in serum calcium levels that often result in neuromuscular tetany

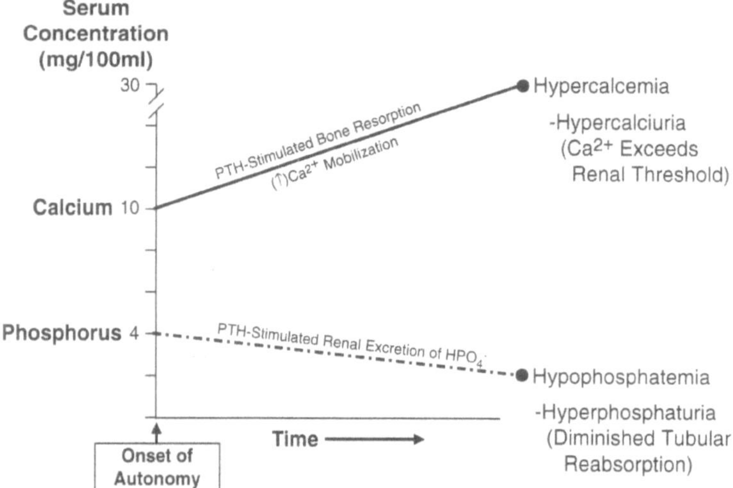

Fig. 340. Alterations in serum calcium and phosphorus in response to an autonomous secretion of parathyroid hormone in primary hyperparathyroidism

thyroidism. Hormone secretion is autonomous, and the parathyroid produces excessive hormone in spite of the increased blood calcium (Fig. 340). PTH acts initially on cells in the renal tubules to promote the excretion of phosphorus and retention of calcium. A prolonged increased secretion of PTH results in accelerated bone resorption and increased renal production of 1,25-$(OH)_2$ cholecalciferol. The lesion in the parathyroid gland responsible for the excessive secretion of PTH usually is an adenoma composed of active chief cells (Capen 1990).

Nonneoplastic Proliferative Lesions of Parathyroid Chief Cells

Diffuse Hyperplasia. Parathyroid hyperplasia as seen with chronic renal failure and long-term dietary imbalances results in a uniform enlargement of all parathyroid glands. In rats with chronic renal failure diffusely hyperplastic parathyroid glands may be detected macroscopically as 1–2 mm nodules projecting from the surface of each thyroid lobe. The uniform enlargement of parathyroid glands in diffuse hyperplasia is due to both hypertrophy and hyperplasia of chief cells. There is not a peripheral rim of compressed atrophic parathyroid parenchyma as around a functional adenoma, but rather a uniform population of hyperplastic chief cells extending to the capsule of the gland (Fig. 341). The chief cells are closely packed together often with indistinct cell boundaries. The expanded cytoplasmic area of chronically stimulated chief cells is lightly eosinophilic with occasional distinct vacuoles. A more prominent fibrovascular stroma in some diffusely hyperplastic parathyroids may

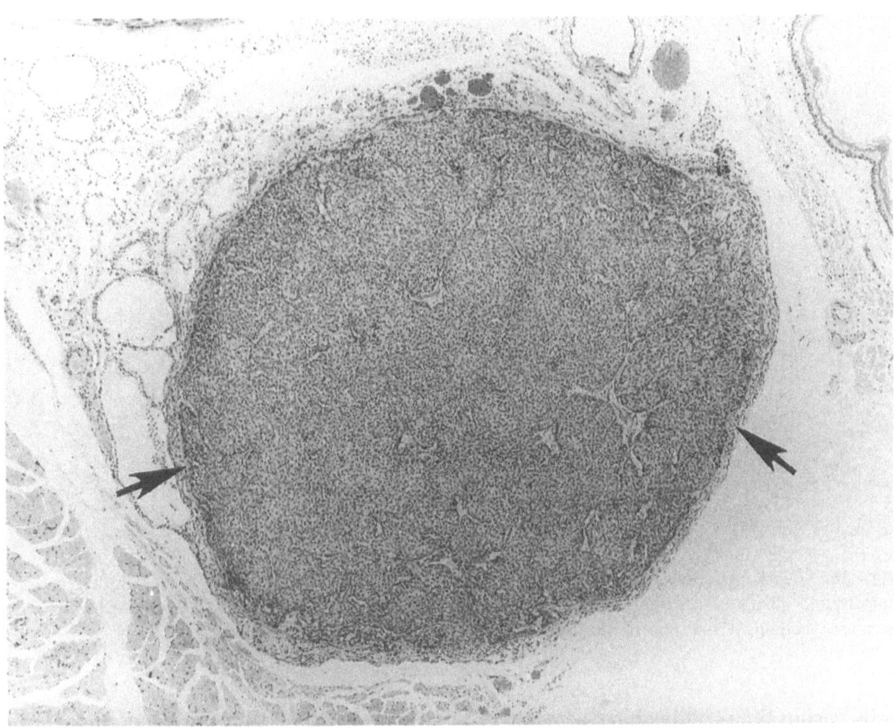

Fig. 341. Diffuse hyperplasia of chief cells with enlargement of parathyroid gland in an F344 rat. There is a uniform increase in cellularity due to hypertrophy and hyperplasia of chief cells. *Arrows*, parathyroid capsule. *Bar*, 100 µm. (From Rosol and Capen 1989)

result in a lobulated appearance (Fig. 341). In other hyperplastic parathyroids the chief cells form distinct acinuslike structures in the gland.

Secondary hyperparathyroidism as a complication of chronic renal failure is characterized by an excessive, but not autonomous, rate of PTH secretion (Capen and Rosol 1989). The secretion of hormone by the hyperplastic parathyroid gland usually remains responsive to fluctuations in blood calcium. The primary etiologic mechanism in this disorder is long-standing progressive renal disease resulting in severely impaired function. When the renal disease progresses to the point at which there is significant reduction in glomerular filtration rate, phosphorus is retained and progressive hyperphosphatemia develops. Although the concentration of blood phosphorus has no direct regulatory influence on the synthesis and secretion of PTH, when elevated, it contributes to parathyroid stimulation by virtue of its ability to lower blood calcium levels.

Parathyroid stimulation associated with chronic renal disease can be attributed directly to the hypocalcemia. An impaired intestinal absorption of calcium due to an acquired defect in vitamin D metabolism plays an important role in the development of persistent hypocalcemia associated with renal insufficiency. Chronic renal disease interferes with the production of 1,25-dihydroxycholecalciferol by the kidney, thereby diminishing intestinal calcium transport. All parathyroids are considerably enlarged as a result initially of hypertrophy of chief cells and, subsequently, by hyperplasia as compensatory mechanisms to increase hormonal synthesis and secretion in response to the long-term hypocalcemic stimulus.

Focal (Multifocal) Hyperplasia. Chief cell hyperplasia may affect the parathyroid in a distinctly focal or multifocal distribution. In focal parathyroid hyperplasia there are single or multiple nodules in one or both glands where there is an increased number of closely packed chief cells often with an expanded cytoplasmic area (Fig. 342). The focal area(s) of chief cell hyperplasia is (are) poorly demarcated and not encapsulated from adjacent parenchyma. Chief

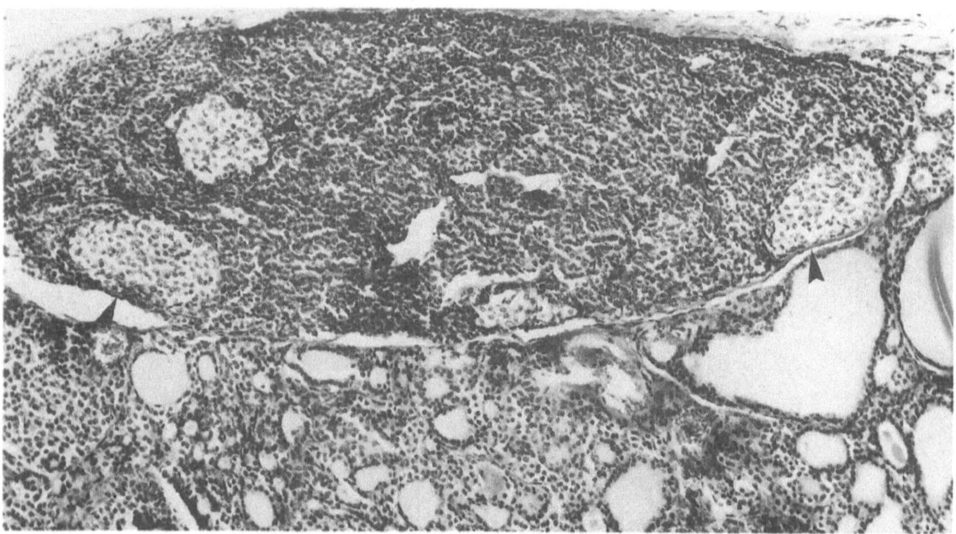

Fig. 342. Focal hyperlasia (*arrowhead*) of chief cells in parathyroid glands of a Long-Evans rat. The focal areas of increased cellularity are poorly demarcated and not encapsulated from adjacent parathyroid parenchyma. *Bar*, 100 μm. (From Rosol and Capen 1989)

cells within the nodules have a relatively uniform composition with a high cytoplasm-to-nuclear ratio and a slightly more hyperchromatic nucleus than adjacent normal chief cells. There may be slight compression of adjacent chief cells around larger focal areas of hyperplasia. Focal chief cell hyperplasia is often difficult to separate from a chief cell adenoma using only morphologic criteria. The presence of multiple nodules of varying sizes and uniform cellularity in one or both parathyroids with minimal compression and no encapsulation is more compatible with an interpretation of focal hyperplasia than chief cell adenoma.

Fluoride-Associated Parathyroid Hyperplasia. Drinking water containing large doses of fluoride (200 ppm) has been reported to cause parathyroid hyperplasia in sheep (Faccini and Care 1965). Chief cells were primarily in the active stage of the secretory cycle after 1 month exposure. The endoplasmic reticulum was aggregated into lamellar arrays and the Golgi apparatus was well developed in chief cells. iPTH levels in the blood were elevated fivefold after 1 week and remained elevated over the experimental period of 1 month. Faccini (1969) interpreted these changes to suggest stimulation of chief cells by fluoride as a response to an increased PTH demand, resulting from decreased mobilization of calcium from fluoroapatite-containing bone. Apatite crystals in fluorotic bone are known to be of larger size than in normal bone and appear more stable and less reactive in surface exchange reactions.

Secondary hyperparathyroidism has been reported in patients with skeletal fluorosis (Teotia and Teotia 1973). The parathyroid glands have morphologic evidence of hyperactivity, and the patients have elevated circulating levels of iPTH. Ream and Principato (1981) reported increased glycogen accumulation in hyperactive chief cells of rats following the ingestion of large doses (150 ppm) of fluoride in drinking water.

Neoplasms of Parathyroid Gland

Chief Cell Adenoma. The size of parathyroid adenomas varies in adult-aged rats from microscopic to unilateral nodules several millimeters in diameter located in the cervical region by the thyroids or infrequently in the thoracic cavity near the base of the heart. Parathyroid neoplasms in the precardiac mediastinum are derived from ectopic parathyroid tissue displaced into the thorax with the expanding thymus during embryonic development. Tumors of parathyroid chief cells do not appear to be a sequela of longstanding secondary hyperparathyroidism of either

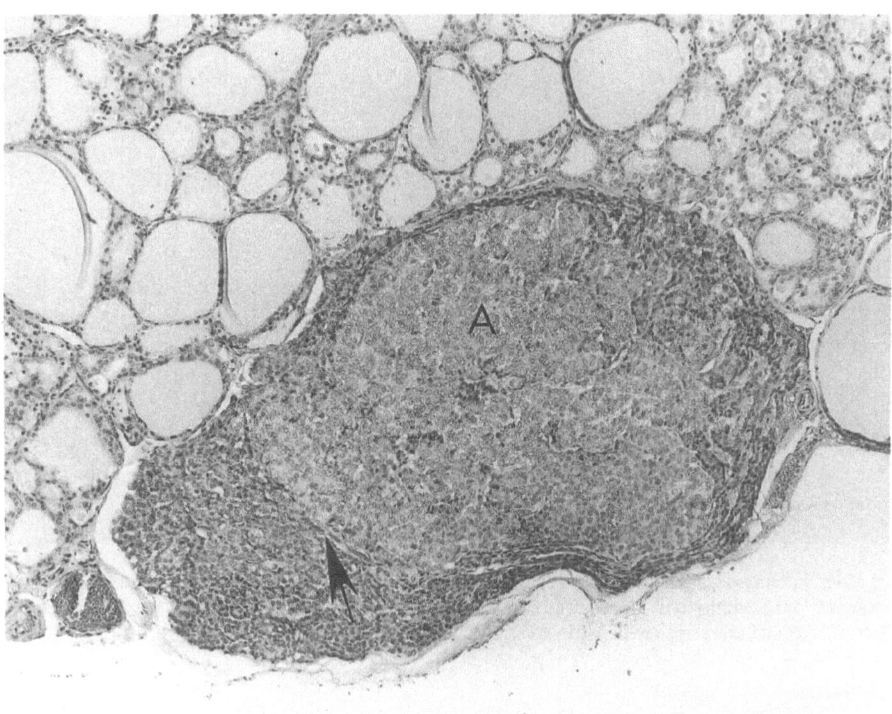

Fig. 343. Chief cell adenoma (*A*) illustrating sharp demarcation and partial encapsulation (*arrow*) from adjacent parathyroid in Fischer rat. Chief cells in the adenoma have a larger cytoplasmic area than those in the compressed rim of the parathyroid gland. *Bar*, 100 µm. (From Rosol and Capen 1989)

renal or nutritional origin. The unaffected parathyroid glands may be atrophic if the adenoma is functional, normal if the adenoma is nonfunctional, or enlarged if there is concomitant hyperplasia. In functional adenomas the normal mechanism by which PTH secretion is controlled by the concentration of blood calcium is lost, and hormone secretion is excessive in spite of an increased level of blood calcium. However, PTH secretion is not completely autonomous since secretion can be reduced by extracellular calcium in vitro.

Adenomas are solitary nodules that are sharply demarcated from adjacent parathyroid parenchyma (Fig. 343). Since the adenoma compresses the rim of surrounding parathyroid to varying degrees depending upon its size, there may be a partial fibrous capsule either from compression of existing stroma or proliferation of fibrous connective tissue.

Adenomas are usually nonfunctional (endocrinologically inactive) in adult-aged rats. Chief cells in nonfunctional adenomas are cuboidal or polyhedral and arranged either in a diffuse sheet, lobules, or acini with or without lumens. Nuclei are round-to-oval, often vesicular, and mitotic figures may be present; however, they are usually infrequent. Chief cells from functional adenomas often are closely packed into small groups by fine connective tissue septae. The chief cells are cuboidal, and the cytoplasm stains lightly eosinophilic. The cytoplasmic area varies from normal size to an expanded area. There is a much lower density of cells in functional parathyroid adenoma compared to the adjacent rim with atrophic chief cells.

Some parathyroid adenomas in the rat become cystic. The cystadenomas contain solid areas of tumor cells and large cystic areas lined by neoplastic chief cells. The cysts contain a densely eosinophilic proteinaceous fluid. As the cystic spaces enlarge, the tumor cells lining the cysts become flattened. Interspersed between the cysts are solid islands of growth of tumor cells.

Chief cells comprising functional parathyroid adenomas ultrastructurally are in the actively synthesizing stage of the secretory cycle. Multiple large lamellar arrays of rough endoplasmic

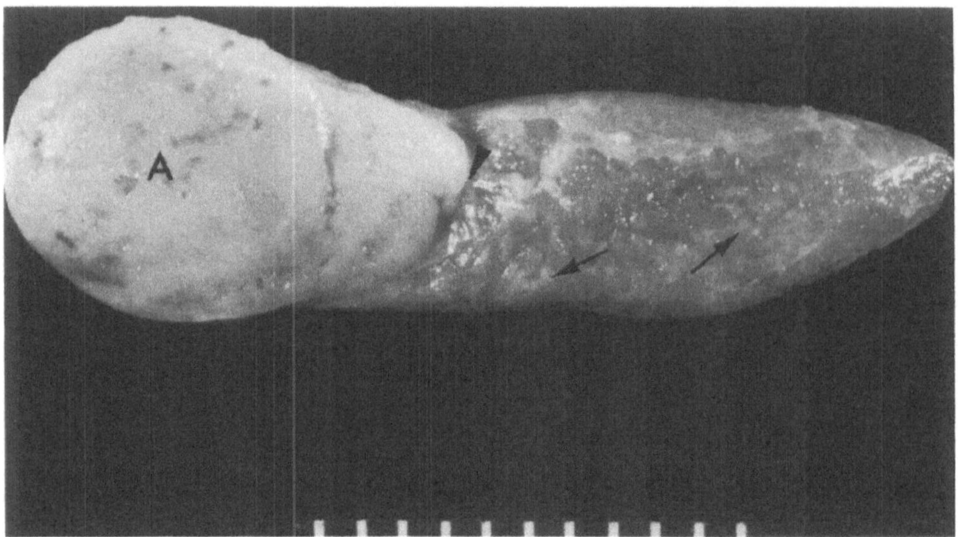

Fig. 344. Parathyroid adenoma (*A*) causing extensive enlargement of one parathyroid gland. Tumor is encapsulated (*arrowhead*) and there are multicentric areas of C cell hyperplasia in the thyroid (*arrows*) as a response to long-term hypercalcemia. *Scale*, centimeters

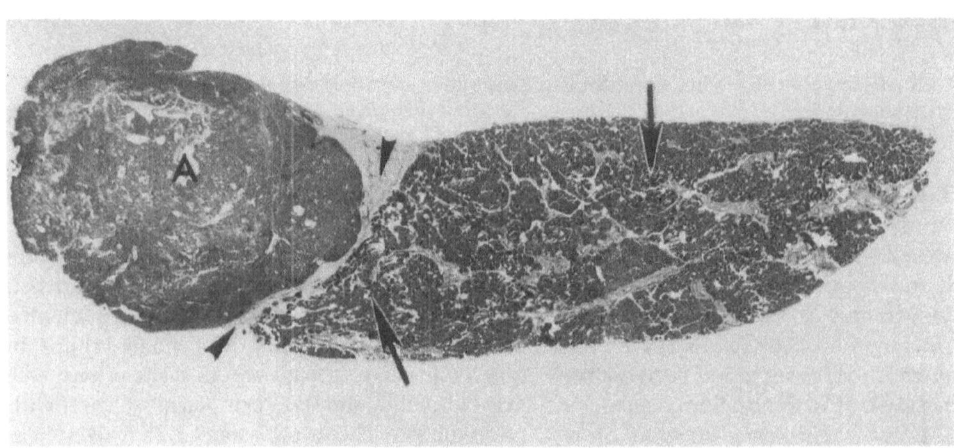

Fig. 345. Chief cell adenoma (*A*) in an external parathyroid gland, from a dog with primary hyperparathyroidism. The adenoma is sharply demarcated and encapsulated (*arrowheads*) from the adjacent thyroid gland. Cranial pole of thyroid is compressed and there are multifocal areas of C cell hyperplasia (*arrows*)

reticulum and clusters of free ribosomes are present in the cytoplasm. Few mature secretory granules are present in autonomous chief cells, suggesting that the rate of PTH secretion is faster than synthesis and storage. Chief cell adenomas usually result in considerable enlargement of a single parathyroid gland (Fig. 344). They are light brown to red and are located either in the cervical region by the thyroids or, infrequently, within the thoracic cavity near the base of the heart (Cheville 1972; Krook 1957). Parathyroid neoplasms in the precardiac mediastinum are derived from ectopic parathyroid tissue, displaced into the thorax with the expanding thymus during embryonic development. The adenomas are sharply demarcated and encapsulated from the adjacent thyroid gland (Fig. 345). Multiple white foci may be seen in the thyroids of dogs with functional parathyroid tumors. These represent areas of C cell hyperplasia in response to the long-term hypercalcemia (Figs. 344, 345).

Larger parathyroid adenomas, such as those

detected macroscopically, often incorporate nearly the entire affected gland. A narrow rim of compressed parenchyma may be detected at one side of the gland, or the affected parathyroid may be completely incorporated by the adenoma. Chief cells in this rim often are compressed and atrophic due to pressure and the persistent hypercalcemia. Peripherally situated follicles in the adjacent thyroid lobe may be compressed to a limited extent by larger parathyroid adenomas. The parathyroid glands that do not contain a functional adenoma also undergo trophic atrophy in response to the hypercalcemia and become smaller.

Influence of Age on Parathyroid Tumors. There are relatively few chemicals or experimental manipulations reported in the literature that significantly increase the incidence of parathyroid tumors. Long-standing renal failure with intense diffuse hyperplasia does not appear to increase the development of chief cell tumors in rats. The historical incidence of parathyroid adenomas in untreated control male F344 rats in studies conducted by the National Toxicology Program (NTP) was 4/1315 (0.3%) and that for female F344 rats 2/1330 (0.15%). Parathyroid adenomas in F344 rats are an example of a neoplasm whose incidence increases dramatically when comparing 2-year studies to life-span data. Solleveld et al. (1984) reported that the incidence of parathyroid adenomas increased in males from 0.1% at 2 years to 3.1% in lifetime studies. Corresponding data for female F344 rats was 0.1% at 2 years and 0.6% in lifetime studies.

Influence of Gonadectomy on Parathyroid Tumors. Oslapas et al. (1982) reported an increased incidence of parathyroid adenomas in female (34%) and male (27%) rats of the Long-Evans strain administered 40 µCi sodium ^{131}I and saline at 8 weeks of age. There were no significant changes in serum calcium, phosphorus, or PTH compared to controls. Gonadectomy performed at 7 weeks of age decreased the incidence of parathyroid adenomas in irradiated rats (7.4% in gonadectomy vs. 27% in intact controls), but there was little change in incidence of parathyroid adenomas in irradiated females. X-irradiation of the thyroid-parathyroid region also increased the incidence of parathyroid adenomas. When female Sprague-Dawley rats received a single absorbed dose of X-rays at 4 weeks of age, they subsequently developed a 24% incidence of parathyroid adenomas after 14 months (Oslapas et al. 1981).

Influence of Xenobiotics on Parathyroid Tumors. Parathyroid adenomas have been encountered infrequently following the administration of a variety of chemicals in 2-year bioassay studies in Fischer rats. In a study in F344 rats on the pesticide Rotenone there appeared to be an increased incidence of parathyroid adenomas in high-dose (75 ppm) males (4 of 44 rats) compared to either low-dose (38 ppm) males, control males (1 of 44 rats) or NTP historical controls (0.3%; Abdo et al. 1988). It was uncertain whether the increased incidence of this uncommon tumor was a direct effect of Rotenone feeding or the increased survival in high-dose males. Chief cell hyperplasia was not present in parathyroids that developed adenomas.

Influence of Irradiation and Hypercalcemia Induced by Vitamin D on Parathyroid Tumors. Wynford-Thomas et al. (1982) reported that irradiation significantly increases the incidence of parathyroid adenomas in inbred Wistar albino rats, and that the incidence could be modified by feeding diets with variable amounts of vitamin D. Neonatal Wistar rats were given either 5 or 10 µCi radioiodine (^{131}I) within 24 h of birth. In rats 12 months of age and older parathyroid adenomas were found in 33% of rats administered 5 µCi ^{131}I and in 37% of rats given 10 µCi ^{131}I compared to 0% in unirradiated controls. The incidence of parathyroid adenomas was highest (55%) in normocalcemic rats fed a low vitamin D diet and lowest (20%) in irradiated rats fed a high vitamin D diet (40000 IU/kg) that had a significant elevation in plasma calcium.

Chief Cell Carcinoma. In laboratory rats chief cell carcinomas are rarely encountered. Carcinomas result in a macroscopically detectable enlargement of one gland. Parathyroid carcinomas are often more fixed in position than chief cell adenomas due to invasion of either the adjacent thyroid lobe or adjacent cervical skeletal muscle. Some of the enlargement may be due to central necrosis and hemorrhage in the carcinoma.

The malignant chief cells either are arranged in solid sheets subdivided into lobules by a fibrovascular stroma, palisade along blood sinusoids, or form acinar structures. There is usually complete incorporation of the affected gland and evidence of invasion through the parathyroid capsule. Evidence of vascular invasion and formation of tumor cell emboli is observed infrequently. Malignant chief cells may be more pleomorphic than those comprising adenomas, but mitotic figures are infrequent. The cytoplasmic area stains lightly eosinophilic, and boundaries of adjacent chief cells are indistinct.

Parathyroid Changes with Cancer-Associated Hypercalcemia

Humoral Hypercalcemia of Malignancy in Dogs. Humoral hypercalcemia of malignancy (HHM) is a common clinical syndrome in dogs with several forms of cancer. The two most common malignancies that induce HHM are lymphoma and adenocarcinomas derived from apocrine glands of the anal sac (Rosol and Capen 1992). The apocrine adenocarcinoma of the anal sac occurs in the perirectal area of predominantly older female dogs and results in persistent hypercalcemia in 90% of tumor-bearing animals but rarely metastasizes to bone (Meuten et al. 1981; Rijnberk et al. 1978). Tumor excision results in a return to normocalcemia. Tumor recurrence is associated with a return of hypercalcemia due to secretion of PTHrP by the neoplastic cells (Rosol et al. 1990, 1992).

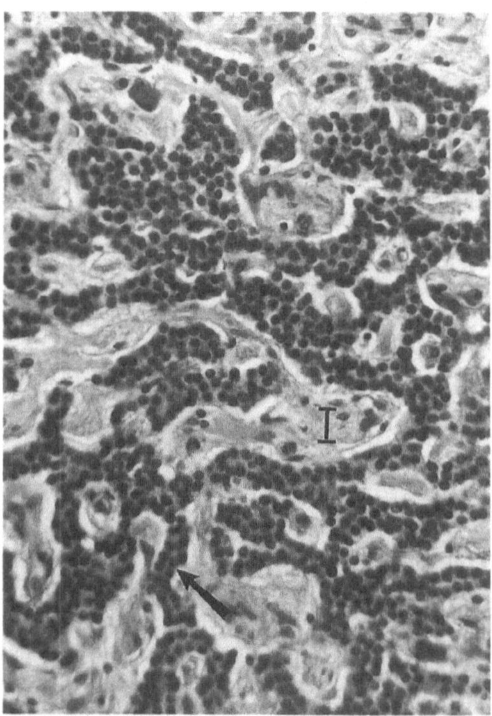

Fig. 346. Parathyroid gland from dog with hypercalcemia (15.8 mg/dl) and apocrine adenocarcinoma of the anal sac. Inactive chief cells have reduced cytoplasmic area and clumped nuclear chromatin. Narrow cords of chief cells (*arrow*) are separated by wide bands of collagen and prominent perivascular spaces (*I*). H&E, ×315. (From Meuten et al. 1983b)

Parathyroid glands from dogs with hypercalcemia and apocrine adenocarcinomas were composed of inactive or atrophic chief cells (Meuten et al. 1983b). They were arranged in narrow cords with prominent perivascular and interstitial spaces containing collagen fibers. Nuclei of inactive chief cells had clumped chromatin and the cytoplasm was lightly eosinophilic (Fig. 346). Ultrastructurally the reduced cytoplasmic area of chief cells, straight cell borders with uncomplicated interdigitations between adjacent cells, and the poorly developed synthetic and secretory organelles suggested that chief cells in dogs with persistent hypercalcemia were either inactive or atrophic (Fig. 347). Inactive chief cells had short profiles of rough endoplasmic reticulum, infrequent secretory granules, and a small Golgi apparatus. Intracytoplasmic lipid droplets were common in inactive chief cells. Parathyroid glands from control dogs had numerous active chief cells interspersed with inactive but no atrophic chief cells.

Lymphoma induces HHM in about 30% of the affected dogs and is usually associated with the T-cell phenotype (Weir et al. 1988). Hypercalcemia is induced by the secretion of PTHrP and other lymphokines that are capable of stimulating bone resorption (Rosol et al. 1992; Rosol and Capen 1992). Parathyroid glands ultrastructurally were composed predominately of inactive chief cells in hypercalcemic dogs with lymphosarcoma (Meuten et al. 1983a). Chief cells interpreted to be inactive had a reduced cytoplasmic area, straight plasma membranes, and increased intracytoplasmic lipid. The Golgi apparatus was small and associated with a few small granules. The rough endoplasmic reticulum consisted of dispersed short profiles and widely scattered mature secretory granules. Although similar chief cells were present in parathyroid glands from normocalcemic lymphosarcoma dogs they were admixed with other chief cells that were in various stages of secretory activity. Chief cells that were interpreted to be active had a larger Golgi apparatus, lamellar arrays of rough endoplasmic reticulum, more numerous secretory granules, an expanded cytoplasmic area, and more complex interdigitations of plasma membranes between

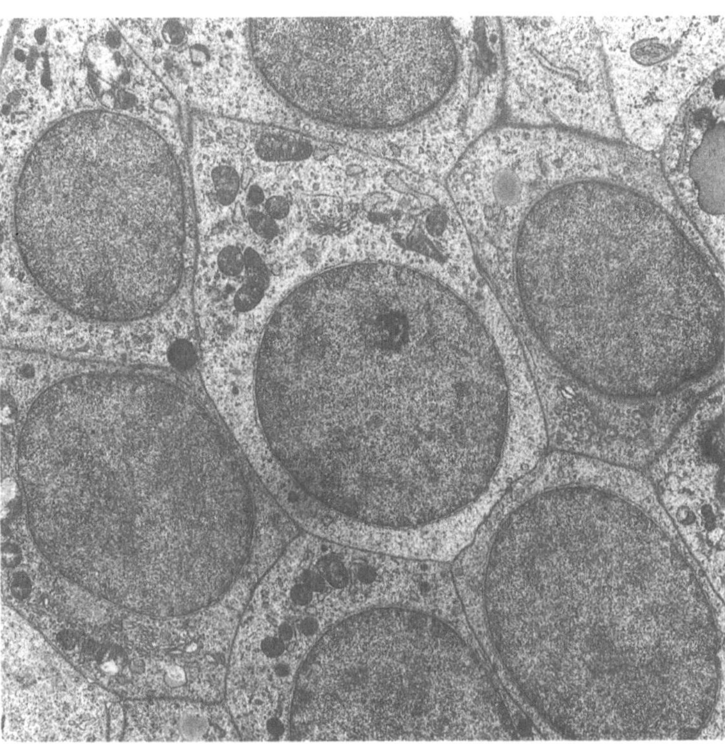

Fig. 347. Chief cells in parathyroid gland from dog with hypercalcemia (20.8 mg/dl), hypophosphatemia (1.8 mg/dl), and an apocrine adenocarcinoma of the anal sac. Inactive chief cells have reduced cytoplasmic area, straight plasma membranes with few uncomplicated interdigitations, lipid bodies, and electron-lucent cytoplasm cotaining few secretory organelles. ×4500. (From Meuten et al. 1983b)

adjacent cells. Parathyroid glands from control dogs had more numerous active chief cells interspersed with a few inactive chief cells.

The ultrastructure of parathyroid chief cells was examined from four groups of nude mice (NIH : Swiss) with different serum calcium concentrations (Gröne et al. 1992). A tumor line designated CAC-8 derived from an adenocarcinoma of the apocrine glands of the anal sac of a hypercalcemic dog was transplanted into eight male mice (Rosol et al. 1986). The mice were euthanatized when the transplanted adenocarcinoma CAC-8 induced hypercalcemia (6–8 weeks posttransplantation). CAC-8 induces HHM in mice, and has been reported to produce PTHrP and transforming growth factors-α and -β (Merryman et al. 1989; Rosol et al. 1990). The mean serum PTH concentration in CAC-8 bearing hypercalcemic mice has been reported to be decreased and serum 1,25-dihydroxyvitamin D increased compared to control mice (Rosol et al. 1988a). To evaluate the effects of PTHrP on chief cells eight female mice were infused with synthetic PTHrP (1–40) for 7 days (Rosol et al. 1988b). To evaluate the effect of low calcium intake on chief cells six male mice were fed a low-calcium diet (0.01% Ca, 0.55% phosphorus) for 14 days (Rosol and Capen 1987). These mice had access to distilled water only to exclude water as a possible calcium source. Ten male control mice were fed an identical diet containing 0.85% Ca.

Parathyroid glands were fixed in cold (4°C) 3% glutaraldehyde in 0.1 *M* sodium cacodylate buffer (pH 7.4), postfixed in 1.33% OsO_4 in s-collidine buffer (pH 7.4), dehydrated through ascending concentrations of ethanol, and embedded in epoxy resin. Thin sections were stained with uranyl acetate and lead citrate and examined with a Philips 300 electron microscope. Electron micrographs were taken randomly of chief cells at magnifications of ×3200–6400. Chief cells from each mouse were evaluated quantitatively and qualitatively. Serum calcium concentrations were significantly different for CAC-8 tumor bearing

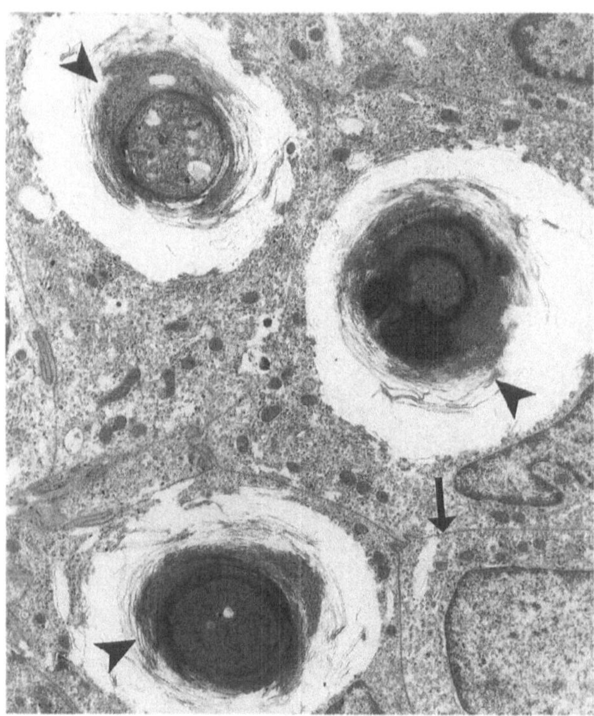

Fig. 348. Parathyroid gland from a hypercalcemia tumor (CAC-8) bearing mouse. Large cytoplasmic membranous whorls are present in cytoplasm of chief cells. The plasma membranes of adjacent cells are straight with uncomplicated interdigitations (*thick arrow*). ×7000. (From Gröne et al. 1992)

mice and PTHrP-infused mice as compared to controls. Tumor CAC-8 bearing mice were markedly hypercalcemic (17.0 ± 3.1 mg/dl) and mice infused with PTHrP (1–40) for 7 days developed less severe hypercalcemia (13.6 ± 1.5) when compared to the control group (9.3 ± 0.8) or mice fed a low-calcium diet (8.6 ± 0.6)

Tumor CAC-8 bearing and PTHrP-infused mice had significantly larger mean area (48 ± 18μm^2, 45 ± 12) of chief cells than the control mice (40 ± 18) and mice fed a low-calcium diet (37 ± 13). The majority of chief cells in tumor CAC-8 bearing mice had decreased tortuosity of plasma membranes and had only a few membranous interdigitations between adjacent cells (Fig. 348). The plasma membranes of the PTHrP-infused mice were similar to the tumor CAC-8 bearing group, whereas the control mice had many chief cells with tortuous cell membranes (Fig. 349). Mice fed a low-calcium diet had more prominent interdigitations of plasma membranes of adjacent chief cells than controls (Fig. 350).

Mature secretory granules had diameters of 150–200 nm, a narrow submembranous space, and an electron-dense core (Fig. 349). They were usually concentrated in one area of the cytoplasm, depending on the plane of section through the cell, and their numbers varied considerably between chief cells. The greatest number of secretory granules was present in chief cells from control mice (5.2 ± 2.8/cell). PTHrP-infused mice (4.3 ± 2.6), CAC-8 bearing mice (2.1 ± 1.3), and mice fed a low-calcium diet (1.7 ± 1.8) had significantly fewer secretory granules than control mice.

Prosecretory granules were larger (200–250 nm) and had a wider submembranous space and a more electron-lucent core than mature secretory granules (Fig. 350). Prosecretory granules often were located in the vicinity of a Golgi apparatus, and their numbers were variable between chief cells. They were most numerous in chief cells of mice fed a low-calcium diet (6.3 ±3.8/cell) followed by the control group (5.3 ± 3.3). The PTHrP-infused mice (4.1 ± 2.7) and the tumor CAC-8 bearing mice (1.8 ± 1.5) had significantly fewer prosecretory granules than control mice.

Chief cells in mice developed unique membranous whorls associated with hypercalcemia induced by PTHrP (Figs. 352, 353). The highest incidence of cytoplasmic membranous whorls was present in severely hypercalcemic tumor CAC-8 bearing mice that had a mean of 24 whorls per 500 chief cells (range 1–45). In PTHrP-infused mice there

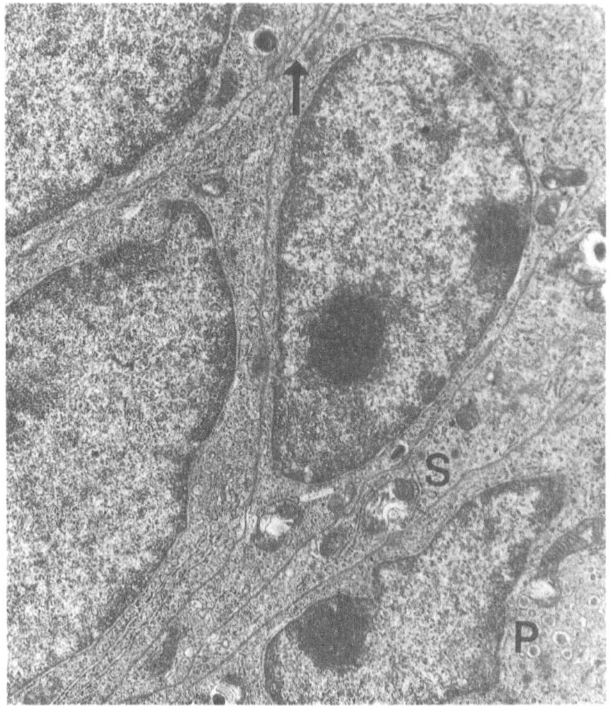

Fig. 349. Parathyroid gland from a normocalcemia control nude mouse. Chief cells have oval nuclei, tortuous cell membranes (*thick arrow*), mature secretory granules (*S*), and prosecretory granules (*P*). ×8000. (From Gröne et al. 1992)

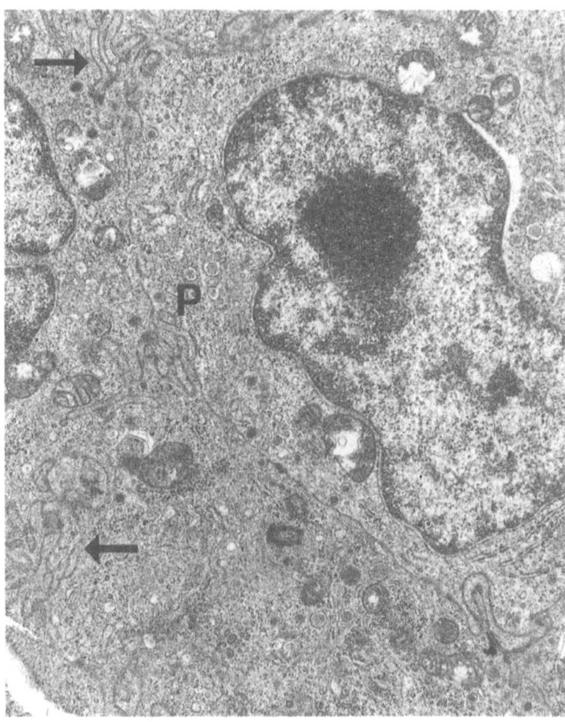

Fig. 350. Parathyroid gland from a nude mouse fed a low calcium diet. Chief cells have tortuous cell membranes (*thick arrows*), mature secretory granules, prosecretory granules (*P*), and well developed profiles of rough endoplasmic reticulum. ×10 000. (From Gröne et al. 1992)

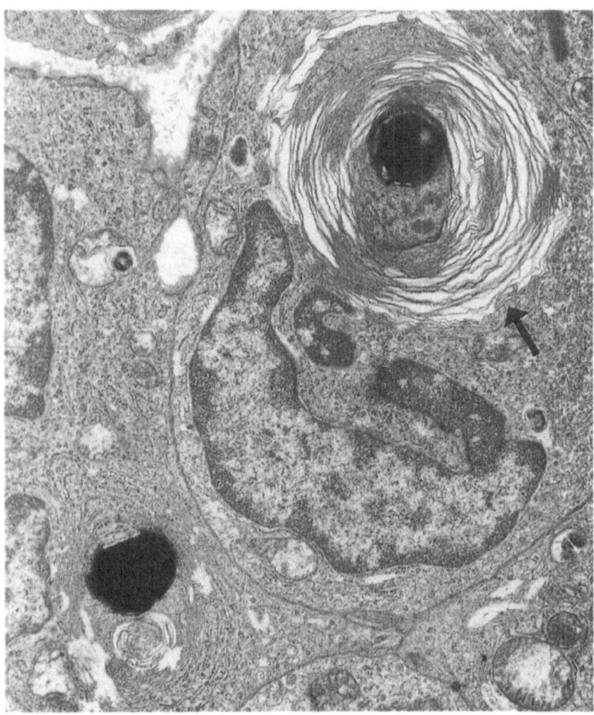

Fig. 351. Parathyroid gland from a hypercalcemic tumor (CAC-8) bearing mouse. Chief cell has a large membranous whorl (*thin arrow*) surrounding a lipid droplet and a markedly irregular nucleus. ×10 000. (From Gröne et al. 1992)

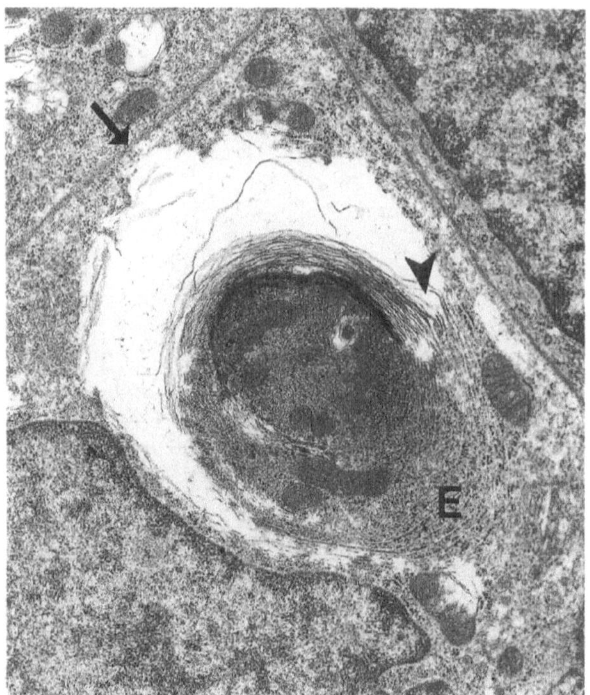

Fig. 352. Parathyroid gland from a hypercalcemic nude mouse infused with PTHrP (1–40). Chief cell illustrates initial stage of whorl formation associated with membranes of the rough endoplasmic reticulum (*E*) and straight plasma membranes between adjacent cells (*thick arrow*). ×12 000. (From Gröne et al. 1992)

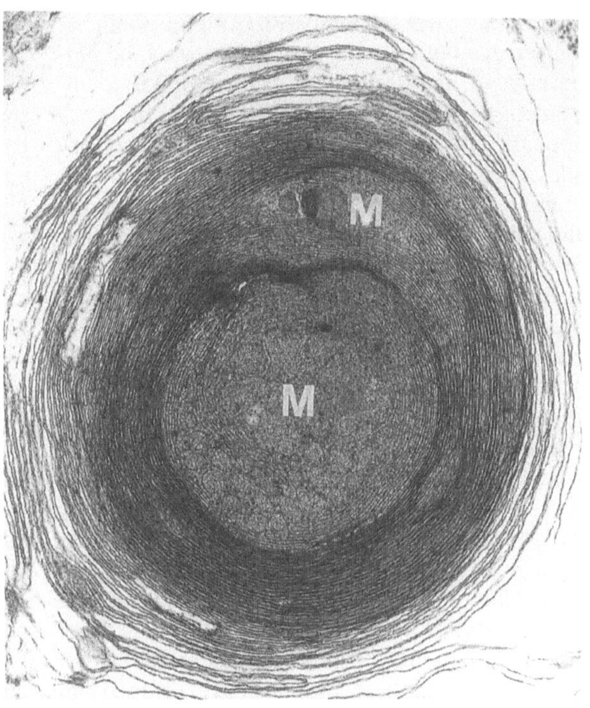

Fig. 353. Parathyroid gland from a hypercalcemic tumor (CAC-8) bearing nude mouse. Cytoplasmic membranous whorl in chief cell with agranular membranes surrounding occasional mitochondria (*M*). ×16000. (From Gröne et al. 1992)

was a mean of 8 whorls per 500 chief cells (range 0–16). Only one whorl was found in chief cells from mice fed a low-calcium diet, and whorls were not observed in the chief cells from control mice. The cytoplasmic area occupied by membranous whorls ranged from 9 to 39 μm^2 in tumor CAC-8 bearing mice and from 7 to 14 μm^2 in PTHrP-infused mice.

The formation of membranous whorls appeared to be similar in all affected mice. The unique whorls consisted of membranes, presumably derived from rough endoplasmic reticulum, plus entrapped cytoplasmic organelles. They often contained lipid droplets near the center of the whorl (Figs. 348, 351). The formation of membranous whorls appeared to begin with a circular aggregation of membranes from the rough endoplasmic reticulum (Fig. 350). Membranes that made up larger whorls did not contain attached ribosomes (Fig. 351). The initial stages of membranous whorl formation were observed most often in the PTHrP-infused mice but were observed infrequently in tumor CAC-8 bearing mice.

One frequently reported ultrastructural change in parathyroid chief cells of mice, with and without hypercalcemia, is the development of unique cytoplasmic membranous whorls under varied conditions such as starvation or after the administration of glucocorticoids, reserpine, and vitamin D (Isono et al. 1981, 1983, 1985; Latta and Rutz 1968; Stoeckel and Porte 1966). These myelinlike structures do not resemble the lamellar bodies found in human parathyroid chief cells in chronic renal failure or in parathyroid adenomas (Elliot and Arhelger 1966; Ellis and Coaker 1989; Hasleton and Ali 1980). In contrast, a parathyroid autograft from a human patient with chronic renal failure was reported to have myelinlike structures in about 5% of the chief cells (Ellis and Coaker 1989) similar to those described in mice. Membranous whorls also have been reported in a parathyroid adenoma from a patient with acute hyperparathyroidism (Boquist et al. 1971).

Membranous whorls in the chief cells of hypercalcemic nude mice did not appear to be the result of enhanced endocytosis of plasma membranes as has been reported in rats after vitamin D_3 administration (Wild et al. 1985) but rather to originate from coiling and condensation of rough endoplasmic reticulum with a gradual loss of ribosomes. Detachment of ribosomes from rough endoplasmic reticulum membranes and subsequent formation of intracellular myelinlike whorls is a common ultrastructural change in injured cells. Fragmentation of intracellular membranes with accumulation of phospholipids and reassembling with cholesterol may be important in the formation of myelinlike membranous whorls. Formation of whorls in chief cells appears to be an indicator of suppressed secretory activity and results from the accumulation of membranous material derived from endoplasmic reticulum. Whorling of cytoplasmic membranes in parathyroid cells of mice appears to be associated with suppression of secretory activity independent of cause rather than only with elevated serum calcium concentrations (Isono et al. 1983, 1985).

Myelinlike structures have been reported in hypocalcemic mice (Isono et al. 1981) and one whorl was observed in a mouse fed a low-calcium diet in this investigation. Either preexisting endoplasmic reticulum accumulated in the form of membranous whorls or, more likely, membrane flow from the secretory apparatus to the cell membrane was blocked in suppressed chief cells. The amount of membranous material that accumulated in these whorls appeared to be in excess of that amount of membranes found in chief cells from normocalcemic mice.

Chief cells of hypercalcemic mice showed evidence of suppression of secretory activity including a decrease in the number of secretory and prosecretory granules. Suppression of chief cells in hypercalcemic mice was also suggested by the straight plasma membranes of adjacent cells with uncomplicated interdigitations. Chief cells in hypercalcemic rats and cows have been reported to be inactive or atrophic (Capen and Roth 1971; Stoeckel and Porte 1966) and dogs with hypercalcemia of malignancy had reduced cytoplasmic area of chief cells (Meuten et al. 1983b). In contrast, our ultrastructural (Fig. 353) and morphometric evaluation revealed that chief cell area in tumor CAC-8 bearing hypercalcemic mice was increased significantly compared to control mice. There was no corresponding increase in nuclear area, indicating that the enlargement was due primarily to an increase in cytoplasmic volume. This finding was unexpected and is without satisfactory explanation at present. The increased cytoplasmic area in hypercalcemic mice was not due to the presence of membranous whorls since only a low percentage of chief cells contained membranous whorls. These findings suggest that chief cells of mice appear to react differently to long-standing hypercalcemia than other species.

Mice infused with PTHrP had similar changes in chief cells compared to tumor-bearing mice with HHM, but to a less severe degree. This suggests that a longer duration and greater magnitude of hypercalcemia results in more profound ultrastructural changes in parathyroid chief cells.

Chief cells of mice fed a low-calcium diet had ultrastructural changes consistent with stimulation of PTH synthesis and secretion. The number of prosecretory granules was increased, suggesting increased synthesis of PTH in response to demand created by feeding a low-calcium diet. The infrequent presence of mature secretory granules suggested that the immediate need for PTH did not permit storage of hormone in the form of mature secretory granules, due to rapid release of hormone after synthesis and processing. Previous studies have reported that animals fed a low-calcium diet for one week had an increased chief cell area (Capen 1971; Wernerson et al. 1991). In contrast, in this study mice fed a low-calcium diet for 2 weeks had a numerically reduced chief cell area as compared to control mice, but this difference was not statistically significant. The feeding of a low-calcium diet for two weeks appeared to be too short an interval to induce either hypocalcemia or hypertrophy of chief cells in mice.

References

Abdo KM, Eustis SL, Haseman J, Huff JE, Peters A, Persing R (1988) Toxicity and carcinogenicity of rotenone given in the feed to F344/N rats and B6C3F1 mice for up to two years. Drug Chem Toxicol 11:225–235

Armbrecht HJ, Wongsurawat N, Zenser TV, Davis BB (1982) Differential effects of parathyroid hormone on the renal 1,25-dihydroxyvitamin D_3 and 24,25-dihydroxyvitamin D_3 production of young and adult rats. Endocrinology 111: 1339–1344

Atwal OS (1979) Ultrastructural pathology of ozone-induced experimental parathyroiditis. IV. Biphasic activity in the chief cells of regenerating parathyroid glands. Am J Pathol 95:611–632

Atwal OS, Pemsingh RS (1981) Morphology of microvascular changes and endothelial regeneration in experimental ozone-induced parathyroiditis. III. Some pathologic considerations. Am J Pathol 102:297–307

Atwal OS, Wilson T (1974) Parathyroid gland changes following ozone inhalation. A morphologic study. Arch Environ Health 28:91–100

Atwal OS, Samagh BS, Bhatnagar MK (1975) A possible autoimmune parathyroiditis following ozone inhalation. II. A histopathologic, ultrastructural, and immunofluorescent study. Am J Pathol 80:53–68

Ayer LM, Szarka RJ, Mortimer ST, Alexander FJ, Martin JM, Andersen MA, Hanley DA (1989) Analysis of parathyroid hormone in bovine parathyroid cysts. J Bone Miner Res 4:335–340

Barbosa JA, Gill BM, Takiyyuddin MA, O'Connor DT (1991) Chromogranin A: posttranslational modifications in secretory granules. Endocrinology 128:174–190

Beck N, Singh H, Reed SW, Davis BB (1974) Direct inhibitory effect of hypercalcemia on renal actions of parathyroid hormone. J Clin Invest 53:717–725

Boquist L, Bergdahl L, Andersson A (1971) Parathyroid adenoma complicated by acute hyperparathyroidism. Ann Surg 173:593–603

Bourdeau AM, et al. (1987) Parathyroid response to aluminum in vitro: ultrastructural changes and PTH release. Kidney Int 31:15–24

Brown EM (1982) PTH secretion in vivo and in vitro. Regulation by calcium and other secretagogues. Miner Electrolytes Metab 8:130–150

Capen CC (1971) Fine structural changes of parathyroid glands in response to experimental and spontaneous alterations of extracellular fluid calcium. Am J Med 50:598–611

Capen CC (1983) Structural and biochemical aspects of parathyroid gland function in animals. In: Jones TC, Mohr U, Hunt RD (eds) (Monographs on pathology of laboratory animals) Endocrine system. Springer, Berlin Heidelberg New York, pp 217–247

Capen CC (1985a) Calcium-regulating hormones and metabolic bone disease. In: Newton CD, Nunamaker DM (eds) Textbook of small animal orthopaedics. Lippincott, Philadelphia, pp 673–722

Capen CC (1985b) The endocrine glands. In: Jubb KVF, Kennedy PC, Palmer N (eds) Pathology of domestic animals, 3rd edn. Academic, Orlando, pp 238–305

Capen CC (1990) Tumors of the endocrine glands. In: Moulton JE (ed) Tumors in domestic animals, 3rd edn. University of California Press, Berkeley, pp 553–639

Capen CC (1993) The endocrine glands. In: Jubb KVF, Kennedy PC, Palmer N (eds) Pathology of domestic animals, 4th edn. Academic, San Diego, pp 238–305

Capen CC, Martin SL (1974) Hyperparathyroidism in animals. In: Kirk RW (ed) Current veterinary therapy. V. Small animal practice. Saunders, Philadelphia, pp 797–805

Capen CC, Rosol TJ (1989) Calcium regulating hormones and diseases of mineral (calcium, phosphorus, magnesium) metabolism. In: Kaneko JJ (ed) Clinical biochemistry of domestic animals. Academic, San Diego, pp 682–766

Capen CC, Roth SI (1971) Ultrastructural and functional relationships of normal and pathologic parathyroid cells. In: Ioachim HL (ed) Pathobiology annual. Appleton, New York, pp 129–175

Capen CC, Rowland GN (1968) Ultrastructural evaluation of the parathyroid glands of young cats with experimental hyperparathyroid SM. Z Zellforsch 90:495–506

Chambers TJ (1980) The cellular basis of bone resorption. Clin Orthop 151:283–293

Chambers TJ, Revell PA, Fuller K, Athanasou NA (1984) Resorption of bone by isolated rabbit osteoclasts. J Cell Sci 66:383–399

Cheville NF (1972) Ultrastructure of canine carotid body and aortic body tumors. Comparison with tissues of thyroid and parathyroid origin. Vet Pathol 9:166–189

Chisari FV, et al. (1972) Parathyroid necrosis and hypocalcemic tetany induced in rabbits by L-asparaginase. Am J Pathol 68:461–468

Chu LLH, MacGregor RR, Anast CS, Hamilton JW, Cohn DV (1973) Studies on the biosynthesis of rat parathyroid hormone and proparathyroid hormone: adaptation of the parathyroid gland to dietary restriction of calcium. Endocrinology 93:915–924

Cole JA, Eber SL, Poelling RE, Thorne PK, Forte LR (1987) A dual mechanism for regulation of kidney phosphate transport by parathyroid hormone. Am J Physiol 253: E221–E227

de Vernejoul M-C, Horowitz M, Demignon J, Neff L, Baron R (1988) Bone resorption by isolated chick osteoclasts in culture is stimulated by murine spleen cell supernatant fluids (osteoclast-activating factor) and inhibited by calcitonin and prostaglandin E_2. J Bone Miner Res 3:69–80

Delaisse J-M, Eeckhout Y, Sear C, Galloway A, McCullagh K, Vaes G (1985) A new synthetic inhibitor of mammalian tissue collagenase inhibits bone resorption in culture. Biochem Biophys Res Commun 133:483–490

Donahue HJ, Fryer MJ, Eriksen EF, Heath H III (1988) Differential effects of parathyroid hormone and its analogues on cytosolic calcium ion and cAMP levels in cultured rat osteoblast-like cells. J Biol Chem 263:13522–13527

Eeckhout Y, Delaisse J-M, Ladent P, Vaes G (1988) The proteinases of bone resorption. In: Glauert AM (ed) The control of tissue damage. Elsevier, Amsterdam, pp 297–313

Elliot RL, Arhelger RB (1966) Fine structure of parathyroid adenomas with special reference to annulate lamellae and septate desmosomes. Arch Pathol 81:200–212

Ellis HA, Coaker T (1989) Ultrastructure of parathyroid autografts in chronic renal failure including the occurrence of concentric membraneous bodies and intermediate filaments. Histopathology 14:401–407

Faccini JM (1969) Fluoride-induced hyperplasia of the parathyroid glands. Proc R Soc Med 62:241

Faccini JM, Care AD (1965) Effect of sodium fluoride on the ultrastructure of the parathryoid glands of the sheep. Nature 207:1399

Farndale RW, Sandy JR, Atkinson SJ, Pennington SR, Meghi S, Meikle MC (1988) Parathyroid hormone and prostaglandin E_2 stimulate both inositol phosphates and cyclic AMP accumulation in mouse osteoblast cultures. Biochem J 252:263–268

Fasciotto BH, Gorr S-U, Bourdeau AM, Cohn DV (1990) Autocrine regulation of parathyroid secretion: Inhibition of secretion by chromogranin-A (secretory protein-I) and potentiation of secretion by chromogranin-A and pancreastatin antibodies. Endocrinology 127:1329–1335

Forte LR, Langeluttig SG, Poelling RE, Thomas ML (1982) Renal parathyroid hormone receptors in the chick: downregulation in secondary hyperparathyroid animal models. Am J Physiol 242 (Endocrinol Metab 5):E154–E163

Fox J (1991) Regulation of parathyroid hormone secretion by plasma calcium in aging rats. Am J Physiol 260 (Endocrinol Metab 23):E220–E225

Goldring SR, Tyler GA, Krane SM, Potts JT Jr, Rosenblatt M (1984) Photoaffinity labeling of parathyroid hormone receptors: comparison of receptors across species and target tissues and after desensitization to hormone. Biochemistry 23:489–502

Goltzman D, Bennett HP, Koutsilieris M, Mitchell J, Rabbani SA, Rouleau MF (1986) Studies of the multiple molecular forms of bioactive parathyroid hormone and parathyroid hormone-like substances. Recent Prog Horm Res 42: 665–703

Gröne A, Rosol TJ, Baumgärtner W, Capen CC (1992) Effects of humoral hypercalcemia of malignancy on the parathyroid gland in nude mice. Vet Pathol 29:343–350

Habener JF (1981) Recent advances in parathyroid hormone research. Clin Biochem 14:223–229

Hanai H, Ishida M, Liang CT, Sacktor B (1986) Parathyroid hormone increases sodium/calcium exchange activity in renal cells and the blunting of the response in aging. J Biol Chem 261:5419–5425

Hanai H, Liang CT, Cheng L, Sacktor B (1989) Desensitization to parathyroid hormone in renal cells from aged rats is associated with alterations in G-protein activity. J Clin Invest 83:268–277

Hanai H, Brennan DP, Cheng L, Goldman ME, Chorev M, Levine MA, Sacktor B, Liang CT (1990) Downregulation of parathyroid hormone receptors in renal membranes from aged rats. Am J Physiol 259 (Renal Fluid Electrolyte Physiol 28):F444–F450

Hasleton PS, Ali HH (1980) The parathyroid in chronic renal failure – a light and electron microscopical study. J Pathol 132:307–323

Henry HL (1985) Parathyroid hormone modulation of 25-hydroxyvitamin D_3 metabolism by cultured chick kidney cells is mimicked and enhanced by forskolin. Endocrinology 116:503–510

Henry HL, Cunningham NS, Noland TA Jr (1983) Homologous desensitization of cultured chick kidney cells to parathyroid hormone. Endocrinology 113:1942–1949

Herrmann-Erlee MP, van der Meer JM, Lowik CW, van Leeuwen JP, Boonekamp PM (1988) Different roles for calcium and cyclic AMP in the action of PTH: studies in bone explants and isolated bone cells. Bone 9:93–100

High WB, Black HE, Capen CC (1981) Histomorphometric evaluation of the effects of low dose parathyroid hormone administration on cortical bone remodeling in adult dogs. Lab Invest 44:449–454

Hruska KA, Moskowitz D, Esbrit P, Civitelli R, Westbrook S, Huskey M (1987) Stimulation of inositol trisphosphate and diacylglycerol production in renal tubular cells by parathyroid hormone. J Clin Invest 79:230–239

Isono H, Shoumura S, Ishizaki N, Emura S, Hayashi K, Yamahira T, Iwasaki Y (1981) Electron microscopic study of the parathyroid gland of the reserpine-treated mouse. J Clin Electron Microscopy 14:113–120

Isono H, Shoumura S, Ishizaki N, Emura S, Iwasaki Y, Yamahira T, Kitamura Y (1985) Effects of starvation on the ultrastructure of the mouse parathyroid gland. Acta Anat 121:46–52

Isono H, Shoumura S, Ishizaki N, Emura S, Hayashi K, Iwasaki Y, Yamahira T, Kitamura Y (1983) Effects of glucocorticoid on the ultrastructure of the mouse parathyroid gland. Arch Histol Jpn 46:293–305

Jaffe N, et al. (1972) Comparison of daily and twice-weekly schedule of L-asparaginase in childhood leukemia. Pediatrics 49:590–595

Jüppner H, Abou-Samra A-B, Freeman M, Kong XF, Schipani E, Richards J, Kolakowski LF Jr, Hock J, Potts JT Jr, Kronenberg HM, Segre GV (1991) A G protein-linked receptor for parathyroid hormone and parathyroid hormone-related protein. Science 254:1024–1026

Kalu DN, Hardin RR, Murata I, Huber MB, Roos BA (1982) Age-dependent modulation parathyroid hormone action. Age 5:25–29

Kiebzak GM, Sacktor B (1986) Effect of age on renal conservation of phosphate in the rat. Am J Physiol 251(Renal Fluid Electrolyte Physiol 20):F399–F407

Knox FG, Haramati A (1985) Renal regulation of phosphate excretion. In: Seldin DW, Giebisch G (eds) The kidney: physiology and pathophysiology. Raven, New York

Kronenberg HM, Igarashi T, Freeman MW, Okazaki T, Brand SJ, Wiren KM, Potts JT Jr (1986) Structure and expression of the human parathyroid hormone gene. Rec Prog Horm Res 42:641–663

Krook L (1957) Spontaneous hyperparathyroidism in the dog. A pathologic-anatomical study. Acta Pathol Microbiol Scand 41 [Suppl 122]:1–88

Latta JS, Rutz TJ (1968) Special ultrastructural features of parathyroid cells from Swiss mice bearing Ehrlich's ascites tumor. Anat Rec 160:255,260–290

Lee DBN, Yanagawa N, Jo O, Yu BP, et al. (1984) Phosphaturia of aging: studies on mechanisms. Adv Exp Med Biol 178:103–108

Loveridge N, Dean V, Goltzman D, Hendy GN (1991) Bioactivity of parathyroid hormone and parathyroid hormone-like peptide: agonist and antagonist activities of amino-terminal fragments as assessed by the cytochemical bioassay and in situ biochemistry. Endocrinology 128: 1938–1946

Lupulescu A, et al. (1968) Experimental investigation on immunology of the parathyroid gland. Immunology 14:475

Mahoney CA, Nissenson RA (1983) Canine renal receptors for parathyroid hormone. Down-regulation in vivo by exogenous parathyrid hormone. J Clin Invest 72:411–421

Mayer GP, Hurst JG (1978) Comparison of the effects of calcium and magnesium on parathyroid hormone secretion rate in calves. Endocrinology 102:1803–1814

McSheehy PM, Chambers TJ (1986) Osteoblastic cells mediate osteoclastic responsiveness to parathyroid hormone. Endocrinology 118:824–828

Merryman JI, Rosol TJ, Brooks CL, Capen CC (1989) Separation of parathyroid hormone-like activity from transforming growth factor-α and -β in the canine adenocarcinoma (CAC-8) model of humoral hypercalcemia of malignancy. Endocrinology 124:2456–2563

Meuten DJ, Cooper BJ, Capen CC, Chew DJ, Kociba GJ (1981) Hypercalcemia associated with an adenocarcinoma derived from the apocrine glands of the anal sac. Vet Pathol 18:454–471

Meuten DJ, Kociba GJ, Capen CC, Chew DJ, Segre GV, Levine L, Tashjian AHJ, Voelkel EF, Nagode LA (1983a) Hypercalcemia in dogs with lymphosarcoma. Biochemical, ultrastructural, and histomorphometric investigations. Lab Invest 49:553–562

Meuten DJ, Segre GV, Capen CC, Kociba GJ, Voelkel EF, Levine L, Tashjian AH, Chew DJ, Nagode LA (1983b) Hypercalcemia in dogs with adenocarcinoma derived from apocrine glands of the anal sac. Biochemical and histomorphometric investigations. Lab Invest 48:428–435

Morrissey J, Slatopolsky E (1986) Effect of aluminum on parathryoid hormone secretion. Kidney Int [Suppl] 29: S41–S44

Morrissey J, et al. (1983) Suppression of parathryoid hormone secretion by aluminum. Kidney Int 23:699–704

Norman AW (1986) Parathyroid hormone stimulates calcium transport in perfused duodena from normal chicks: comparison with the rapid (transcaltachic) effect of 1,25-dihydroxyvitamin D3. Endocrinology 119:1406–1408

Oettgen HF, et al. (1970) Toxicity of E coli L-asparaginase in man. Cancer 25:253–278

Oslapas R, et al. (1981) Incidence of radiation-induced parathyroid tumors in male and female rats. Clin Res 29:734A

Pliam NB, Nyiredy KO, Arnaud CD (1982) Parathyroid hormone receptors in avian bone cells. Proc Natl Acad Sci USA 79:2061–2063

Raisz LG, Kream BE (1983) Regulation of bone formation (second of two parts). N Engl J Med 309:83–89

Ream LJ, Principato R (1981) Glycogen accumulation in the parathyroid gland of the rat after fluoride ingestion. Cell Tissue Res 220:125–130

Rijnberk A, Elsinghorst TA, Koeman JP, Hackeng WHL, Lequin RM (1978) Pseudohyperparathyroidism associated with perirectal adenocarcinomas in elderly female dogs. Tijdschr Diergeneeskd 103:1069–1075

Rodan GA, Martin TJ (1981) Role of osteoblasts in hormonal control of bone resorption – a hypothesis. Calcif Tissue Int 33:349–351

Rosol TJ, Capen CC (1987) The effect of low calcium diet, mithramycin, and dichlorodimethylene bisphosphonate on humoral hypercalcemia of malignancy in nude mice transplanted with the canine adenocarcinoma tumor line (CAC-8). J Bone Miner Res 2:395–405

Rosol TJ, Capen CC (1989) Tumors of the parathyroid glands and circulating parathyroid hormone-like protein associated with persistent hypercalcemia. Toxicol Pathol 17:346–356

Rosol TJ, Capen CC (1992) Mechanisms of cancer-induced hypercalcemia. Lab Invest 67:680–702

Rosol TJ, Capen CC, Weisbrode SE, Horst RL (1986) Humoral hypercalcemia of malignancy in nude mouse model of a canine adenocarcinoma derived from apocrine glands of the anal sac. Biochemical, histomorphometric, and ultrastructural studies. Lab Invest 54:679–688

Rosol TJ, Capen CC, Deftos LJ, Horst RL (1988a) Nude mouse model (CAC-8) of humoral hypercalcemia of malignancy with increased serum levels of 1,25-dihyroxycholecalciferol: in vivo and in vitro studies. In: Norman AW, Schaefer K, Grigoleit HG, Herrath DV (eds) Vitamin D: molecular, cellular and clinical endocrinology. De Gruyter, Berlin, pp 867–868

Rosol TJ, Capen CC, Horst RL (1988b) Effects of infusion of human parathyroid hormone-related protein (1–40) in nude mice: histomorphometric and biochemical investigations. J Bone Miner Res 3:699–706

Rosol TJ, Capen CC, Danks JA, Suva LJ, Steinmeyer CL, Hayman J, Ebeling PR, Martin TJ (1990) Identification of parathyroid hormone-related protein in canine apocrine adenocarcinoma of the anal sac. Vet Pathol 27:89–95

Rosol TJ, Nagode LA, Couto CG, Hammer AS, Chew DJ, Peterson JL, Ayl RD, Steinmeyer CL, Capen CC (1992) Parathyroid hormone (PTH)-related protein, PTH, and 1,25-dihydroxyvitamin D in dogs with cancer-associated hypercalcemia. Endocrinology 131:1157–1164

Roth SI, Raisz LG (1964) Effect of calcium concentration on the ultrastructure of rat parathyroid in organ culture. Lab Invest 13:331–345

Silve CM, Hradek GT, Jones AL, Arnaud CD (1982) Parathyroid hormone receptor in intact embryonic chicken bone: characterization and cellular localization. J Cell Biol 94:379–386

Solleveld HA, Haseman JK, McConnell EE (1984) National history of body weight gain, survival and neoplasia in the F344 rat. J Natl Cancer Inst 72:929–940

Stoeckel ME, Porte A (1966) Ultrastructural studies on the mouse parathyroid gland II. Experimental studies (in French). Zellforsch Mikrosk Anat 73:503–520

Sutton RAL, Dirks JH (1978) Renal handling of calcium. Fed Proc 37:2112–2119

Teitelbaum AP, Silve CM, Nyiredy KO, Arnaud CD (1986) Down-regulation of parathyroid hormone (PTH) receptors in cultured bone cells is associated with agonist-specific intracellular processing of PTH-receptor complexes. Endocrinology 118:595–602

Teotia SPS, Teotia M (1973) Secondary hyperparathyroidism in patients with endemic skeletal flurosis. BMJ 1: 637–640

Tettenborn D, Hobik HP, Luckhaus G (1970) Hypoparathyroidism following application of L-asparaginase in the rabbit (in German). Arzneimittelforschung 20:1753–1755

Uden P, Halloran B, Daly R, Duh QY, Clark O (1992) Setpoint for parathyroid hormone release increases with postmaturational aging in the rat. Endocrinology 131: 2251–2256

Vaes G (1988) Cellular biology and biochemical mechanism of bone resorption. A review of recent developments on the formation, activation, and mode of action of osteoclasts. Clin Orthop 231:239–271

Wada L, Daly R, Kern D, Halloran B (1992) Kinetics of 1,25-dihydroxyvitamin D metabolism in the aging rat. Am J Physiol 262 (Endocrinol Metab 25):E906–E910

Weir EC, Norrdin RW, Matus RE, Brooks MB, Broadus AE, Mitnick M, Johnston SD, Insogna KL (1988) Humoral hypercalcemia of malignancy in canine lymphosarcoma. Endocrinology 122:602–608

Wernerson A, Mengarelli Widholm SM, Svensson O, Reinholt FP (1991) Parathyroid cell number and size in hypocalcemic young rats. APMIS 99:1096–1102

Wild P, Gloor S, Vetsch E (1985) Quantitative aspects of membrane behavior in rat parathyroid cells after depression or elevation of serum calcium. Lab Invest 52:490–496

Wong GL (1986) Skeletal effects of parathyroid hormone. In: Peck WA (ed) Bone and mineral research, 4th edn. Elsevier, Amsterdam, pp 103–129

Wongsurawat N, Armbrecht HJ (1987) Comparison of calcium effect on in vitro calcitonin and parathyroid hormone release by young and aged thyroparathyroid glands. Exp Gerontol 22:263–269

Wynford-Thomas V, Wynford-Thomas D, Williams ED (1982) Experimental induction of parathyroid adenomas in the rat. J Natl Cancer Inst 70:127–134

Yamaguchi DT, Kleeman CR, Muallem S (1987) Protein kinase C-activated calcium channel in the osteoblast-like clonal osteosarcoma cell line UMR-106. J Biol Chem 262:14967–14973

Young DM, et al. (1973) Clinicopathologic and ultrastructural studies of L-asparaginase-induced hypocalcemia in rabbits. An experimental animal model of acute hypoparathyroidism. Lab Invest 29:374–386

Anatomy, Histology, and Ultrastructure, Parathyroid, Syrian Hamster

Birgit Kittel, Heinrich Ernst, and Kenji Kamino

Gross Appearance

In hamsters, as in rats and mice, only one pair of parathyroids is present. The oval or lens-shaped organs are small and variable in size (0.7–1 mm × 0.3–0.5 mm; Michel 1957; Pour 1983b) and usually located at the anteriolateral margin of the thyroid gland (Fig. 354). In the Syrian hamster *Mesocricetus auratus* major parts of the glands are frequently surrounded by thyroid tissue, and they are therefore difficult to detect grossly. In some instances the parathyroids of Syrian hamsters possess a slender "tail" which extends laterally and caudally into the thyroid (Pour 1983b).

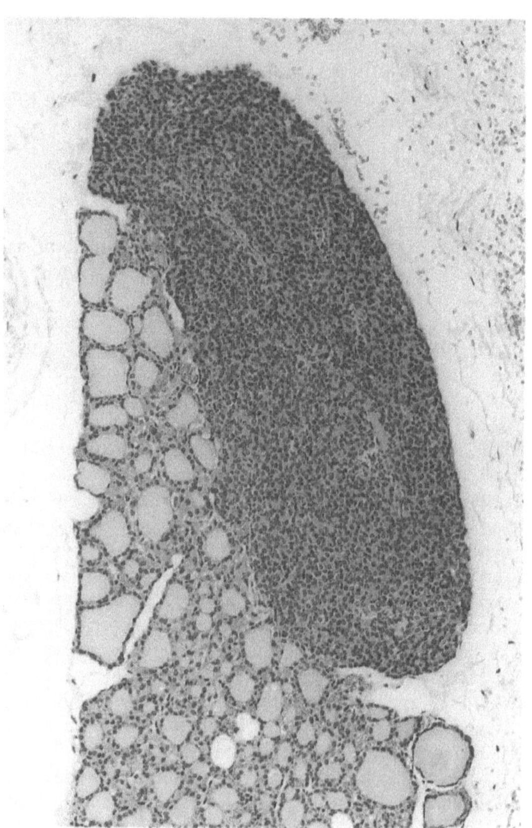

Fig. 354. Parathyroid (*right*) and thyroid gland of a 4-week-old Syrian Hamster. H&E, ×120

Microscopic Features

Because of the small size and variations in localization and shape of the parathyroids it is recommended for histological processing that the larynx be separated from the trachea vertically at the level of the third or fourth tracheal ring, fixed in toto, and embedded in a horizontal position with the hyoid facing up. Sections of three or more steps usually make it possible to find the parathyroid glands as well as any ectopic parathyroid tissue (Pour 1983a). The parathyroid gland of the golden hamster is enclosed in a thin fibrous capsule. Fine strands of delicate connective tissue containing nerves and vessels run between cords or solid masses of chief cells (Figs. 355, 356). Oxyphilic cells which are common in humans, monkeys, bovidae, equidae, and turtles (Roth and Capen 1974), but which are absent in rats and mice have been observed only in the hamster by Pour (1983b), with an extremely low frequency (0.01%). Nevertheless, as in rats and mice, light and dark staining chief cells can frequently be found (Fig. 355). Chief cells in parathyroid glands of hamsters have indistinct cell borders surrounding a faintly eosinophilic, granular cytoplasm. The cells have round or oval nuclei with one or more prominent nucleoli and aggregates of chromatin mostly at the nuclear periphery (Fig. 356).

Ultrastructure

The plasma membranes of adjacent chief cells pursue a tortuous course with occasional inter-

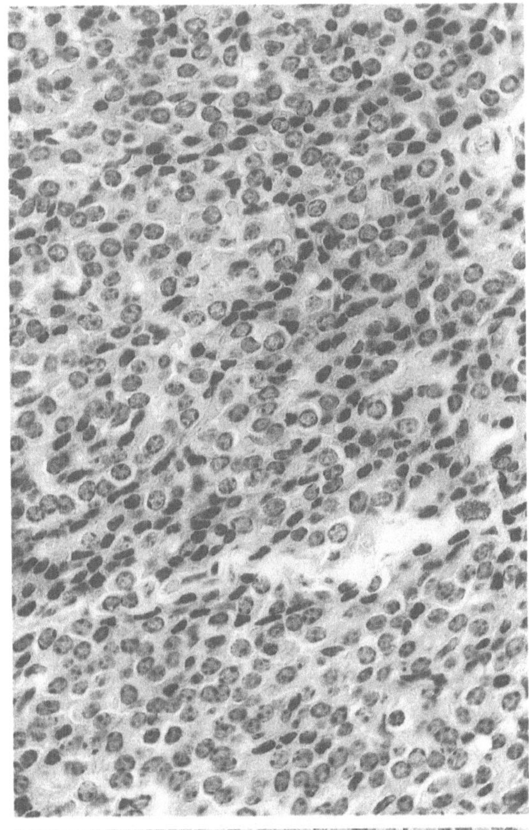

Fig. 355. (*above*) Parathyroid gland of a 4-week-old Syrian Hamster. Light and dark staining chief cells. H&E, ×300

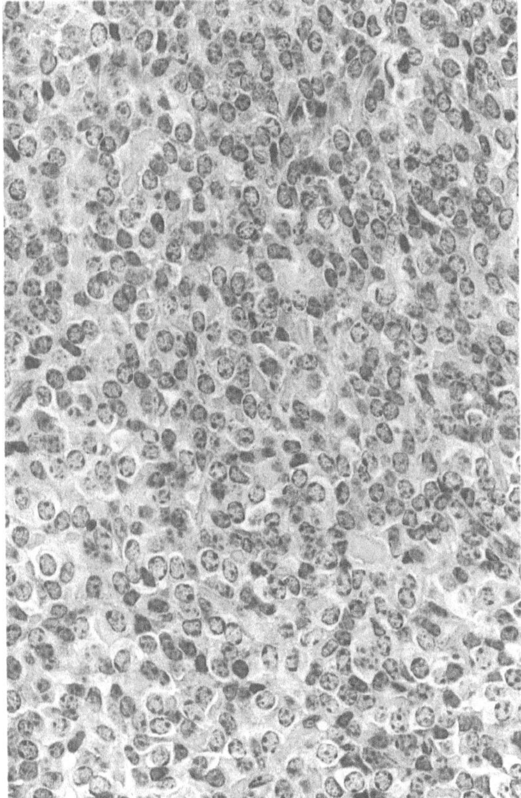

Fig. 356. (*below*) Parathyroid gland of a 4-week-old Syrian Hamster. Chief cells with indistinct cell borders and round to ovoid nuclei with prominent nucleoli. H&E, ×300

digitations. They are rich in free ribosomes and mitochondria. The rough endoplasmic reticulum is randomly distributed or arranged in parallel arrays. Most Golgi complexes are relatively well developed and contain a few small coated vesicles, 70 nm in diameter. Secretory granules 150–300 nm in diameter can be found in Golgi areas or in the peripheral cytoplasm. Sometimes large secretory granules of 350–600 nm diameter can be observed (Emura et al. 1984; Chen et al. 1991; Shoumura et al. 1992).

A marked seasonal variation occurs in parathyroid chief cell ultrastructure of *Cricetus cricetus* with an increased number of dark, secretory granule-rich chief cells in the winter months and more light chief cells in summer. This has been interpreted as indicative of increased parathyroid activity in winter (Kayser et al. 1961, cited by Roth and Capen 1974).

References

Chen H, Shoumura S, Emura S, Utsumi M, Yamahira T, Isono H (1991) Effects of melatonin on the ultrastructure of the golden hamster parathyroid gland. Histol Histopathol 6:1–7

Emura S, Shoumura S, Ishizaki N, Hayashi K, Iwasaki Y, Yamahira T, Kitamura Y, Isono H (1984) Effects of ovariectomy on the ultrastructure of the parathyroid gland of the golden hamster. Acta Anat 119:224–230

Michel G (1957) Beitrag zur Anatomie der Schilddrüse, der Epithelkörperchen und der Nebennieren des Syrischen Goldhamsters (Mesocricetus auratus W). Zentralbl Veterinärmed 4:497–508

Pour P (1983a) Parathyroid glands, hamster, introduction. In: Jones TC, Mohr U, Hunt RD (eds) Monographs on pathology of laboratory animals, endocrine system, 1st edn. Springer, Berlin Heidelberg New York, p 248

Pour P (1983b) Anatomy, histology, parathyroid, hamster. In: Jones TC, Mohr U, Hunt RD (eds) Monographs on pathology of laboratory animals, endocrine system, 1st edn. Springer, Berlin Heidelberg New York, pp 249–252

Roth S, Capen C (1974) Ultrastructural and functional correlations of the parathyroid gland. Int Rev Exp Pathol 13:161–221

Shoumura S, Emura S, Utsumi M, Chen H, Hayakawa D, Yamahira T, Terasawa K, Tamada A, Arakawa M, Isono H (1992) Ultrastructure of the parathyroid gland of fetal and pregnant golden hamsters subjected to hypergravity environment. Acta Anat 145:112–118

Anatomy, Histology, and Ultrastructure, Parathyroid, Mouse

Birgit Kittel, Heinrich Ernst, and Kenji Kamino

Embryology and Anatomy

As in the rat and hamster, the parathyroid glands are derived from the third pharyngeal pouch. The fourth pharyngeal pouch does not develop, and therefore only one pair of glands is found. Because of the close embryologic relationship between thymus and parathyroids ectopic parathyroid tissue can sometimes occur in the thymus or close to the larynx and ectopic thymic tissue can occasionally be observed close to the parathyroid (Fig.357). In aged OF1 mice ectopic parathyroid tissue which is embedded within the thyroid gland can sometimes be found (Pour et al. 1983; see p. 333 this volume). Cysts lined by cuboidal or columnar (ciliated) epithelium and filled with eosinophilic or mucinous basophilic material (Fig. 358) seen to be remnants of embryonic ducts between primordial thymus and parathyroids.

The ovoid-shaped glands are located at the anteriolateral aspect of the thyroid, often lying in a depression and sometimes with focal extension into the thyroid (Fig. 359). They are difficult to detect macroscopically. The parathyroids are separated by delicate strands of connective tissue from the thyroid gland.

Histology

The mouse parathyroid consists of only one cell type, the chief cell. Oxyphilic cells, as in human beings, are absent in mice. Light and dark cell variants (see below) can be distinguished within routinely processed tissue: smaller, spindle-shaped dark cells (6–7 μm) with scanty cytoplasm and a dark nucleus, and larger, ovoid light cells (10–12 μm) with abundant faintly eosinophilic and finely granular cytoplasm. This cell variant has a large, ovoid nucleus with one or more nucleoli and indistinct cell borders. The parenchyma consists of closely packed, branching, and folded cords of chief cells that are arranged in a trabecular structure (Fig. 360), separated by delicate fibrous stroma which contains capillaries, lymphatics, and nerves.

Ultrastructure

The ultrastructure of the normal parathyroid gland in the mouse has been reported by Isono et al. (1983), Coleman and Silbermann (1978), Latta and Rutz (1968), and Pour et al. (1983). The closely packed chief cells possess a smooth plasma membrane with occasional interdigitations. Desmosomes can be seen at the lateral cell wall. The nucleus is polygonal or oval in shape and may have indentations. The cytoplasm contains abundant mitochondria and free ribosomes, a well-developed Golgi complex, and a rough endoplasmic reticulum which occasionally is arranged in parallel arrays. Secretory granules of 150–200 nm in diameter are located in the periphery close to the apical cell membrane. Larger secretory granules 300–600 nm in diameter are believed to be storage granules by some authors (Isono et al. 1983, 1985). The presence of light and dark cells and of a transitional cell type is, at least in the rat, probably provoked during fixation (Wild et al. 1986, 1987; Wild and Schraner 1989; Marti et al. 1987) or due to different functional stages (Moreira et al. 1985; Moreira and Goncalves 1985).

References

Coleman R, Silbermann M (1978) Ultrastructure of parathyroid glands in triamcinolone-treated mice. J Anat 126:181–192

Isono H, Shoumura S, Ishizaki N, Emura S, Hayashi K, Iwasaki Y, Yamahira T, Kitamura Y (1983) Effects of glucocorticoid on the ultrastructure of the mouse parathyroid gland. Arch Histol Jpn 46:293–305

Isono H, Shoumura S, Ishizaki N, Emura S, Iwasaki Y, Yamahira T, Kitamura Y (1985) Effects of starvation on the ultrastructure of the mouse parathyroid gland. Acta Anat 121:46–52

Latta JS, Rutz TJ (1968) Special ultrastructural features of parathyroid cells from Swiss mice bearing Ehrlichs ascites tumor. Anat Rec 160:255–259

Marti R, Wild P, Schraner EM, Mueller M, Moor H (1987) Parathyroid ultrastructure after aldehyde fixation, high-pressure-freezing, or microwave irradiation. J Histochem Cytochem 35:1415–1424

Moreira JE, Gonalves RP (1985) Ultrastructural changing of the rat parathyroid gland under various fixation methods. Anat Anz 158:413–423

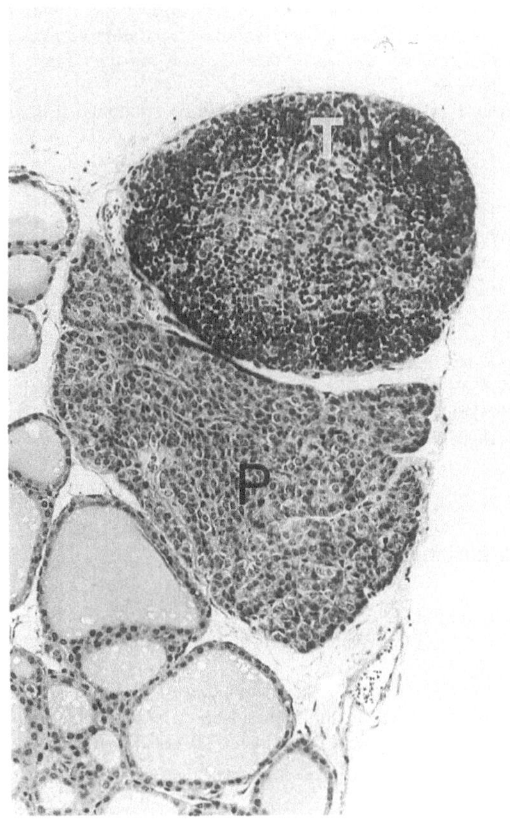

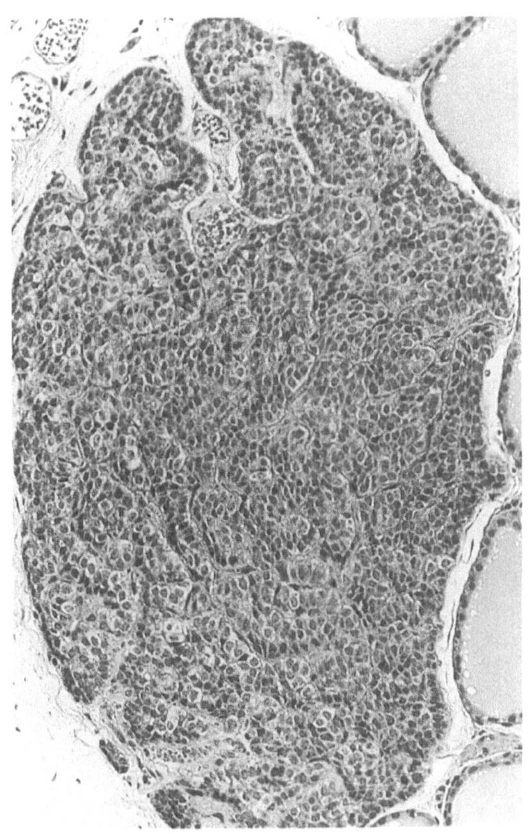

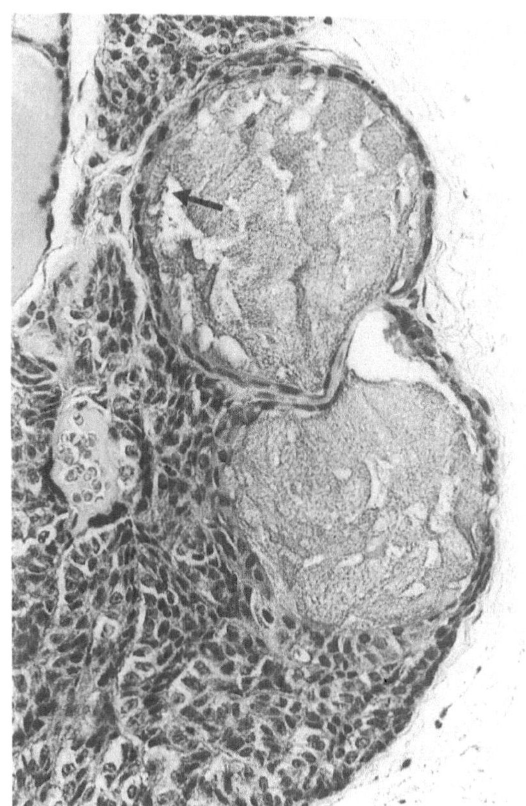

Fig. 357. (*upper left*) C57 Black mouse, 3 months. Ectopic thymic tissue (*T*) located in close proximity to parathyroid tissue (*P*); *left*, thyroid. H&E, ×200

Fig. 358. (*below*) Parathyroid, C57 Black mouse, 3 months. Mucus-filled cysts lined by cuboidal and ciliated epithelium (*arrow*). H&E, ×400

Fig. 359. (*upper right*) Parathyroid gland, C57 Black mouse, 3 months. Parathyroid gland lying in a depression of the thyroid gland. H&E, ×200

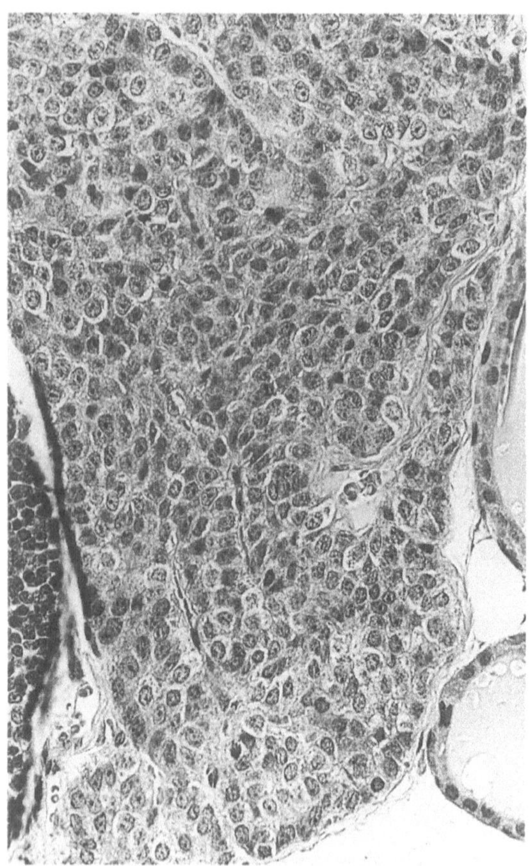

Fig. 360. Parathyroid gland, C57 Black mouse, 3 months. Strands of chief cells with indistinct cell borders, a finely granular cytoplasm and nuclei with prominent nucleoli. H&E, ×400

Moreira JE, Gonalves RP, Acosta AH (1985) Light- and electron microscopic observations on parathyroid glands in different age groups of rats. Gegenb Morphol Jahrb 131: 869–882

Pour P, Qureshi SR, Salmasi S (1983) Anatomy, histology, ultrastructure, parathyroid, mouse. In: Jones TC, Mohr U, Hunt RD (eds) Monographs on the pathology of laboratory animals: endocrine system, 1st edn. Springer, Berlin Heidelberg New York, pp 252–257

Wild P, Schraner EM (1989) Quantitative assessment of cellular changes provoked by microwave enhanced fixation of parathyroids. Histochemistry 92:69–72

Wild P, Kellner SJ, Schraner EM (1987) Parathyroid cell variants may be provoked during immersion fixation. Histochemistry 87:263–271

Wild P, Schraner EM, Augsburger H, Beglinger R, Pfister R (1986) Ultrastructural alterations in mammalian parathyroid glands induced by fixation. Acta Anat 126:87–96

Additional Reading

Coporale LH, Rosenblatt M (1986) Parathyroid hormone secretion: molecular events and regulation. Contr Nephrol 50:73–95

Inoue Y, Setoguti T (1986) Immunocytological localization of parathormone in the mammalian parathyroid gland using the protein A-gold technique. Cell Tissue Res 243:3–7

Anatomy, Histology, Ultrastructure, Parathyroid, Rat

Birgit Kittel, Kenji Kamino, and Heinrich Ernst

Anatomy

The parathyroid glands of rats are oval or lens-shaped, paired organs that derive from the third pharyngeal pouch and correspond to the lateral parathyroid glands of other mammals. A second pair of parathyroids comparable to the medial parathyroid glands of other mammals is not present in the rat, but the occurrence of accessory parathyroid tissue has been frequently reported (see p. 333, this volume).

In the rat the parathyroids are embedded in the lateral aspect of the thyroid glands near their anterior pole, separated by a fibrous capsule which even in young animals may be relatively thick (Fig. 361, 362).

Histology

The parathyroid gland of the rat is composed of only a single cell type, the chief cell. The presence

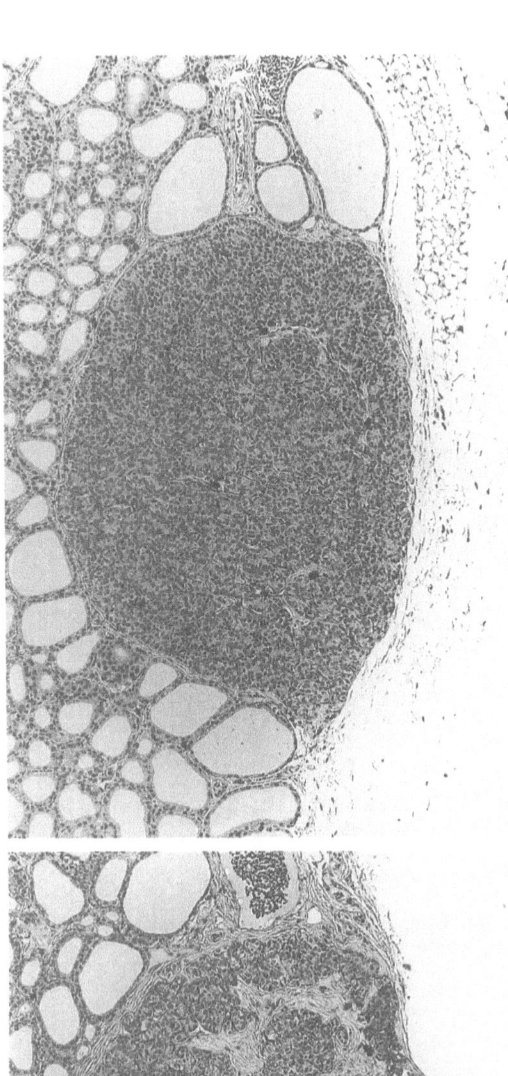

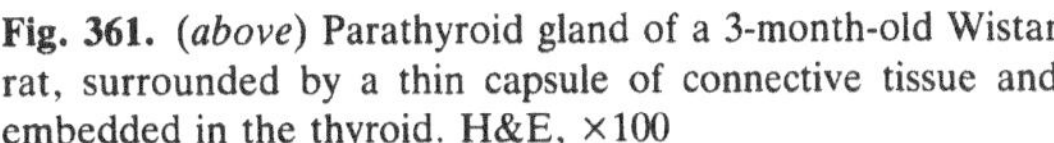

Fig. 361. (*above*) Parathyroid gland of a 3-month-old Wistar rat, surrounded by a thin capsule of connective tissue and embedded in the thyroid. H&E, ×100

Fig. 362. (*below*) Parathyroid gland of a 3-month-old Wistar rat. Fibrous thickening of the collagenous stroma and of the capsule. H&E, ×100

of light and dark staining chief cells is associated with different functional stages (Zawistowski 1966; Moreira et al. 1985; Moreira and Goncalves 1985), artifacts induced by fixation (Stoeckel and Porte 1966; Wild and Manser 1985; Wild et al. 1987) or in areas incompletely perfused by the fixative (Setoguti et al. 1981). No dark or light cell differentiation is seen in parathyroids of newborn animals (Moreira et al. 1985).

The polygonal chief cells are arranged in cords or sheets and surrounded by a thin stroma of connective tissue and a capillary network. In routinely fixed paraffin sections the cytoplasm of the faintly staining chief cells is granulated and surrounded by an indistinct cell border. The nuclei appear round or oval with finely dispersed chromatin (Fig. 363).

Ultrastructure

By transmission electron microscopy, the plasma membrane of chief cells is smooth at the basal side. Laterally cells are connected by desmosomes or tight junctions, whereas in the inner part of the cords both smooth areas and interdigitations between cells can be observed. The basally located nuclei are often indented and of medium electron density. The Golgi complex is well developed and situated, as are the secretory granules, in the apical part of the cell. Among the secretory granules, two types can be distinguished (Altenähr 1970; Wild and Manser 1985; Setoguti et al. 1981): (a) a smaller type with a large halo (100–400 nm in diameter) and (b) larger granules (500–700 nm in diameter) with a smaller halo and a more electron-dense core.

Mitochondria, rough endoplasmatic reticulum, and free ribosomes are evenly dispersed throughout the chief cells. Mitochondria of rat parathyroids have been described as long and undulating structures winding about in the cytoplasm (Svensson et al. 1989). Scanning electron microscopic studies of corrosion casts demonstrate that the rat parathyroid glands contain a rich capillary

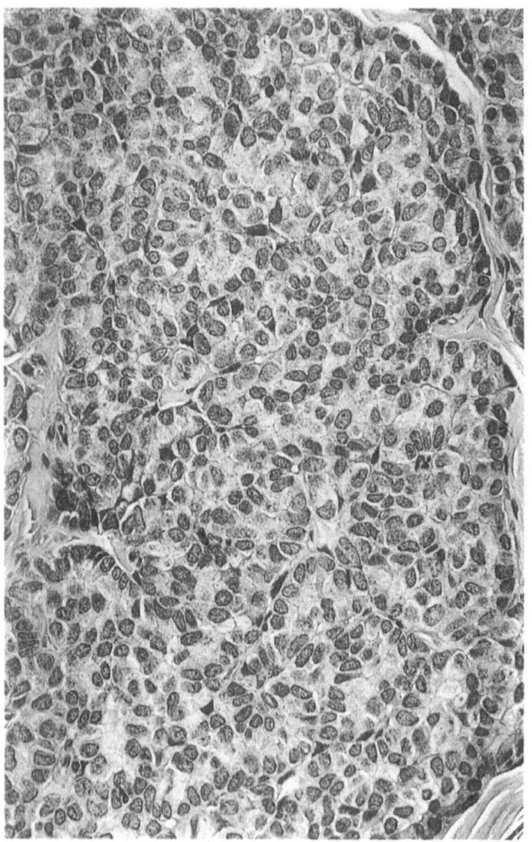

Fig. 363. Parathyroid gland of a 3-month-old Wistar rat. Cords of chief cells with granular cytoplasm and indistinct cell borders and finely dispersed nuclear chromatin. H&E, ×400

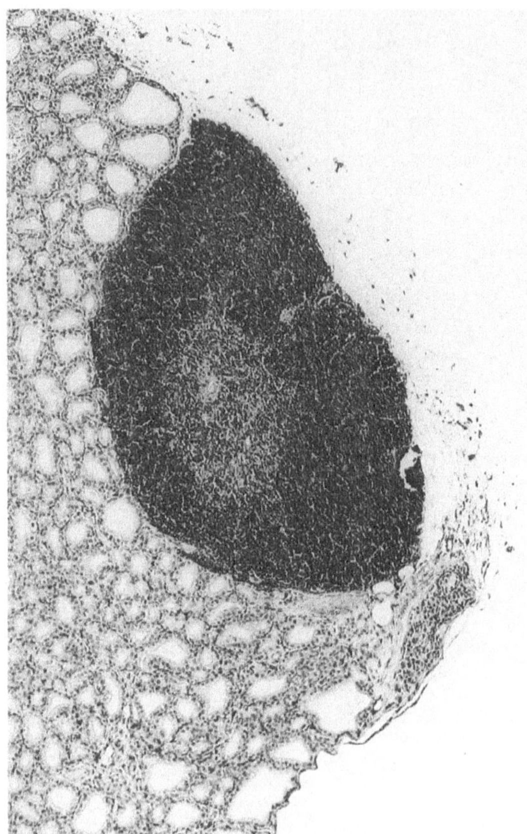

Fig. 364. Ectopic thymic tissue in close proximity to thyroid. H&E, ×100

network that is completely isolated from the capillary plexus of the thyroid gland (Murakami et al. 1987).

Accessory and Ectopic Tissue

Ectopic parathyroids were found in about 3% of MCR rats and were located anywhere from between the pharynx-larynx to the mediastinum. They can also occur as solid masses within the thyroid gland (Pour et al. 1983). Ectopic parathyroid glands are reported to be more common in aged rats and in the thymus of several other rat strains (Van Dyke 1959; Dunlay et al. 1969, cited after Pour et al. 1983). As in mice, ectopic thymic tissue can also be found in close proximity to the parathyroid gland (Fig. 364).

References

Altenähr A (1970) Zur Ultrastruktur der Rattenepithelkrperchen bei Normo-, Hyper- und Hypocalcämie. Virchows Arch [A] 351:122–141

Moreira JE, Gonçalves RP (1985) Ultrastructural changing of the rat parathyroid gland under various fixation methods. Anat Anz Jena 158:413–423

Moreira JE, Gonçalves RP, Acosta AH (1985) Light- and electron microscopic observations on parathyroid glands in different age groups of rats. Gegenb Morphol Jahrb 131: 869–882

Murakami T, Hinenoya H, Taguchi T, Ohtsuka A, Uno Y (1987) Blood vascular architecture of the rat parathyroid glands: a scanning electron microscopic study of corrosion casts. Arch Histol Jpn 5:495–504

Pour PM, Wilson JT, Salmasi S (1983) Anatomy, histology, ultrastructure, parathyroid, rat. In: Jones TC, Mohr U, Hunt RD (eds) Monographs on pathology of laboratory animals, 1st edn. Springer, Berlin Heidelberg New York, pp 257–262

Setoguti T, Inoue Y, Kato K (1981) Electron-microscopic studies on the relationship between the frequency of parathyroid storage granules and serum calcitonin levels in the rat. Cell Tissue Res 219:457–467
Stoeckel ME, Porte A (1966) Observations ultrastructurales sur la parathyreoide de souris. II. Etude experimentale. Z Zellforsch 73:65–84
Svensson O, Wernerson A, Reinholt FP (1989) The parathyroid glands in the rat as seen by ultrathin step and serial sectioning. Bone Miner 6:237–248
Van Dyke JH (1959) Aberrant parathyroid tissue and the thymus: postnatal development of accessory parathyroid gland in the rat. Anat Rec 134:185–205
Wild P, Manser EM (1985) Ultrastructural morphometry of parathyroid cells in rats of different ages. Cell Tissue Res 240:585–591
Wild P, Kellner S, Schraner EM (1987) Parathyroid cell variants may be provoked during immersion fixation. Histochemistry 87:263–271
Zawistowki S (1966) Ultrastructure of the parathyroid gland of the albino rat. Folia Histochem Cytochem (Krakow) 4:273–278

Additional Reading

Bjerneroth G, Juhlin C, Åkerström G, Rastad J (1992) Immunelectron microscopical evidence of a calcium receptor function in parathyroid, placenta and kidney. J Submicrosc Cytol Pathol 24:179–186
Capen CC (1976) Functional and fine structural relationships of parathyroid glands. Adv Vet Sci Comp Med 19:249–286
Caporale LH, Rosenblatt M (1986) Parathyroid hormone secretionMolecular events and regulation. Contr Nephrol 50:73–95
Inoue Y, Setoguti T (1986) Immunocytological localization of parathormone in the mammalian parathyroid gland using the protein A-gold technique. Cell Tissue Res 243:3–7
Keller B, Schraner EM, Wild P (1991) Morphometric analysis of compartments concerned with secretion of parathormone in male and female rats. Acta Anat 141:324–328
Kristie R (1980) Three dimensional organization of the rat parathyroid glands. Z Mikrosk Anat Forsch 94:445–450
Marti R, Wild P, Schraner EM, Mueller M, Moor H (1987) Parathyroid ultrastructure after aldehyde fixation, high-pressure-freezing, or microwave irradiation. J Histochem Cytochem 35:1415–1424
Raybuck HE (1952) The innervation of the parathyroid glands. Anat Rec 112:117–123
Roth SI, Capen CC (1974) Ultrastructural and functional correlations of the parathyroid gland. Int Rev Exp Pathol 13:161–221
Wild P, Schraner EM (1989) Quantitative assessment of cellular changes provoked by microwave enhanced fixation of parathyroids. Histochemistry 92:69–72
Wild P, Schraner EM, Ausburger H, Beglinger R, Pfister R (1986) Ultrastructural alterations in mammalian parathyroid glands induced by fixation. Acta Anat 126:87–96
Zabel M, Dietel M (1987) S-100 protein and neuron-specific enolase in parathyroid glands and C-cells of the thyroid. Histochemistry 86:389–392

Ectopic Parathyroid, Mouse

Charles H. Frith and Judith Fetters

Synonyms. Aberrant or ectopic parathyroid tissue.

Gross Appearance

Ectopic parathyroid tissue in the mouse is not visible grossly.

Microscopic Features

Ectopic parathyroid tissue in the mouse may be found in the septa, or surface connective tissue, of the thymus. It is surrounded by a delicate fibrous capsule which extends into and separates the tissue into small lobules (Fig. 365). Small capillaries are present in the septa. Lobules are composed of polygonal cells with prominent vesicular nuclei and scant, lightly basophilic cytoplasm.

Ultrastructure

The structures recognized in aberrant locations with the light microscope closely resemble normal parathyroid tissue; their ultrastructural characteristics have not been demonstrated.

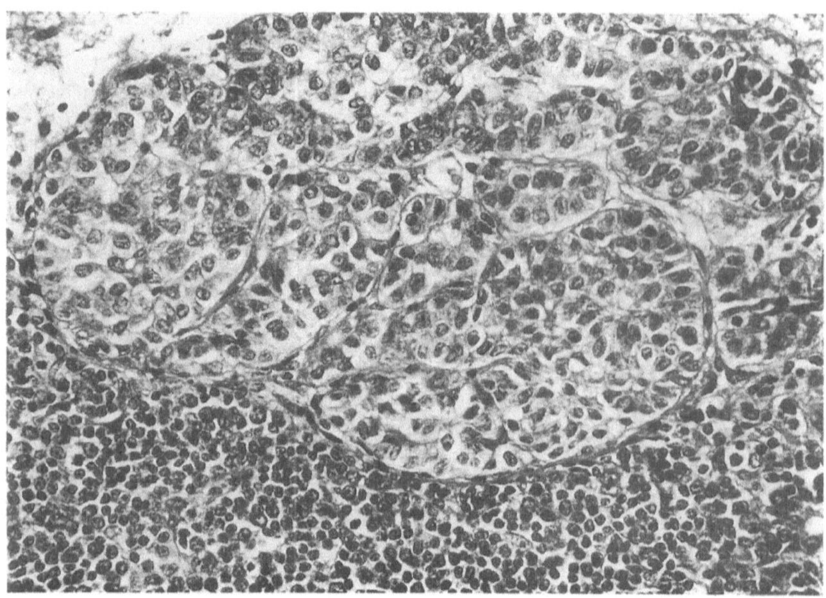

Fig. 365. Ectopic parathyroid tissue located in thymus. H&E, ×300

Differential Diagnosis

No specific differential diagnostic problem arises concerning this entity.

Biologic Features

Ectopic parathyroid tissue is usually encountered in the course of histopathologic studies of the mouse. In one study (Pour et al., this volume) these were found in the thyroid and adjacent to the caudal part of the trachea in 1% of Swiss mice. The biologic significance of this distribution of parathyroid cells is not clear at this time.

Comparison with Other Species

Ectopic parathyroid has been described in the mouse (Smith and Clifford 1962; Dunn 1954), rat (Van Dyke 1959), and man (Ficarra 1958; Brewer 1934; Kurtay and Crile 1969).

References

Brewer LA (1934) The occurrence of parathyroid tissue within the thymus. Endocrinology 18:397–408

Dunn TB (1954) Normal and pathologic anatomy of the reticular tissue in laboratory mice. JNCI 14:1281–1433

Ficarra BJ (1958) Diseases of the thyroid and parathyroid glands. Intercontinental, New York, pp 211–222

Kurtay M, Crile G (1969) Aberrant parathyroid glands in relationship to the thymus. Am J Surg 117:705

Smith C, Clifford CP (1962) Histochemical study of aberrant parathyroid glands associated with the thymus of the mouse. Anat Rec 143:229–238

Van Dyke JH (1959) Aberrant parathyroid tissue and the thymus. Postnatal development of accessory parathyroid glands in the rat. Anat Rec 134:185–205

Hyperplasia, Parathyroid: Syrian Hamster

Heinrich Ernst, Birgit Kittel, and Kenji Kamino

Gross Appearance

Due to the small size of the parathyroids in hamsters only severely enlarged glands can be identified grossly. Marked diffuse parathyroid hyperplasia may be visible as uniform enlargement of both glands. Less severe diffuse hyperplasia may be detectable only by weighing the parathyroids and comparing them with normal glands. Focal (nodular) hyperplasia may appear as a focal poorly demarcated nodule in an otherwise normal or diffusely enlarged gland.

Microscopic Features

Diffuse hyperplasia affects both glands (Fig. 366) and consists of increased numbers of slightly enlarged (hypertrophic) chief cells with increased eosinophilic or clear cytoplasm and more vesicular nuclei than normal (Fig. 367). There is no peripheral rim of compressed normal parathyroid tissue. In severe cases the adjacent thyroid tissue may be compressed. The acinar arrangement of the chief cells is normal or slightly more prominent. Stromal tissue is not increased in amount and is therefore inconspicuous. Mitotic figures are rarely seen.
Focal (nodular) hyperplasia (Figs. 368, 369) may be observed in an otherwise normally appearing or in a diffusely hyperplastic gland. The cytological and architectural characteristics of focal hyperplasia do not differ from those seen in diffuse hyperplasia. The boundaries of the hyperplastic areas are more discrete, but there is no or only minimal compression of the surrounding tissue (Figs. 368, 369).

Differential Diagnosis

The differentiation between focal or nodular hyperplasia and adenoma of the parathyroids is based on morphological criteria. The two types of proliferative lesion usually have comparable cytological characteristics. The main criteria for adenoma are the presence of sharp peripheral demarcation with definite compression of adjacent parenchyma and possible formation of a capsule or pseudocapsule. Nodular hyperplasia (Figs. 368, 369) is seen as a somewhat more densely cellular, circumscribed area in a normal or hyperplastic parathyroid gland. It is not encapsulated and does not compress or displace adjacent tissues, features which differentiate it from adenomas (see 345, this volume).
Diffuse hyperplasia involves both parathyroid glands which are very much enlarged (Fig. 366) and filled with large clear cells intermingled with normal appearing "chief" cells (Fig. 367). Renal disease and fibrous osteodystrophy of bones usually accompany diffuse hyperplasia.

Biologic Features

Hyperplasia of the parathyroids may develop either as a primary or as a secondary disorder. Depending on the ability of the chief cells to secrete parathyroid hormone, parathyroid hyperplasia can also be either functional or nonfunctional. In aged hamsters secondary hyperplasia due to chronic nephropathy (amyloidosis, nephrocalcinosis) and/or long-term dietary imbalances is a common finding (Pour 1983). Renal failure with retention of phosphorus, calcium deficiency, and phosphorus excess in the diet are etiologic factors that lead to decreased serum ionized calcium concentration and subsequent, usually diffuse hyperplasia and secondary hyperparathyroidism.

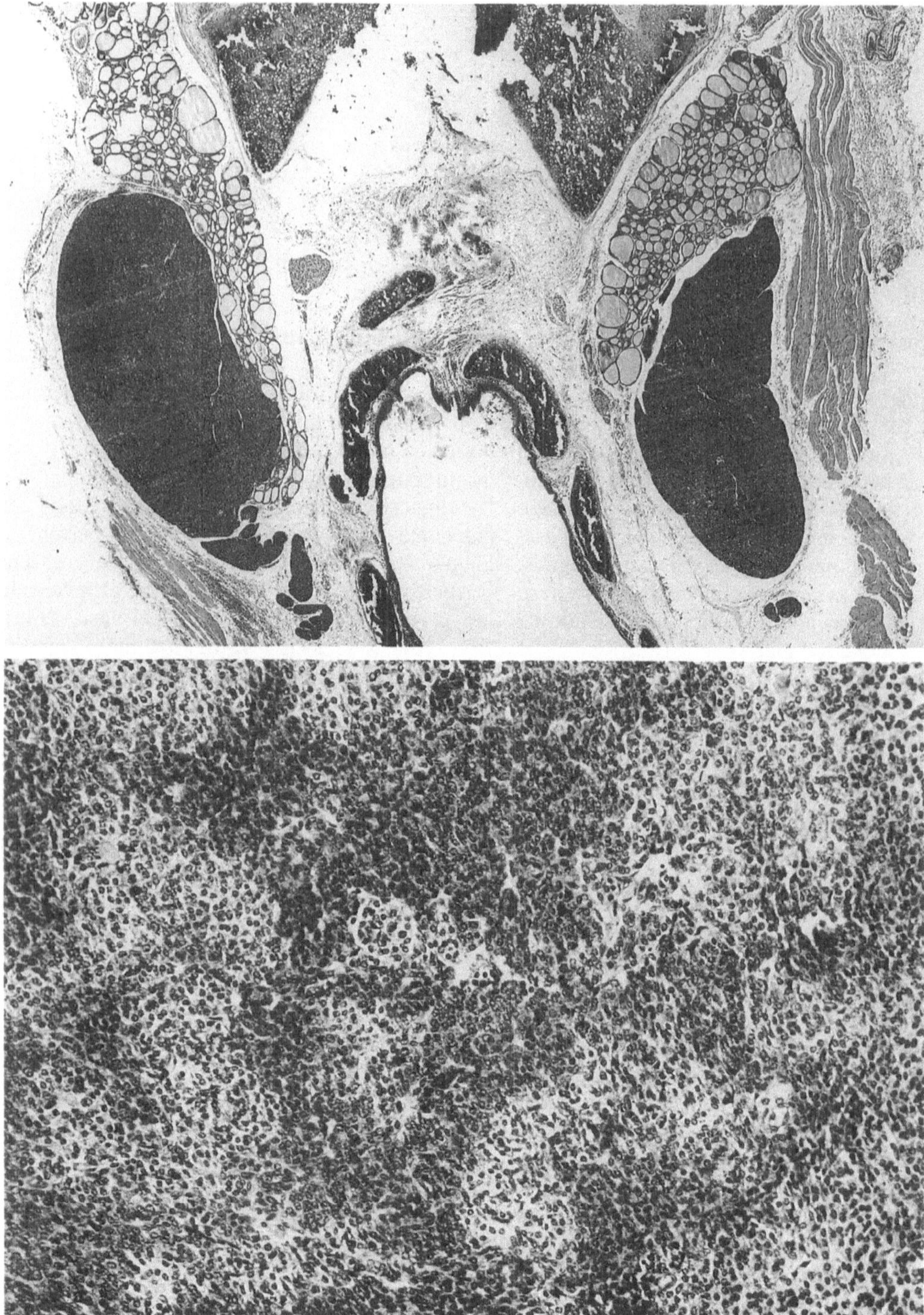

Fig. 366. (*above*) Diffuse hyperplasia of parathyroids, Syrian hamster. Note small "islands" or "tails" at the caudal pole of each gland. H&E, ×20

Fig. 367. (*below*) Diffuse hyperplasia of parathyroid, Syrian hamster. Uniform clear cells with indistinct borders intermingle with normally looking chief cells. H&E, ×160

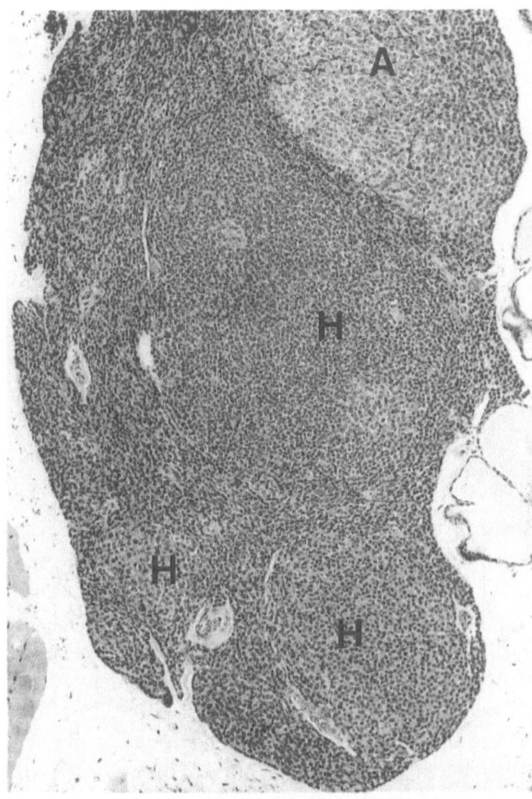

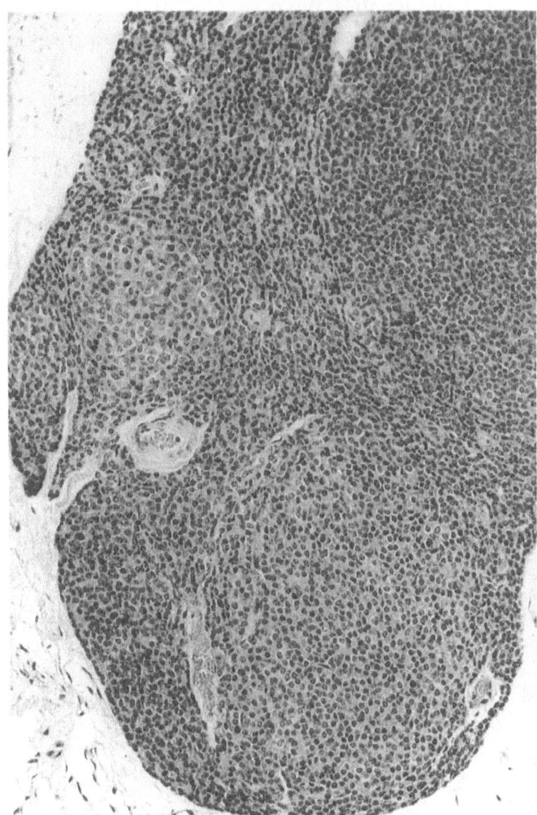

Fig. 368. (*above*) Multifocal hyperplasia (*H*) and adenoma (*A*) of parathyroid, Syrian hamster. Note variation in cellular appearance and degree of compression of surrounding tissue between hyperplastic areas and adenoma. H&E, ×70

Fig. 369. (*below*) Higher magnification of Fig. 368. The cells of the hyperplastic areas contain increased cytoplasm but do not or only minimally compress the adjacent parathyroid tissue. H&E, ×135

Focal hyperplasia is uncommon in laboratory animals and is usually nonfunctional (Rosol and Capen 1989). As a further diagnostic aid, parathyroid hyperplasia may be associated with fibrous osteodystrophy in the skeletal system. The frequency of parathyroid hyperplasia varies significantly between different hamster strains. Frequencies ranging from 2%–3% in Eppley-derived cream hamsters and albino hamsters to 83% in aged hamsters of the Eppley colony have been reported (Pour et al. 1976; Pour 1983). In aged male hamsters of various unspecified commercial sources 5.3% of the animals had parathyroid hyperplasias (Schmidt et al. 1983).

Comparison with Other Species

Hyperplasia of the parathyroid is also observed in other animal species. In hamsters it seems to be more common than in rats and mice, and may be due to a greater sensitivity of hamsters to the dietary composition (Pour 1983). In humans some familial forms of diffuse parathyroid hyperplasia associated with multiple endocrine neoplasia are recognized. A plasma-related mitogenic activity for parathyroid cells has been identified in these patients (Brandi et al. 1986). In dogs renal disease often leads to parathyroid hyperplasia and secondary hyperparathyroidism, which ultimately produces generalized fibrous osteodystrophy (Jones and Hunt 1985).

References

Brandi ML, Aurbach GD, Fitzpatrick LA, Quarto R, Spiegel AM, Bliziotes MM, Norton JA, Doppman JL, Marx SJ (1986) Parathyroid mitogenic activity in plasma from patients with familial multiple endocrine neoplasia type I. N Engl J Med 314:1287–1293

Jones TC, Hunt RD (1985) Veterinary pathology, 5th edn. Lea and Febiger, Philadelphia, pp 1615–1619

Pour PM (1983) Hyperplasia, parathyroid, hamster. In: Jones TC, Mohr U, Hunt RD (eds) ILSI monographs on pathology of laboratory animals: endocrine system. Springer, Berlin Heidelberg New York, pp 265–268

Pour PM, Mohr U, Althoff J, Cardesa A, Kmoch N (1976) Spontaneous tumors and common diseases in two colonies of Syrian hamsters. III. Urogenital system and endocrine glands. J Natl Cancer Inst 56:949–961

Rosol TJ, Capen CC (1989) Tumors of the parathyroid gland and circulating parathyroid hormone-related protein associated with persistent hypercalcemia. Toxic Pathol 17: 346–356

Schmidt RE, Eason RL, Hubbard GB, Young JT, Eisenbrandt DL (1983) Pathology of aging Syrian hamsters. CRC Press, Boca Raton, pp 141–174

Hyperplasia, Parathyroid, Rat

Kenji Kamino, Birgit Kittel, and Heinrich Ernst

Gross Appearance

In moderate to severe diffuse parathyroid hyperplasia both glands may be found macroscopically as 1- to 2-mm, opaque, sometimes grayish nodules projecting from the surface of each thyroid lobe (Fig. 370). In focal or multifocal hyperplasia the lesions are not visible grossly.

Microscopic Features

The uniform enlargement of parathyroid glands in diffuse hyperplasia is due to both hypertrophy and hyperplasia of chief cells. Figures 371 and 372 show a diffusely hyperplastic parathyroid gland composed of a homogeneous cell population of chief cells. The chief cells are packed closely together, often with indistinct cell boundaries. An acinar or trabecular disposition of the chief cells is sometimes evident, or they may appear to consist of several cell layers in a finely lobulated pattern. These features are subtle, however, since the fibrovascular stroma is scanty. The cells are also hypertrophic; they have slightly more abundant, pale cytoplasm and larger, more vesicular nuclei than normal.

In some cases hyperplastic parathyroid glands are composed of a heterogeneous cell population of chief cells (Fig. 373). In such lesions some cells

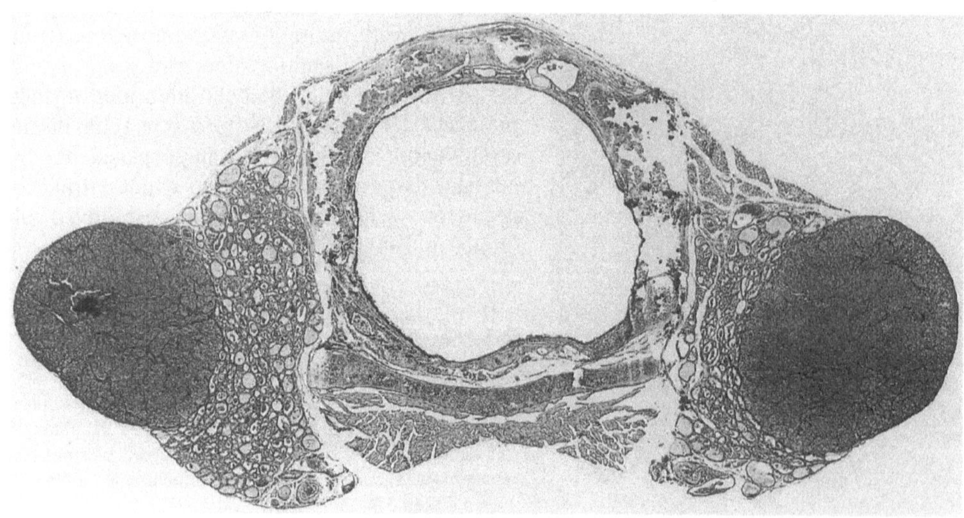

Fig. 370. Diffuse parathyroid hyperplasia, rat. Uniform enlargement of both glands. Note lobular structure. Han: Wistar rat. H&E, ×20

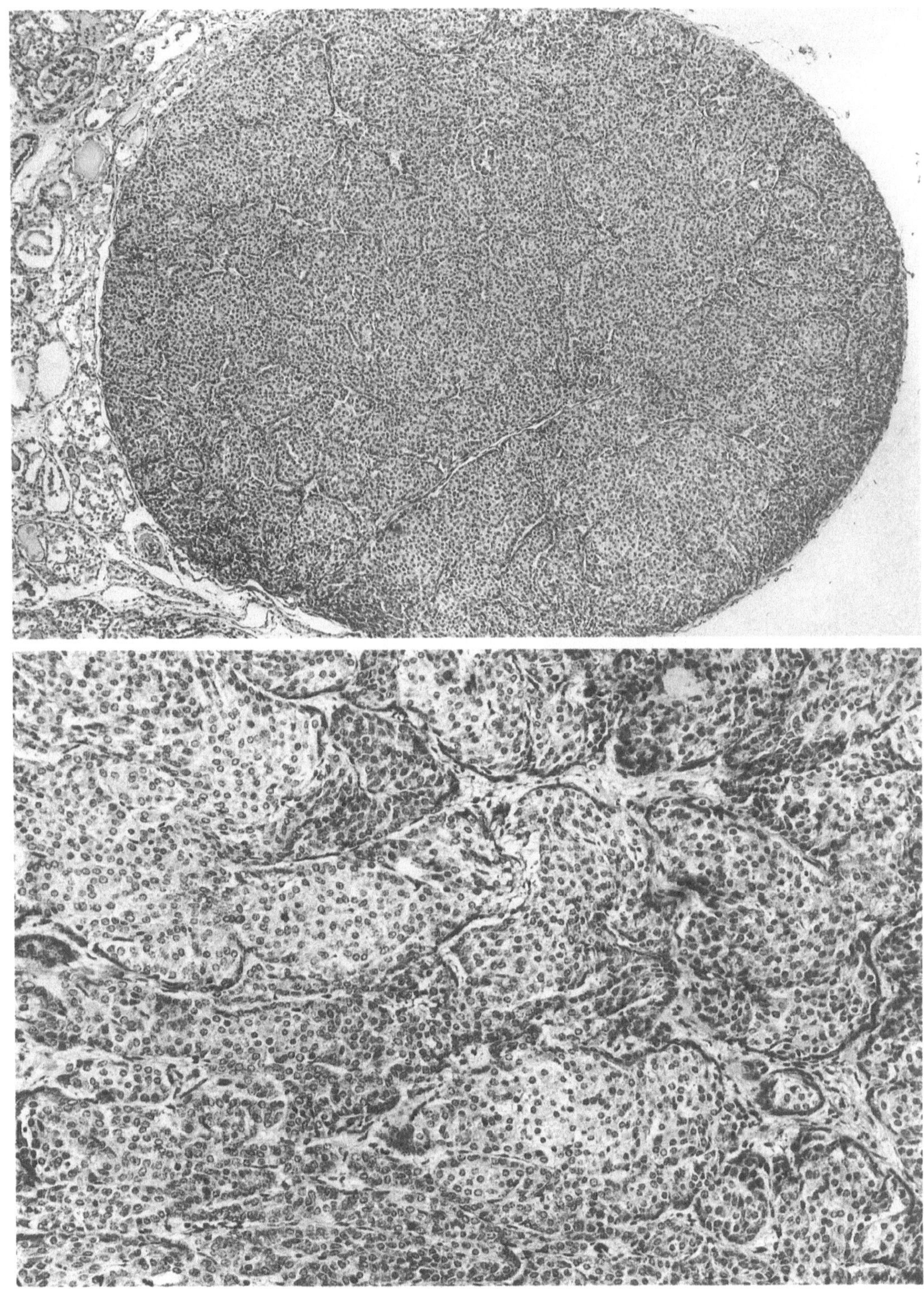

Fig. 371. (*above*) Enlarged parathyroid gland, rat, consisting of hyperplastic chief cell population. Note uniformly distributed vascular system. OFA rat. H&E, ×30

Fig. 372. (*below*) Diffuse parathyroid hyperplasia, rat. Lobulation with slightly increased perivascular connective tissue. Rat. H&E, ×120

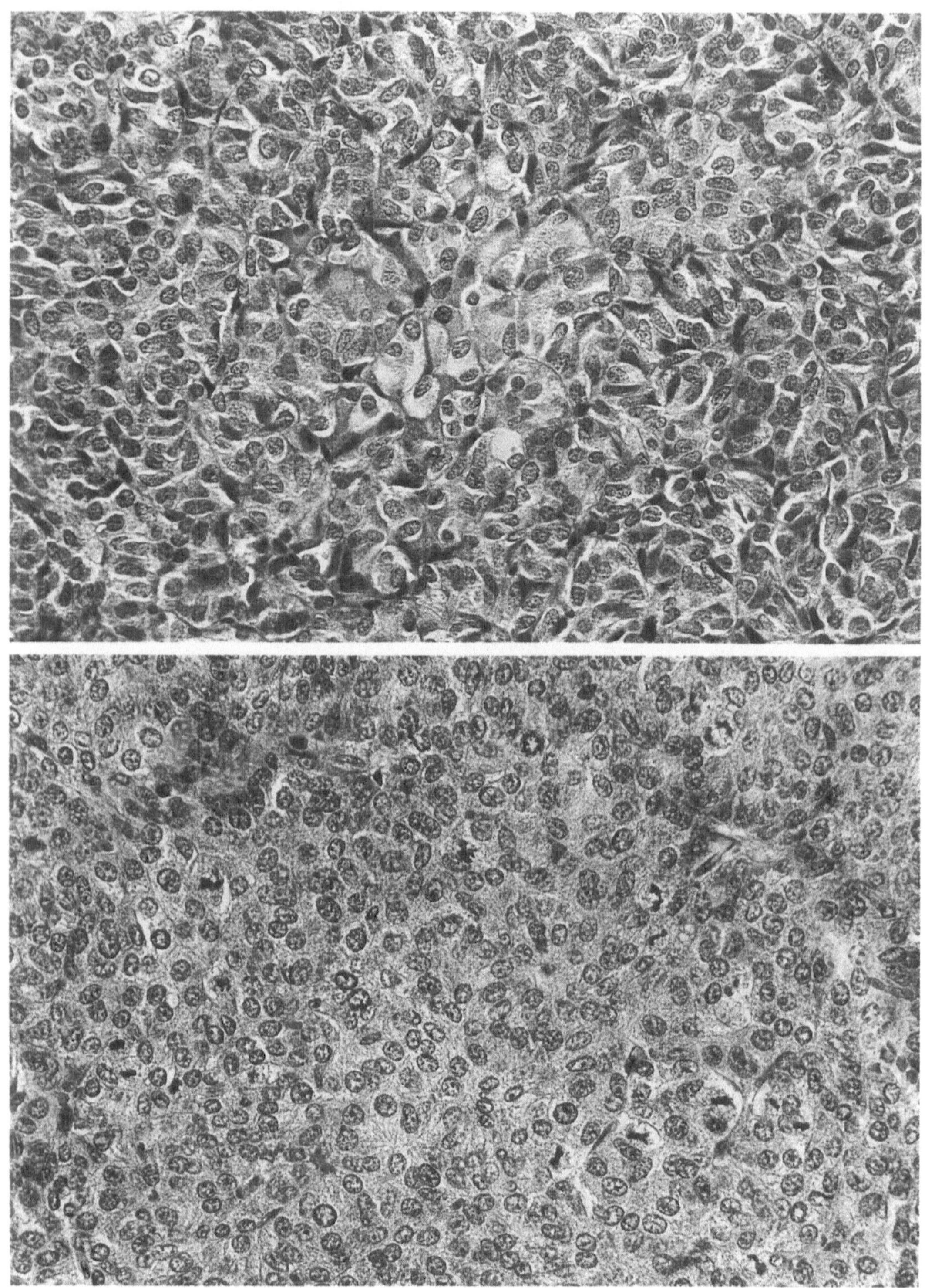

Fig. 373. (*above*) Hyperplastic parathyroid gland, rat, composed of heterogenous chief cell population. Some cells have distended cytoplasm. OFA rat. H&E, ×300

Fig. 374. (*below*) Diffuse parathyroid hyperplasia, rat. Note numerous mitotic figures. Rat. H&E, ×300

have faintly stained eosinophilic cytoplasm; others have clear cytoplasm and elongated hyperchromatic nuclei. In a few cases foci of oxyphilic cells with abundant cylindrical cytoplasm are present. All of these cell types appear to represent different stages of function of the chief cells. Mitotic figures are sometimes observed, but they are not consistent and when present are not an indicator of neoplasia (Fig. 374). The diagnosis of diffuse hyperplasia depends upon: (a) the uniform enlargement of both parathyroids, (b) the absence of any peripheral rim of compressed atrophic parathyroid parenchyma, (c) the hyperplastic chief cell population extending to the capsule of the gland (Fig. 371). Occasionally inflammation in the capsule presents a picture suggesting capsular invasion or penetration by hyperplastic parathyroid cells (Figs. 375, 376). Injury to the capsule may allow hyperplastic cells to push out or escape into the capsule (Fig. 376). Inflammatory reactions, calcification (Fig. 376), or increased numbers of mast cells (Fig. 377) may also be seen.

In focal parathyroid hyperplasia, single or multiple nodular lesions are present in one or both glands. The hyperplastic areas are poorly demarcated and not encapsulated from surrounding parenchyma. Closely packed chief cells within the nodular lesions have a relatively uniform composition with abundant cytoplasm and a slightly enlarged nucleus. Focal hyperplasia causes no compression of the adjacent tissue and merges imperceptibly with the surrounding normal chief cells (Fig. 378). Focal chief cell hyperplasia is often difficult to separate from a chief cell adenoma.

Ultrastructure

The ultrastructural features of hyperplasia include increased interdigitations of the cell membranes between contiguous cells, enlarged mitochondria, an increased number of ribosomes, a prominent Golgi apparatus, and numerous Golgi vesicles (Shimamura and Morrison 1971).

Differential Diagnosis

The following histologic criteria are used to diagnose parathyroid hyperplasia:

- Diffuse hyperplasia
  - Diffuse enlargement of both glands
  - Uniform pattern of cellular arrangement in both glands
  - Uniform population of enlarged cells
  - No rim of compressed normal parathyroid parenchyma
  - No compression of adjacent tissue
- Focal hyperplasia
  - Poorly demarcated nodular lesion of enlarged cells
  - Similar pattern of cellular arrangement to that of normal parenchyma
  - No compression of surrounding tissue
- Aenoma
  - Usually is a single lesion
  - Compresses adjacent parathyroid gland
  - Partially or completely encapsulated

Biologic Features

Etiology. Spontaneous parathyroid hyperplasia may be either primary or secondary. Primary parathyroid hyperplasia may be functional (endocrinologically active) or nonfunctional, depending on the ability of chief cells to secrete parathyroid hormone. Primary hyperparathyroidism is the disorder that results from excessive and autonomous secretion of parathyroid hormone from chief cell hyperplasia. Atrophy of the remaining normal parathyroid tissue is present with functional focal or multifocal parathyroid hyperplasia (Capen et al. 1991). Parathyroid hyperplasia, as is seen with chronic renal failure and long-term dietary imbalances, results in a uniform enlargement of all parathyroid glands (secondary parathyroid hyperplasia) and secondary hyperparathyroidism (Capen 1988). Experimental hyperplasia and hyperparathyroidism can be induced by or associated with the following: experimental chronic renal disease (Shimamura and Morrison 1971); transplantation of parathyroid glands (Gittes and Radde 1966a,b; Fisher and Gittes 1969); administration of deoxycorticosterone acetate (Hansson and Angervall 1966a), alloxan (Hansson and Angervall 1966b; Schneider et al. 1974), and calcitonin (Sorensen et al. 1972); large doses of inorganic phosphate (Haase 1978); irradiation (Sommers and Berdjis 1970); Leydig's cell tumor (Petrea and Gueritee 1976); hypergastrinemia (Grimelius et al. 1977); adrenalectomy (Hansson 1966) and nephrectomy (Hansson 1967); and castration (Setoguchi et al. 1981).

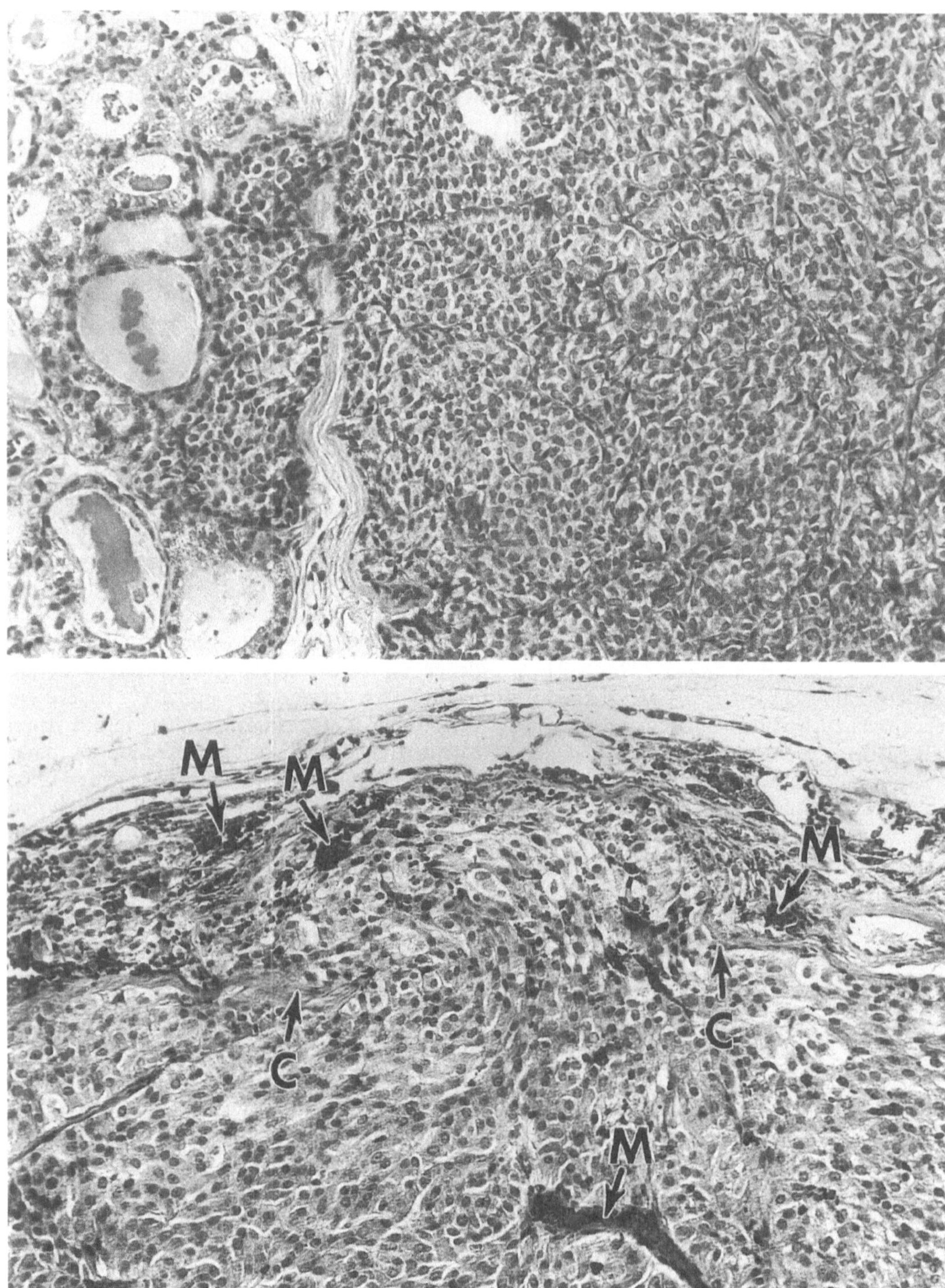

Fig. 375. (*above*) Diffuse parathyroid hyperplasia, rat. Uniform chief cells seem to have penetrated the capsule into the thyroid gland, probably due to prolapse. Rat. H&E, ×150

Fig. 376. (*below*) Diffuse parathyroid hyperplasia, rat. Prolapse of hyperplastic chief cells through capsule (*C*). Mineralization of interstitium (*M*). Rat. H&E, ×120

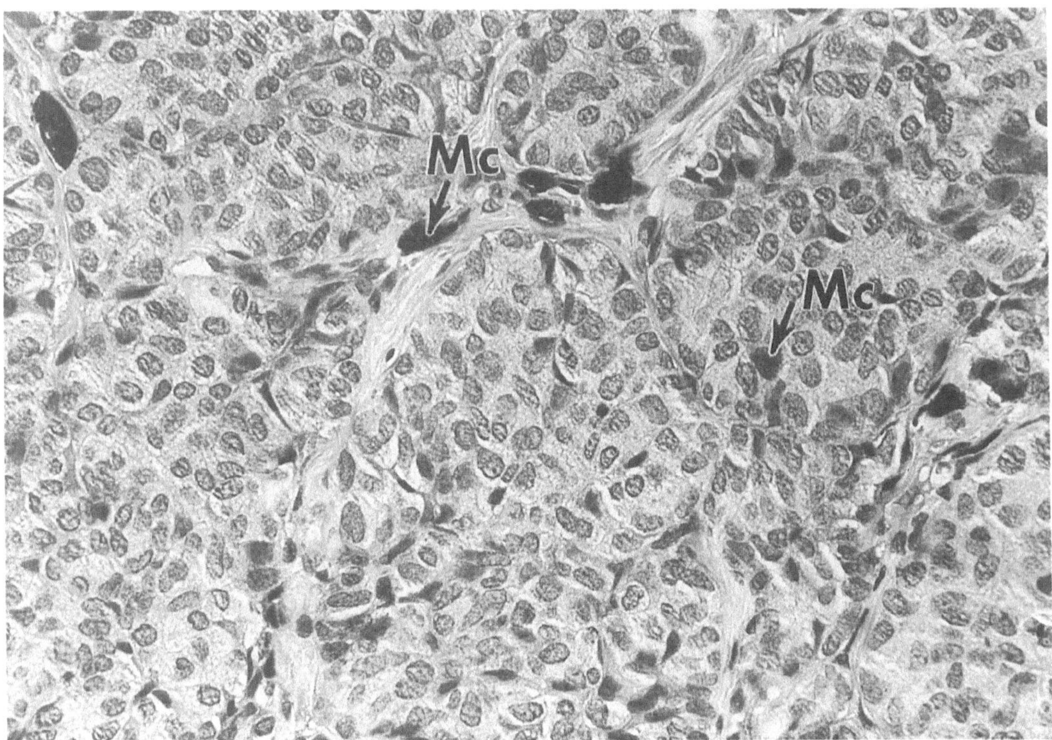

Fig. 377. Diffuse parathyroid hyperplasia, rat. Lobular structure and mast cells (*Mc*). Rat. H&E, ×300

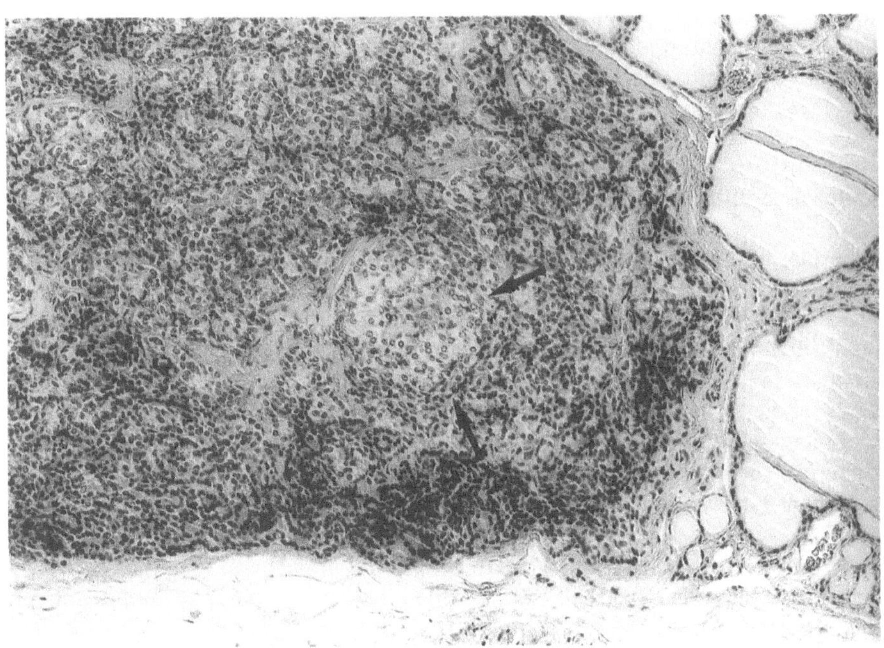

Fig. 378. Focal parathyroid hyperplasia (*arrows*), rat. Note no compression of the adjacent tissue. Han:Wistar rat. H&E, ×120

Frequency. Diffuse parathyroid hyperplasia is described as a frequent occurrence in aging rats and is almost always bilateral and secondary to severe chronic nephropathy or dietary imbalances (Seely and Hildebrandt 1990; MacKenzie and Garner 1973). On the other hand, Haley (1978) and Lindsay and Nichols (1969) reported remarkably varied frequencies of the lesion in different strains of rats, that is: Osborne-Mendel, 30%; Long-Evans, 20.4%; Wistar, 13.0%; Sprague-Dawley, 6.0%; Buffalo, 4.0%; and Fischer 344, 1.0%. In addition, Pour et al. (1983) reported that the frequency in OFA rats is about 12%, in Han:Wistar 8.0%, and in MRC rats 4.0%. Spontaneous diseases, especially of the kidneys, and dietary factors are obvious causes. These factors may explain the differences in the frequency of parathyroid hyperplasia among various strains of rats. Focal parathyroid hyperplasia is uncommon in laboratory animals, including rats, and is usually nonfunctional (Rosol and Capen 1989). Parathyroid hyperplasia may also be associated with neoplasms of the thyroid gland. This kind of association has been seen in 40% of cases of parathyroid hyperplasia in OFA rats (Pour et al. 1983). Similar coexisting parathyroid and thyroid lesions have been reported by Lindsay and Nichols (1969) and Haley (1978). However, according to Lindsay and Nichols (1969) coincidental finding of parathyroid hyperplasia and thyroid neoplasms did not imply a special relationship between them.

Comparison with Other Species

Hyperplasia of the parathyroids occurs in many species including humans, rats, Syrian hamsters, dogs, and mice. Some species are discussed in detail in other parts of this volume. It is more common in the hamster than in rats or mice (Pour et al. 1983). In contrast to the usually nonfunctional focal hyperplasia in rats, this focal lesion is a cause of primary hyperparathyroidism in humans (Brown and LeBoff 1986).

Acknowledgement. We acknowledge the contribution of Dr. Parvis M. Pour who provided the illustrations which are reproduced here from the first edition.

References

Brown EM, LeBoff MS (1986) Pathophysiology of hyperparathyroidism. Prog Surg 18:13–22

Capen CC (1988) Endocrine system. In: Thompson RG (ed) Special veterinary pathology. Decker, Philadelphia, pp 369–436

Capen CC, DeLellis RA, Yarrington JT (1991) Endocrine system. In: Haschek WM, Rousseaux CG (eds) Handbook of toxicologic pathology. Academic, San Diego, pp 675–760

Fischer JE, Gittes RF (1969) Experimental hyperparathyroidism. Effects on gastric secretion. J Surg Res 9:49–53

Gittes RF, Radde IC (1966a) Experimental hyperparathyroidism from multiple isologous parathyroid transplants: homeostatic effect of simultaneous thyroid transplants. Endocrinology 78:1015–1023

Gittes RF, Radde IC (1966b) Experimental model for hyperparathyroidism: effect of excessive numbers of transplanted isologous parathyroid glands. J Urol 95:595–603

Grimelius L, Johansson H, Lindquist G, Olazabal A, Polak JH, Pearse GE (1977) The parathyroid glands in experimentally induced hypergastrinemia in the rat. Scand J Gastroenterol 12:739–744

Haase P (1978) Parathyroid stimulation in phosphate-induced nephrocalcinosis. J Anat 125:299–311

Haley TJ (1978) Retrospective analysis of control animal data–the rat. Clin Toxicol 12:249–263

Hansson CG (1966) Effects of adrenalectomy on the parathyroids in nephrectomized rats. Acta Endocrinol (Copenh) 51:350–358

Hansson CG (1967) Nephrectomy of pregnant rats. Effects on the parathyroids in mother and offspring. Acta Endocrinol (Copenh) 54:166–172

Hansson CG, Angervall L (1966a) The parathyroids in corticosteroid-treated pregnant rats and their offspring. II. Effect of deoxycorticosterone acetate (DOCA). Acta Endocrinol (Copenh) 53:553–560

Hansson CG, Angervall L (1966b) The parathyroids in pregnant alloxan diabetic rats and their offspring. Acta Endocrinol (Copenh) 52:633–640

Lindsay S, Nichols CW (1969) Medullary thyroid carcinoma and parathyroid hyperplasia in rats. Arch Pathol 88:402–406

MacKenzie WF, Garner FM (1973) Comparison of neoplasms in six sources of rats. J Natl Cancer Inst 50:1243–1257

Petrea I, Gueritee N (1976) Hyperplasia of the parathyroids and the pituitary in rats with experimental leydigiomas and inhibitory effect of several steroids. Cancer Res 36: 3748–3760

Pour PM, Wilson JT, Salmasi S (1983) Hyperplasia, parathyroid, rat. In: Jones TC, Mohr U, Hunt RD (eds) Monographs on pathology of laboratory animals, endocrine system, 1st edition. Springer, Berlin Heidelberg New York, pp 268–274

Rosol TJ, Capen CC (1989) Tumors of the parathyroid gland and circulating parathyroid hormone-related protein associated with persistent hypercalcemia. Toxicol Pathol 17(2):346–356

Schneider LE, Hargis GK, Schedl HP, Williams GA (1974) Parathyroid function in the alloxan diabetic rat. Endocrinology 95:749–752

Seely JC, Hildebrandt PK (1990) Parathyroid gland. In: Boorman GA, Eustis SL, Elwell MR, Montgomery CA Jr, MacKenzie WF (eds) Pathology of the Fischer rat: reference and atlas. Academic, San Diego, pp 537–543

Setoguchi T, Inoue Y, Kato K (1981) Electron-microscopic studies on the relationship between the frequency of parathyroid storage granules and serum calcium levels in the rat. Cell Tissue Res 219:457–467

Shimamura T, Morrison AB (1971) Secondary hyperparathyroidism in rats with an experimental chronic renal disease. Exp Mol Pathol 15:345–353

Sommers S, Berdjis CC (1970) Effects of ionizing radiation upon endocrine glands. In: Berdjis CC (ed) Pathology of irradiation. Williams and Wilkins, Baltimore, pp 409–446

Sorensen OH, Hindberg I, Madsen SN (1972) Secondary hyperparathyroidism in young rats given prolonged treatment with calcitonin. Acta Endocrinol (Copenh) 71:313–320

Additional Reading

Boorman GA, Hollander CF (1973) Spontaneous lesions in the female WAG/Rij (Wistar) rat. J Gerontol 28:152–159

Boquist L (1973) Follicles in human parathyroid glands. Lab Invest 28:313–320

Capen CC (1989) Neoplasms of the parathyroid glands. In: Stinson SF, Reznik G (eds) Atlas of tumor pathology in the F344 rat. CRC Press, Boca Raton, pp 367–378

Fujita T, Ohata M, Ota K, Tsuda T, Uezu A, Okano K, Yoshikawa M (1976) Aging and parathyroid hormone secretion. J Gerontol 31:523–526

Geertinger P (1967) Cot deaths associated with congenital anomalies of the parathyroids of infants. Experimental production of parathyroid abnormalities in the offspring of rats. J Forensic Med 14:46–59

Handler AH (1965) Spontaneous lesions of the hamster, chap 9. In: Ribelin WE, McCoy JR (eds) The pathology of laboratory animals. Thomas, Springfield

Hansson CG, Angervall L (1966c) The parathyroids in corticosteroid-treated pregnant rats and their offspring. I. Effect of cortisone. Acta Endocrinol (Copenh) 53:547–552

Hara J, Hatta T (1967) Histological and histochemical changes of the parathyroid gland by the injection of parathormone in the rat. Okajimas Folia Anat Jpn 43:235–251

Kooh SW, Fraser D (1968) Experimental parathyroid hormone deficiency produced by injection of antibodies to bovine parathyroid hormone. Can J Physiol Pharmacol 46:441–448

Mizumoto R, Nishio I, Honjo I (1965) Parathyroid hormone and metastasis of experimental tumor. II. Effect of parathyroid hormone on lymph node and production of antibody. Gan 56:425–428

Monchik JM, Gemma FE, Bond H, Wray H (1976) Experimental induction of hypoparathyroidism with parathyroid hormone antibodies. Am J Surg 131:471–475

Okano K, Fujita T, Yoshikawa M (1974) A radioimmunoassay for parathyroid hormone in rat parathyroid gland. J Lab Clin Med 83:665–672

Ravazzola M (1976) Golgi complex alterations induced by X537A in chief cells of rat parathyroid gland. Lab Invest 35:425–429

Rogers MC, Bergstrom WH (1971) Diet-induced hypoparathyroidism: a model for neonatal tetany. Pediatrics 47 [Suppl 2]:207–210

Roth SI (1970) The ultrastructure of primary water-clear cell hyperplasia of the parathyroid glands. Am J Pathol 61: 233–248

Roth SI (1971) Recent advances in parathyroid gland pathology. Am J Med 50:612–622

Roth SI, Raisz LG (1966) The course and reversibility of the calcium effect on the ultrastructure of the rat parathyroid gland in organ culture. Lab Invest 15:1187–1211

Roth SI, Capen CC (1974) Ultrastructure and function of the parathyroid. Int Rev Exp Pathol 13:179–181

Sevastik JA, Mattsson S (1971) Osteoporosis and parathyroid glands. Isr J Med Sci 7:346–349

Strebel RF, Wagner BM (1969) Experimental tissue calcification. V. Effect of parathyroidectomy on spontaneously occurring calcific arteriosclerosis in female breeder rats. Arch Pathol 87:93–99

Weisbrode SE, Capen CC (1974) Effects of uremia and vitamin D on bone and the ultrastructure of thyroid parafollicular cells and parathyroid chief cells in the rat. Virchows Arch Cell Pathol 16:231–241

Wells SA, Christiansen C (1974) The transplanted parathyroid gland: evaluation of cryopreservation and other environmental factors which affect its function. Surgery 75:49–55

Adenoma, Parathyroid, Syrian Hamster

Heinrich Ernst, Paul-Georg Germann, and Kenji Kamino

Gross Appearance

Parathyroid adenomas vary from grossly undetectable to nodules several millimeters in diameter and originate primarily in the median portion of the gland. They usually occur unilaterally (Fig. 379). Bilateral tumors are very rarely observed (Fig. 380).

Microscopic Features

Parathyroid adenomas develop as solitary nodules which are sharply demarcated from the adjacent parenchyma. A size-dependent degree of compression of the surrounding parathyroid or thyroid tissue is an essential criterion for the diagnosis (Fig. 381). Formation of a

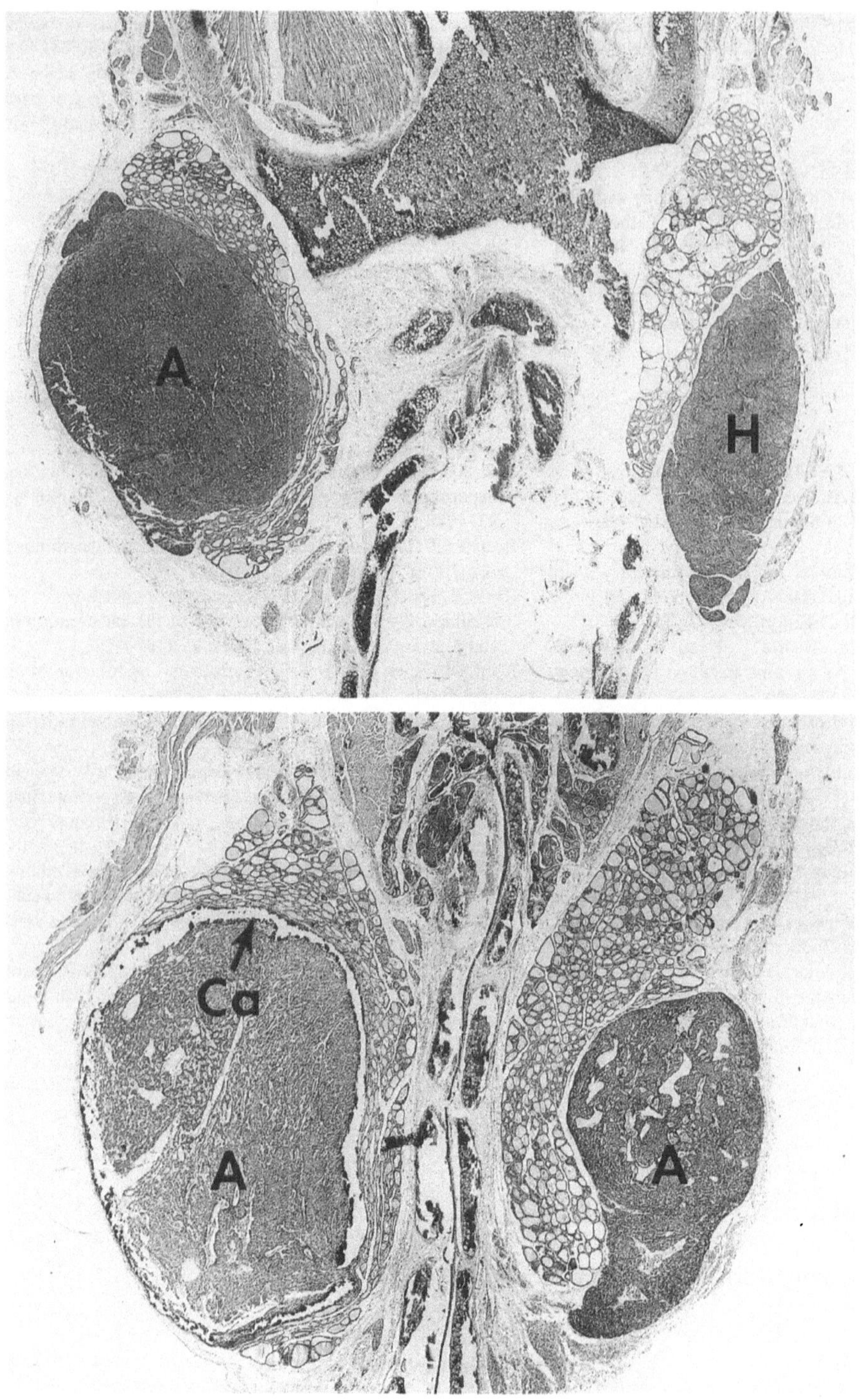

Fig. 379. (*above*) Adenoma (*A*) ansd hyperplastic parathyroid (*H*), Syrian hamster. H&E, ×20

Fig. 380. (*below*) Bilateral parathyroid adenomas (*A*), Syrian hamster. Note unilateral subcapsular calcification (*Ca*). H&E, ×20

pseudocapsule or capsule (Fig. 382) as a result of compression of preexisting stromal tissue or proliferation of collagen, respectively, is not always observed. The cellular composition of parathyroid adenomas is generally similar to that seen in hyperplastic lesions and consists of uniformly enlarged chief cells with eosinophilic or clear cytoplasm and prominent vesicular nuclei (Fig. 383). Mitotic figures are infrequent. Especially in larger adenomas the cells may be arranged in cords, clusters, or rosettes (Figs. 384, 385). Connective tissue is usually scanty within the tumor and forms fine capillary-rich septa that surround groups of tumor cells. Occasionally psammoma bodies are observed (Fig. 386).

Differential Diagnosis

Adenomas often develop within a background of focal or diffuse parathyroid hyperplasia. The main criterion for distinguishing adenoma from focal (nodular) hyperplasia is the absence of distinct compression of surrounding parenchyma in hyperplasia. Parathyroid carcinomas show definite signs of invasion and a high degree of cellular pleomorphism and atypia. So far, fewer than ten cases of parathyroid carcinoma in Syrian hamsters have been reported in the literature (Kirkman 1962, 1972; Kirkman and Algard 1968; Pour 1983), with only one case being documented photographically (Cardesa et al. 1982). This case occurred in a 760-day-old, ovariectomized female after treatment with stilbestrol for 248 days, the tumor metastasized into the cervical lymph nodes. C-cell tumors of the thyroid sometimes present diagnostic difficulty since they may show some morphological similarity to parathyroid adenomas. This applies especially to sections in which the parathyroids are missing. Demonstration of follicles within the tumor and immunohistochemical detection of calcitonin help to identify thyroid C-cell tumors.

Biologic Features

As with hyperplasia, parathyroid adenoma may be either functional or nonfunctional. In functional adenomas the normal, unaffected parathyroid tissue may become atrophic. In contrast to hyperplasia, parathyroid tumors seem not to be a sequela to long-lasting secondary hyperparathyroidism of renal or nutritional origin (Rosol and Capen 1989). It is also uncertain whether adenomas develop from focal (nodular) hyperplasias. In humans the monoclonality of parathyroid adenomas has been confirmed, whereas parathyroid hyperplasia is likely to be polyclonal in origin (Arnold et al. 1988; Rosol and Capen 1989). Similarly to parathyroid hyperplasia, the frequency of neoplasms of the parathyroid varies between different hamster strains. In most strains about 2% of older animals develop parathyroid adenomas (Cardesa et al. 1982). Pour et al. (1976, 1979), in two studies, observed adenomas in 7.7% and 1.5%, respectively, of white and albino hamsters in the Eppley colony, whereas no parathyroid tumor was found in Eppley-derived cream colored hamsters. In aged male hamsters of various unspecified commercial sources parathyroid adenomas were detected in 2.3% of the animals (Schmidt et al. 1983).
The frequency of parathyroid adenomas in hamsters has been reported to be not significantly influenced by hormonal imbalances (Pour 1983). The composition of the diet, however, seems to effect parathyroid tumorigenesis. In hamsters fed a high-fat diet the incidence of parathyroid adenomas increased up to 15% (Birt and Pour 1985).

Comparison with Other Species

As with parathyroid hyperplasia, adenomas seem to be more frequent in hamsters than in rats and mice what may be due to a greater sensitivity of hamsters to the dietary composition (Pour 1983). For most rat strains frequencies below 2% have been reported (see 356, this volume). In mice parathyroid neoplasms are extremely rare. To our knowledge, only six cases of parathyroid adenoma in mice have been reported in the literature (Dunn 1979; Frith and Ward 1988; Lang 1989; Maita et al. 1988; Ward et al. 1979).

Acknowledgment. We acknowledge the contribution of Dr. Parviz Pour who provided some illustrations which are reproduced here from the first edition.

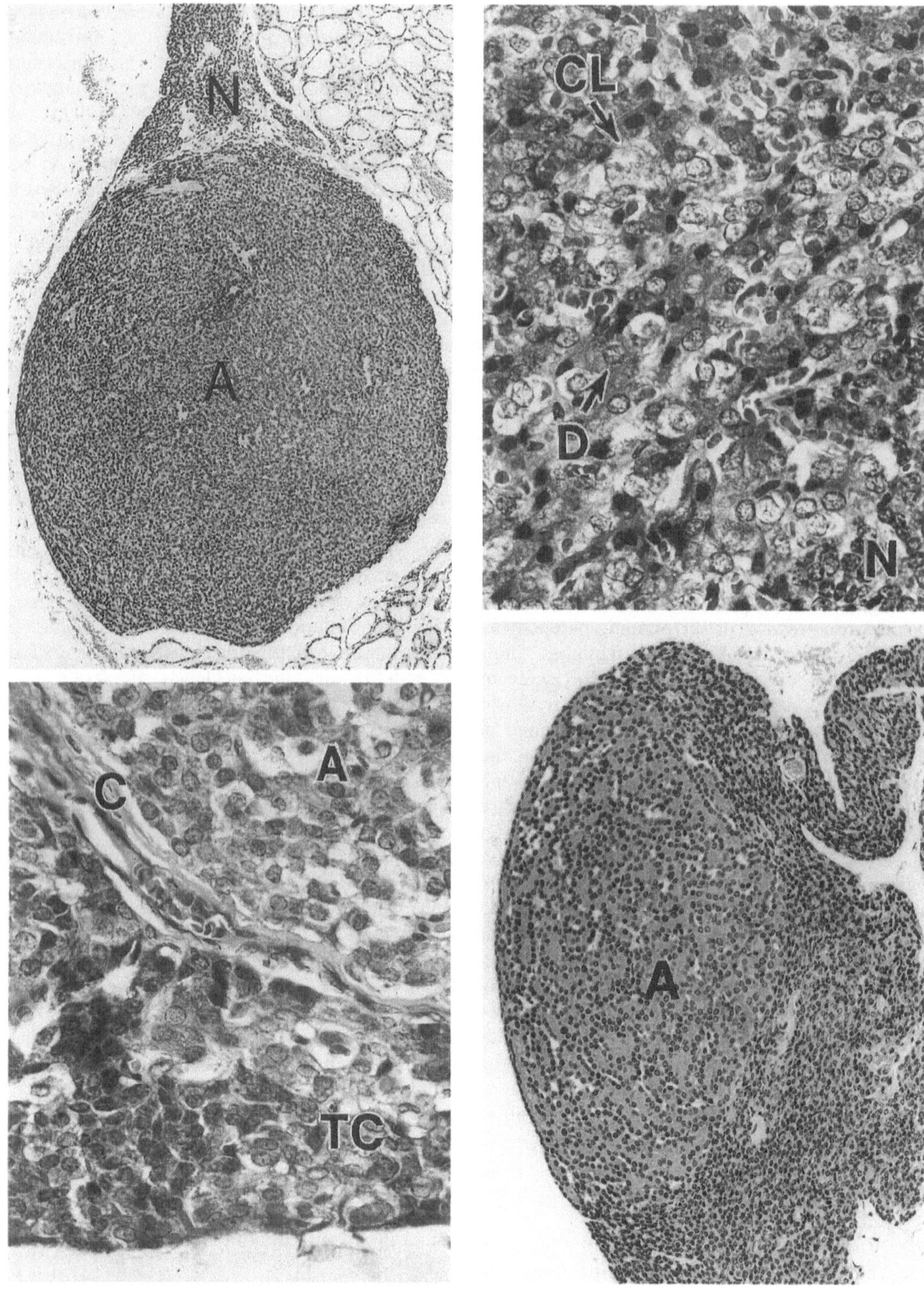
N
A
CL
D
N
C
A
TC
A

◀
Fig. 381. (*upper left*) Parathyroid adenoma (*A*), Syrian hamster. Note distinct compression of adjacent thyroid and normal parathyroid tissue (*N*). H&E, ×75

Fig. 382. (*lower left*) Parathyroid adenoma (*A*), Syrian hamster. Note tumor capsule (*C*) and tumor cells outside of capsule (*TC*). H&E, ×400

Fig. 383. (*upper right*) Parathyroid adenoma, Syrian hamster. Three cell types: normal (*N*), large clear (*CL*), and dark cells (*D*). Same cells in different functional stages. H&E, ×400

Fig. 384. (*lower right*) Parathyroid adenoma (*A*), Syrian hamster. Note trabecular arrangement of tumor cells. H&E, ×120

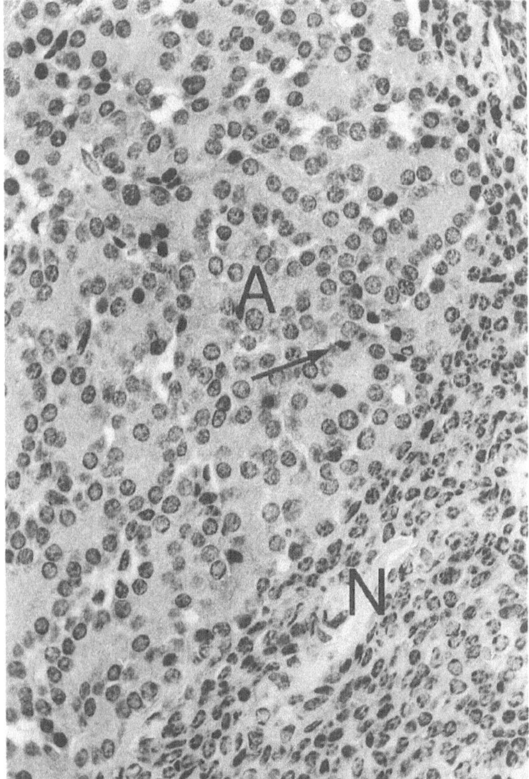

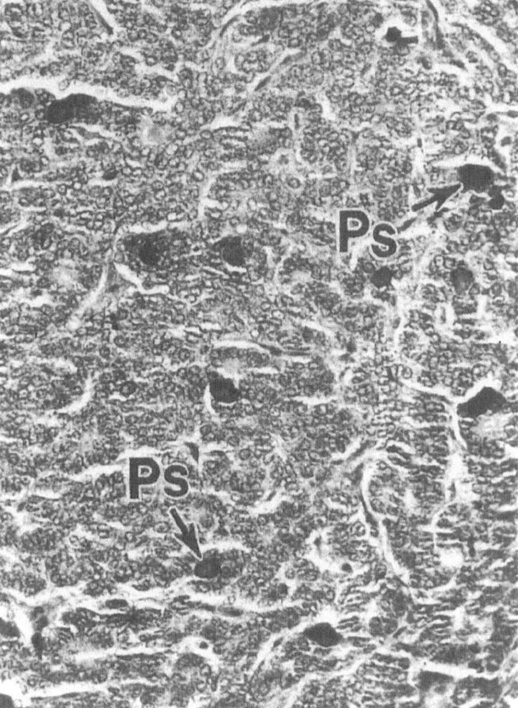

▶
Fig. 385. (*above*) Higher magnification of Fig. 384. Note sharp demarcation of tumor (*A*), difference in cell size between tumor and normal cells (*N*), and mitotic figure (*arrow*). H&E, ×350

Fig. 386. (*below*) Parathyroid adenoma, Syrian hamster. Note numerous psammoma bodies (*Ps*) within tumor tissue. H&E, ×160

References

Arnold A, Staunton CE, Kim HG, Gaz RD, Kronenberg HM (1988) Monoclonality and abnormal parathyroid hormone genes in parathyroid adenomas. N Engl J Med 318:658–662

Birt DF, Pour PM (1985) Interaction of dietary fat and protein in spontaneous diseases of Syrian golden hamsters. J Natl Cancer Inst 75:127–133

Cardesa A, Handler AH, Kelman AD (1982) Tumours of the parathyroid gland. In: Turusov VS et al (eds) Pathology of tumours in laboratory animals, vol III. Tumours of the hamster. IARC Sci Publ 34:275–280

Dunn TB (1979) Tumours of the parathyroid gland. In: Turusov VS et al (eds) Pathology of tumours in laboratory animals, vol II. Tumours of the mouse. IARC Sci Publ 23:469–474

Frith CH, Ward JM (1988) Color atlas of neoplastic and non-neoplastic lesions in aging mice. Elsevier, Amsterdam, pp 33–48

Kirkman H (1962) A preliminary report concerning tumors observed in Syrian hamsters. Stanford Med Bull 20:163–166

Kirkman H (1972) Hormone-related tumors in Syrian hamsters. Prog Exp Tumor Res 16:201–240

Kirkman H, Algard FT (1968) Spontaneous and nonviral-induced neoplasms. In: Hoffman RA, Robinson PF, Magalhaes H (eds) The golden hamster: its biology and use in medical research. Iowa State University Press, Ames, pp 227–240

Lang PL (1989) Spontaneous neoplastic lesions in the B6C3F1/CrlBR mouse. Charles River Laboratories, Wilmington

Maita K, Hirano M, Harada T, Mitsumori K, Yoshida A, Takahashi K, Nakashima N, Kitazawa T, Enomoto A, Inui K, Shirasu Y (1988) Mortality, major cause of moribundity, and spontaneous tumors in CD-1 mice. Toxicol Pathol 16:340–349

Pour PM (1983) Hyperplasia, parathyroid, hamster. In: Jones TC, Mohr U, Hunt RD (eds) ILSI Monographs on pathology of laboratory animals: endocrine system, 1st edition. Springer, Berlin Heidelberg New York, pp 265–268

Pour PM, Althoff J, Salmasi SZ, Stepan K (1979) Spontaneous tumors and common diseases in three types of hamsters. J Natl Cancer Inst 63:797–809

Pour PM, Mohr U, Althoff J, Cardesa A, Kmoch N (1976) Spontaneous tumors and common diseases in two colonies of Syrian hamsters. III. Urogenital system and endocrine glands. J Natl Cancer Inst 56:949–961

Rosol TJ, Capen CC (1989) Tumors of the parathyroid gland and circulating parathyroid hormone-related protein associated with persistent hypercalcemia. Toxicol Pathol 17:346–356

Schmidt RE, Eason RL, Hubbard GB, Young JT, Eisenbrandt DL (1983) Pathology of aging Syrian hamsters. CRC Press, Boca Raton, pp 141–174

Ward JM, Goodman DG, Squire RA, Chu KC, Linhart MS (1979) Neoplastic and nonneoplastic lesions in aging (C57BL/6N × C3H/HeN)F1 (B6C3F1) mice. J Natl Cancer Inst 63:849–854

Adenoma, Carcinoma, Parathyroid, Rat

Kenji Kamino, Heinrich Ernst, and Birgit Kittel

Synonyms. Adenoma: adenoma of chief cells, parathyroid; carcinoma: adenocarcinoma of chief cells, parathyroid.

Gross Appearance

Adenoma. Parathyroid adenomas vary from grossly undetectable to unilateral nodules several millimeters in diameter. They are located in the cervical region embedded under the capsule of the thyroid (Fig. 387) and appear as soft, grayish white, opaque, or pink tissue. Adenomas derived from ectopic parathyroid tissue may be seen infrequently in the thoracic cavity near the base of the heart or in the precardiac mediastinum (Capen et al. 1991).

Carcinoma. Chief cell carcinomas result in a macroscopically detectable unilateral enlargement. They appear as grayish white, ill-defined masses and are more fixed in position than adenomas due to invasion of the adjacent tissue. Carcinomas may include necrotic and/or hemorrhagic areas.

Microscopic Features

Adenoma. Small adenomas are solitary nodules which are clearly demarcated from adjacent parathyroid parenchyma. The adenomas compress the surrounding parathyroid or thyroid tissue to varying degrees, depending upon their size; however, even small neoplasms have this effect. Focal bulging into the adjacent parathyroid tissue may sometimes occur (Fig. 388). Adenomas generally are not encapsulated, but there may be a partial fibrous capsule, either from compression of existing stroma or from

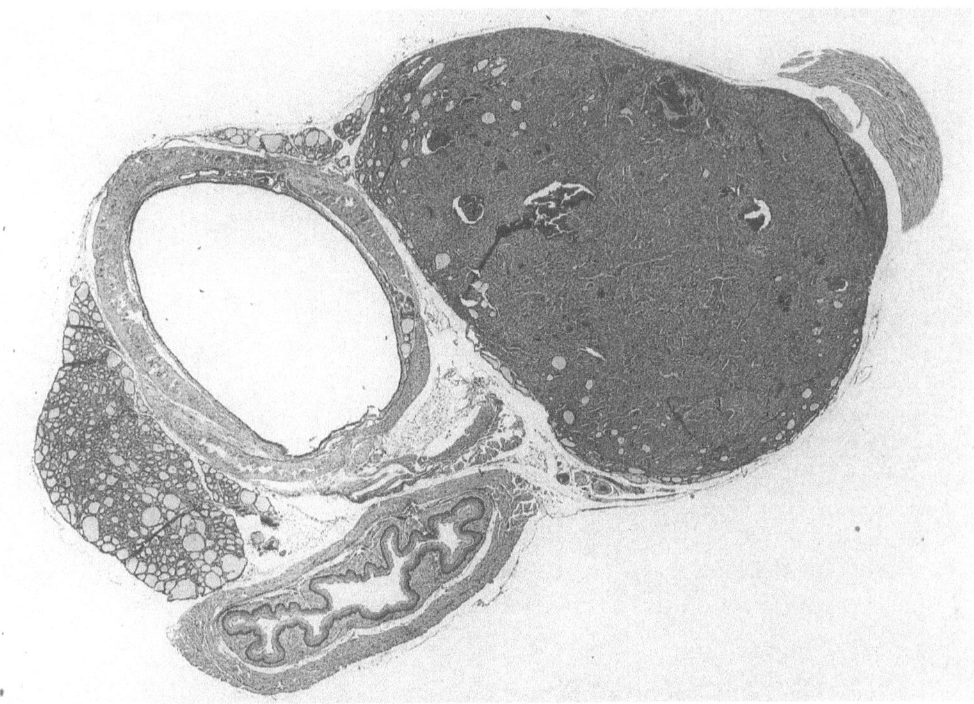

Fig. 387. Parathyroid adenoma occurring as a large unilateral nodule, Han:Wistar rat. Contralateral gland could not be found, even in step section. H&E, ×20

proliferation of connective tissue. Figure 389 shows the usual solid pattern of small adenomas, but they may have various architectural features such as papillary, pseudoglandular, or acinar patterns (Pour et al. 1983).

Larger, macroscopically detectable parathyroid adenomas often involve almost the entire gland. A narrow rim of residual compressed parenchyma may be seen at one side of the adenoma (Fig. 390). Adenomas are usually nonfunctional in rats. Chief cells in nonfunctional adenomas are cuboidal or polyhedral and have round to oval, often vesicular nuclei and vacuolated or clear cytoplasm (Figs. 391, 392). Mitotic figures may be present, but they are infrequent and usually are associated with slight nuclear pleomorphism (Fig. 392).

Chief cells from functional adenomas are closely packed into small groups by fine connective tissue septa. They are cuboidal and their cytoplasm stains lightly eosinophilic. Occasional oxyphil cells, water-clear cells, and transitional forms are distributed throughout the adenoma. The contralateral parathyroid gland which does not contain a functional adenoma undergoes atrophy in response to hypercalcemia. Some parathyroid adenomas in rats become cystic (cystadenomas; Rosol and Capen 1989). The cystadenomas consist of solid areas of tumor cells and large cystic areas lined by neoplastic chief cells. The cysts contain eosinophilic proteinaceous fluid.

Carcinoma. Carcinomas usually completely incorporate the affected gland and show evidence of invasion through the parathyroid capsule. Desmoplasia and inflammatory cell infiltration often accompany penetration of the parathyroid capsule by malignant chief cells. Infiltrations of perithyroidal connective tissue, lymphatics, and blood vessels (Fig. 393) are observed infrequently. Small pulmonary tumor cell emboli are also occasionally seen. Malignant chief cells are either arranged in solid sheets, palisade along blood sinusoids, or form acinar structures. The solid sheets are often subdivided into lobules by a fibrovascular stroma. The tumor cells are more pleomorphic than those comprising adenomas. Mitoses, however, are less frequent than in adenomas or hyperplasia. Elongated or spindle-shaped tumor cells may be also observed (Fig.

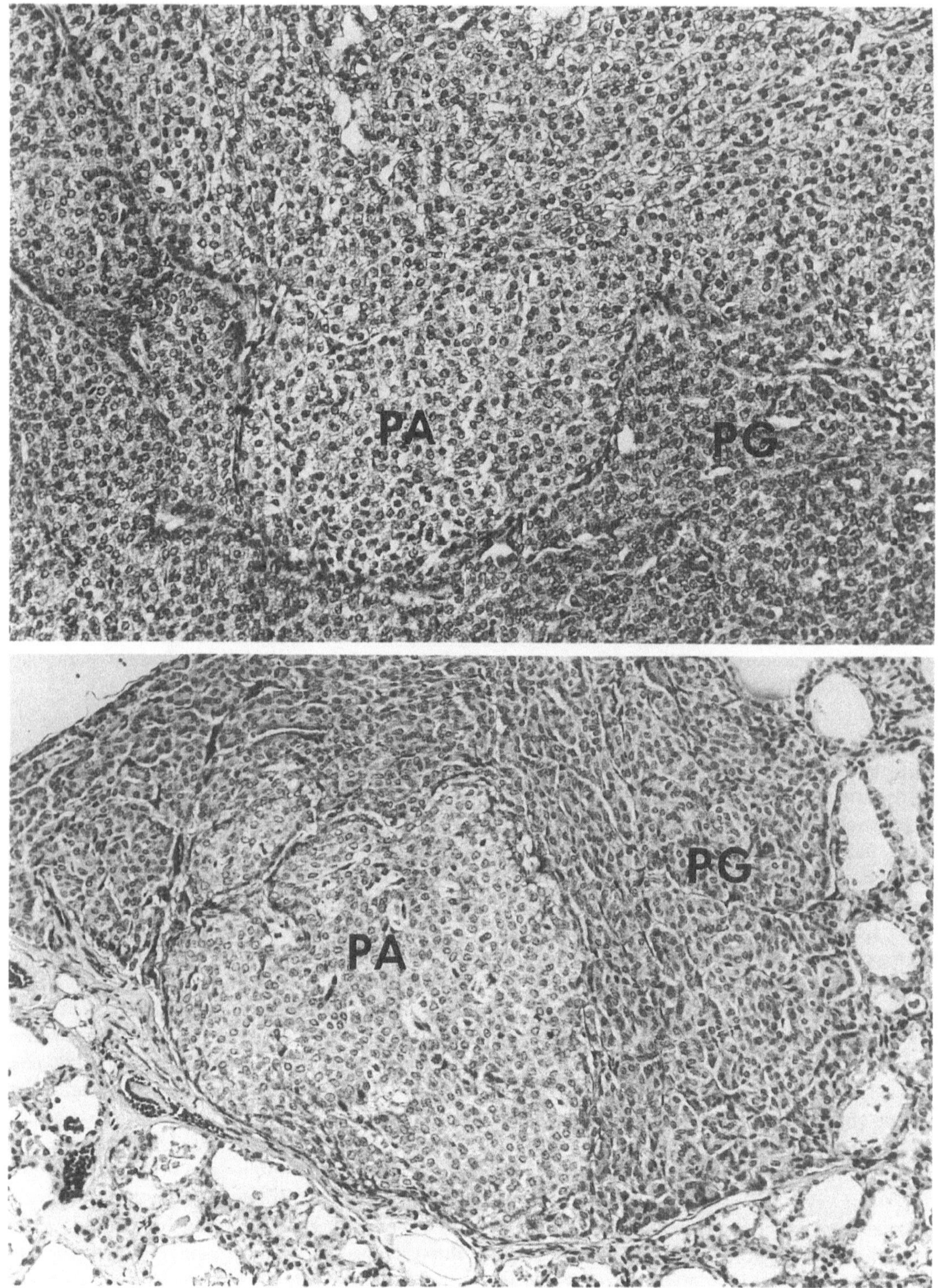

Fig. 388. (*above*) Parathyroid adenoma, clear cell type, OFA rat. Tumor cells (*PA*) protrude into adjacent hyperplastic parathyroid tissue (*PG*). H&E, ×120

Fig. 389. (*below*) Parathyroid adenoma (*PA*). Normal parathyroid gland (*PG*), rat. H&E, ×120

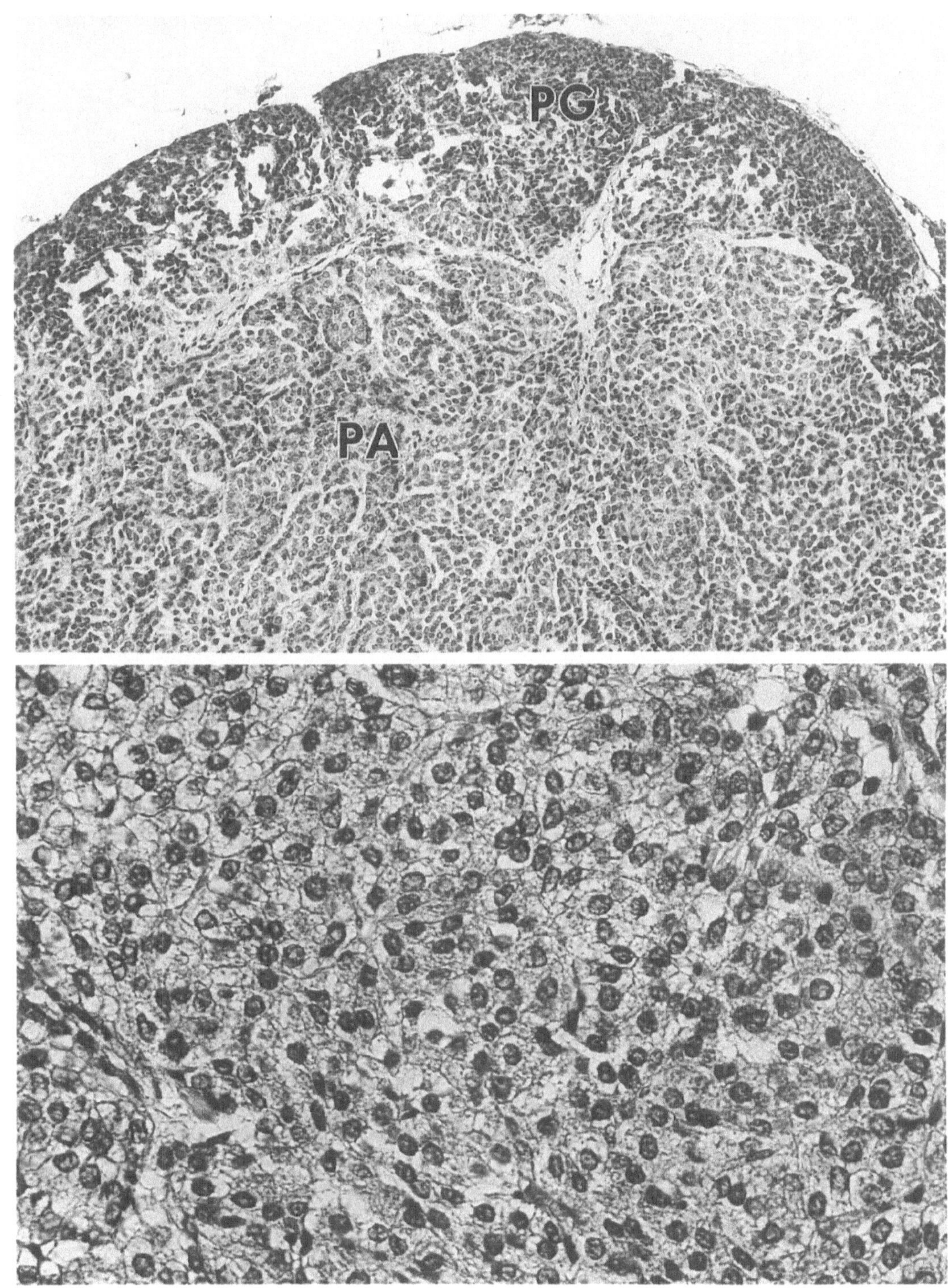

Fig. 390. (*above*), Parathyroid adenoma (*PA*), Rat. Parathyroid tissue (*PG*) around border. H&E, ×60

Fig. 391. (*below*) Parathyroid adenoma, clear cell type, MCR rat. Note vesicular nuclei and clear cytoplasm. H&E, ×300

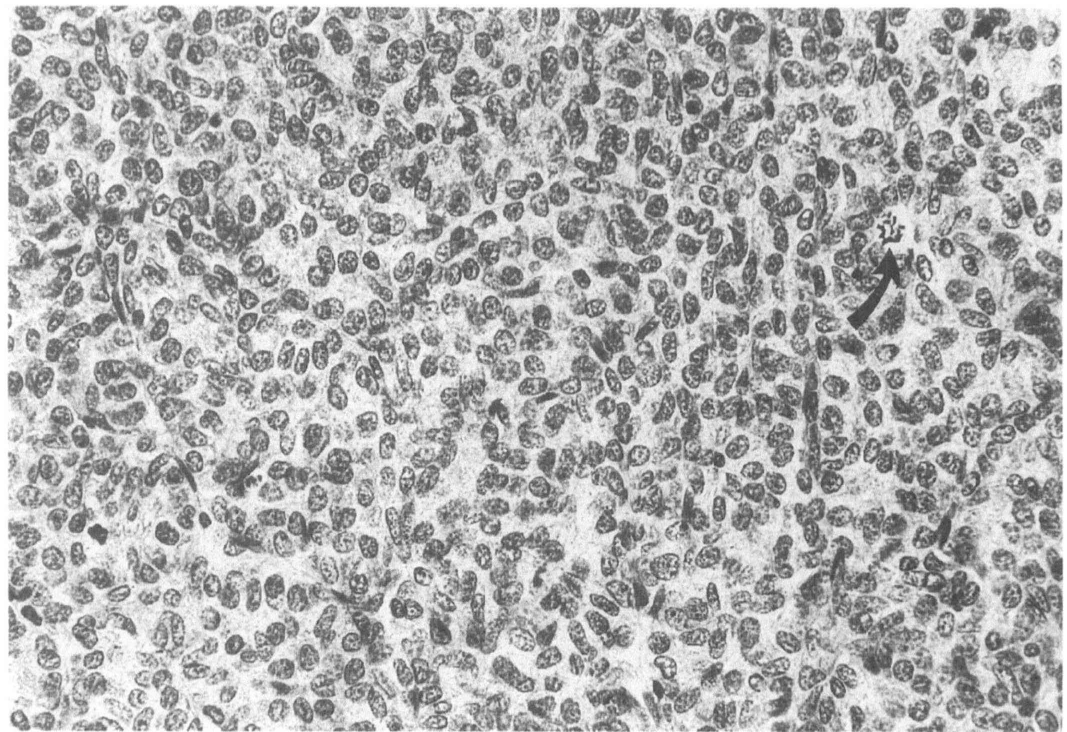

Fig. 392. Parathyroid adenoma, rat. Note slightly pleomorphic nuclei and a mitosis (arrow). H&E, ×300

394). The malignant chief cells have an ill-defined, slightly eosinophilic cytoplasm.

Ultrastructure

Chief cells comprising functional parathyroid adenomas are usually in the actively synthesizing stage of the secretory cycle (Capen 1983). Multiple large lamellar arrays of rough endoplasmic reticulum and clusters of free ribosomes are present in the cytoplasm. Additionally, large mitochondria, prominent Golgi apparatuses, and a few mature secretory ("storage") granules are present in neoplastic chief cells. The annulate lamellae which occur frequently in parathyroid adenoma chief cells have not been reported in normal chief cells (Rosol and Capen 1989).

Differential Diagnosis

Criteria for distinguishing neoplastic lesions of the parathyroid glands are:

- Adenoma
  - Unilateral enlargement of parathyroid gland with the normal or atrophic contralateral gland (Fig. 387)
  - Solitary well-demarcated nodule or mass
- A rim of normal or compressed atrophic parathyroid parenchyma at one pole of the lesion (Fig. 390)
  - Variable compression of thyroid and/or adjacent tissue
  - Usually no capsule; occasionally large lesions with a pseudocapsule of compressed stroma
  - Cells usually arranged in solid clusters; occasionally papillary, pseudoglandular or acinar pattern
  - Uniform but enlarged cells with enlarged nuclei and slightly prominent nucleoli
- Carcinoma
  - Large mass displacing thyroid
  - Solid, papillary or glandular growth pattern
  - Cellular pleomorphism and atypia
  - Invasion of adjacent tissue, lymphatics and/or blood vessels (Fig. 393)
  - Metastases

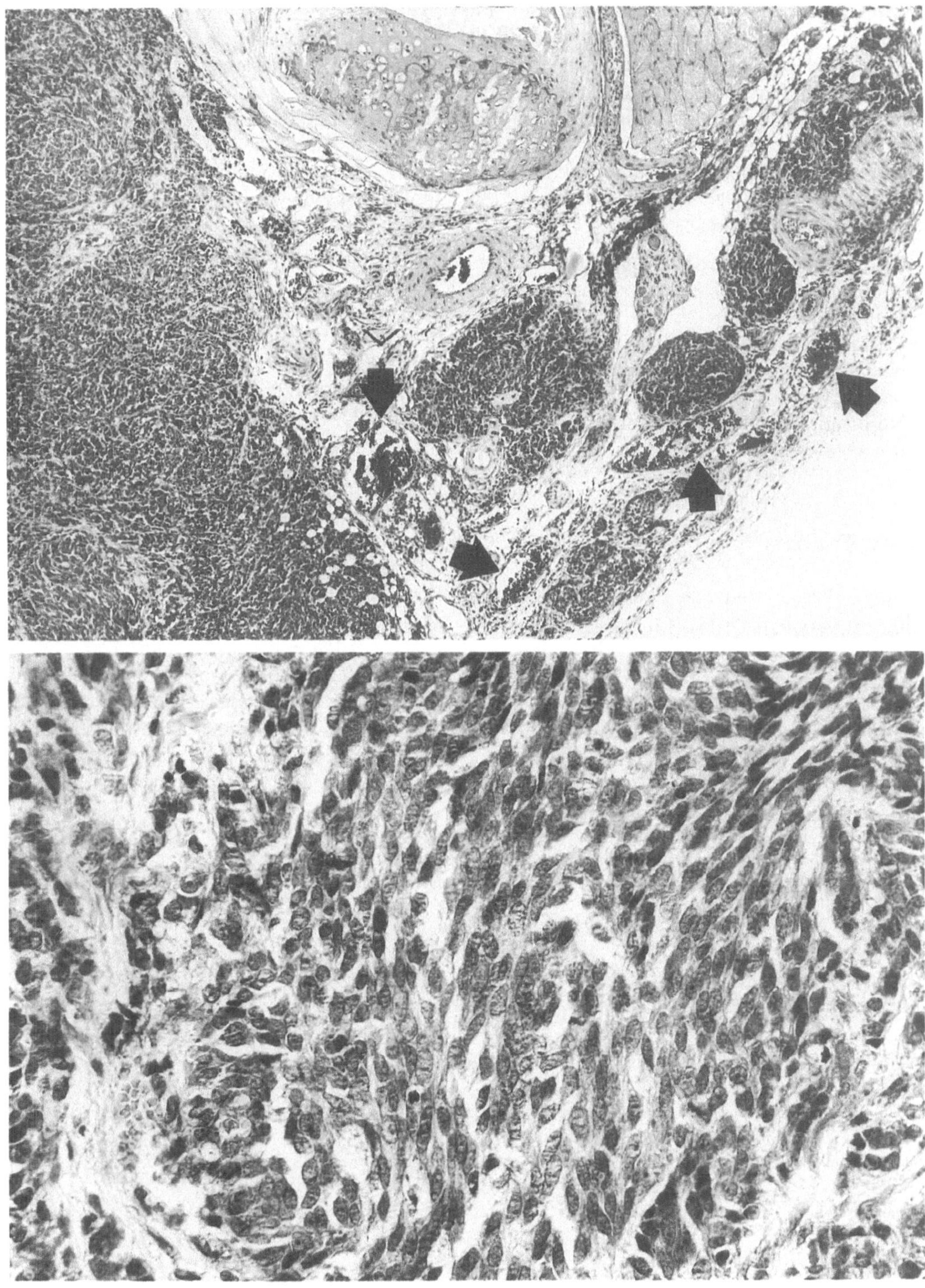

Fig. 393. (*above*) Parathyroid carcinoma, OFA rat. Infiltration of adjacent soft tissue, lymphatics, and vessels (*arrow*). H&E, ×48

Fig. 394. (*below*) Parathyroid carcinoma, OFA rat. Large pleomorphic tumor cells with elongated to spindle-shaped or oval nuclei. H&E, ×300

Differential diagnosis from the more common medullary (C-cell) tumors of the thyroid could cause a problem. Tumors of C-cell origin should be clearly identified through identification of intracellular calcitonin using the immunoperoxidase method.

Parathyroid hyperplasia, a relatively frequent lesion in the rat, may be differentiated by the following characteristics:

- Diffuse enlargement of both glands
- Uniform pattern of cellular arrangement in both glands
- Uniform population of enlarged cells
- No rim of compressed normal parathyroid parenchyma
- No compression of adjacent tissue (see p. 338 this volume)

Biologic Features

Etiology. Parathyroid adenomas occur sporadically in parathyroid glands, with or without hyperplasia. It is not known whether adenomas develop as a progression of focal hyperplasia. They have not been associated with a response to a physiological stimulus (Seely and Hildebrandt 1990). According to Capen et al. (1991), they do not appear to be a result of long-standing secondary hyperparathyroidism of renal or nutritional origin. On the other hand, Pour et al. (1983) presented cases in which the alteration of calcium metabolism was considered an etiologic factor. Namely, in OFA rats with frequent spontaneous vascular diseases such as periarteritis nodosa, renal damage appeared to be a primary cause of parathyroid hyperplasia, and this presumably could have led to development of adenoma. Bone lesions seemed most frequently to be associated with either adenoma or carcinoma, but osteitis fibrosa (fibrous osteodystrophy) has been observed in rats with parathyroid hyperplasia (Berdjis 1972).

Frequency. Spontaneous parathyroid adenomas are rare and are most commonly found in Long-Evans rats (Lindsay et al. 1957). The data in the literature show the following tumor incidences in different strains (Table 24). Solleveld et al. (1984) reported that the incidence of parathyroid adenomas increased in male F344 from 0.1% at 2 years to 3.1% in life span studies. Corresponding data for female F344 was 0.1% at 2 years and 0.6% in life span studies. The preponderance in males is very noticeable in almost all cases. Para-

Table 24. Frequency of parathyroid adenomas in rats

Strain	Sex	Frequency (%)	Reference
OFA	M	1.0	Pour et al. 1983
Han : Wistar	M	2.0	
MRC	M	3.0	
Han : Wistar	M	3.0	Deerberg et al. 1980
Han : Wistar	F	0.7	
WAG/Rij	M	2.0	Burek 1978
WAG/Rij	F	2.0	
BN/B	F	<1.0	
Holtzman-SD	F	0.4	MacKenzie and Garner 1973; Prejean et al. 1973
Charles River-SD	F	0.2	
Osborne-Mendel	F	0.8	
Oregon	F	0.3	
Sprague-Dawley	F	1.2	
Diablo-SD	F	0	
Fischer 344	F	0.3	Goodman et al. 1979
WAG/Rij	F	0.7	Boorman and Hollander 1973
M520	M	*	Snell 1965
WN	M	*	

* Sporadic.

thyroid adenomas can be induced by irradiation (Triggs and Williams 1977; Fjälling et al. 1981; Oslapas et al. 1981; Wynford-Thomas et al. 1983). Dietary vitamine D and/or plasma calcium may be of importance in determining the tumorigenic effect of irradiation (Wynford-Thomas et al. 1983). Chief cell carcinomas are encountered rarely in laboratory rats, and few have been reported in the literature (Warren and Chute 1962; Berdjis 1972; Pour et al. 1983). Adenomas are usually nonfunctional in rats (Capen et al. 1991). In functional adenomas, there is loss of the normal mechanism by which parathyroid hormone secretion is controlled by the concentration of blood calcium, and hormone secretion is excessive in spite of an increased level of blood calcium. Pour et al. (1983) presented a case of parathyroid carcinoma with severe generalized osteitis fibrosa, indicating functional activity of this tumor.

Comparison with Other Species

Rat parathyroid adenomas do not have the wide histologic variations which are seen in human cases (Pour et al. 1983). In contrast to those in cats, dogs, and humans, adenomas in rats are usually nonfunctional (Brown and LeBoff 1986, Capen 1978, 1983, 1989). Spontaneous remission of primary hyperparathyroidism has been reported in dogs and humans, associated with infarction of functional adenomas (Rosol et al. 1988). In the mouse parathyroid adenomas are very rare (see p. 347, this volume). Arnold et al. (1988) presented data on human parathyroid adenomas indicating that the adenomas are of monoclonal origin. The presence of identical DNA mutations in chief cells of the adenomas implied that the mutation originated from one common ancestral cell. In contrast to adenomas, parathyroid hyperplasia is likely to be polyclonal and may follow a hereditary basis (Arnold et al. 1988). Therefore the pathogenesis of parathyroid adenoma and idiopathic hyperplasia may be different, at least in humans. As in humans and other vertebrates, parathyroid carcinoma is a rare disease in rats. The carcinoma presented by Pour et al. (1983) was morphologically and biologically similar to those found occasionally in hamsters.

Acknowledgement. We acknowledge the contribution of Dr. P.M. Pour who provided the illustrations which are reproduced here from the first edition.

References

Arnold A, Staunton CE, Kim HG, Gaz RD, Kronenberg HM (1988) Monoclonality and abnormal parathyroid hormone genes in parathyroid adenomas. N Engl J Med 318:658–662

Berdjis CC (1972) Parathyroid diseases and irradiation. Strahlentherapie 143:48–62

Boorman GA, Hollander CF (1973) Spontaneous lesions in the female Wag/Rij (Wistar) rat. J Gerontol 28:152–159

Brown EM, LeBoff MS (1986) Pathophysiology of hyperparathyroidism. Prog Surg 18:13–22

Burek JD (1978) Pathology of aging rats. CRC Press, West Palm Beach, pp 38–41

Capen CC (1978) Tumors of the endocrine glands. In: Moulton JE (ed) Tumors in domestic animals, 2nd edn. University of California Press, Berkeley, pp 372–429

Capen CC (1983) Structural and biochemical aspects of parathyroid gland function in animals. In: Jones TC, Mohr U, Hunt RD (eds) Monographs on pathology of laboratory animals, endocrine system, 1st edition. Springer, Berlin Heidelberg New York, pp 217–247

Capen CC (1989) Neoplasms of the parathyroid glands. In: Stinson SF, Reznik G (eds) Atlas of tumor pathology in the F344 rat. CRC Press, Boca Raton, pp 367–378

Capen CC, DeLellis RA, Yarrington JT (1991) Endocrine system. In: Haschek WM, Rousseaux CG (eds) Handbook of toxicologic pathology. Academic, San Diego, pp 625–760

Deerberg F, Rapp KP, Pittermann W, Rehm S (1980) Zum Tumorspektrum der Han: WIST-Ratte. Z Versuchstierkd 22:267–280

Fjälling M, Hansson G, Hedman I, Ragnhult I, Tisell LE (1981) Radiation-induced parathyroid adenomas and thyroid tumors in rats. Acta Pathol Microbiol Scand [A] 89:425–429

Goodman DG, Ward JM, Squire RA, Chu KC, Linhart MS (1979) Neoplastic and non-neoplastic lesions in aging F344 rats. Toxicol Appl Pharmacol 48:237–248

Lindsay S, Potter GD, Chaikoff IL (1957) Thyroid neoplasms in the rat: a comparison of naturally occurring and I-131-induced tumors. Cancer Res 17:183–189

MacKenzie WF, Garner FM (1973) Comparison of neoplasms in six sources of rats. J Natl Cancer Inst 50:1243–1257

Oslapas R, Prinz R, Ernst K, Smith M, Greenlee W, Hofmann C, Lawrence AM, Paloyan E (1981) Incidence of radiation-induced parathyroid tumors in male and female rats. Clin Res 29:734A

Pour PM, Wilson JT, Salmasi S (1983) Adenoma, Carcinoma, Parathyroid, Rat. In: Jones TC, Mohr U, Hunt RD (eds) Monographs on pathology of laboratory animals, endocrine system, 1st edition. Springer, Berlin Heidelberg New York, pp 281–287

Prejean JD, Peckham JC, Casey AE, Griswold DP, Weisburger EK, Weisburger JH (1973) Spontaneous tumors in Sprague-Dawley rats and Swiss mice. Cancer Res 33: 2768–2773

Rosol TJ, Capen CC (1989) Tumors of the parathyroid gland and circulating parathyroid hormone-related protein associated with persistent hypercalcemia. Toxicol Pathol 17:346–356

Rosol TJ, Chew DJ, Capen CC, Sherding RG (1988) Acute hypocalcemia associated with infarction of parathyroid gland adenomas in two dogs. J Am Vet Med Assoc 192: 212–214

Seely JC, Hildebrandt PK (1990) Parathyroid gland. In: Boorman GA, Eustis SL, Elwell MR, Montgomery CA Jr, MacKenzie WF (eds) Pathology of the Fischer rat, reference and atlas. Academic, San Diego, pp 537–543

Snell KC (1965) Spontaneous lesions of the rat. In: Ribelin WE, McCoy JR (eds) The pathology of laboratory animals. Thomas, Springfield, pp 284–287

Solleveld HA, Haseman JK, McConnell EE (1984) Natural history of body weight gain, survival, and neoplasia in the F344 rat. J Natl Cancer Inst 72:929–940

Triggs SM, Williams ED (1977) Irradiation of the thyroid as a cause of parathyroid adenoma. Lancet 1:593–594

Warren S, Chute R (1962) Parathyroid carcinoma in parabiont rats. Science 135:927–928

Wynford-Thomas V, Wynford-Thomas D, Williams ED (1983) Experimental induction of parathyroid adenomas in the rat. J Natl Cancer Inst 70:127–134

Pancreatic Islets

Hyperplasia, Adenoma, and Carcinoma of Pancreatic Islets, Mouse

Charles H. Frith and Winslow D. Sheldon

Synonyms. Hyperplasia: none; islet-cell adenoma: pancreatic endocrine adenoma, islet-cell carcinoma, islet-cell adenocarcinoma, pancreatic endocrine adenocarcinoma.

Gross Appearance

Islet-cell hyperplasia and islet-cell adenomas are often not visible grossly. Islet-cell carcinomas appear as hard reddish masses in the parenchyma of the pancreas.

Microscopic Features

Hyperplasia of the pancreatic islets usually involves more than one islet, and may involve all of the visible islets within a histologic section. These islets are much larger due to an increased number of cells (Figs. 396, 398), but morphologically they are similar to the smaller normal islets. (Figs. 395, 397). The specific cell type is difficult to identify at the light microscopic level, and histochemistry and electron microscopy are often needed.

Islet-cell adenomas commonly involve a single islet within a histologic section. The cells form ribbons along sinusoidal, thin-walled vessels, and the adenomas are quite often more vascular in appearance (Figs. 399, 400). The cells stain lightly eosinophilic with H&E; the nuclei demonstrate a delicate chromatin pattern. The cells are well differenticated, and the mitotic index is low or nonexistent.

Islet-cell carcinomas are invariably larger than adenomas and are commonly visible grossly. The cells vary from being well-differentiated to extremely pleomorphic and anaplastic. Well-differentiated islet-cell carcinomas may metastasize or invade locally. Figures 401 and 402 demonstrate a well-differentiated islet-cell carcinoma which metastasized to the liver (Fig. 403). The cytoplasm of the neoplastic cells is eosinophilic and the nuclei are vesicular. Nucleoli are prominent and may be multiple. Mitotic figures are evident and pleomorphism may be prominent. Anaplastic islet-cell carcinomas may be difficult to accurately identify as islet cell in orign.

Ultrastructure

Ultrastructural features have rarely been reported in murine islet-cell hyperplasia and islet-cell tumors owing to their scarcity, as well as to the inability to recognize the hyperplasia and adenomas grossly. Like et al. (1965) reported ultrastructural features of enlarged islets in (C3H × I)F-1 mice. The cells contained increased rough endoplasmic reticulum, polysomes and free ribosomes, mitochondria, an enlarged Golgi apparatus, and depletion of beta granules.

Differential Diagnosis

Islet-cell hyperplasia and islet-cell adenomas are similar morphologically, and the specific diagnosis is somewhat subjective. Islet-cell carcinomas may be difficult to distinguish from islet-cell adenomas if they are well differentiated and do not invade other organs or metastasize.

Biologic Features

Islet-cell lesions are generally considered to be rare in mice, and may be functional or nonfunctional, as in humans (Jones 1964; Cardesa et al. 1979). Like et al. (1965) reported that enlarged islets were associated with glycosuria and clinical

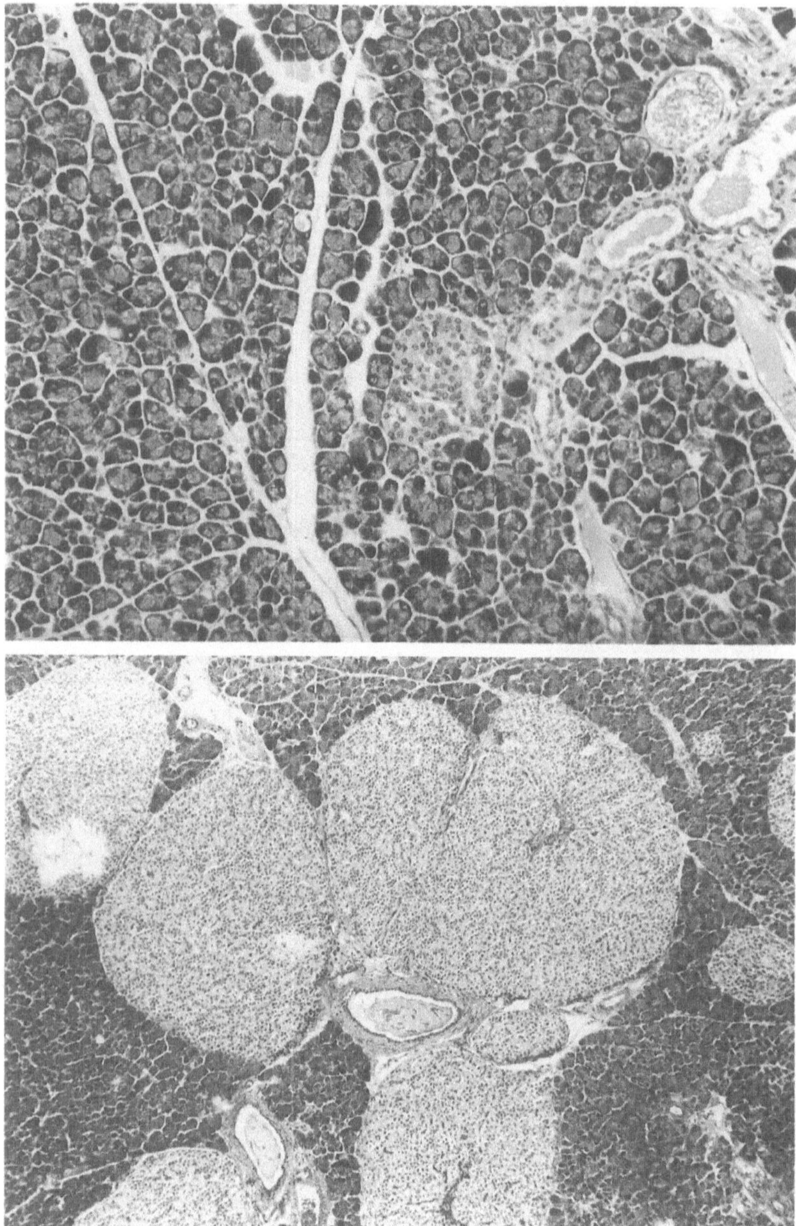

Fig. 395. (*above*) Pancreatic islet, normal mouse. H&E, ×120

Fig. 396. (*below*) Pancreatic islets, hyperplasia. Yellow A^{vy}/A hybrid mouse. H&E, ×150

diabetes in mice, but the investigators were not sure if the lesions were hyperplastic or neoplastic. They demonstrated that the islet-cell lesions were almost exclusively composed of beta cells. Rowlatt (1967) stated that, unless the islets differ morphologically from that of a normal islet, the diagnostic interpretation is entirely subjective.

Hueper (1936) reported a single case of an islet cell adenoma, and Cloudman (1941) described two islet-cell tumors in mice. Deringer (1951, 1956) recorded a frequency of 2% for islet-cell tumors in HR/DE mice. Murphy (1966) also reported a frequency of 2% for islet-cell adenomas in untreated HR/DE mice. Sass et al. (1978) observed 12 islet-cell adenomas in a total of 127 $C3H/A^{vy}$

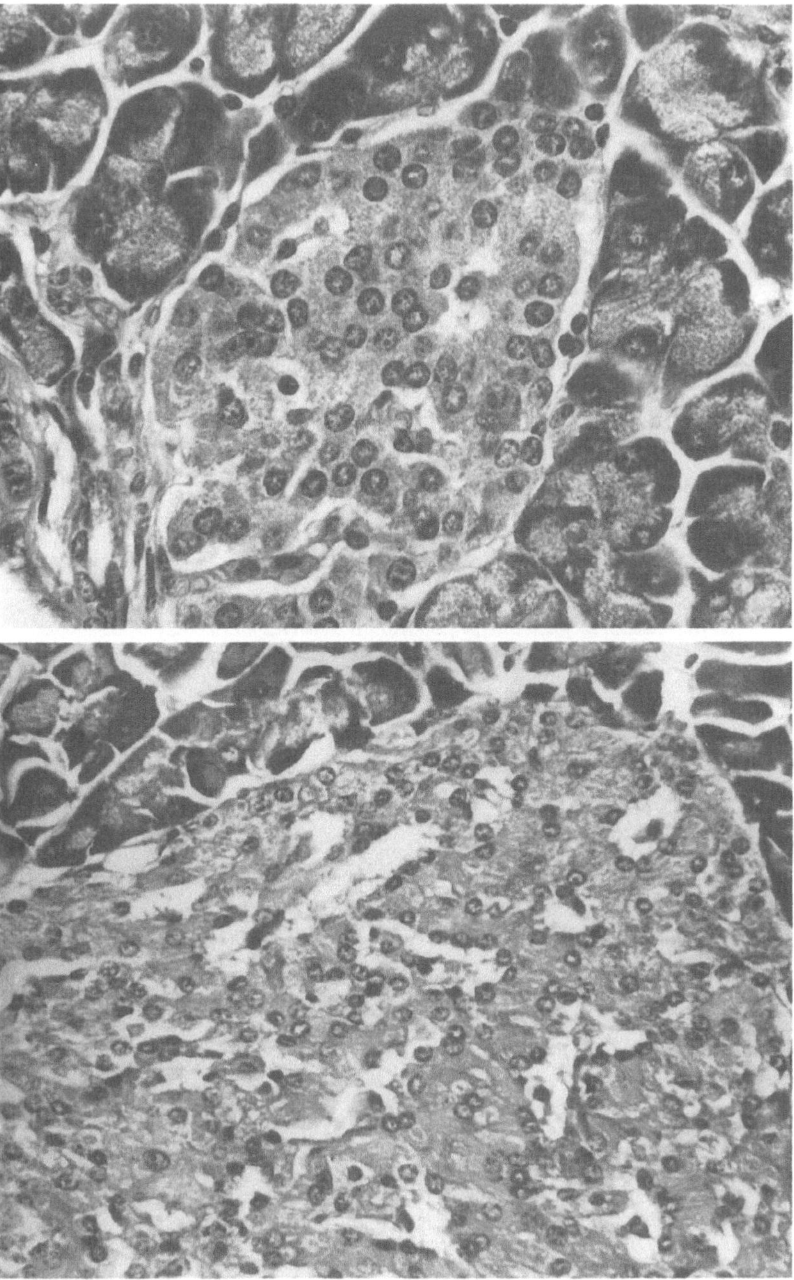

Fig. 397. (*above*) Pancreatic islet, normal, mouse. H&E, ×384

Fig. 398. (*below*) Pancreatic islet, hyperplasia, mouse. H&E, ×96

mice (9.4%). Jones (1964) found a high frequency of B-cell hyperplasia and islet-cell tumors in (C3H × I)F-1 hybrids. Belkin (1942) described an exocrine adenocarcinoma of the pancreas in one of 800 Bagg-albino mice injected with benz(a) pyrene subcutaneously; and Rowlatt (1967) reported a pancreatic cystadenoma in a C-strain mouse treated with 7,12-dimethylbenz(a)anthracine (DMBA), and an adenocarcinoma in an ICI mouse following skin painting with cigarette-smoke condensate. All of these were nevertheless considered to be spontaneous tumors.

Islet-cell hyperplasia has rarely been encountered in most strains of mice at the National Center for

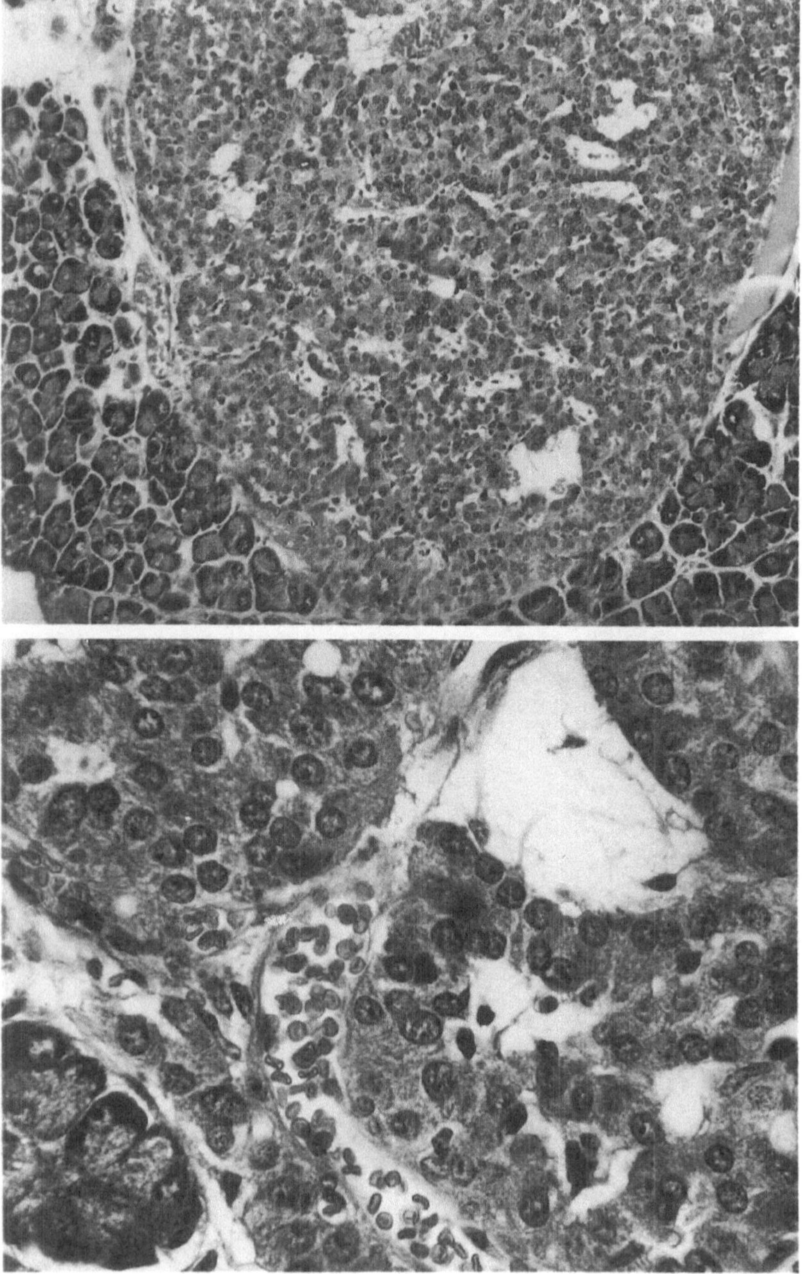

Fig. 399. (*above*) Adenoma, islet-cell, mouse. H&E, ×96

Fig. 400. (*below*) Adenoma, pancreatic islet cell, mouse. H&E, ×384

Toxicological Research (NCTR), and appears to be slightly more common in 12-month-old mice than in older mice. Islet-cell hyperplasia, however, is very common in the yellow (C3H × VY-A^{vy}) hybrid F-1 female (C3H/HeNIcrWf females × A^{vy}/A males), and occurs at an early age (Table 25). In one study at NCTR involving yellow (C3H × VY-A^{vy}) hybrid F-1 females, islet-cell hyperplasia was noted in over 90%. Many enlarged islets were often visible in each section of pancreas. The cells of the hyperplastic islets were morphologically similar to those of the normal

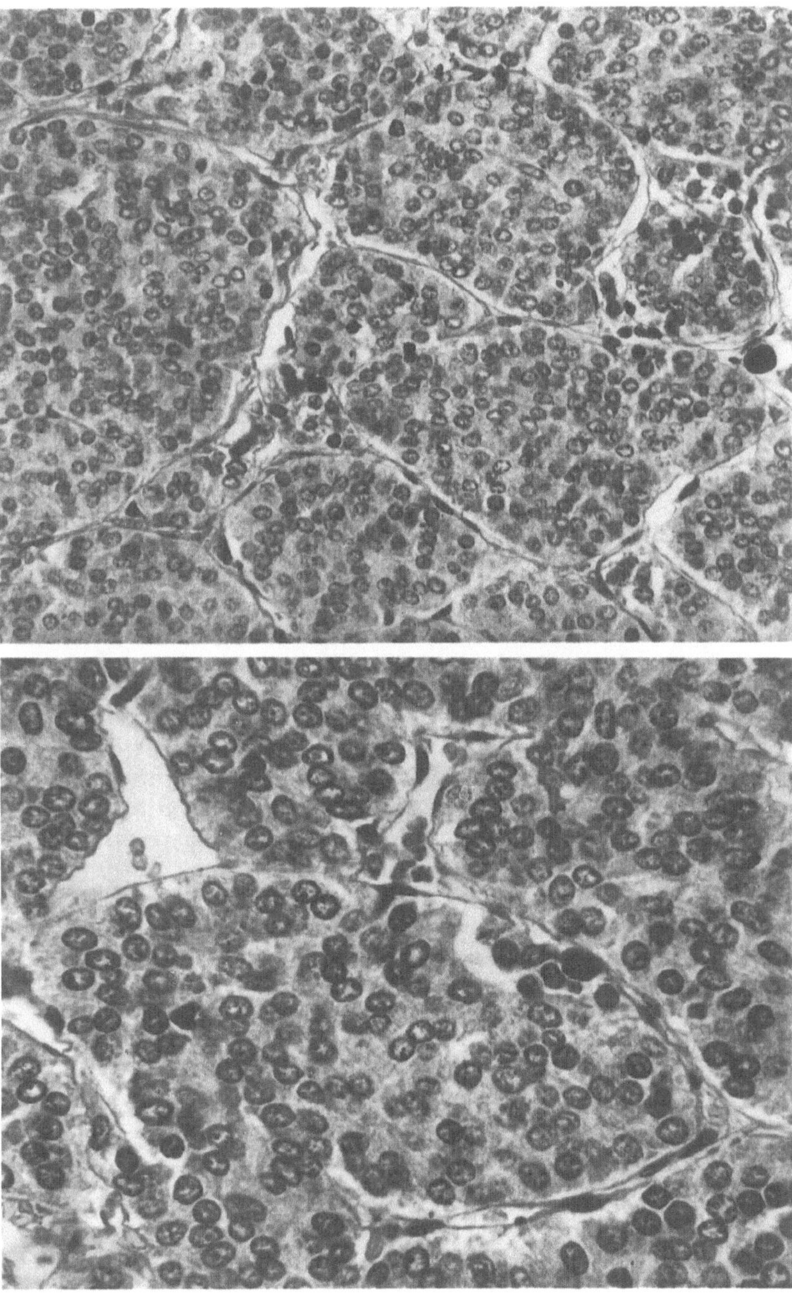

Fig. 401. (*above*) Carcinoma, islet cell, mouse. H&E, ×240

Fig. 402. (*below*) Carcinoma, islet cell, mouse; higher magnification of Fig. 401. H&E, ×384

islets except for their increase in number and size. The islets of almost 50% of these mice contained cystic degenerative changes, and the changes were more prevalent in the larger islets. The etiology and pathogenesis of this cystic degenerative change is not known. No clinical chemical tests were done on these mice, and it is not known if the islets were functional.

Islet-cell adenomas were much less frequent and seldom occurred before one year of age at NCTR (Table 26). Islet-cell carcinomas were rare in all strains and only five have been reported in the

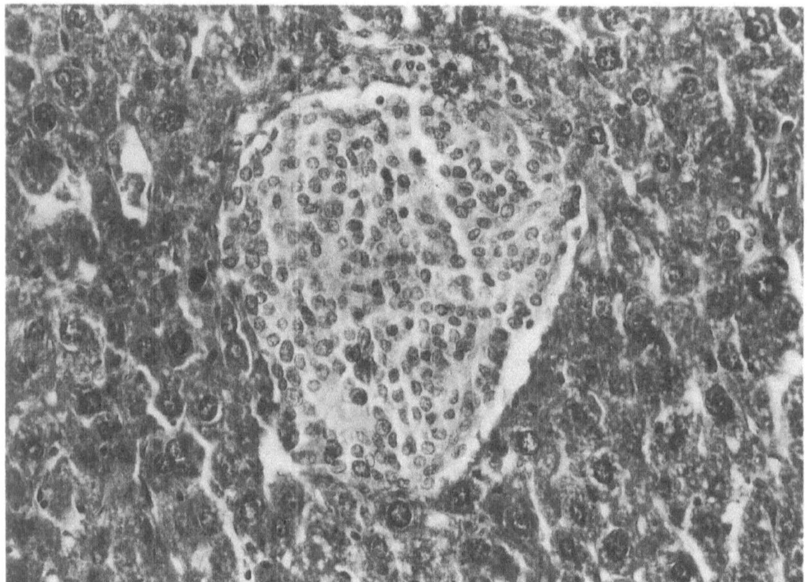

Fig. 403. Carcinoma, islet-cell, mouse, metastasis in liver. H&E, ×300

NCTR control data base to date. All mice with islet-cell carcinomas were older than 13 months of age (Table 27). Cardesa et al. (1979) stated that the only reliable criterion of malignancy in an islet-cell tumor is metastasis, since the histologic appearance can be misleading. Local invasion into the intestinal wall is also evidence of malignancy. At NCTR the diagnosis of carcinoma may be made without local invasion or metastasis if cytologic features suggestive of malignancy are present. These incluce plemorphism, anaplasia, and increased mitotic index.

Comparison with Other Species

Since the frequency of islet-cell tumors is relatively low in most mouse strains and only reported in isolated cases in the literature, it is difficult to compare them with other species. The identification of such strains as the F-1 yellow hybrid and the (C3H × I)F-1 hybrid with high frequencies of islet-cell hyperplasia and islet-cell tumors respectively provides a possible model for studying the lesions and comparing them with those occurring in humans.

Table 25. Spontaneous islet-cell hyperplasia in mice

Strain	Sex	Age (months)			
		≤6 (%)	7–12 (%)	13–18 (%)	>24 (%)
BALB/c	M	1/3368 (0.03)*	0/1120	3/767 (0.4)	3/720 (0.4)
BALB/c	F	1/3508 (0.03)	1/5360 (0.02)	1/13033 (0.01)	10/11025 (0.09)
C57BL/6	M	3/1415 (0.02)	44/1172 (3.8)	2/311 (0.6)	7/424 (1.7)
C57BL/6	F	0/999	0/370	1/387 (0.3)	6/386 (1.6)
F-1 hybrid	M	0/61	1/706 (0.1)	1/373 (0.3)	12/863 (1.4)
F-1 hybrid	F	0/40	0/716	2/466 (0.4)	7/771 (0.9)
Monohybrid	M	0/65	2/732 (0.3)	1/440 (0.2)	16/715 (2.2)
Monohybrid	F	0/22	0/729	0/518	5/683 (0.7)
C3H-MTV−	F	4/689 (0.6)	23/831 (2.8)	28/758 (3.7)	19/839 (2.3)
C3H-MTV+	F	10/3507 (0.3)	7/1290 (0.5)	0/15	ND
Yellow A^{vy}/A	F	7/7 (100)	356/394 (90.4)	ND	ND

F-1 hybrid, C57BL/6 females × BALB/c males; monohybrid, F-1 females × F-1 males; ND, no data.

Table 26. Spontaneous adenomas of islet cells in mice

Strain	Sex	Age (months)			
		≤6	7–12 (%)	13–18 (%)	>24 (%)
BALB/c	M	0/3368*	0/1120	0/767	1/720 (0.1)
BALB/c	F	0/3508	1/5360 (0.02)	4/13033 (0.03)	10/11025 (0.09)
C57BL/6	M	0/1415	1/1172 (0.09)	0/311	1/424 (0.2)
C57BL/6	F	0/999	0/370	1/387 (0.3)	0/386
F-1 hybrid	M	0/61	0/706	0/373	2/863 (0.2)
F-1 hybrid	F	0/40	0/716	0/466	3/771 (0.4)
Monohybrid	M	0/65	0/732	0/440	1/715 (0.1)
Monohybrid	F	0/22	0/729	1/518 (0.2)	1/683 (0.1)
C3H-MTV−	F	0/689	0/831	2/758 (0.3)	7/839 (0.8)
C3H-MTV+	F	0/3507	0/1290	0/15	ND
Yellow A^{vy}/A	F	0/7	0/394	ND	ND

F-1 hybrid, C57BL/6 females ×BALB/c males; monohybrid, F-1 females × F-1 males; ND, no data.

Table 27. Spontaneous carcinomas of islet cells in mice

Strain	Sex	Age (months)			
		≤6	7–12 (%)	13–18 (%)	≤24 (%)
BALB/c	M	0/3368	0/1120	0/767	0/720
BALB/c	F	0/3508	0/5360	0/13033	0/11025
C57BL/6	M	0/1415	0/1172	0/311	0/424
C57BL/6	F	0/999	0/370	0/387	0/386
F-1 hybrid	M	0/61	0/706	0/373	1/386 (0.1)
F-1 hybrid	F	0/40	0/716	0/466	0/771
Monohybrid	M	0/65	0/732	0/440	0/715
Monohybrid	F	0/22	0/729	0/518	0/683
C3H-MTV−	F	0/689	0/831	2/758 (0.3)	2/839 (0.2)
C3H-MTV+	F	0/3507	0/1290	0/15	ND
Yellow A^{vy}/A	F	0/7	0/394	ND	ND

F-1 hybrid, C57BL/6 females × BALB/c males; monohybrid, F-1 females × F-1 males; ND, no data.

References

Belkin M (1942) The lack of influence of di-(hydroxymethyl) peroxide on the incidence and growth of transplanted, induced and spontaneous mouse tumors. Cancer Res 2:264–279

Cardesa A, Bullon-Ramirez A, Levitt MH (1979) Tumours of the pancreas. In: Turosov VS (ed) Pathology of tumours in laboratory animals. Vol. II IARC Scientific Publications No. 23, Lyon, pp 235–241

Cloudman AM (1941) Spontaneous neoplasms in mice. In: Snell GD (ed) Biology of the laboratory mouse. Blakiston, Philadelphia, pp 168–233

Deringer MK (1951) Spontaneous and induced tumors in haried and hairless strain HR mice. JNCI 12:437–445

Deringer MK (1956) The effect of subcutaneous inoculation of 4-0-tolylazo-toluidine in strain HR mice. JNCI 17:533–539

Hueper WC (1936) Islet-cell adenoma in the pancreas of a mouse. Arch Pathol 22:220–221

Jones EE (1964) Spontaneous hyperplasia of the pancreatic islets associated with glucosuria in hybrid mice. In: Brolin SE (ed) The structure and metabolism of the pancreatic islets. Pergamon, New York, pp 189–191

Like AA, Steinke J, Jones EE, Cahill GF Jr (1965) Pancreatic studies in mice with spontaneous diabetes mellitus. Am J Pathol 46:621–644

Murphy ED (1966) Characteristic tumors. In: Biology of the laboratory mouse, 2nd edn. McGraw-Hill, New York, Chapter 17, pp 521–567

Rowlatt UF (1967) Pancreatic neoplasms of rats and mice. In: Cotchin E, Roe FJC (eds) Pathology of laboratory rats and mice. Blackwell Scientific, Oxford Edinburgh, pp 85–103

Sass B, Vernon ML, Peters RL, Kelloff GJ (1978) Mammary tumors, hepatocellular carcinomas, and pancreatic islet cell changes in C3H/A^{vy} mice. JNCI 60:611–621

Pancreatic Islet-Cell Hyperplasia, Golden Hamster

J.K. Frenkel

Synonym. Nesidioblastosis.

Gross Appearance

Enlarged islets of Langerhans may be visible grossly as clear, hyperemic, or hemorrhagic nodules 1–2 mm in diameter, embedded in opaque, gray acinar tissue.

Microscopic Features

Islets undergo varying degrees of enlargement with an increase in the number of cells. In some of the islet cells the nuclei appear polarized, and are arranged at the side of the cell opposite the capillary. Comori's aldehyde fuchsin stain indicates an increased number of beta cells with granules, which are generally situated next to the capillary. When the islets reach about twice normal size cystic spaces develop, arising from hydropic changes which lead to cytolysis. In still larger islets, the cystic spaces are often filled with extravasated red blood cells. Acinar cells surrounding the islets are compressed and atrophied, new acinar tissue sometimes arises from acinar ductules, and adjacent islets become confluent (Frenkel 1960, 1972; Figs. 404–406).

Ultrastructure

Studies with the electron microscope have not been done on this lesion.

Differential Diagnosis

Hyperplastic enlarged islets are diffusely distributed throughout the pancreas. Hemorrhage, if present, is associated with islets, and inflammation is negligible or absent. In acute hemorrhagic pancreatitis, hemorrhage is associated with acinar tissue and generally accompanied by necrosis and inflammation. Islet cell neoplasms have not been found in hamsters, but presumably would involve only one or two islets.

Biologic Features

Natural History. Islet-cell hyperplasia has not been seen in untreated hamsters, but slight-to-moderate islet-cell hyperplasia has been observed in hamsters treated with adrenocorticosteroids. Hyperplasia becomes pronounced after treatment with corticosteroids when chlorothiazide (a mild diuretic) is added. Chlorothiazide administered alone has no effect on islet size. If spontaneous islet-cell hyperplasia is found in animals, their diet and whatever drugs have been administered should be examined for possible diabetogenic effects.

Pathogenesis. Islet-cell hyperplasia appears to be a compensatory reaction to the diabetogenic effects of glucocorticosteroids, and an inhibitory effect of chlorothiazide on insulin activity in hypercorticoid hamsters.

Etiology. Islet-cell hyperplasia was found in hypercorticoid hamsters and was more pronounced in groups that had also been treated with chlorothiazide. Blood glucose levels were elevated in these two groups of hamsters. In acute tolerance tests, the administration of chlorothiazide, glucose, and epinephrine may be followed by highter blood glucose levels in hypercorticoid hamsters than in chlorothiazide-treated or normal hamsters. Exogenous insulin was effective in hypercorticoid hamsters treated with chlorothiazide, but its effect was shorter with higher cortisol doses. Tolbutamide (an orally active antidiabetic sulfonylurea compound) stimulated insulin release in hypercorticoid hamsters injected with chlorothiazide. The degrees of islet-cell hyperplasia and blood glucose elevations are proportional to the degree of hypercorticism and to the dose of clorothiazide added (Frenkel 1972).

The gluconeogenic effect of glucocorticoids on proteins is well known. Hyperglycemia and glycosuria are commonly associated with hypercorticism in many animal species (Hausberger and Ramsay 1953; Lazarus and Bencosme 1955; Conn 1958). Rare among animal species, however, is the capacity for islets of Langerhans to become markedly hyperplastic (Volk and Lazarus 1963),

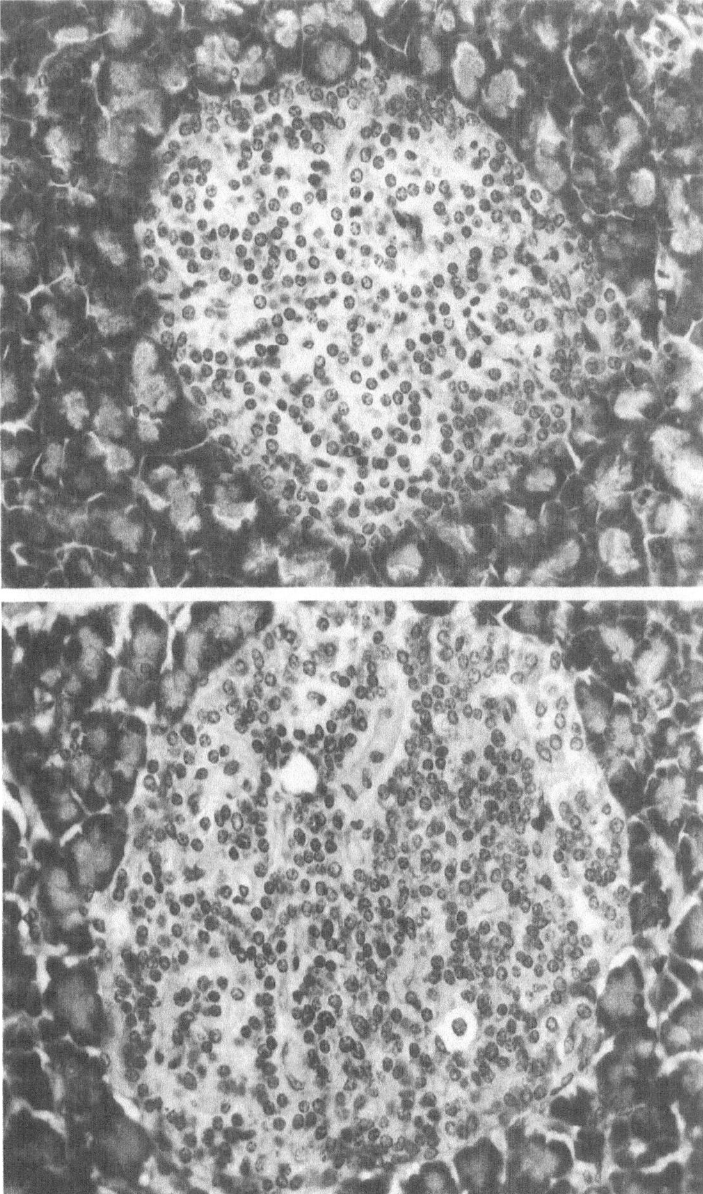

Fig. 404. Islet of Langerhans, untreated normal Golden hamster. Nuclei separated by unstained cytoplasm. Periodic acid–Schiff hematoxylin (PASH), ×320

Fig. 405. Islet of Langerhans, Golden hamster treated with cortisone acetate (10 mg/week for 33 days). Nuclei are more closely spaced and larger. PASH, ×320

and to compensate for the corticosteroid effects seen in golden hamsters. It is especially notable that the capacity for undergoing hyperplasia is maintained by beta cells of adult hamsters.

Chlorothiazide is known to give rise to carbohydrate intolerance in some patients, especially those with diabetes (Goldner et al. 1960; Runyan 1962). It appears to inhibit insulin release by beta cells; however, its hyperglycemic effect in pancreatectomized and alloxan treated diabetic rats indicates the participation of extrapancreatic mechanism (Staquet et al. 1965). While insulin receptor affinity was reduced in corticosteroid treated rats (Kahn et al. 1978), I have seen no data on the effects of chlorothiazide in rats or hamsters. The hyperglycemic effects of diazoxide, a related thiazide, has been attributed to suppression of insulin release (Fajans et al. 1968).

Whereas earlier studies compared the acute response of corticosteroid-treated, chlorothiazide-treated, or doubly treated hamsters with that of untreated hamsters (Frenkel 1972; Visser et al.

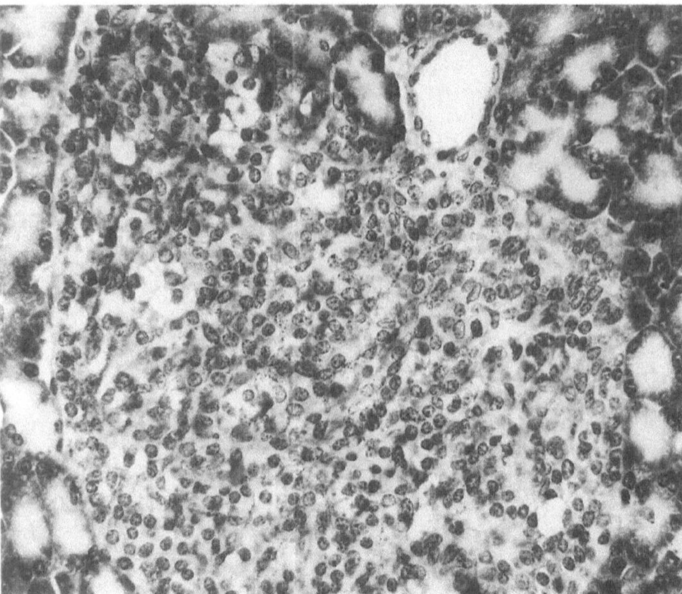

Fig. 406. Islet of Langerhans, Golden hamster given cortisone acetate (10 mg/week) and chlorothiazide (10 mg/day p.o.) for 34 days. Nuclei are closely spaced and larger. Active hyperplasia originates from ductule. PASH, ×320

1979), Tomita et al. (1984) have recently followed the dynamics of doubly treated hamsters for a period of 8 weeks. Serum glucose levels started at 123 mg/dl, increased to a maximum of 412 mg/dl after 2 weeks, fell to mild hyperglycemic levels (130–160 mg/dl) between 3 and 6 weeks, and then rose to about 200 mg/dl. Serum insulin levels started at 35 µg/ml, rose to 122 µg/ml after 1 week, and to 500 µg/ml after 3 weeks, remaining generally over 700 µg/ml for 4–8 weeks. Pancreatic insulin levels increased from 40 to 85 µg/g after 1 week, dropped to 30 µg/g after 2 weeks, rose to 100–150 µg/g between the 3rd and 5th weeks, falling again to 70–80 µg/g in the 6th–8th weeks. Using the normal islet cell area as one unit as measured by an MOP-3 (Carl Zeiss), it increased six- to eightfold after 2–4 weeks, 28-fold after 5 weeks, and 15- to 20-fold between the 6th and 8th weeks. These data indicate that following maximal hyperglycemia after 2 weeks, the compensatory hyperplasia of beta calls mitigated diabetes successfully for 5 weeks. Coincident with the appearance of hydropic changes and necrosis of beta cells at 6 weeks, pancreatic insulin levels decreased, blood insulin levels fluctuated, and glucose levels started to rise again.

The authors conclude that the relatively short time course of islet cell hyperplasia and necrosis in hamsters may provide an excellent model for the study of islet cell regeneration and degeneration in the experimentally induced diabetic syndrome, and as a model for the type 2 or adult-onset diabetes in humans who present glucose intolerance and relative insulin hypersecretion because of resistance to insulin at the target organs.

Comparison with Other Species

Hyperglycemic effects of administration of glucocorticosteroids and chlorothiazides have been observed in animals and man. "Steroid diabetes" was studied in guinea pigs (Hausberger and Ramsay 1953), rabbits (Lazarus and Bencosme 1955; Volk and Lazarus 1963), and in humans (Conn 1958). The hyperglycemic effects of chlorothiazides were studied mainly in humans with diabetes (Goldner et al. 1960; Runyan 1962). This was complemented by studies of the related thiazide and diazoxide in several animals (Tabachnik and Gulbenkian 1968).

Golden hamsters appear uniquely able to respond with significant islet-cell hyperplasia even as adults. Rats, mice, dogs, and rabbits are capable of only limited islet-cell hyperplasia after corticosteroid loading (Volk and Lazarus 1963). Humans appear to be similar in this respect, with islet hypertrophy seen principally in babies born to diabetic mothers (Potter et al. 1941). Review of sections of the pancreas of several adult patients treated with corticosteroids and chlorothiazide prior to and during their final illness only rarely revealed islets with increased diameters.

Of collateral interest is the spontaneous tendency of Chinese hamsters to develop diabetes (Meier and Yerganian 1959); slight islet hypertrophy precedes development of diabetes in Chinese hamsters (Carpenter et al. 1967).

References

Carpenter AM, Gerritsen GC, Dulin WE, Lazarow A (1967) Islet and beta cell volumes in diabetic Chinese hamsters and their nondiabetic siblings. Diabetologia 3:92–96

Conn JW (1958) Prediabetic state in man: definition, interpretation and implications. Diabetes 7:347–357

Fajans SS, Floyd JC, Thiffault CA, Knopf RF, Harrison TS, Conn JW (1968) Further studies on diazoxide suppression of insulin release from abnormal and normal islet tissue in man. Ann N Y Acad Sci 150:261–280

Frenkel JK (1960) Pancreatic islet cell hyperplasia in hamsters treated with cortisone and chlorothiazide (Diuril). Fed Proc 19:160

Frenkel JK (1972) Dissecting aneurysms of the aorta, and pancreatic islet cell hyperplasia with diabetes in corticosteroid and chlorothiazide-treated hamsters. Prog Exp Tumor Res 16:300–324

Goldner MG, Zarowitz H, Akgun S (1960) Hyperglycemia and glycosuria due to thiazide derivatives administered in diabetes mellitus. N Engl J Med 262:403–405

Hausberger FX, Ramsay AJ (1953) Steroid diabetes in guinea pigs: effects of cortisone administration on blood and urinary glucose, nitrogen excretion, fat depositon, and islets of Langerhans. Endocrinology 53:423–435

Kahn CR, Goldfine ID, Neville DM Jr, DeMeyts P (1978) Alterations in insulin binding induced by changes in vivo in the levels of glucocorticoids and growth hormone. Endocrinology 103:1054–1066

Lazarus SS, Bencosme SA (1955) Alterations of pancreas during cortisone diabetes in rabbit. Proc Soc Exp Biol Med 89:114–118

Meier H, Yerganian GA (1959) Spontaneous hereditary diabetes mellitus in Chinese hamster (*Cricetulus griseus*). I. Pathological findings. Proc Soc Exp Biol Med 100:810–815

Potter EL, Seckel HPG, Stryker WA (1941) Hypertrophy and hyperplasia of the islets of Langerhans of the fetus and of the newborn infant. Arch Pathol 31:467–482

Runyan JW Jr (1962) Influence of thiazide diuretics on carbohydrate metabolism in patients with mild diabetes. N Engl J Med 267:541–543

Staquet MJ, Nabwangu J, Wolff F (1965) The effect of thiazides on the blood sugar of alloxanized and suballoxanized rats. Metabolism 14:1307–1310

Tabachnick IIA, Gulbenkian A (1968) Mechanism of diazoxide hyperglycemia in animals. Ann N Y Acad Sci 150:204–218

Tomita T, Visser P, Friesen S, Doull V (1984) Cortisone induced islet cell hyperplasia in hamsters. Virchows Arch [B] 45:85–95

Visser PA, Pierce GE, Tomita T, Friesen SR (1979) Stimulation of pancreatic islet hypertrophy and beta cell hyperplasia in Syrian hamsters. Surg Forum 30:310–311

Volk BW, Lazarus SS (1963) Ultramicroscopic studies of rabbit pancreas during cortisone treatment. Diabetes 12: 162–173

Adenoma and Carcinoma, Pancreatic Islets, Rat

James E. Heath

Synonyms. Islet cell adenoma; islet cell carcinoma; islet cell tumor, benign and malignant; pancreatic endocrine tumor, benign and malignant; insulinoma; gastrinoma; apudoma; alpha cell tumor; beta cell tumor.

Gross Appearance

Adenomas of the pancreatic islets may not be visible grossly, or they may occur as pale to reddish, usually spherical nodules 3–5 mm or more in diameter within the pancreas. Carcinomas may appear grossly as round or irregular flesh-colored to dark red nodules up to 10 mm or more in diameter. Larger and more aggressive carcinomas on rare occasions may present as diffusely infiltrative masses which involve the duodenum or other abdominal organs.

Microscopic Features

Adenomas are composed of round cells with pale, eosinophilic cytoplasm and round to ovoid nuclei that resemble the cells of normal islets, and the smaller tumors may be difficult to distinguish from islet cell hyperplasia. Adenomas usually

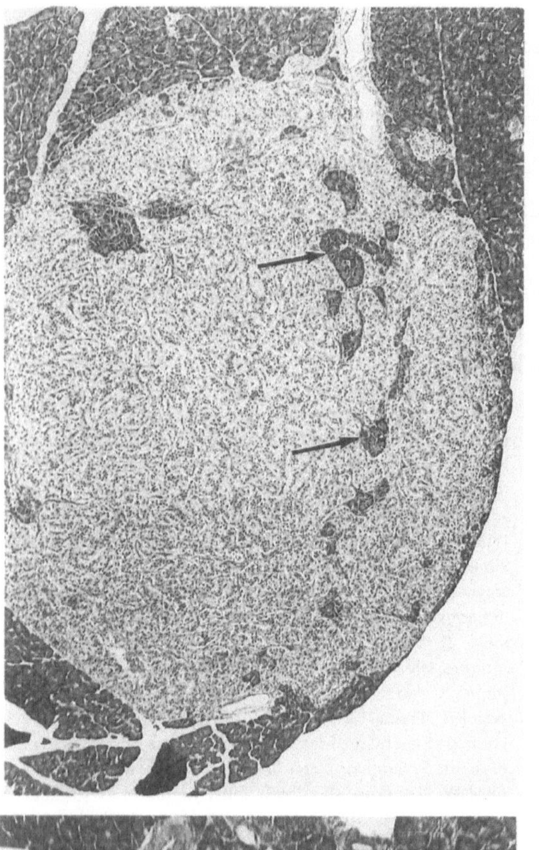

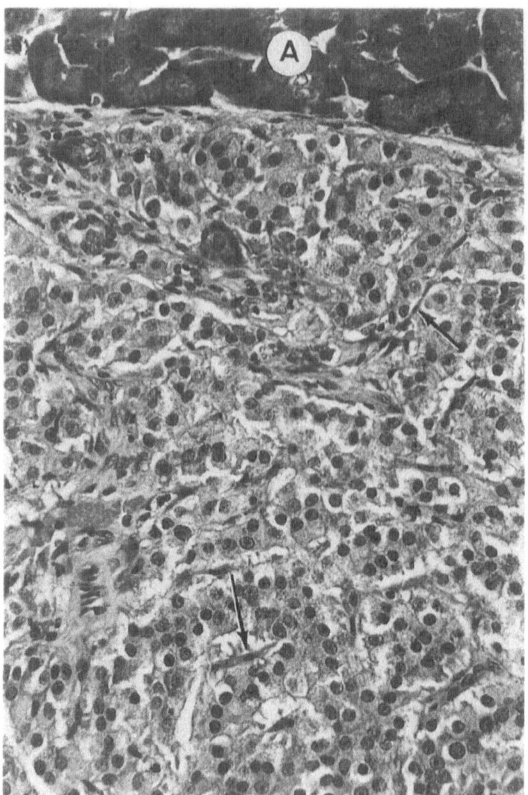

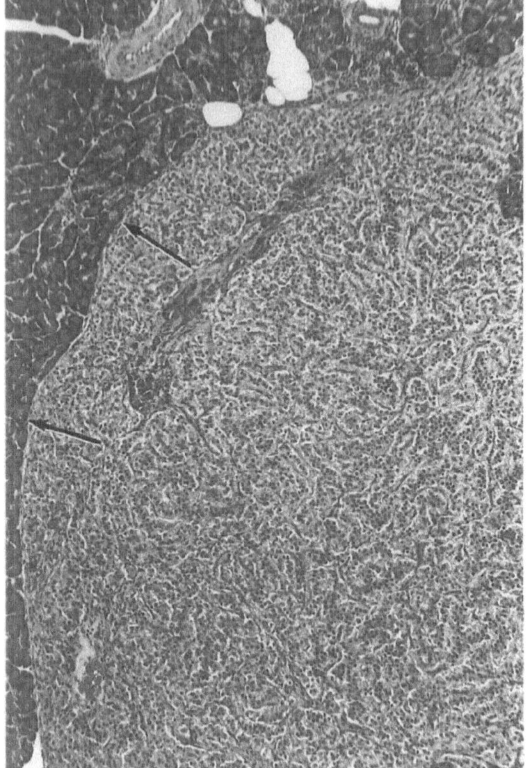

Fig. 407. (*upper left*) Islet cell adenoma, rat, with characteristic, well circumscribed appearance. Islands of acinar tissue (*arrows*) are entrapped among the neoplastic islet cells. H&E, ×40

Fig. 408. (*lower left*) Islet cell adenoma, rat, with compression of adjacent acinar tissue (*arrows*). H&E, ×63

Fig. 409. (*upper right*) Islet cell adenoma, rat, with cords of neoplastic cells separated by thin fibrovascular septa (*arrows*). The tumor abuts the adjacent acinar tissue (*A*). H&E, ×250

consist of a single, well-circumscribed aggregate of islet cells at least three or four times the size of normal islets and which often compress the adjacent pancreatic acinar tissue and may be bordered by a fibrous capsule (Figs. 407, 408). The cells comprising the nodule are usually slightly larger than those of the normal islets and are arranged in cords two to several cell layers thick which are separated by fibrovascular septa (Fig. 409). Occasional mitotic figures may be present. Islands of entrapped acinar tissue often occur among the neoplastic islet cells, and rarely a combination of neoplastic endocrine and acinar elements is seen within a mass (Figs. 410, 411). All of these mixed endocrine-exocrine tumors seen by the present author have been benign. In contrast to adenomas, islet cell hyperplasia usually exists as multiple, enlarged, often confluent islets two or three times normal size. The individual cells comprising the hyperplastic islets are occasionally hypertrophied, but they are arranged in random fashion rather than in cords along blood sinusoids, as usually occurs in adenomas. Islet cell hyperplasia in aging rats often occurs in conjunction with atrophy and fibrosis of the adjacent acinar tissue.

Islet cell carcinomas vary considerably in appearance (Figs. 412–415). The more differentiated tumors appear similar to adenomas and are made up of cells easily recognizable by individual morphology and architecture as being of islet cell origin but contain areas of atypia that indicate transformation to carcinoma. The degree of anaplasia is not always a good indicator of the infiltrative character and aggressiveness of islet cell tumors in that some neoplasms which are morphologically similar to adenomas invade surrounding tissue. The cells of the more anaplastic carcinomas differ from those of adenomas in having larger and more pleomorphic nuclei, and mitotic figures may be frequent. The orderly, cordlike arrangement of cells observed in adenoma is diminished or lost, and palisading of cells and pseudorosette formations may be present. The tumor cells may be densely packed in solid sheets,

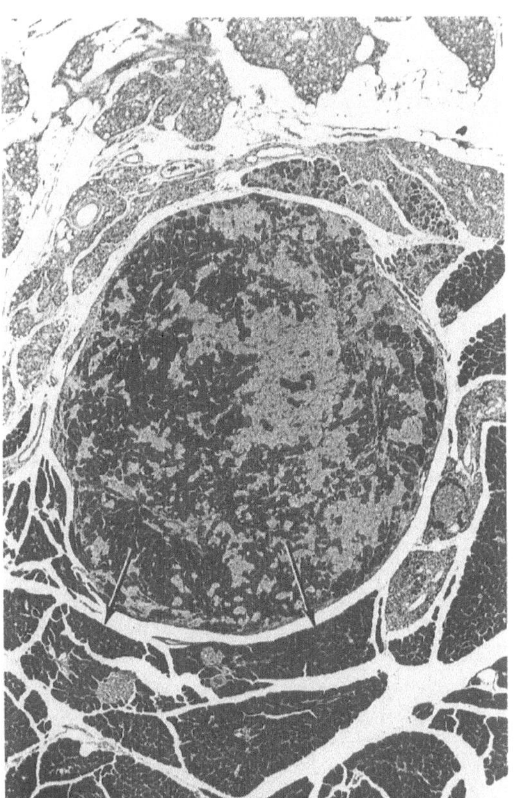

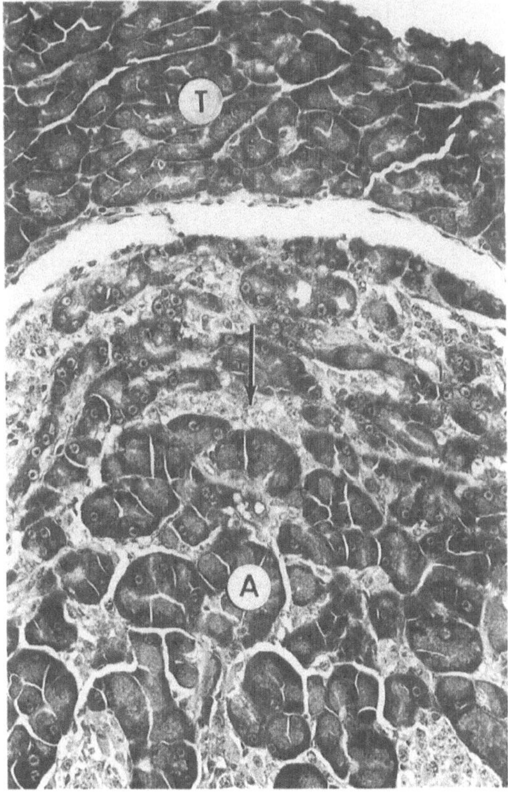

Fig. 410. (*above*) Mixed pancreatic tumor, rat, containing both islet and acinar elements with compression of adjacent nonneoplastic acinar tissue (*arrows*). H&E ×40

Fig. 411. (*below*) Mixed pancreatic tumor, rat, containing both acinar (*A*) and islet cells (arrow) and bordering nonneoplastic acinar tissue (*T*). H&E, ×200

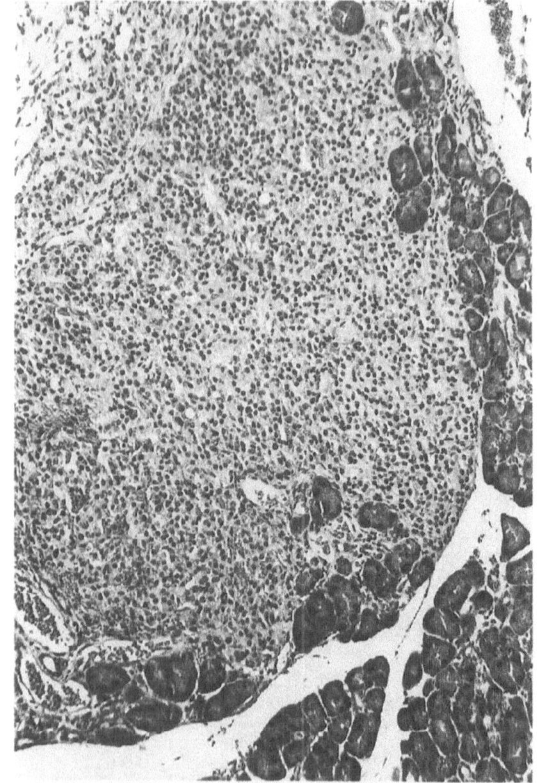

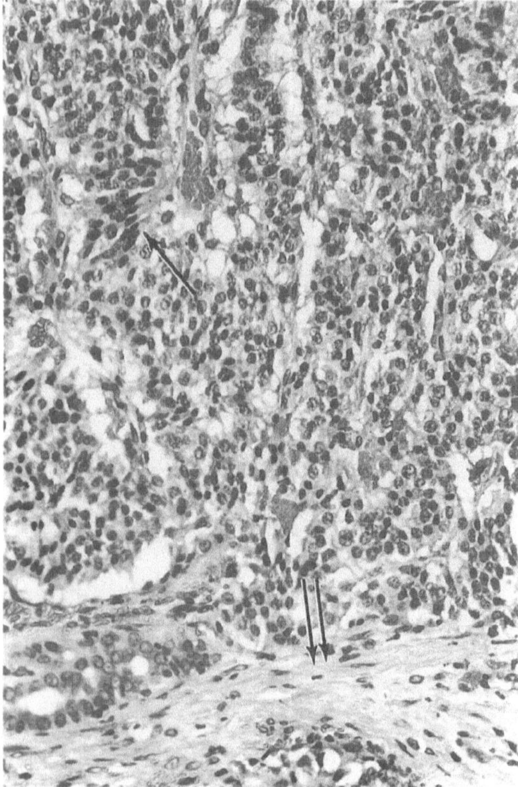

often with little or no resemblance to islet architecture. Variable vascularization, necrosis, and/or sclerosis are commonly present within the larger neoplasms. There is usually at least some infiltration into the adjoining acinar tissue, and the more aggressive tumors may result in obliteration of the acinar pancreas with invasion of the small intestine, stomach, regional lymph nodes, and other abdominal tissues. The more highly undifferentiated carcinomas may assume a mesenchymal appearance and contain fusiform cells with or without a scirrhous reaction. Metastasis to lung or liver occurs in rare cases (Figs. 416, 417).

Ultrastructure

Spontaneously occurring pancreatic islet cell tumors in Fischer 344 rats were evaluated with electron microscopy, and two types of islet cells were recognized (Stromberg et al. 1983). One type had numerous electron-dense secretory granules while the other cell type had fewer electron-dense granules but more mitochondria. In another report a transplantable insulinoma, the original tumor having been induced by total body X-irradiation, was composed of cells with increased quantities of endoplasmic reticulum and secretory granules indistinguishable from non-neoplastic β cells (Chick et al. 1977). A mixed ductal-squamous-islet cell carcinoma induced in a Fischer 344 rat with tobacco-specific carcinogen revealed endocrine cells with electron-dense granules of heterogenous shape, a large number of mitochondria, and cytoplasmic vacuoles possibly representing lipid inclusions (Pour and Rivenson 1989). In all three of these reports the tumor cells were shown with immunocytochemical methods to be predominantly or exclusively β cells.

Differential Diagnosis

Islet cell adenomas must be differentiated from islet cell hyperplasia and islet cell carcinomas;

Fig. 412. (*above*) Islet cell carcinoma, rat. Note the infiltration of adjacent exocrine pancreas. H&E, ×100

Fig. 413. (*below*) Islet cell carcinoma, rat, with fibroplasia (*double arrow*) and cellular atypia including palisading (*single arrow*). H&E, ×200

distinguishing features of these entities are discussed above. An additional diagnostic aid in separating islet cell hyperplasia from adenoma is the distribution of cell types within the proliferative lesion by means of immunocytochemistry (Spencer et al. 1986). In contrast to hyperplastic islets, in which most of the glucagon-containing cells are concentrated near the periphery of the nodule, glucagon-containing cells when present in islet cell adenomas are scattered haphazardly throughout the mass.

The two neoplasms most likely to require differentiation from islet cell carcinoma are undifferentiated pancreatic acinar cell carcinoma and malignant carcinoid. Although some acinar cell carcinomas of the rat are very anaplastic and show marked cellular atypia including mesenchymal differentiation, areas can usually be found which contain cells showing a transition from the more typical exocrine morphology. Identification of islet cell tumors might also be aided by the use of electron microscopy or immunocytochemistry to demonstrate cytoplasmic neurosecretory granules. Carcinoid tumors are extremely rare in rats and when present, usually originate in the stomach. Carcinoids and islet cell tumors both arise from cells of the neuroendocrine system and could be expected to have similar light and electron-microscopic morphologies and perhaps common immunohistochemical characteristics. Differentiation could be difficult with a large, aggressive neoplasm for which the site of origin has been obscured.

Biologic Features

Natural History and Pathogenesis. The cells that comprise the pancreatic islets are part of the dispersed neuroendocrine or amine precursor uptake and decarboxylation system (DeLellis and Wolfe 1981). Also included in this system are the thyroid gland C cells, cutaneous Merkel's cells, and adrenal medullary cells as well as neuroendocrine tissue within the lung, liver, thymus, and gastrointestinal tract. The neuroendocrine cells,

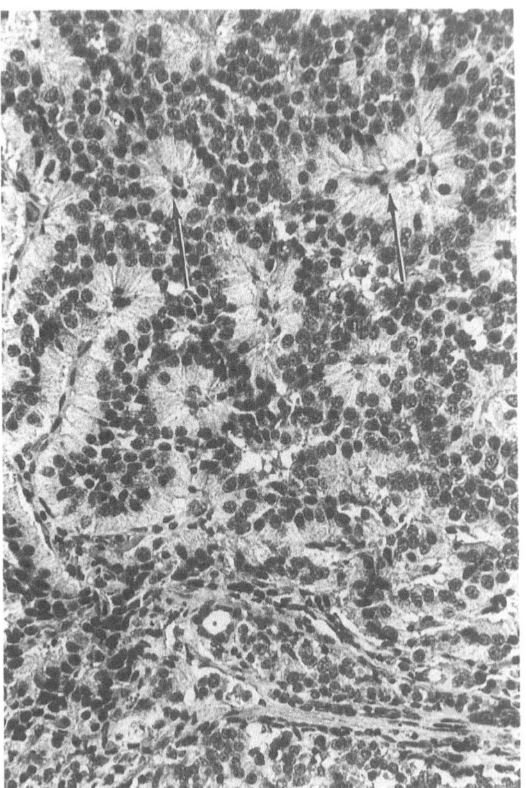

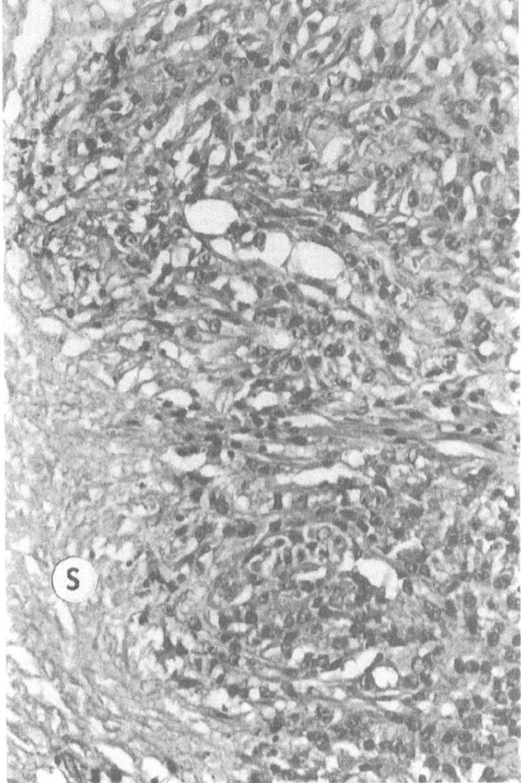

Fig. 414. (*above*) Islet cell carcinoma, rat, containing pseudorosette formations (*arrows*). H&E, ×200

Fig. 415. (*below*) Islet cell carcinoma, rat, with mesenchymal differentiation and sclerosis (*S*). H&E, ×250

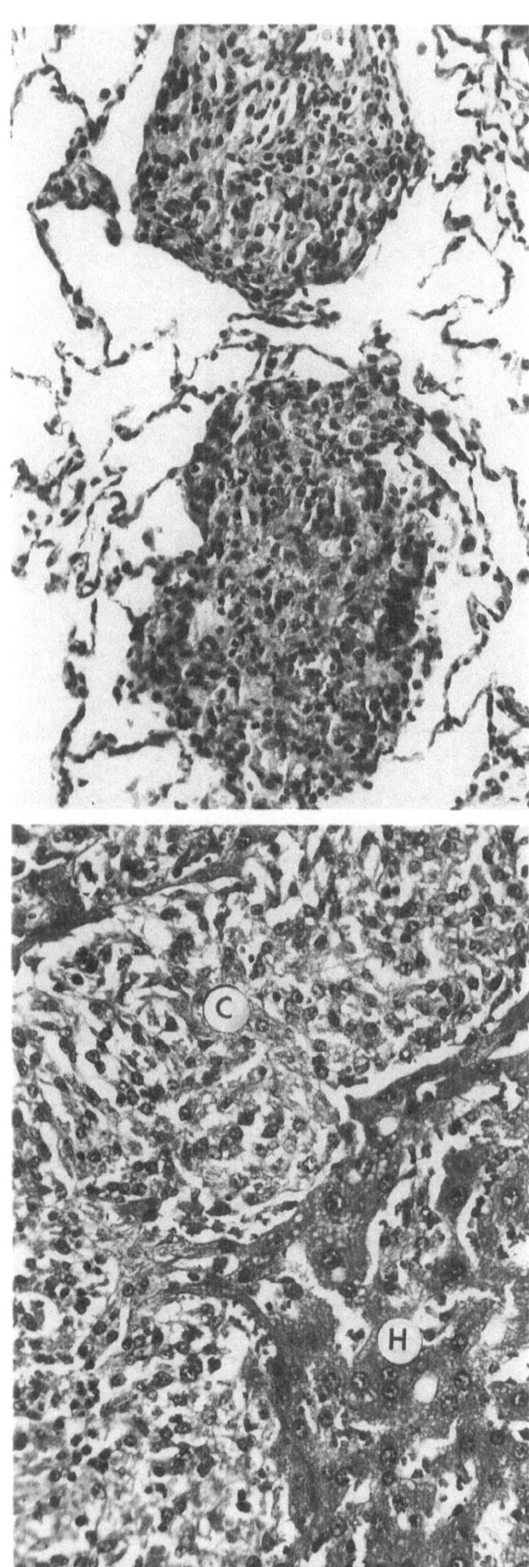

regardless of location, are capable of synthesis and secretion of a variety of polypeptide hormones which are responsible for the normal function of a variety of metabolic processes. Hyperplasia or neoplasia of any of the dispersed endocrine cell types may result in polypeptide hormone excess with the potential for adverse clinical effects. Many islet cell neoplasms in human beings are multihormonal, and immunohistochemical staining has demonstrated the presence of insulin, glucagon, somatostatin, and gastrin within the same tumor. Islet cell tumors in rats are composed primarily of β cells, although scattered α and δ cells may occur (Stromberg et al. 1983; Longnecker and Wilson 1991). Spontaneously occurring islet cell neoplasms in aging Sprague-Dawley and Long-Evans rats were composed principally of insulin-containing β cells but had additional and variable small proportions of cells that stained immunohistochemically for somatostatin, glucagon, or, rarely, pancreatic polypeptide (Spencer et al. 1986). Although clinical signs and altered clinical pathology values resulting from these tumors are not widely recognized in rodents, weight loss and hypoglycemia due to insulin excess have been reported in rats with transplanted insulinoma (Chick et al. 1977). Weight loss and cachexia in F344 rats with spontaneous islet cell adenomas have been observed by the author at the Southern Research Institute, although blood glucose levels were not measured.

Etiology. Islet cell tumors have been induced in rats using a variety of xenobiotics. Two agents widely used in endocrine pancreatic research, streptozotocin and alloxan, cause islet cell tumors after approximately 7 months administration (Longnecker and Wilson 1991). Other chemicals known to induce islet cell neoplasms include heliotrine, azinophosmethyl, 6-diethylamino-methyl-4-hydroxyaminoquinoline 1-oxide, and pyrrolizidine alkaloids (Hayashi et al. 1972; Longnecker and Wilson 1991; Schoental et al. 1970). A mixed ductal-squamous-islet cell carcinoma occurred in a F344 rat following long term administration of tobacco-specific N-nitrosamines

Fig. 416. (*above*) Metastasis to lung of islet cell carcinoma, rat. H&E, ×250

Fig. 417. (*below*) Liver metastasis of islet cell carcinoma. Bundles of neoplastic islet cells (*C*) are infiltrating the hepatocytes (*H*). H&E, ×250

Table 28. Incidences of spontaneous islet-cell tumors in various rat strains

Strain	Sex	Experimental Period (Weeks)	Incidence		Reference
			Adenoma	Carcinoma	
Wistar	Male	Life span	16/553 (2.9)	1/553 (0.2)	Gilbert et al. 1958
	Female	Life span	6/542 (1.1)	0/542 (0.0)	
BN/Bi	Male	Life span	11/74 (14.8)	0/74 (0.0)	Burek 1978
	Female	Life span	25/236 (10.6)	0/236 (0.0)	
WAG/Rij	Male	Life span	1/124 (0.8)	0/124 (0.0)	Burek 1978
	Female	Life span	3/101 (3.0)	0/101 (0.0)	
F344	Male	0–104	59/1868 (3.2)	39/1868 (2.1)	Haseman et al. 1990
	Female	0–104	19/1934 (1.0)	5/1934 (0.3)	
Sprague-Dawley	Male	0–104	44/583 (7.5)	11/583 (1.9)	McMartin et al. 1992
	Female	0–104	23/585 (3.9)	6/585 (1.0)	

in the drinking water (Pour and Rivenson 1989). Islet cell tumors can also be induced in rats using X-irradiation (Berdjis 1963; Chick et al. 1977).

Frequency. Spontaneous islet cell neoplasms are relatively infrequent in rats, and they occur more commonly in male rats of most strains than in females (Table 28). The incidence is somewhat higher for Sprague-Dawley than for Fischer 344 rats, two strains used extensively in safety and carcinogenicity assays. The incidence appears to increase with age; in a study with BN/Bi rats allowed to live out their life span, the mean age of rats with islet cell tumors was 132 weeks for both sexes (Burek 1978). Adenomas occur more frequently than carcinomas in both sexes for all strains for which incidence data are available.

Comparison with Other Species

Islet cell tumors are rare in most strains of mice commonly used in safety and carcinogenicity studies, but islet cell hyperplasia and/or neoplasia occur quite frequently in some strains of genetically obese mice (Jones 1964; Sass et al. 1978). Islet cell tumors are infrequently reported in hamsters, guinea pigs, cats, horses, cattle, swine, sheep, and nonhuman primates (Strandberg 1987; Seibold and Wolf 1973; Jones and Hunt 1983). They are also considered uncommon in dogs, occurring most often in older animals, and there is no sex predilection (Hawkins et al. 1987). Pancreatic endocrine tumors in dogs have most often been associated with insulin excess and hypoglycemia, although some tumors have resulted in gastrin secretion and a Zollinger-Ellison type of syndrome (Caywood et al. 1979; Drazner 1981). Unlike the situation with rats, islet cell carcinomas are more common than adenomas in dogs, and signs of hyperinsulinism are more likely to occur with carcinomas than with adenomas (Capen and Martin 1969; Njoku et al. 1972).

Islet cell tumors are considered rare in human beings and, as in rats, are more likely to be adenomas than carcinomas (Noltenius 1988). The tumors are known to result in hypersecretion of a variety of polypeptide hormones with diverse clinical consequences, although many are nonfunctional or poorly functional and clinically silent (Friesen 1982; Robbins et al. 1984). Functional neoplasms in man, as in rats, are most frequently β cell tumors. Frequency of occurrence for islet cell tumors is similar in men and women, and they occur most commonly in older individuals (4th to 7th decades). In contrast to the case with rats, where they are unreported in very young animals, islet cell neoplasms in humans have been observed in individuals of all ages, including newborns (Noltenius 1988).

References

Berdjis CC (1963) Protracted effects of repeated doses of X-ray irradiation in rats. Exp Mol Pathol 2:157–172

Burek JD (1978) Pathology of aging rats. CRC Press, West Palm Beach, pp 54–58

Capen CC, Martin SL (1969) Hyperinsulinism in dogs with neoplasia of the pancreatic islets: a clinical, pathologic, and ultrastructural study. Pathol Vet 6(4):309–341

Caywood DD, Wilson JW, Hardy RM, Shull RM (1979) Pancreatic islet cell adenocarcinoma: clinical and diagnostic features of six cases. J Am Vet Med Assoc 174:714–717

Chick WL, Warren S, Chute RN, Like AA, Lauris V, Kitchen KC (1977) A transplantable insulinoma in a rat. Proc Natl Acad Sci USA 74(2):628–632

DeLellis RA, Wolfe HJ (1981) The polypeptide hormone-producing cells and their tumors: an immunohistochemical analysis. Methods Achiev Exp Pathol 10:190–220

Drazner FH (1981) Canine gastrinoma: a condition analogous to the Zollinger-Ellison syndrome in man. Calif Vet 11: 6–11

Friesen SR (1982) Tumors of the endocrine pancreas. N Engl J Med 306:580–590

Gilbert C, Gillman J (1958) Spontaneous neoplasms in the albino rat. S Afr J Med Sci 23:257–272

Haseman JK, Arnold J, Eustis SL (1990) Tumor incidences in Fischer 344 rats: NTP historical data. In: Boorman GA, Eustis SL, Elwell MR, Montgomery CA, McKenzie WF (eds) Pathology of the Fischer rat: reference and atlas. Academic, San Diego, pp 555–564

Hawkins KL, Summers BA, Kuhajda FP, Smith CA (1987) Immunocytochemistry of normal pancreatic islets and spontaneous islet cell tumors in dogs. Vet Pathol 24:170–177

Hayashi Y, Furukawa H, Hasegawa T (1972) Pancreatic tumors in rats induced by 4-nitroquinoline 1-oxide. In: Nakahara W, Takayama S, Sugimura T, Odashima S (eds) Topics in chemical carcinogenesis. University Park Press, Baltimore, pp 53–72

Jones EE (1964) Spontaneous hyperplasia of the pancreatic islets associated with glucosuria in hybrid mice. Wenner Gren Cent Int Symp Ser 3:189–191

Jones TC, Hunt RD (1983) Veterinary pathology, 5th edn. Lea and Febiger, Philadelphia, pp 1633–1635

Longnecker DS, Wilson GL (1991) Pancreas. In: Haschek WM, Rousseaux CG (eds) Handbook of toxicologic pathology. Academic, San Diego, pp 253–278

McMartin DN, Sahota PS, Gunson DE, Hsu HH, Spaet RH (1992) Neoplasms and related proliferative lesions in control Sprague-Dawley rats from carcinogenicity studies. Historical data and diagnostic considerations. Toxicol Pathol 20(2): 212–225

Njoku CO, Strafuss AC, Dennis SM (1972) Canine islet cell neoplasia: a review. J Am Anim Hosp Assoc 8:284–290

Noltenius H (1988) Human oncology. Pathology and clinical characteristics, 2nd edition, vol I. Urban and Schwarzenberg, Baltimore, pp 425–449

Pour PM, Rivenson A (1989) Induction of a mixed ductal-squamous-islet cell carcinoma in a rat treated with a tobacco-specific carcinogen. Am J Pathol 134(3):627–631

Robbins SL, Cotran RS, Kumar V (1984) Pathologic basis of disease, 3rd edn. Saunders, Philadelphia, pp 986–989

Sass B, Vernon ML, Peters RL, Kelloff GJ (1978) Mammary tumors, hepatocellular carcinomas and pancreatic islet changes in C3H-A^{vy} mice. J Natl Cancer Inst 60:611–621

Schoental R, Fowler ME, Coady A (1970) Islet cell tumors of the pancreas found in rats given pyrrolizidine alkaloids from Amsinckia intermedia Fisch and Mey and from Heliotropium supinum L. Cancer Res 30:2127–2131

Seibold HR, Wolf RH (1973) Neoplasms and proliferative lesions in 1065 nonhuman primate necropsies. Lab Anim Sci 23:533–539

Spencer AJ, Andreu M, Greaves P (1986) Neoplasia and hyperplasia of pancreatic endocrine tissue in the rat: an immunocytochemical study. Vet Pathol 23:11–15

Strandberg JD (1987) Neoplastic diseases. In: Van Hoosier GL, McPherson CW (eds) Laboratory hamsters. Academic, Orlando, pp 157–168

Stromberg PC, Wilson F, Capen CC (1983) Immunocytochemical demonstration of insulin in spontaneous pancreatic islet cell tumors of Fischer rats. Vet Pathol 20:291–297

Adrenals

Embryology, Adrenal Gland, Mouse

Bernard Sass

Knowledge concerning the embryogenesis of the adrenal is essential to the correct interpretation of the pathologic processes which affect this gland. The following review is offered to augment the few reports in the literature on the adrenal of the mouse (Waring 1935; Politzer 1936; McPhail and Read 1942; Rugh 1968; Fernholm 1971; Theiler and Müntener 1974). The most detailed studies are those of Theiler and Müntener (1974), who examined embryos of C57BL/6 and CBA mice. The embryos ranged in age from 10.5 days post gestation to birth; the specimens were serially sectioned. Theiler (1972) also reported on the embryogenesis of other organs of the laboratory mouse based on studies in which serial sectioning techniques were used. In his study, embryogenesis of the adrenal gland cortex and medulla were discussed in relation to the embryogenesis of the other organs.

Adrenal Gland Cortex

The period from conception to birth of the mouse ranges from 18 to 21 days, but the mean gestation period of C57BL/6 mice is 19 days (Snell 1966). The analge of the cortex first forms on the 11th day, appearing as an area of budding of the coelomic epithelium, located between the mesogastrium and urogenital fold. This bud has been termed the "anterior splanchnic plate" (Green 1967). Using closely spaced serial sections, Theiler and Müntener (1974) observed that the connection between the adrenal cortical anlage and the coelomic epithelium is lost early, as the anlage pushes the urogenital ridge forward. Based on these findings, they concluded that the cortical cells complete their migration within a few hours. Having observed that mesenchymal cells with a high mitotic rate are located just beneath the coelomic epithelium, these workers postulated that such cells could also convert directly to cortical cells. At this stage the cortical cells appear as a population of dark cells arising medial to the developing gonad. The cortical anlage is then pushed dorsally to lie between the mesonephros and the aorta. In the 12-day mouse embryo, the pale adrenal cortical cells are in close proximity to the dark-staining sympathoblasts. The adrenal gland connective tissue begins when branches of veins bud to form fields.

Gonocytes, the precursor cells of the sexually neutral gonad, are identifiable by means of the alkaline phosphatase stain. They may be found both within the adrenal cortical anlage and in the gonad up to the 13th day (Figs. 418, 419). After the 13th day of intrauterine life, these cells have disappeared from the adrenal cortex (Theiler and Müntener 1974).

In the 13-day embryo, the cortical anlage has enlarged and contains single capillaries. By this time the anlage's contact with coelomic epithelium has been in great part lost and is difficult to distinguish from the medulla.

In the 14-day embryo, the cortex is arranged as a meshwork subdivided by capillaries. The capsular anlage now surrounds the largest part of the organ. The outer surface of the cortex contains only a few undifferentiated cells, whereas the cortex proper has a wide zone of small undifferentiated cells.

On the 15th day, the cortical cells are much larger than the medullary cells. The cells of the peripheral cortex stain less intensely and are smaller than the more deeply located cells, and the capsule is now more prominent.

From the 16th day until birth no further changes occur in the cortex. According to Dunn (1970) the "x-cell zone," located between the cortex and medulla, is made up of a layer of small cells. This x-cell zone regresses in males at sexual maturity

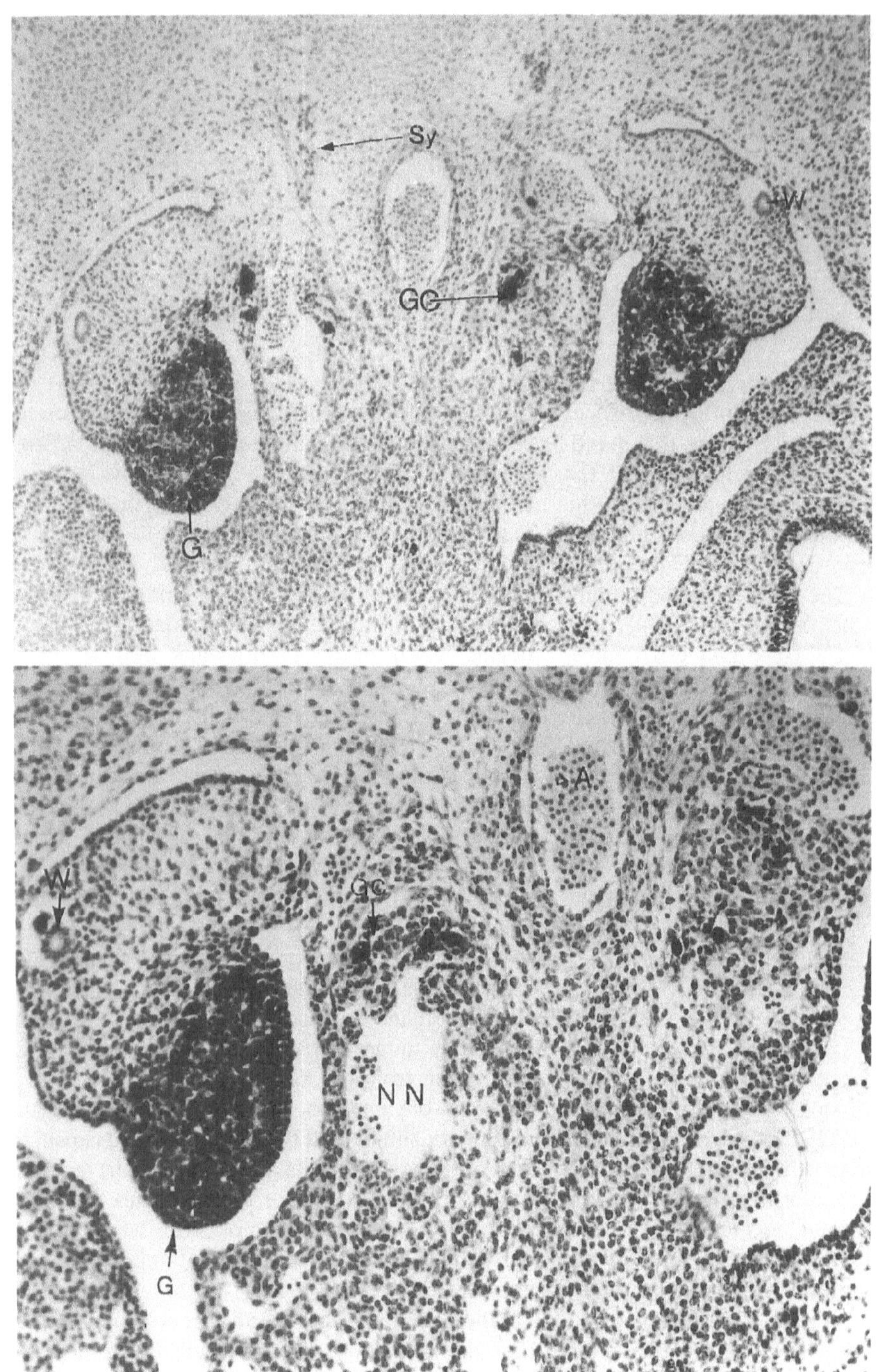

Fig. 418. (*above*) Cross section of 12-day mouse embryo, alkaline phosphatase stain. *G*, Gonad; *GC*, gonocytes; *Sy*, sympathetic trunk; *W*, Wolffian duct. (Courtesy of Prof. K. Theiler, University of Zurich)

Fig. 419. (*below*) Enlargement of portion of Fig. 418, with heavier background staining, better demonstrating the adrenal (*NN*). *A*, Aorta; *G*, gonad; *GC*, gonocytes; *W*, Wolffian duct (Courtesy of Prof. K. Theiler, University of Zurich)

and in females following the first pregnancy; in virgin females it regresses slowly.

Dunn (1970) believes the x-cell zone of mice to be analogous to the fetal adrenal cortex. This fetal adrenal cortex is also found in humans, nonhuman primates, armadillos, and perhaps sloths (Anderson and Capen 1978), and disappears after birth.

Adrenal Gland Medulla

The earliest phase of medullary development is discernible at the end of the 11th day of gestation and takes the form of two chains of sympathoblasts, one on either side of the aorta. At 11.5 days, clusters of sympathoblasts are distributed between the dorsal sympathetic trunk and the ventrally migrating mass of sympathoblasts (Figs. 420, 421). Some of these ventral sympathoblasts surround the circumference of the cranial aorta; others lie in close proximity to the cortical anlage. Thus, most of the smpathoblasts are in intimate contact with the caudal cardinal veins. Sympathetic nerve fibers extend from the sympathetic trunk (rami communicans) and continue ventrally to the cortical anlage. According to Theiler and Müntener (1974), these sympathetic nerve fibers constitute the pathway utilized by sympathoblasts in their migration to the cortical anlage.

In the 12-day embryo the small, deeply stained sympathoblasts are close to the less densely stained cells of the cortical anlage (Figs. 422, 423). Cells destined to become medullary cells are still in close contact with the anlage of paravertebral ganglia. The first of the developing nerve fibers may now be seen emerging from around the sympathoblasts.

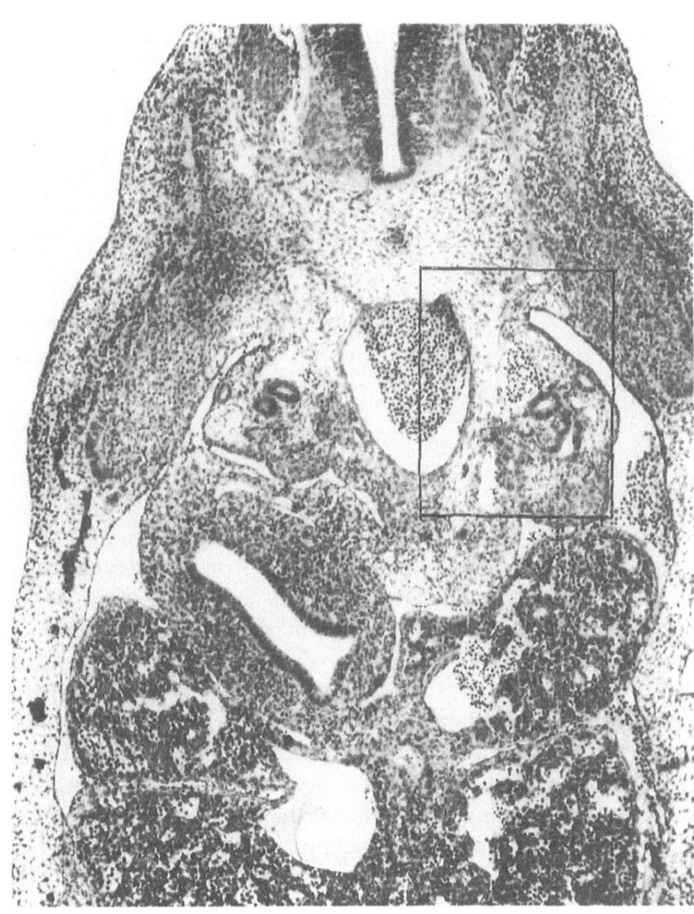

Fig. 420. Cross section of 11-day- 10-h mouse embryo; adrenal anlage in *rectangle*. (Courtesy of Prof. K. Theiler, University of Zurich)

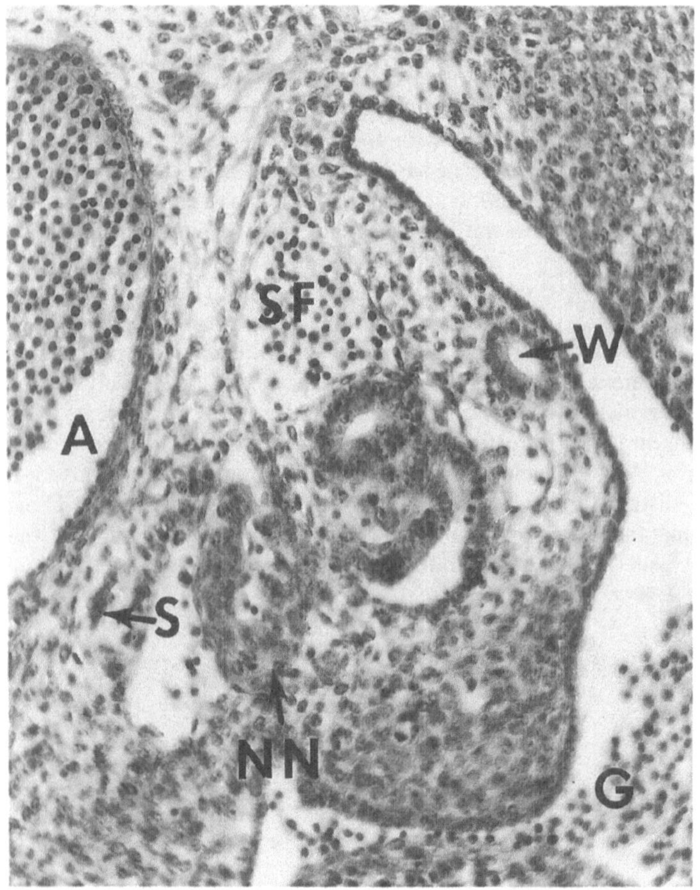

Fig. 421. Enlargement of area in box, Fig. 420. *A*, Aorta; *S*, sympathoblasts; *SF*, sympathetic nerve fibers; *W*, Wolffian duct; *G*, gonad; *NN*, adrenal gland cortical anlage. (Courtesy of Prof. K. Theiler, University of Zurich)

In the 14-day embryo the medullary cells, appearing as small dense aggregates, are centrally located in the developing adrenal gland. The coeliac ganglion is greatly enlarged.

In the 15-day embryo the medullary cells begin to enlarge. Their pale cytoplasm is in marked contrast to the acidophilic cytoplasm of the cortical cells.

During the interval between birth and the 16th day, the chromaffin reaction of the medullary cells becomes more pronounced. Kohno (1925) reviewed the comparative aspects of the development of the adrenal gland medulla in various species. He made a distinction between those species of mammals, including the mouse, which have a well-developed adrenal medulla at birth and other mammals, including man and some nonhuman primates, which do not. It is believed that in the latter, the organs of Zuckerkandl (aortic paraganglia) assume the function of the developing adrenal medulla. Since the mouse and some other mammals do not possess the organs of Zuckerkandl, it is believed that an adrenal medulla fully functional at birth is essential to life in these species. In 18-mm human embryos, which correspond to 14- to 15-day mouse embryos (13–14 mm) with recognizable adrenal medullas, sympathoblasts have not yet penetrated the cortical anlage and no medulla is evident (Uotila 1940).

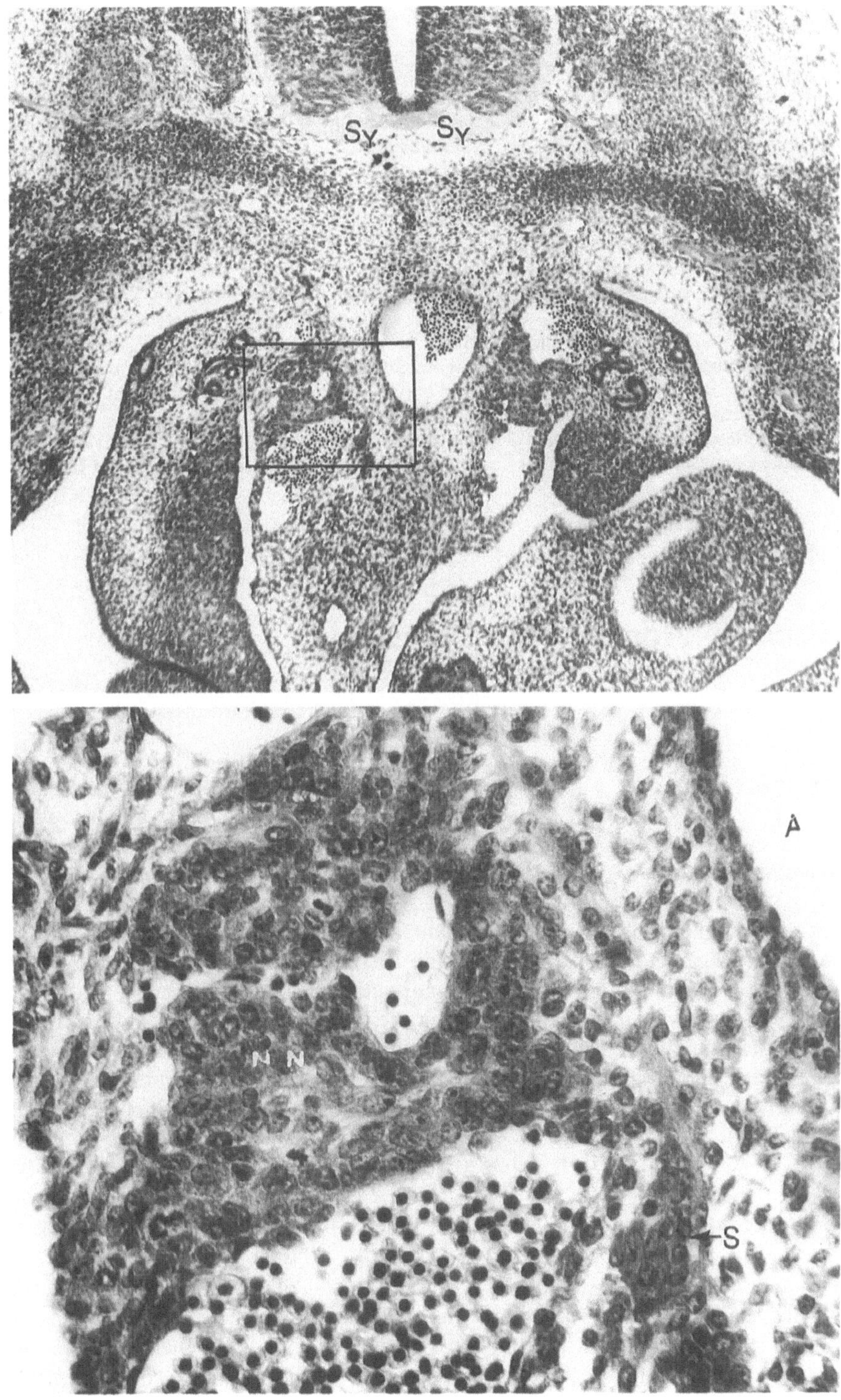

Fig. 422. (*above*) Cross section of 12-day (8-mm) mouse embryo. *Sy*, Sympathetic trunk. (Courtesy of Prof. K. Theiler, University of Zurich)

Fig. 423. (*below*) Enlargement of area shown in box of Fig. 422. *A*, Aorta; *NN*, adrenal gland; *S*, sympathoblasts. (Courtesy of Prof. K. Theiler, University of Zurich)

References

Anderson MP, Capen CC (1978) The endocrine system. In: Benirschke K, Garner FM, Jones TC (eds) Pathology of laboratory animals, vol I. Springer, Berlin Heidelberg New York, chapter 6

Dunn TB (1970) Normal and pathologic anatomy of the adrenal gland of the mouse, including neoplasms. J Natl Cancer Inst 44:1323–1389

Fernholm M (1971) On the development of the sympathetic chain and the adrenal medulla in the mouse. Z Anat Entwicklungsgesch 133:305–317

Green MC (1967) A defect of the splanchnic mesoderm caused by the mutant gene dominant hemimelia in the mouse. Dev Biol 15:62–89

Kohno S (1925) Zur vergleichenden Histologie und Embryologie der Nebenniere der Sauger und des Menschen. Z Anat Entwicklungsgesch 77:419–486

McPhail MK, Read HC (1942) The mouse adrenal. I. Development, degeneration and regeneration of the x zone. Anat Rec 84:51–73

Politzer G (1936) Über die Entwicklung der Nebenniere beim Menschen. Z Anat Entwicklungsgesch 106:40–48

Rugh R (1968) The mouse, its reproduction and development. Burgess, Minneapolis, Minn

Snell GD (1966) Reproduction. In: Green EL (ed) Biology of the laboratory mouse, 2nd edn. McGraw-Hill, New York

Theiler K (1972) The house mouse, development and normal stages from fertilization to 4 weeks of age. Springer, Berlin Heidelberg New York

Theiler K, Müntener M (1974) Die Entwicklung der Nebennieren der Maus. Z Anat Entwicklunsgesch 144:195–203

Uotila U (1940) The early embryologic development of the fetal and permanent adrenal cortex in man. Anat Rec 76:183–204

Waring H (1935) The development of the adrenal gland of the mouse. Q J Microb Sci 78:329–366

Histology, Adrenal Gland, Mouse

Charles H. Frith

Synonym. Suprarenal.

Gross Appearance

The adrenal glands of the mouse are small, paired endocrine organs situated on either side of the anterior pole of the kidneys. The right adrenal is more closely attached to the kidney than the left adrenal (Dunn 1970). The glands are ovoid, and are slightly larger and more opaque in female mice due to the presence of more lipid (Hummel et al. 1966).

Microscopic Features

The adrenal gland of the mouse, as of other species, consists of the cortex and the medulla (Fig. 424). The cortex is surrounded by a thin fibrous capsule. The zone glomerulosa and the zone fasciculata are distinguishable in the mouse adrenal cortex at the light microscopic level (Fig. 425); the zone reticularis is not discernible. The zone glomerulosa consists of small cells that form indistinct arches and become columns of cells in the fascicular zone. The cells have relatively large nuclei, and slightly basophilic cytoplasm. Although they are well vascularized with small capillaries, these are not conspicuous in ordinary histologic preparations unless distended with blood. The zona fasciculata extends to the medulla and is composed of columns of cells with centrally located nuclei. The nuclei are vesicular and the cytoplasm is eosinophilic.

The adrenal medulla is composed of homogeneous polyhedral cells arranged in small irregular packets separated by sinusoids (Fig. 426). The cytoplasm is finely granular and more basophilic than the cytoplasm of the cortical cells, and the nuclei are large and centrally located. The medulla is usually completely surrounded by the cortex, but may extend to the capsular surface at the hilus.

An unusual feature of the adrenal glands of young mice is the transient X zone (Fig. 427) that surrounds the medulla. The cytoplasm of the cells in this X zona is conspicuously more basophilic than the cytoplasm of cells of the zona fasciculata. The X zona appears about 10 days post-partum and disappears rapidly without undergoing vacuolization in the male mouse as sexual maturity is reached at approximately 5 weeks of age. In female mice, the zone disappears at first preg-

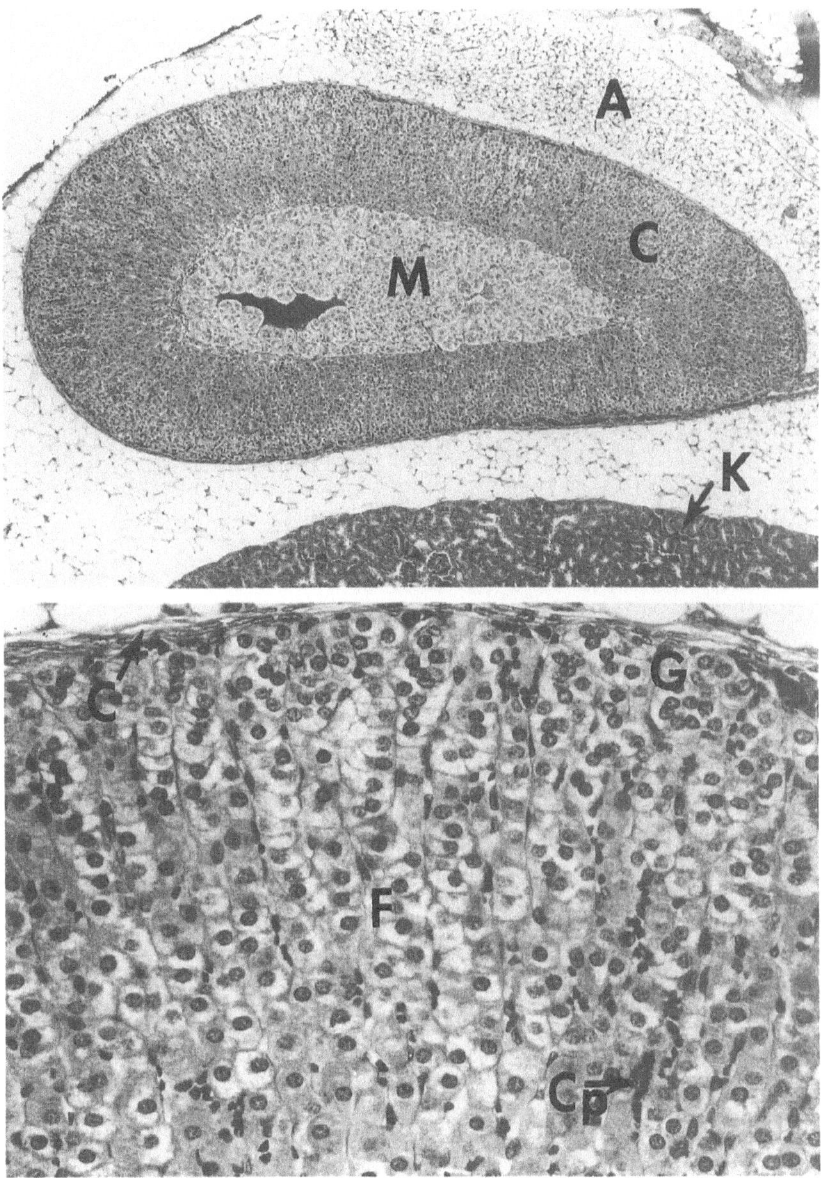

Fig. 424. (*above*) Adrenal gland, mouse. In perirenal adipose tissue, (*A*), closely related to right kidney (*K*). *C*, Cortex; *M*, medulla. H&E, ×48

Fig. 425. (*below*) Adrenal cortex, mouse. *C*, Capsule; *G*, glomerulosa; *F*, fascicular zone; *Cp*, capillary. H&E, ×300

nancy, but in virgin female mice it may be visible for up to 30 weeks. The zone undergoes prominent vacuolization in the female, in contrast to events that occur in the male (Fig. 428). It is important to be aware of this entity and not mistake it for a pathologic lesion. The X zone appears to be analogous to the fetal cortex in humans (Howard-Miller 1926).

Ultrastructure

The ultrastructural features of the adrenocortical epithelial cells are dependent upon the area of the cortex examined. The zones are not sharply demarcated, but gradually merge into one another (Zelander 1959; Sato 1967, 1968). The epithelial cells in the glomerular zone contain round, homo-

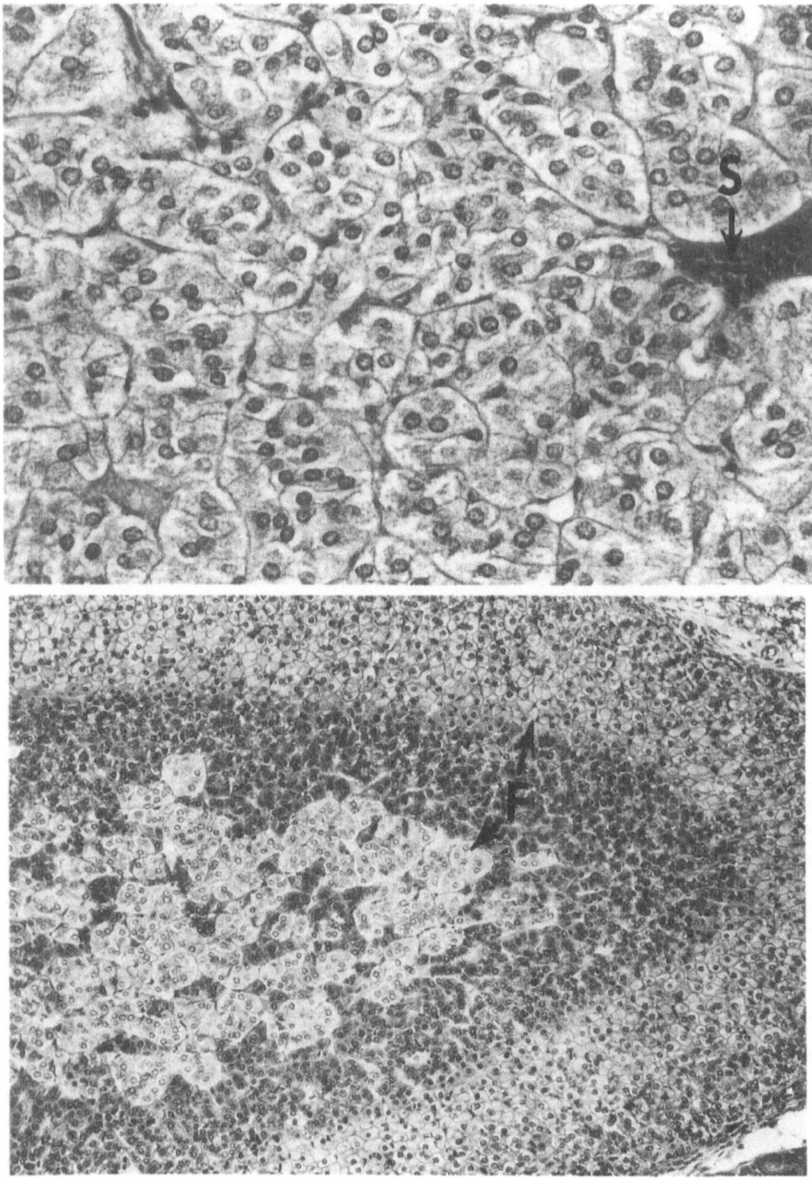

Fig. 426. (*above*) Adrenal medulla, mouse; packets of polyhedral cells. Sinusoid (*S*) seen when distended with blood. H&E, ×300

Fig. 427. (*below*) Adrenal, young female mouse. *F*, X or fetal zone. H&E, ×120

geneously osmiophilic lipid droplets centered around the nucleus (Fig. 429). Round or ovoid mitochondria are present in large numbers and are uniformly dispersed throughout the cytoplasm. Their cristae are often tubular in form. The most characteristic features of the epithelial cells in the fascicular zone include irregular, somewhat osmiophilic lipid droplets, and an abundance of round mitochondria. Elongated and round mitochondria are present in the innermost part of the cortex, and the cytoplasm also contains a small number of dense granules, features which suggest an otherwise indistinguishable reticular zone.

Sato (1968) examined ultrastructural features of the adrenal X zone in 14 female SMA mice ranging in age from 40 to 70 days. Within this range the X zone showed no degeneration. The cells of the X

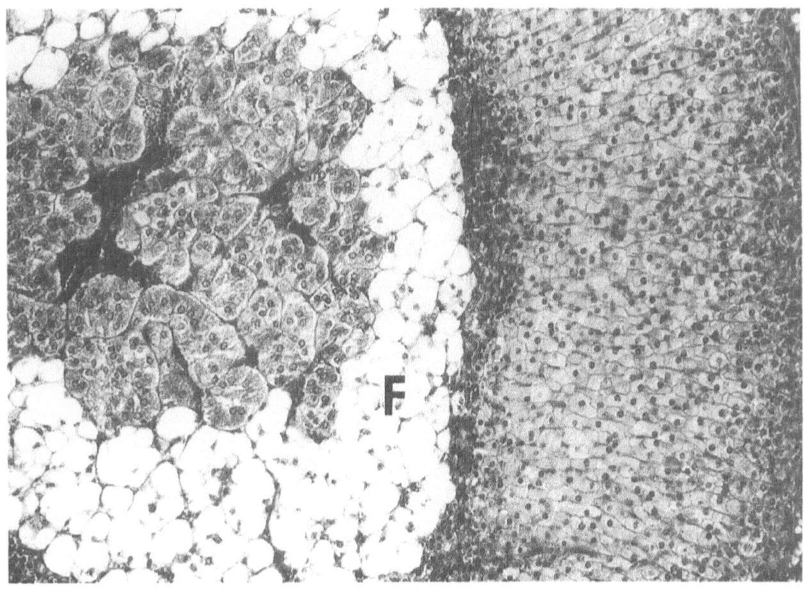

Fig. 428. Adrenal, female mouse. Vacuolization (lipid) in cells of X-zone (*F*). H&E, ×120

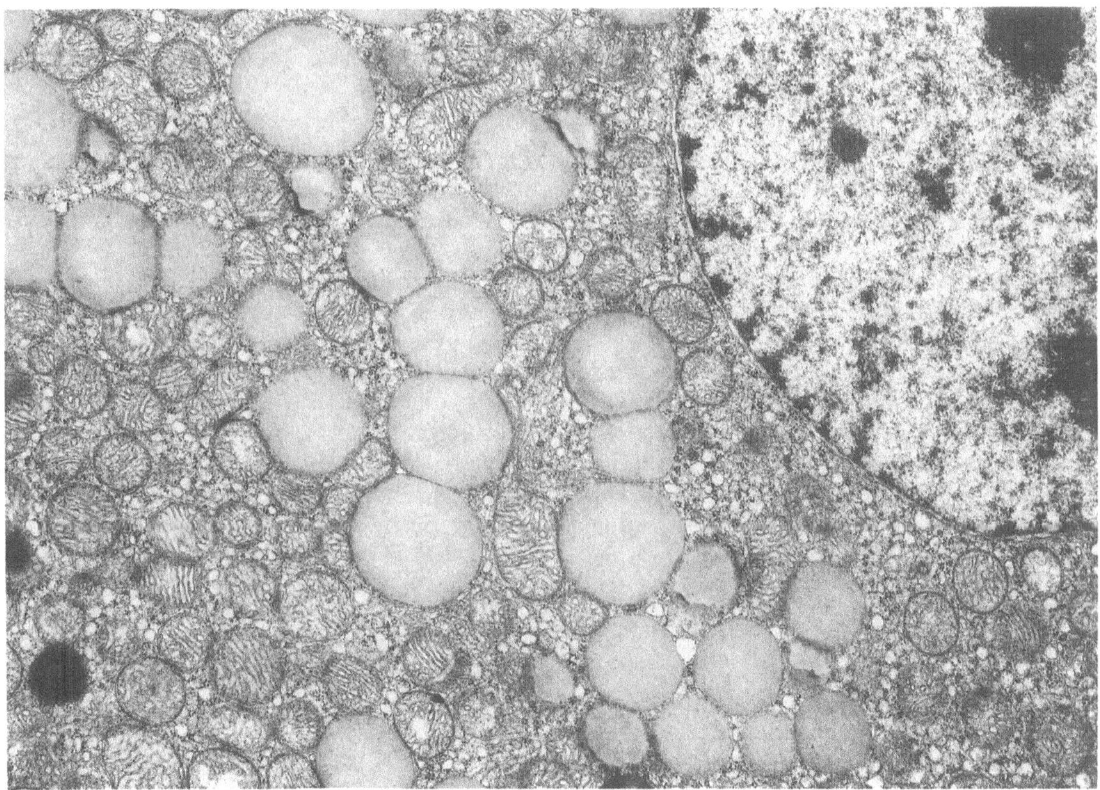

Fig. 429. Adrenal cortex (fasciculata) of mouse. Uranyl acetate–lead citrate, ×15600

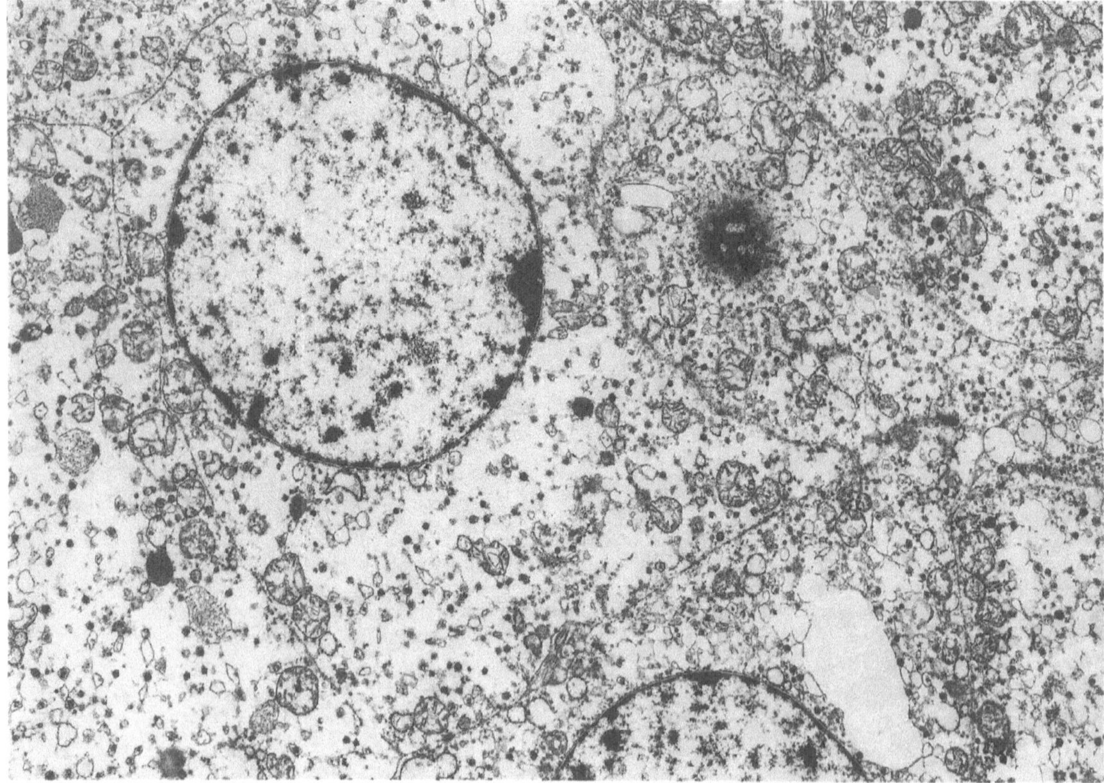

Fig. 430. Adrenal medulla, mouse. Inner zones of fasciculata. Uranyl acetate–lead citrate, ×7800

zone contained an abundance of smooth endoplasmic reticulum and small lipid droplets, and the mitochondria were quite bizarre in shape. In the same article, Sato postulated that the presence of lipid droplets and the abundant smooth endoplasmic reticulum may indicate that these cells are producing steroids.

The ultrastructure of the normal mouse adrenal medulla has been insufficiently investigated. The electron-lucent cytoplasm is abundant and contains rough endoplasmic reticulum, a Golgi apparatus, mitochondria, lysosomal dense bodies, and characteristic secretory granules scattered throughout it at random (Fig. 430).

Biologic Features

Lipids are prominent in the adrenal cortex of the mouse, but vary in amount with sex and strain; the predominant lipid is cholesterol. Alkaline phosphatase is present in the zona fasciculata of the adult males but absent in the glomerulosa. It is much less apparent in female mice (Nicander 1952). Acid phosphatase has also been reported in the adrenal cortex of mice (Gomori 1941).

Comparison with Other Species

The adrenal glands of the mouse are similar to those of other species. Peculiarities of the mouse adrenal include lack of a distinct zona reticularis, accessory adrenocortical nodules (p. 391), and ceroid pigment (p. 458) and proliferation of subcapsular spindle cells (p. 464) in older mice. These features are not completely understood, but they are clearly variations and are therefore described in detail elsewhere in this volume. The transient X zone appears to be analogous with the fetal zone described in man and other species (Moser and Benirschke 1962; Benirschke and Richart 1964).

References

Benirschke K, Richart R (1964) Observations on the fetal adrenals of marmoset monkeys. Endocrinology 74:382–387
Dunn TB (1970) Normal and pathologic anatomy of the adrenal gland of the mouse, including neoplasms. J Natl Cancer Inst 44:1323–1389
Gomori G (1941) Distribution of acid phosphatase in the tissues under normal and under pathologic conditions. Arch Pathol Lab Med 32:189–199
Howard-Miller E (1926) The development of the epinephrine content of the suprarenal medulla in early stages of the mouse. Am J Physiol 75:267–277
Hummel KL, Richardson FL, Fekete E (1966) Anatomy. In: Green EL (ed) Biology of the laboratory mouse, 2nd edn. McGraw-Hill, New York, chapter 13
Moser HG, Benirschke K (1962) Fetal zone of the adrenal gland in the nine-banded armadillo, *Dasypus novemcinctus*. Anat Rec 143:47–88
Nicander L (1952) Histological and histochemical studies on the adrenal cortex of domestic and laboratory animals. Acta Anat 14:1–88
Sato T (1967) Age and sex differences in the fine structure of the mouse adrenal cortex. Nagoya J Med Sci 30:225–251
Sato T (1968) The fine structure of the mouse adrenal X-zone. Z Zellforsch 87:315–329
Zelander T (1959) Ultrastructure of mouse adrenal cortex. An electron microscopic study in intact and hydrocortisone treated male adults. J Ultrastruct Res [Suppl] 2:1–111

Accessory Adrenocortical Tissue, Mouse

Bernard Sass

Synonyms. Accessory adrenal, accessory adrenal cortical nodule, supernumerary adrenal.

Gross Appearance

Hummel (1958) studied the location of accessory adrenal glands with the dissecting microscope. Accessory adrenal cortical nodules on the left side surround the vena cava and renal vein, and on the right are in proximity to the renal vein or the adrenal vessels. Dunn (1970) observed these accessory nodules in the measorchium. They cannot be seen with the unaided eye.

Microscopic Features

This structure consists of single or multiple spherical or ovoid nodules, which are encapsulated, vary in size, and are usually located at one pole of the adrenal. The zones of the adrenal cortex are usually identifiable in the lesion, but medullary tissue is lacking (Figs. 431–434). According to Hummel (1958) accessory adrenal cortical nodules develop the same aging changes as the main body of the adrenal gland. These changes include subcapsular spindle cell hyperplasia and deposition of ceroid. The latter is especially frequent in the accessory nodule as well as in the adrenal gland of aged mice (Figs. 435, 436).

Differential Diagnosis

Accessory adrenal cortical tissue must be differentiated from cortical adenomas which lie within the adrenal cortex and share a common capsule. Accessory adrenal cortical tissue should also be distinguished from cortical carcinomas that have penetrated the capsule. Such carcinomas are characterized by the loss of normal architecture, by cell atypia, and by continuity with a neoplasm within the cortex.

Pathogenesis

According to Hummel (1958), accessory adrenal cortical nodules can arise at any time during embryonic life from the coelomic epithelium, and during adult life from abdominal fat. In strains C3H and C57L, new cortical tissue may differentiate continously.

Frequency

Hummel (1958) studied the occurrence of one or more accessory adrenal cortical nodules in mice

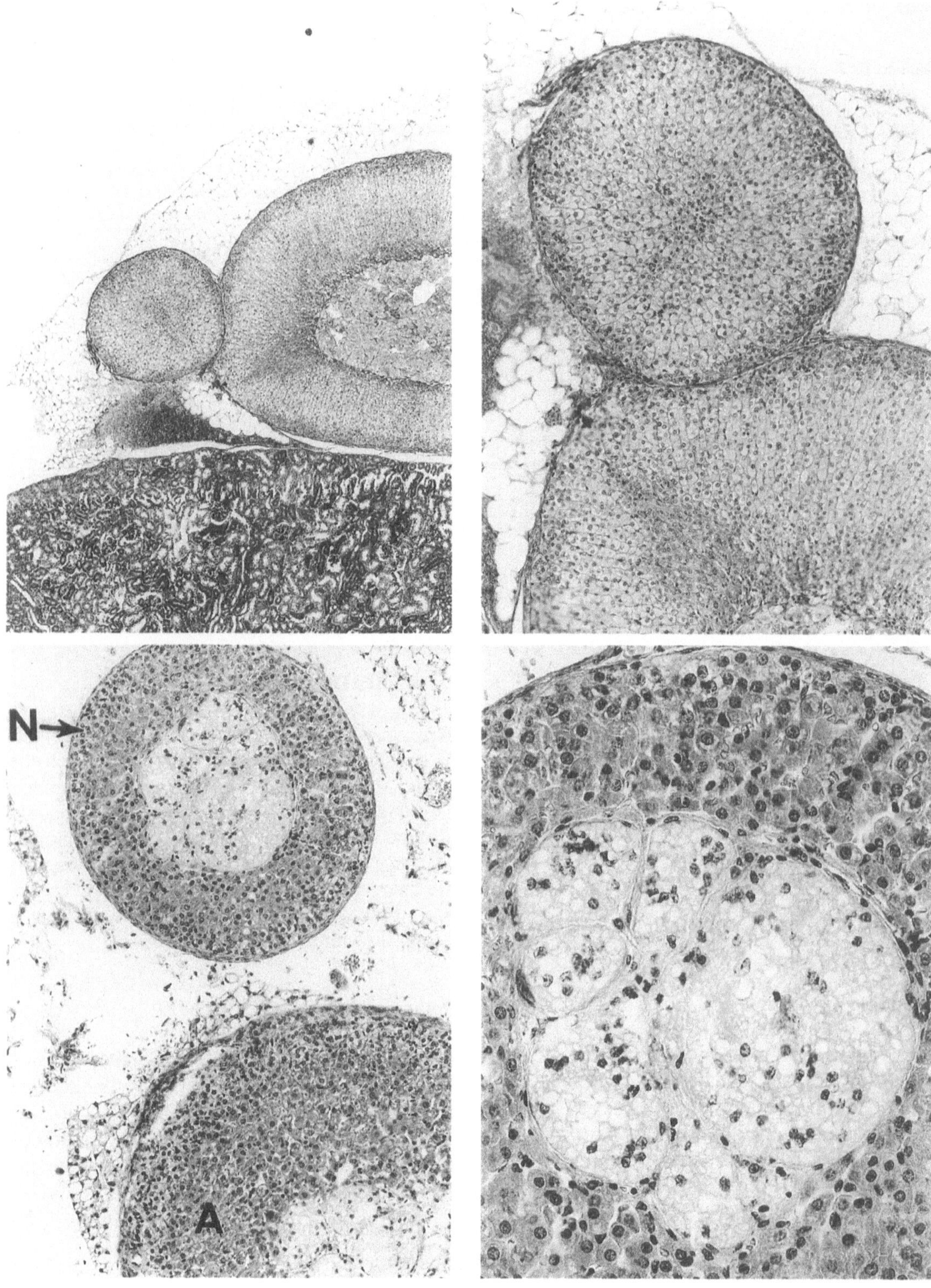

Fig. 431. (*upper left*) Accessory adrenal cortical tissue – a single nodule of cortical tissue is completely encapsulated. H&E, ×54

Fig. 432. (*upper right*) Higher power view of accessory adrenal cortical tissue in Fig. 431; two distinct zones of the cortex are visible. H&E, ×130

Fig. 433. (*lower left*) Accessory adrenal cortical tissue (*N*) with ceroid deposition in zona reticularis. *A*, Adrenal. H&E, ×130

Fig. 434. (*lower right*) Higher magnification of accessory adrenal cortical tissue with ceroid in zona reticularis. H&E, ×330

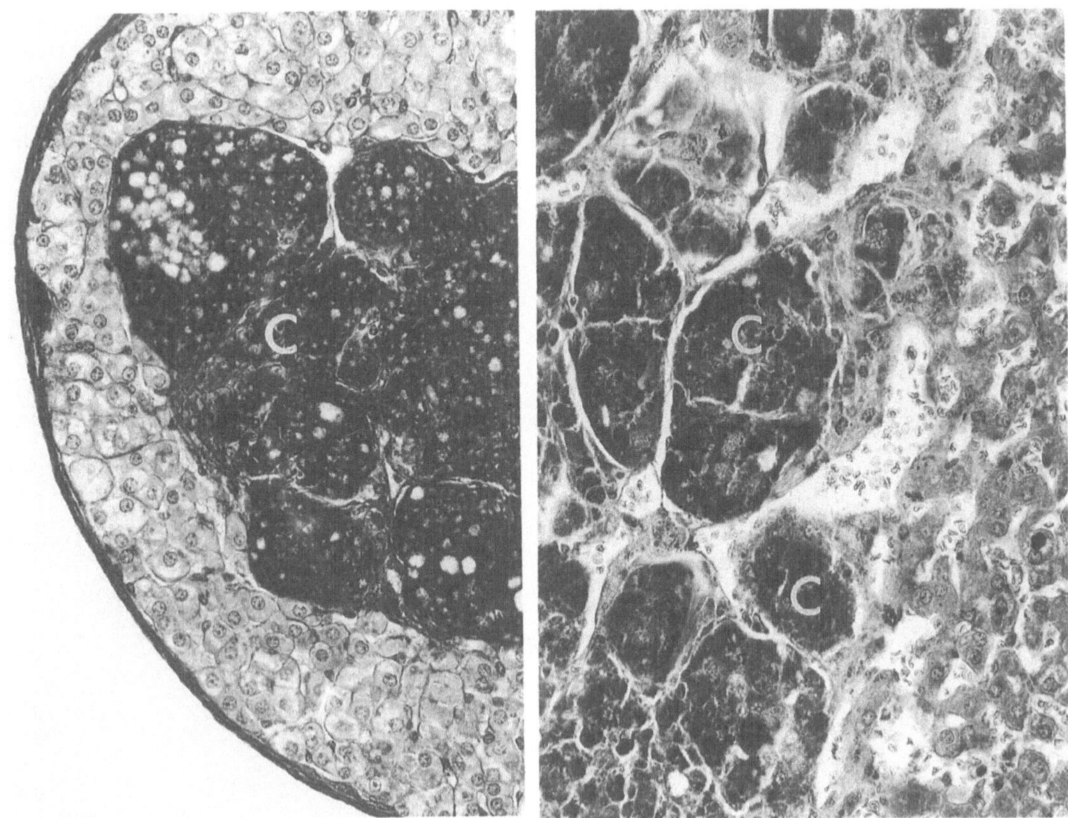

Fig. 435. Accessory adrenal cortical tissue; ceroid (*C*) stained with PAS, ×330

Fig. 436. Accessory adrenal cortical tissue. *C*, ceroid; acid-fast stain, ×540

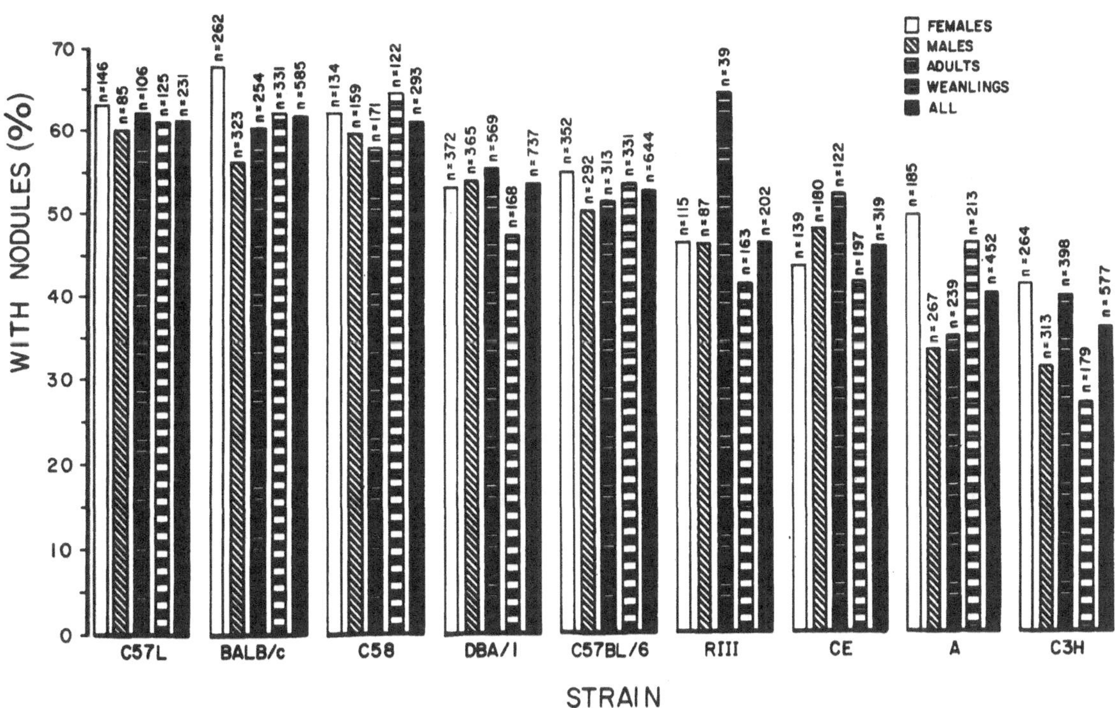

Fig. 437. Accessory adrenal cortical nodules in mice (from Hummel 1958)

of each of nine strains. Mice of strains (C57L, BALB/c, and C58 had the highest percentage (approximately 60%), while strain C3H had the lowest (38%; see Fig. 437). In all strains studied, there was a greater percentage of the accessory nodules on the left than on the right side, with a ratio of 4:1. The nodules often occurred more frequently in females than in males. Multiple nodules were present in 11% of BALB/c mice and at a lower percetage in the other strains studied.

Comparison with Other Species

Accessory adrenal cortical tissue is frequent in dogs, lagomorphs and nonhuman primates, squirrels, moles, and armadillos (Anderson and Capen 1978). It is usually found within or outside of the capsule of the adrenal or in the perirenal adipose tissue. It is frequently found in the vicinity of the equine testis. In patas monkeys, accessory adrenal tissue may be found in the mesovarium, the epoophoron tubules, and the mesosalpinx. See also under accessory adrenocortical tissue, rat (p. 394).

References

Anderson MP, Capen CC (1978) The endocrine system. In: Benirschke K, Garner FM, Jones TC (eds) Pathology of laboratory animals, vol I. Springer, Berlin Heidelberg New York, chapter 6

Dunn TC (1970) Normal and pathologic anatomy of the adrenal gland of the mouse, including neoplasms. J Natl Cancer Inst 44:1323–1389

Hummel KP (1958) Accessory adrenal cortical nodules in the mouse. Anat Rec 132:281–296

Accessory Adrenocortical Tissue, Rat

George A. Parker and Marion G. Valerio

Synonyms. Adrenocortical rests, accessory adrenocortical nodules, extracapsular cortical nodules, ectopic adrenal cortex.

Gross Appearance

Foci of accessory adrenocortical tissue are rarely large enough to be observed grossly in the rat. The identity of those few nodules which are grossly visible must be confirmed microscopically; thus, gross diagnosis is virtually impossible.

Microscopic Features

Accessory adrenocortical tissue most commonly consists of small nests of normally appearing adrenal cortical cells, found in virtually any location in the abdominal cavity. The most common locations are adjacent to the adrenal capsule or in the periadrenal or perirenal fat (Anderson and Capen 1978; Burek 1978; Dribben and Wolfe 1947; Russfield 1967). Large nodules may contain all three layers of the primary adrenal cortex, but medullary cells are rarely present. Extracapsular cortical tissue may be associated with discontinuities in the adrenal capsule, which are most commonly located near the point of entry of blood vessels at the hilus. It can be distinguished from accessory adrenocortical nodules by the presence of a fibrous capsule around the latter (Hamlin and Banas 1990).

Ultrastructure

No information is available on the ultrastructure.

Differential Diagnosis

In most locations accessory adrenocortical tissue is morphologically distinct and presents little diagnostic challenge to the microscopist. Adrenocortical nodules in the hilus of the ovary, a fairly common occurrence in some species, must be distinguished from normal intraovarian endocrine tissue. Immunohistochemical techniques may be useful in definitive identification of such foci. Extracapsular cortical tissue associated with breaks in the adrenal capsule is distinguished from accessory adrenocortical nodules by the presence of a fibrous capsule around the latter (Hamlin and Banas 1990).

Biologic Features

Each adrenal gland has a double origin and in reality is two distinct glands combined in a common capsule. The cortex is derived from mesoderm, and the medulla is derived from ectodermal chromaffin tissue. In lower animals, such as fish, the cortex and medulla appear as separate organs. Progressing up the phylogenetic scale there is an increasingly intimate association of cortex and medulla, until the ultimate is reached in mammals by the cortex fully encapsulating the medulla (Arey 1965).

Accessory adrenocortical tissue is presumed to result from multiple cortical primordia or separated fragments of the primary gland. Separated fragments are seen primarily in organs that arise in the immediate vicinity of the fetal adrenals, for example, the kidney and testes (Arey 1965).

Few data are available concerning the frequency of occurrence of accessory adrenocortical tissue in rats. Burek (1978), Anderson and Capen (1978), and Russfield (1967) indicated that accessory adrenocortical tissue is not an uncommon finding in rats, although the latter authors restricted their observation to rats over 1 year of age. A study of age-related changes in the rat adrenal revealed greater numbers of accessory adrenocortical tissue in old (540–884 days) rats (Dribben and Wolfe 1947). Russfield (1967) reported the frequency to be a strain-related phenomenon in mice, with higher numbers in weanlings of some strains and aged mice of other strains. Given the difficulty in gross diagnosis and the widespread distribution of the foci, an acceptable study of the incidence of accessory adrenocortical tissue would probably require serial sectioning of the entire abdominal cavity.

The significance of accessory adrenocortical tissue lies in its ability to serve as a point of origin of adrenocortical neoplasms in atypical locations, thus posing diagnostic problems. Accessory adrenocortical tissue can partially, and perhaps entirely, replace adrenocortical function in adrenalectomized animals, thus complicating studies of adrenocortical function (Wyman and zum Suden 1937).

Comparison with Other Species

Accessory adrenocortical tissue has been found scattered throughout the body cavities of the majority of mammalian species (Bourne 1949). Accessory adrenocortical nodules in mice were most commonly found related to blood vessels around the kidneys and adrenals (p. 391, this volume; Hummel 1958). Some strains of mice had a higher incidence of accessory adrenocortical tissue, as did females of all strains (p. 393, this volume; Figs. 431–436). Hybrid mice exhibited a lower incidence than the parent strains (Fig. 437). Accessory adrenocortical tissue has been frequently observed in the ovarian hili of several species (Seliger et al. 1966). Adrenocortical rests ranging from 1 to 5 mm in diameter were seen in each of 26 patas monkeys (Conaway 1969). The nodules were larger and more numerous in sexually mature monkeys. Adrenocortical nodules in the ovary are reported to be a nearly constant finding in some species of squirrels (Sciuridae) and moles (Talpidae; Mossman 1946, 1966). Accessory adrenocortical tissue was commonly found in the ovaries of 13-lined ground squirrels (*Citellus tridecemlineatus* Mitchell), and functionally replaced the adrenal in adrenalectomized ground squirrels (Chester-Jones and Henderson 1963; Wyman and zum Suden 1937). Accessory adrenocortical tissue in the ovary also was seen with unspecified frequency in nine-banded armadillos and Rocky Mountain pikas (Duke 1952; Enders and Buchanan 1959).

References

Anderson MP, Capen CC (1978) The endocrine system. In: Benirschke K, Garner FM, Jones TC (eds) Pathology of laboratory animals, vol. 1. Springer, Berlin Heidelberg New York, p 436

Arey LB (1965) Developmental anatomy: a textbook and laboratory manual of embryology, 7th edn. Saunders, Philadelphia, pp 518–519

Bourne GH (1949) The mammalian adrenal gland. Clarendon, Oxford, pp 30–31

Burek JD (1978) Pathology of aging rats. CRC, West Palm Beach, p 42

Chester-Jones I, Henderson IW (1963) The ovary of the 13-lined ground squirrel (Citellus tridecemlineatus Mitchell) after adrenalectomy. J Endocrinol 26:265–272

Conaway CH (1969) Adrenal cortical rests of the ovarian hilus of the patas monkey. Folia Primatol 11:175–180

Dribben IS, Wolfe JM (1947) Structural changes in the connective tissue of the adrenal glands of female rats associated with advancing age. Anat Rec 98:557–585

Duke KL (1952) Ovarian histology of Ochotona princeps, the Rocky Mountain pika. Anat Rec 112:737–760

Enders AC, Buchanan GD (1959) The reproductive tract of the female nine-banded armadillo. Tex Rep Biol Med 17:323–340

Hamlin MH, Banas DA (1990) Adrenal gland. In: Boorman GA, Eustis SL, Elwell MR, Montgomery CA, MacKenzie WF (eds) Pathology of the Fischer rat. Academic, San Diego, p 506

Hummel KP (1958) Accessory adrenal cortical nodules in the mouse. Anat Rec 132:281–295

Mossman HW (1946) Glandular tissues of the adult mammalian ovary. Anat Rec 94:484

Mossman HW (1966) The rodent ovary. In: Rowlands IW (ed) Comparative biology of reproduction in mammals. Academic, London, pp 455–470

Russfield AB (1967) Pathology of the endocrine glands, ovary and testis of rats and mice. In: Cotchin E, Roe FJC (eds) Pathology of laboratory rats and mice. Davis, Philadelphia, pp 425–434

Seliger WG, Blair AJ, Mossman HW (1966) Differentiation of adrenal cortex-like tissue at the hilum of the gonads in response to adrenalectomy. Am J Anat 118:615–629

Wyman LC, zum Suden C (1937) The functional efficiency of transplanted adrenal cortical tissue. Endocrinology 21: 587–593

Immunohistochemical and In Situ Hybridization Analysis of Steroidogenic Enzymes for Study of Steroid Metabolism in Endocrine Organs

Hironobu Sasano

Introduction

Recent advancements in radioimmunoassays, enzyme-linked immunoassays, and a variety of chromatography techniques have made it possible to measure circulating steroid hormones with reasonable accuracy. However, to obtain a better understanding of steroid metabolism it is important to analyze the tissues that synthesize and secrete steroids. Major steroid-producing organs, including adrenal cortex, ovary, and testis, are all associated with complicated morphological features. Therefore it is essential to determine the localization of steroidogenesis, i.e., the steroid hormones produced in specific cells of the tissue. Biochemical studies of steroidogenesis, including tissue concentration of steroids and activity of steroidogenic enzymes, certainly provided important information. However, owing to the nature of invitro biochemical analysis, it is nearly impossible to determine which parts of the tissue have steroidogenic capability. Therefore efforts have been directed toward analysis of steroidogenesis morphologically in tissue sections.

Conventional Morphological Approaches to Steroidogenesis

Conventional light-microscopic analysis defined steroidogenic or steroid-producing cells morphologically, especially by assessing the correlation between histopathologic features and clinical endocrine manifestations in cases in which lesions were associated with abnormalities of steroid metabolism. However, light-microscopic observation has a limited role in assessing the functional status of the tissue, as is evidenced, for instance, by the fact that in most instances histopathologic differentiation is nearly impossible among adrenocortical adenomas associated with Cushing's syndrome, primary aldosteronism, and clinically normal adrenocortical hormonal status without being aware of the clinical or endocrine setting (Lack et al. 1990).

Electron microscopy has made it possible to identify organelles such as smooth endoplasmic reticulum and mitochondria, which are considered to be associated with steroid metabolism. These ultrastructural features are observed in steroid-producing cells in adrenal, testis, ovary, and to some extent hepatocytes, in which steroid hormones are also metabolized. Based on the presence of these characteristic cell organelles, electron microscopy can be used to demonstrate to some extent whether the cells are actively involved in corticosteroidogenesis and, in addition, whether they participate in increased biosynthesis by observing how well these organelles are developed. However, ultrastructural observation cannot demonstrate what types of steroids are being produced in the cells.

Identification of Steroids in Tissue Sections

Attempts have been made both histochemically and immunohistochemically to identify steroid hormones themselves. Histochemical studies to identify steroid hormones (such as the Ashbel-Seligman reaction, which was believed to stain ketosteroids, and the Vine's fuchsinophil stain for androgens) turned out not to be valuable and are of only historical interest at present. The presence of fat, identified by specific stains (oil red O, Sudan III), is still widely employed in many laboratories to estimate steroid hormones in tissue sections. This method is nonspecific for hormones and has marginal value at best. With the development of antibodies against specific steroids, immunohistochemical studies of steroids have been reported by a number of investigators (Kurman et al. 1979; Martinelli et al. 1983). However, immunolocalization of steroids themselves presents numerous technical problems, including fixation of steroids, extraction of steroids into organic solvents, and others. In addition, it is currently not known whether antisteroid antibodies recognize the hormones in the cells in which the hormones are synthesized, stored, or bound to receptors (Kurman et al. 1984). Therefore, the immunoreactivity of steroids in tissue sections has limited biologic significance.

Histochemical Studies of Steroidogenic Enzymes

Attempts to develop methods directed specifically toward staining steroids subsequently gave way to techniques directed toward illustrating the enzyme systems specifically involved in steroidogenesis. Wattenberg (1958) developed a histochemical method to detect the overall activity of the 3β-hydroxysteroid dehydrogenase (3β-HSD) reaction based on the reduction of a neotetrazollium salt. Histochemical analysis can detect 3β-HSD activity with reasonable accuracy if it is carefully performed. However, this method requires relatively thick fresh-frozen sections and is associated with a variety of methodological difficulties, and interpretation of the results can sometimes be very difficult (Sasano 1975). Therefore no success has been obtained in efforts to study steroidogenesis through examining the expression of steroidogenic enzyme molecules themselves.

Cytochrome P-450 and Steroidogenesis

In steroidogenesis, as is shown in the pathway of corticosteroidogenesis in Fig. 438, a series of hydroxysteroid reactions and cleavage of c-c bonds, with the exception of 3β-hydroxysteroid dehydrogenation, are catalyzed by heme-containing enzymes, cytochromes P-450, which generally act as a terminal oxidase of the nicotinamide adenine dinucleotide phosphate (NADPH) dependent electron transfer system (Hall 1985). The protein moiety of the cytochrome P-450 provides the specificity for the specific substrates (Hall 1985). Therefore demonstration of the presence or expression of this cytochrome P-450 and/or 3β-HSD strongly indicate that the steroid hormone catalyzed by the enzyme(s) is produced in the cells where the enzyme(s) is identified. Recent advances in biochemical and molecular biochemical techniques have made it possible to purify all the types of the enzymes including cytochrome P-450 involved in steroidogenesis, and from these purified products specific antibodies have been generated and DNA sequences determined.

Immunohistochemistry and In Situ Hybridization of Steroidogenic Enzymes

Based on the principles described above, Sasano and colleagues studied the distribution of all the steroidogenic enzymes in adrenal and its disorders (Sasano 1992), ovary and its disorders (Sasano and Sasano 1989; Sasano et al. 1990a,b), and testis and its disorders (Sasano et al. 1992a) including insitu hybridization analysis employing cDNA and oligonucleotides against P45Ocl7 (Sasano et al. 1992b; Suzuki et al. 1992). The following summarizes the results of these studies, with particular emphasis upon the findings

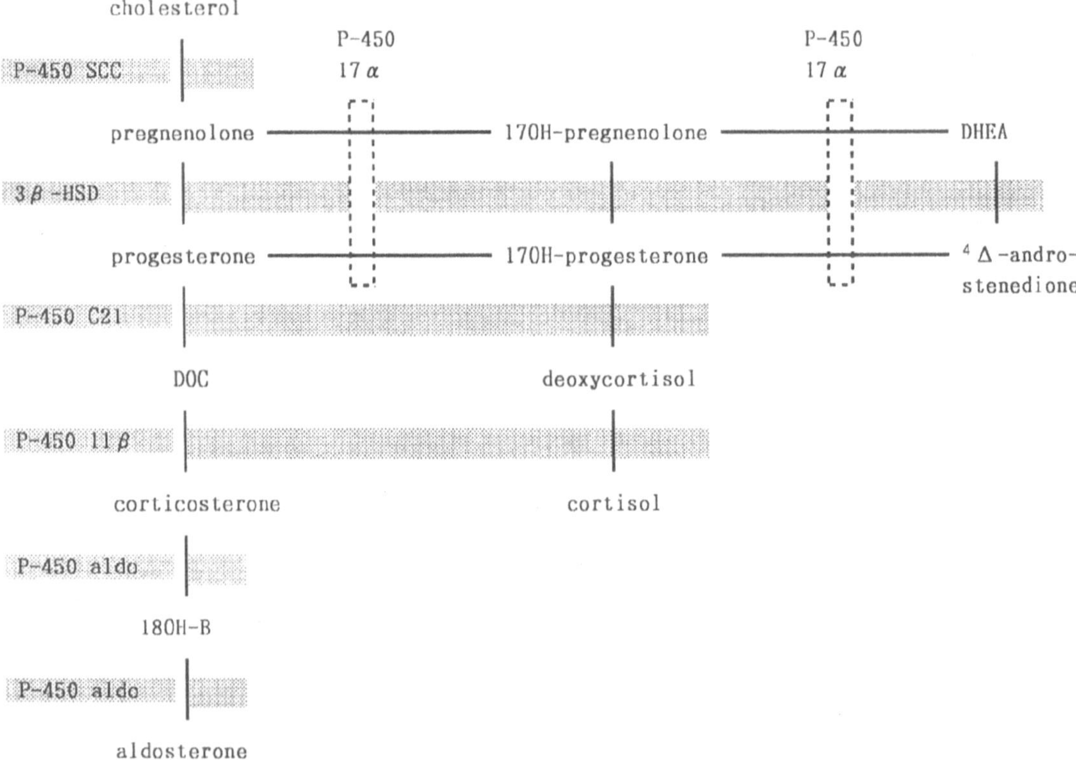

Fig. 438. Pathway of corticosteroidogenesis in humans. *DHEA*, Dehydroepiandrostenedione; *DOC*, deoxycorticosterone

which can be obtained only by applying these techniques.

Adrenal Gland

The question of functional zonation of the adrenal cortex has long been in dispute. It has been postulated that aldosterone or mineralocorticoids synthesis occurs in the zona glomerulosa and cortisol or glucocorticoids is synthesized in the zonae fasciculata and reticularis. However, there had been no convincing data to prove this hypothesis of functional zonation of the adrenal cortex. Immunohistochemistry and in situ hybridization of P45Ocl7, a cytochrome P450 variant required in glucocorticoid and androgen biosynthesis but not in mineralocorticoid biosynthesis, was absent from the zona glomerulosa (Fig. 439A,B; Suzuki et al. 1992; Sasano et al. 1989a,b). This finding demonstrates that the zona glomerulosa cells of the adrenal cortex do not participate in glucocorticoid-biosynthesis. In addition, immunolocalization of P450aldo, which catalyzes the final pathways of aldosterone biosynthesis but not 11β-hydroxylation, revealed its expression in the zona glomerulosa cells (Fig. 440A, B). This finding therefore confirms that aldosterone biosynthesis occurs predominantly in the zona glomerulosa. Steroid biosynthesis associated with adrenocortical carcinoma is generally characterized by excessive secretion of biologically inactive precursor steroids. Recent immunolocalization of steroidogenic enzymes reveals that carcinoma cells do not express all the enzymes required for cortisol or aldosterone biosynthesis, which accounts for ineffective steroidogenesis or accumulation of precursor steroids that are converted to biologically active corticosteroids by normal adrenal cortex and cortical adenoma (Sasano et al. 1993). Immunolocalization and in situ hybridization of steroidogenic enzymes provided new insights into pathogenesis and/or pathophysiology of a variety of adrenocortical disorders, including primary pigmented (nodular adrenocortical disease, hormonally inactive ad-

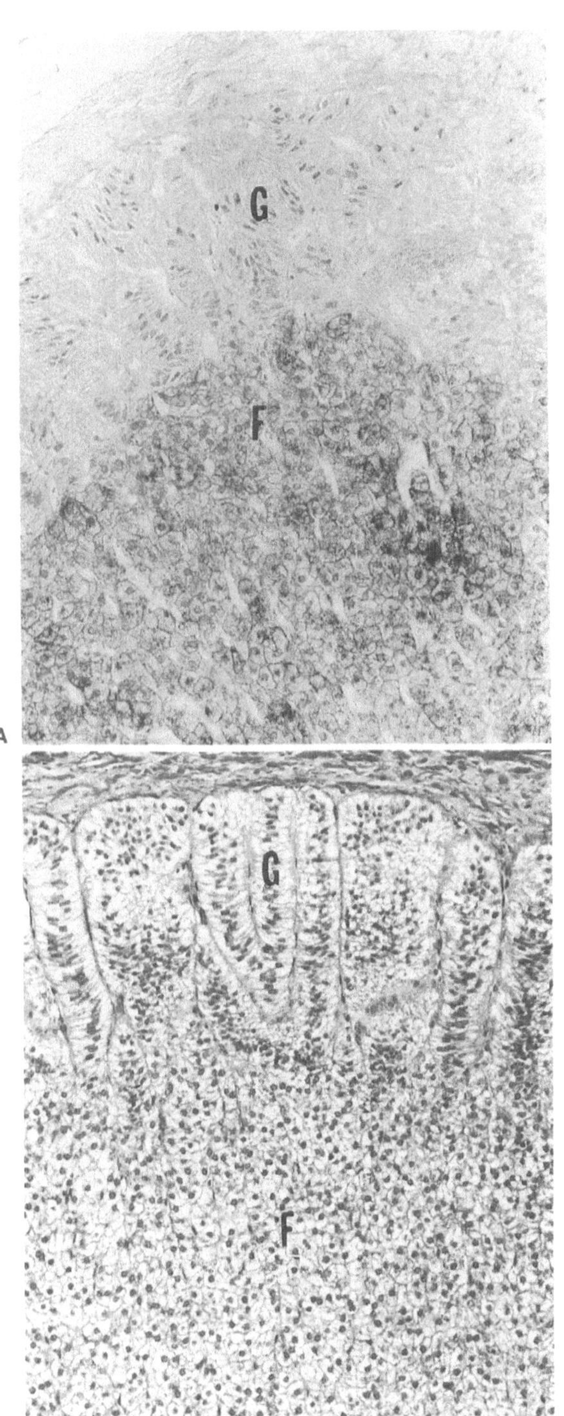

Fig. 439A,B. Immunolocalization of P450c17 (17α-hydroxylase) in the adrenal of dog. **A** Cytochrome P450c17, which plays key steps of cortisol biosynthesis but not involved in aldosterone production, is present in the zona fasciculata (*F*) but absent in the zona glomerulosa (*G*). **B** Dog adrenal. H&E, ×200

renocortical adenoma, functioning adrenocortical adenoma, and other adrenocortical disorders (Sasano 1992).

Ovary

The steroidogenic pathway and the enzymes involved are described in Fig. 441. In the ovary the production rates of various sex steroid hormones change episodically during the ovarian cycle, corresponding to the fluctuation of secretion of pituitary gonadotropin. In parallel with these hormonal changes, the ovarian morphology changes dramatically, with the development of follicles and corpus luteum. Therefore, to obtain a better understanding of ovarian sex steroid metabolism one must account for not only spatial distribution of steroidogenesis, i.e., which types of cells produce what steroids, but also the chronological distribution of steroidogenesis, i.e., at what stages of menstrual cycle these cells produce sex steroids. It has been postulated that at the follicular stage estrogen is synthesized exclusively in the granulosa cells derived from androgens produced in the theca interna (McNatty et al. 1979). This theory has been called the "two-cell theory" but had not been directly confirmed until immunolocalization of cytochromes P450cl7 and P450arom in normal cycling ovary was reported (Sasano et al. 1989c). P450c17, which catalyzes the biosynthesis of androgens, was localized exclusively in the theca interna (Fig. 442) while P450arom, which converts androgens to estrogens, was expressed exclusively in the membrana granulosa (Fig. 443). Similar patterns of immunolocalization were observed in the corpus luteum after ovulation. This finding confirmed the two-cell theory of estrogen biosynthesis. Immunolocalization and in situ hybridization of steroidogenic enzymes also contributed to the identification of the sites of specific steroidogenesis in various ovarian lesions associated with abnormalities of sex steroid metabolism, including ovarian sex cord stromal tumors, hyperthecosis, and Brenner's tumor (Sasano and Sasano 1989).

Testis

Androgen or testosterone production is considered to occur in Leydig's cells. Immunolocalization and in situ hybridization of steroidogenic

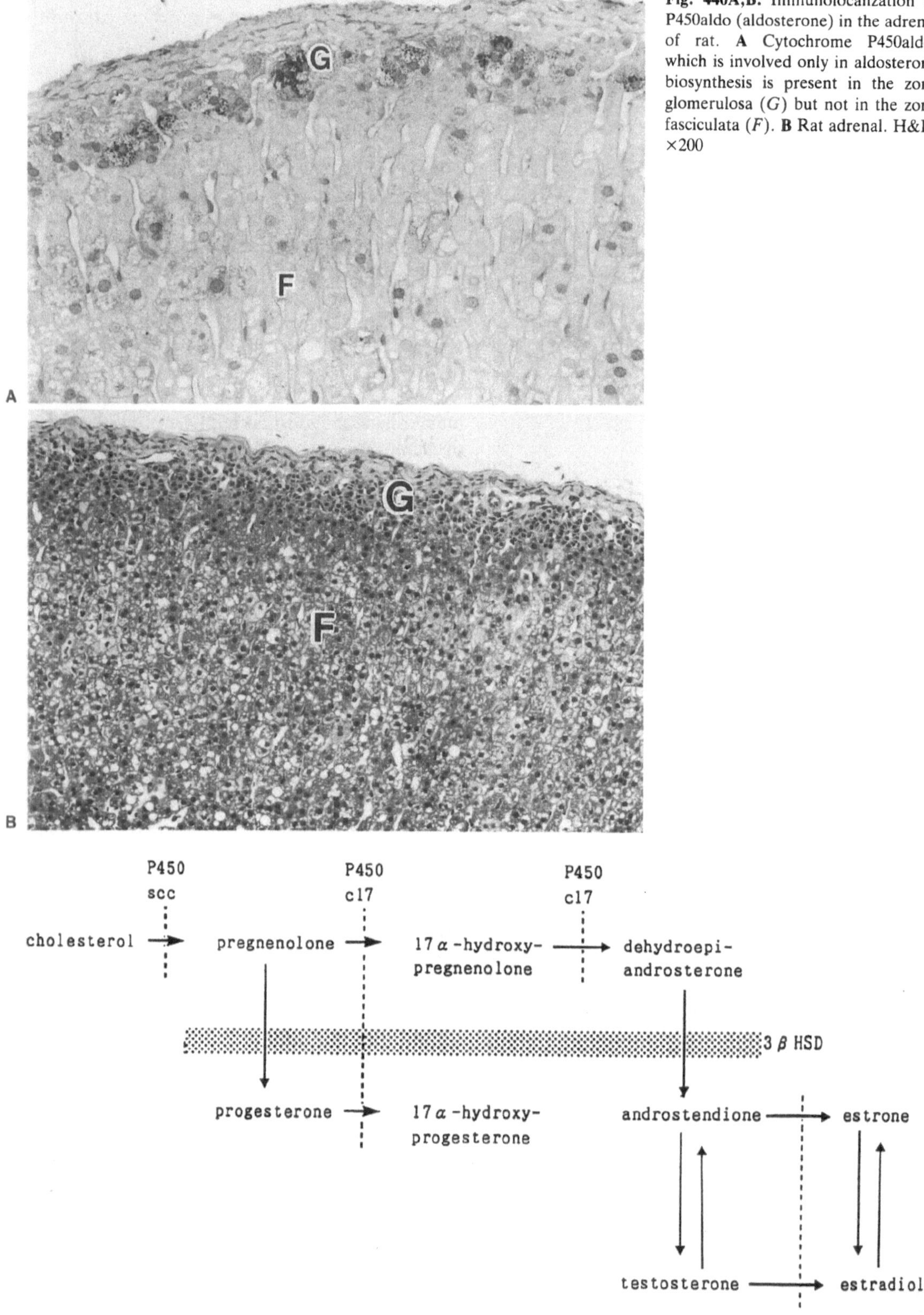

Fig. 440A,B. Immunolocalization of P450aldo (aldosterone) in the adrenal of rat. **A** Cytochrome P450aldo, which is involved only in aldosterone biosynthesis is present in the zona glomerulosa (*G*) but not in the zona fasciculata (*F*). **B** Rat adrenal. H&E, ×200

Fig. 441. Steroidogenic pathway in sex-steroid synthesis (human). *3β-HSD*, 3β-Hydroxysteroid dehydrogenase

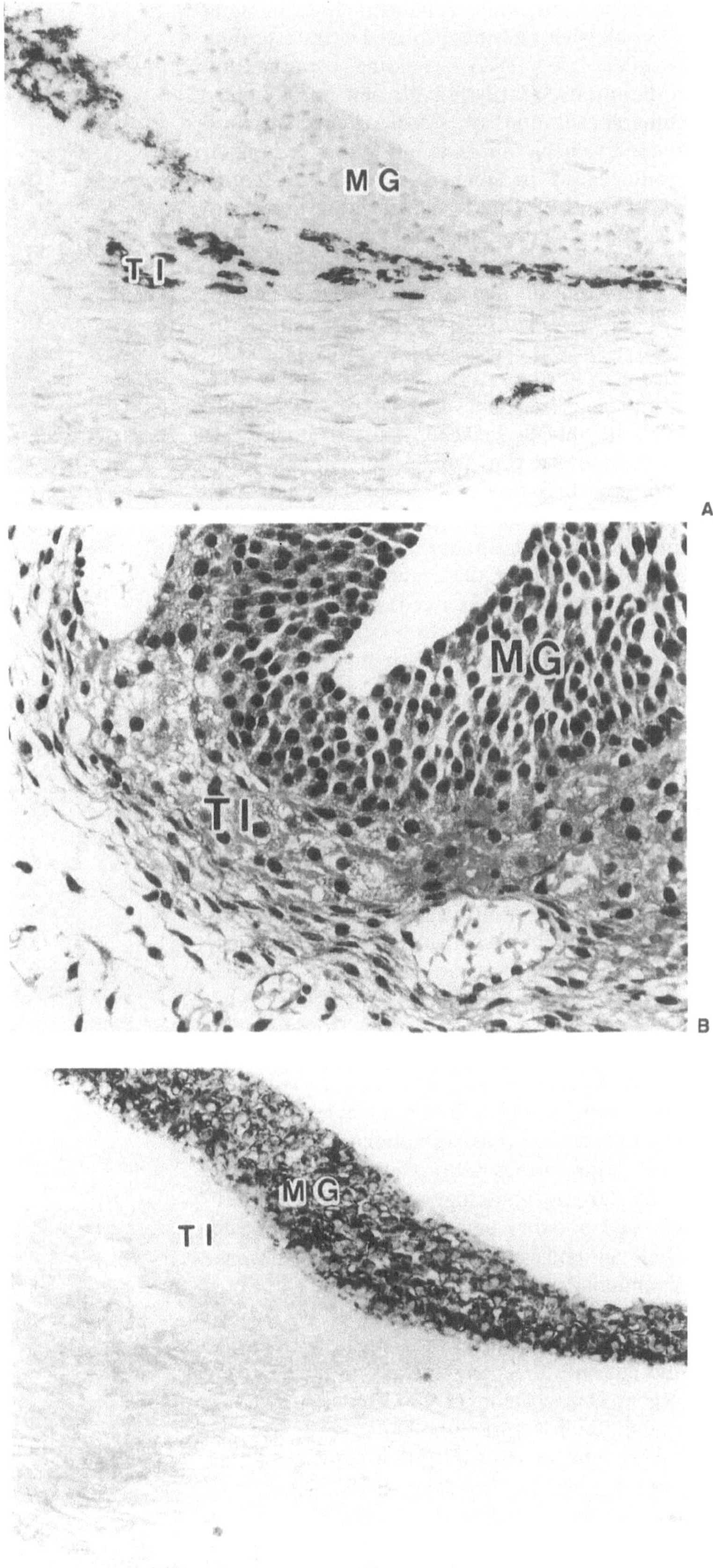

Fig. 442. A Immunolocalization of P450c17 in the ovarian follicle at follicular stage of ovarian cycle (human). P450c17 is exclusively localized in theca interna (*TI*) and absent in the membrana granulosa (*MG*). **B** Human ovary. H&E, ×300

Fig. 443. Immunolocalization of P450arom in the ovarian follicle at follicular stage of ovarian cycle (human). The same case as in Fig. 442. P450arom is exclusively present in the membrana granulosa (*MG*) but absent in the theca interna (*TI*). ×200

enzymes in testis, which demonstrated expression of steroidogenic enzymes involved in testosterone biosynthesis (Fig. 444A,B) is rather confirmatory but did not necessarily provide new information. Immunolocalization of steroidogenic enzymes provided valuable information on the analysis of steroidogenesis of human testicular sex cord-stromal tumors of the testis which are known to be associated with sex steroid abnormalities, but the analysis of neoplastic steroidogenesis has been very difficult due to the complicated histological features and the fact that sufficient preoperative hormonal evaluation is usually not performed. Leydig's cell tumor expressed all four steroidogenic enzymes, P450scc, P45Ocl7, P450arom, and 3β-HSD (Fig. 445A,B), indicating that this tumor can synthesize estrogen from cholesterol. In Sertoli's cell tumor the tumor cells with clear cytoplasm and without Reinke's crystals expressed P450scc, 3β-HSD, and P45Ocl7 (Fig. 446A,B), suggesting the capability of androgen production in these tumor cells.

Conclusion

Immunohistochemistry and in situ hybridization of steroidogenic enzymes demonstrated the capability of the cells to produce steroids which are catalyzed by the enzymes studied in the cells positive for immunoreactivity or mRNA hybridization signals. The availability of substrate and other conditions for enzymatic reactions also play important roles in the active secretion of steroids, and the presence or expression of the enzymes themselves alone may not be sufficient for definitive evidence of steroid secretion. However, the technique is valuable especially in the retrospective analysis of the specimens, endocrine pathological relationship, identification or characterization of steroid-producing cells, correlation of steroidogenesis with various factors and others in both human surgical pathology materials and specimens of laboratory animals. It is worthwhile to include antibodies against steroidogenic enzymes in immunohistochemistry laboratories.

Technical Notes. Antibodies against steroidogenic enzymes are commercially available from Oxygene Dallas, Dallas, TX 75240, USA. Among these antibodies, anti-3β-HSD can recognize the enzyme with accuracy in the specimens of rat, guinea pig, pig, dog, monkey, and human fixed in 10% formalin and embedded in paraffin.

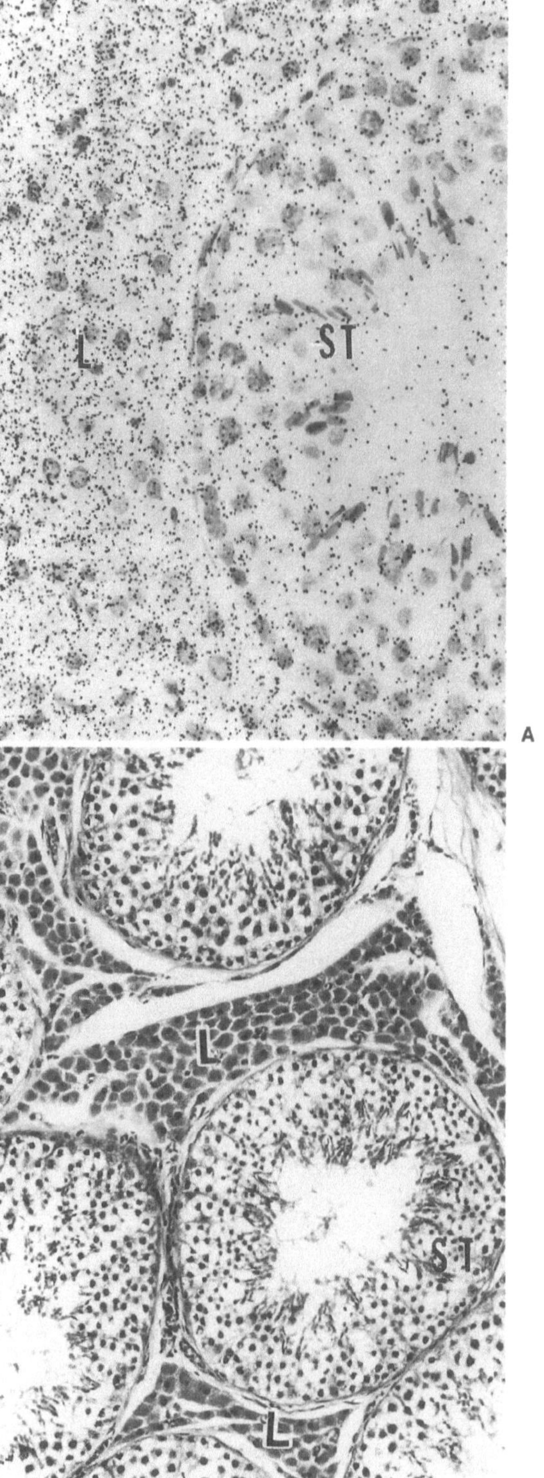

Fig. 444A,B. A In situ hybridization of P450c17 in porcine testis. *Black dots*, hybridization signals (silver grains on autoradiograph). *L*, Leydig's cells; *ST*, seminiferous tubules. **B** Porcine testis. H&E, ×340

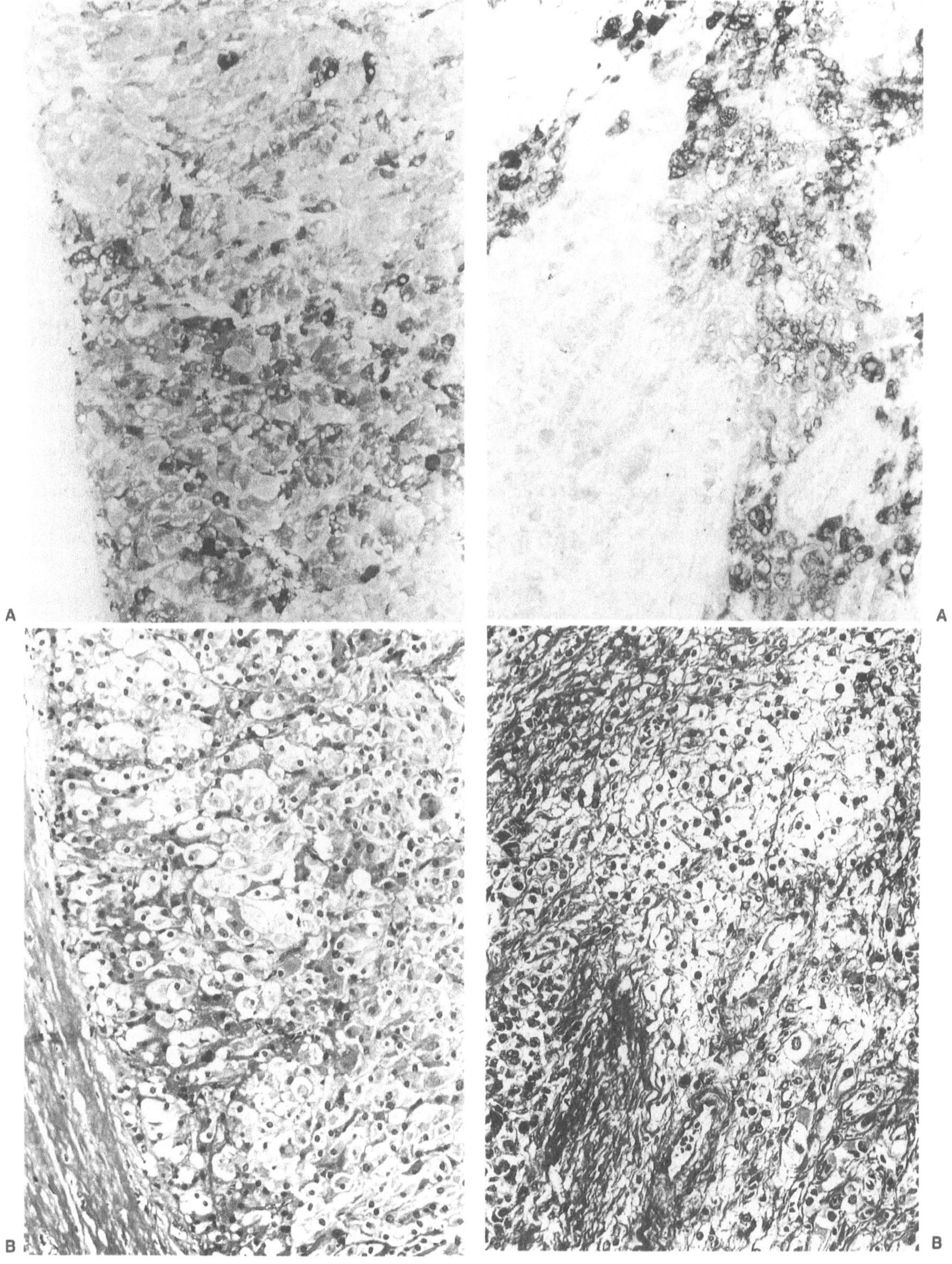

Fig. 445A,B. **A** Immunohistochemistry of 3β-HSD in testicular Leydig's cell tumor. **B** Corresponding section. H&E, ×200

Fig. 446A,B. **A** Immunohistochemistry of P450c17 in testicular Sertoli cell tumor. **B** Corresponding section. H&E, ×300. 3β-HSD, 3-Hydroxysteroid dehydrogenase

References

Hall PF (1985) Cytochrome P-450: physiology of steroidogenesis. Ann N Y Acad Sci 458:203–215

Kurman RJ, Goebelsmann U, Taylor CR (1979) Steroid localization in granulosa-theca tumors of the ovary. Cancer 43:2377–2384

Kurman RJ, Ganjei P, Nadji M (1984) Contributions of immunocytochemistry to the diagnoaia and study of ovarian neoplasms. Int J Gynecol Pathol 3:3–26

Lack EE, Travis WD, Ortel JE (1990) Adrenal cortical neoplasms. In: Lack EE (ed) Pathology of the adrenal glands. Churchill Livingstone, New York, pp 115–171

Martinelli G, Govoni E, Pileri S, Grigione FW, Doglioni C, Pelvsi G (1983) Sclerosing stromal tumor of the ovary. A hormonal, histochemical and ultrastructural study. Virchows Arch [A] 402:155–161

McNatty KP, Makris A, DeGrazia C, Osathmondh R, Ryan KJ (1979) The production of progesterone, androgen and estrogens by granulosa cells, thecal tissue and stromal tissue from human ovaries in vitro. J Clin Endocrinol Metab 49: 687–699

Sasano H (1992) New approaches in human adrenocortical pathology: assessment of adrenocortical function in surgical specimen of human adrenal glands. Endocr Pathol 3: 4–13

Sasano H, Sasano N (1989) What's new in the localization of sex steroids in the human ovary and its tumors? Pathol Res Pract 185:942–948

Sasano H, Mason JI, Sasano N (1989a) Immunohistochemical analysis of cytochrome P-450 17alpha-hydroxylase in pig adrenal cortex, testis and ovary. Mol Cell Endocrinol 62: 197–202

Sasano H, Mason JI, Sasano N (1989b) Immunohistochemical study of cytochrome P-450 17alpha-hydroxylase in human adrenal disorders. Hum Pathol 20:113–117

Sasano H, Okamoto M, Mason JI, Simpson ER, Mendelson CR, Sasano N, Silverberg SG (1989c) Immunolocalization of aromatase, 17alpha-hydroxylase and side-chain cleavage cytochromes P-450 in the human ovary. J Reprod Fertil 85: 163–169

Sasano H, Mason JI, Sasaki E, Yajima A, Kimura N, Namiki T, Sasano N, Nagura H (1990a) Immunohistochemical study of 3–beta hydroxysteroid dehydrogenase in sex cord-stromal tumors of the ovary. Int J Gynecol Pathol 9: 352–362

Sasano H, Mori T, Sasano N, Nagura H, Mason JI (1990b) Immunolocalization of 3beta-hydroxysteroid dehydrogenase in human ovary. J Reprod Fert 89:743–751

Sasano H, Nakashima N, Matsuzaki O, Kato H, Aizawa S, Sasano N, Nagura H (1992a) Testicular sex cord-stromal lesions: immunohistochemical anlysis of cytokeratin, vimentin and steroidogenic enzymes. Virchows Arch [A] 421:163–169

Sasano H, Miyazaki S, Sawai T, Sasano N, Nagura H, Funahashi H, Alba M, Demura H (1992b) Primary pigmented nodular adrenocortical disease (PPNAD): immunohistochemical and in situ hybridization analysis of steroidogenic enzymes in eight cases. Mod Pathol 5:23–29

Sasano H, Suzuki T, Nagura H, Nishikawa T (1993) Steroidogenesis in human adrenocortical carcinoma – biochemical activities, immunohistochemistry and in situ hybridization of steroidogenic enzymes and histopathological study in nine cases. Hum Pathol 24:397–404

Sasano N (1975) Functional pathology of human adrenal cortex. Trans Soc Pathol Jpn 63:31–54

Suzuki T, Sasano H, Sawai T, Mason JI, Nagura H (1992) Immunohistochemistry and in situ hybridization of P-45017α (17alphahydroxylase/17,20–lyase). J Histochem Cytochem 40:903–908

Wattenberg LW (1958) Microscopic histochemical demonstration of steroid 30-01-dehydrogenase in tissue sections. J Histochem Cytochem 6:225–232

Cell Proliferation in the Adult Adrenal Medulla: Chromaffin Cells as a Model for Indirect Carcinogenesis

Arthur S. Tischler

Cell Proliferation in the Rat Adrenal Medulla

Proliferation of chromaffin cells in the adrenal medulla of rats declines rapidly after birth. Mitotic figures are readily identified in histologic sections of postnatal rat adrenals but are rare after the age of 60 days. Adult rat chromaffin cells were generally regarded for many years as essentially postmitotic and terminally differentiated, until Malvaldi et al. (1968) examined serially sectioned adrenal glands of Wistar rats treated with colchicine to arrest dividing cells in mitosis and concluded that small numbers of chromaffin cells do divide in adults. The issue of the proliferative potential of adult chromaffin cells then remained largely dormant for almost two decades, until it was reopened (Tischler et al. 1988) in the course of investigating the pathogenesis of adrenal medullary tumors. These renewed studies were facilitated by the advent of the bromodeoxyuridine (BrdU) labeling technique, which incorporates immunocytochemically detectable BrdU into replicating DNA to label S-phase nuclei (Gratzner 1982; Figs. 447, 448).

Adrenal Medullary Lesions and Toxicological Risk Assessment

Hyperplasia and neoplasia are known to arise frequently in the rat adrenal medulla, either spontaneously in the course of aging or in response to a wide variety of xenobiotic agents. These lesions are rare in humans (Beard et al. 1983), mice (Wright et al. 1990), and other species. Because of their frequent occurrence in rat carcinogenicity studies adrenal medullary proliferative lesions have been an important problem in cancer risk assessment (Diener 1988). Nevertheless, there is at present little scientific basis for understanding their pathogenesis or their relevance to human cancer.
The incidence of adrenal medullary lesions in rats is variable and depends upon both endogenous and exogenous factors, as recently reviewed (Tischler and DeLellis 1988; Tischler and Coupland 1994). The former include the animals' strain, age and sex. For example, spontaneous adrenal medullary hyperplasia and neoplasia are frequent in Wistar, Wistar-derived, and Fischer 344 rats and are less frequent in the Charles River Sprague-Dawley strain. Within any given strain the lesions occur most frequently in older animals and in males. A partial list of exogenous factors associated with adrenal medullary neoplasia includes reserpine, nicotine, growth hormone, estrogen, nonsteroid anti-inflammatory agents, phosphodiesterase inhibitors, antithyroid drugs, retinoids, and neuroleptics. Also implicated are sugars and sugar alcohols that affect absorption of dietary calcium, miscellaneous drugs and toxins, and radiation (Tischler and DeLellis 1988). The diversity of these agents, together with the lack of evidence, in most instances, for ability to cause DNA damage, suggests that many of the agents influence the adrenal medulla indirectly rather than by a direct carcinogenic effect.

Indirect Effects of Xenobiotic Agents on Chromaffin Cell Proliferation: In Vivo and In Vitro Models

A series of in vivo investigations employing mitotic counts and BrdU labeling to study possible mechanisms of adrenal medullary carcinogenesis have shown that the rate of proliferation of rat chromaffin cells is markedly increased by

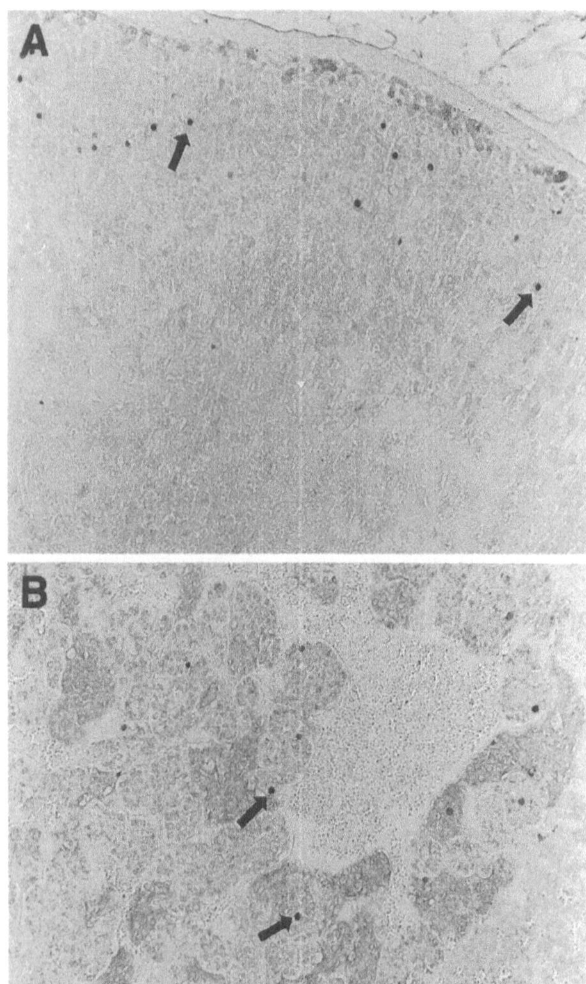

Fig. 447. S-phase nuclei demonstrated by immunocytochemical staining for BrdU in cortex **A** and medulla **B** of an adrenal gland of an adult rat fixed in glutaraldehyde 6 h after injection of BrdU. *Arrows*, representatively labeled nuclei. The thin band of labeled cells in the outer portion of the cortex is characteristic and serves as an internal positive control. The medulla has islands of norepinephrine-containing chromaffin cells with cytoplasm that appears darker than that of adjacent epinephrine cells due to oxidation of norepinephrine insolubilized by glutaraldehyde (Tischler et al. 1989). Occasional BrdU-labeled nuclei are present in both chromaffin cell types. A small area of the inner portion of the adrenal cortex without any labeled nuclei is present (**B**, *lower right*; ×120). Immunocytochemical staining for BrdU may be combined with staining for catecholamine biosynthetic enzymes to discriminate norepinephrine from epinephrine-producing cells in formalin-fixed tissue (Tischler et al. 1989)

short-term administration of reserpine (Tischler et al. 1988, 1989), one of the many agents associated with development of adrenal medullary tumors in long-term experiments. Proliferation is markedly decreased by unilateral adrenal denervation (Tischler et al. 1991). Reserpine is known to directly deplete catecholamine stores and to reflexly increase the activity of the splanchnic nerve endings innervating the adrenal medulla to stimulate both secretion and synthesis of catecholamines and other secretory granule constituents (Sietzen et al. 1987). The effects of reserpine and denervation on chromaffin cell proliferation therefore suggest that neurally derived signals might also normally regulate chromaffin cell number to meet changing phy-

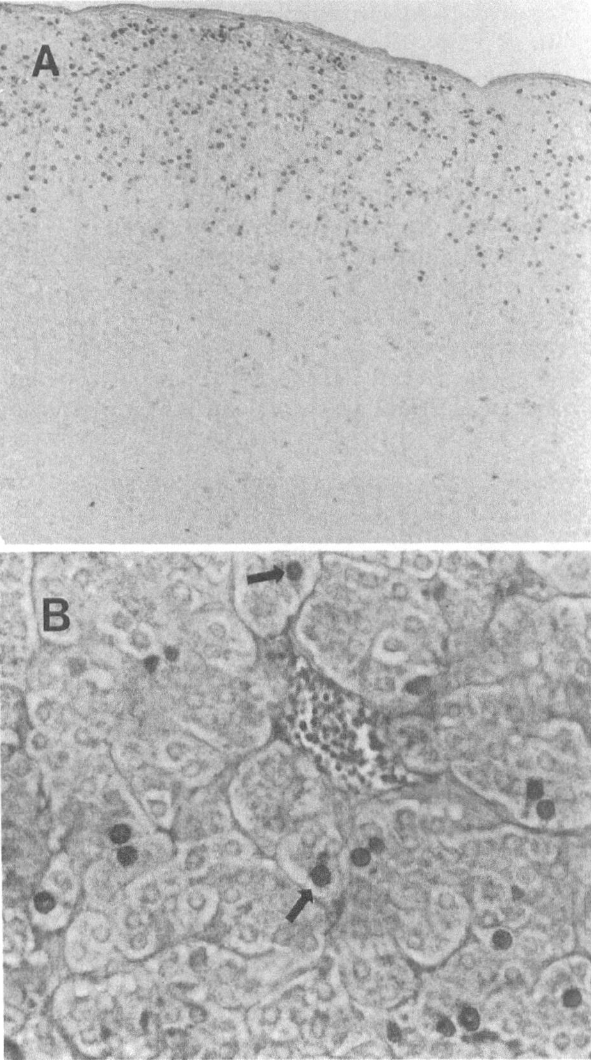

Fig. 448. S-phase nuclei demonstrated by immunocytochemical staining for BrdU in cortex (**A**) and medulla (**B**) of an adrenal gland fixed in buffered formalin after infusion of BrdU for 1 week by osmotic minipump (Tischler et al. 1991). Prolonged administration of BrdU results in accumulation of labelled nuclei, which may facilitate study of cell populations with low turnover. Labeled chromaffin cells can be distinguished from other types of labeled cells by their round nuclei of uniform size. Labeled chromaffin cells often appear as doublets after prolonged labelling. Representative chromaffin cells at high magnification (**B**, *arrows*). **A**, ×100; **B** ×400

siological needs. This regulation might in turn provide a common mechanism permitting pharmacologically diverse substances to produce adrenal medullary tumors secondarily to increased cell turnover, and interspecies differences in signaling pathways may contribute to the different frequencies of adrenal medullary tumors.

Studies attempting to characterize mitogenic signaling pathways in chromaffin cells are currently in progress. Functional innervation of the rat adrenal medulla occurs during the second week after birth (Slotkin et al. 1980). In cell cultures obtained from rats prior to the onset of innervation fetal and neonatal chromaffin cells proliferate in response to peptide growth factors, including nerve growth factor (NGF; Lillien and Claude 1985) and fibroblast growth factor (FGF; Claude et al. 1988; Stemple et al. 1988), suggesting that these or other humoral agents may regulate chromaffin cell number early in life.

Responsiveness to these agents has recently been shown to persist or recur in chromaffin cells cultured from adults (Mahanthappa et al. 1990; Tischler and Riseberg 1993; Fig. 449), providing an opportunity to study interactions of growth factor signaling pathways with pathways that might be activated by innervation.

Adult adrenal chromaffin cells are innervated by nerve endings that release acetylcholine and a variety of neuropeptides. The latter may include "conventional" peptide neurotransmitters such as vasoactive intestinal peptide (Maubert et al. 1990) and the recently described pituitary adenylate cyclase activating polypeptide, which may be a more potent physiological peptide released from the splanchnic nerve (Watanabe et al. 1992). Stimulation of muscarinic cholinergic receptors on chromaffin cells is known to result in activation of protein kinase C (Malhotra et al. 1989), while stimulation of neuropeptide receptors is known in some instances to activate adenylate cyclase and protein kinase A (Tischler et al. 1985; Watanabe et al. 1992).

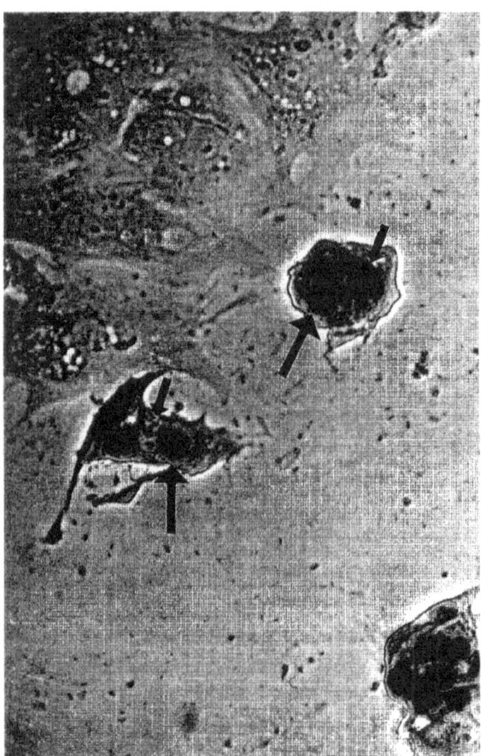

Fig. 449. Phase contrast photomicrograph of cell culture of adult rat adrenal medulla maintained with NGF for 4 days and then pulsed with BrdU. *Large arrows*, labeled chromaffin cell nuclei; *small arrows*, unlabeled nuclei. A cluster of labeled chromaffin cells is present (*bottom right*). Unlabeled fibroblasts are present in background (*top left*). Chromaffin cells in vitro are distinguished from other cell types by double-staining for BrdU and tyrosine hydroxylase, the rate-limiting enzyme in catecholamine synthesis (Tischler et al. 1992). Epinephrine- and norepinephrine-producing chromaffin cells can be discriminated from each other by additional staining for phenylethanolamine *N*-methyltransferase, as illustrated in color for the cells at the center of this figure in the reference by Tischler et al. 1993

Cell culture studies have been designed to mimic the effects of innervation by direct pharmacological activation of intracellular signaling pathways normally activated by neurotransmitters in adrenal medullary nerve endings. In cell cultures prepared from adult rats chromaffin cell proliferation is stimulated either by the peptide growth factors NGF and FGF or by activators of adenylate cyclase or protein kinase C. Differing susceptibilities to inhibitors and potentiators suggest that growth factors, cyclic AMP dependent protein kinases, and protein kinase C act via partially distinct and partially overlapping signaling pathways (Herman et al. 1991; Tischler et al. 1994). Moreover, activators of adenylate cyclase inhibit mitogenic responses to NGF or FGF (Frödin et al. 1993; Tischler et al. 1994).

To further assess the effects of conditions that mimic innervation chromaffin cells in vitro have been depolarized to induce ion fluxes through multiple voltage-gated channels that are normally activated after transsynaptic stimulation. Depolarization inhibits the mitogenic response to NGF, through a mechanism that apparently involves activation of voltage-gated calcium channels while sparing the response to phorbol esters that activate protein kinase C (Tischler et al. 1994). Considered together, currently available data suggest that during normal development neurally derived signals supersede growth factors in regulating proliferation of chromaffin cells by selectively inhibiting or coopting portions of growth factor signaling pathways. This switch from humoral to neural regulation might provide a means of fine-tuning proliferation through both positive and negative control (Tischler et al. 1994). This hypothesis requires further testing.

Interspecies Differences in Mitogenic Signaling: Relation to Tumor Susceptibility

The development of in vitro models for studying chromaffin cell proliferation has facilitated direct comparisons of cells from species with high and low frequencies of pheochromocytomas. Existing data based on studies of BrdU incorporation (Fig. 449) suggest that inability to respond to mitogenic signals or responsiveness to different types of signals may account for the low frequency of pheochromocytomas in species other than rats. These data are summarized in Table 29. Perhaps the most important observation from these studies is that human chromaffin cells show little or no labeling under any conditions thus far tested (Tischler and Riseberg 1993). This finding is important from the standpoint of toxicological risk assessment because it suggests that substances shown to cause pheochromocytomas in rats may pose no risk of pheochromocytoma to normal humans due to the absence of a susceptible population of proliferative cells.

Data related to the influence of sex, strain, and age on the development of pheochromocytomas are less clearcut. There appear to be only small differences or no differences in proliferative responses of rat chromaffin cells cultured from male or female, virgin, or postpartum animals. Likewise, only small differences are seen between cells from young adults or retired breeders or between cells from rats of strains with high or low frequencies of pheochromocytomas (A.S. Tischler and J. Riseberg, unpublished data). However, the significance of these in vitro findings is unclear because the possibility of age-, sex-, or strain-related differences in neural stimulation of chromaffin cells in vivo (McCarty and Kopin 1978; Gilad et al. 1979; Ito et al. 1986) has not been ruled out. An additional consideration is that the adult body weight of male rats continues to increase substantially during the first year of life for some time after the weight of females becomes stationary. It remains to be determined whether this difference is reflected in a higher basal rate of chromaffin cell proliferation in vivo in males than in females during the period of continued growth. An interesting intermediary position with respect to tumor frequency and cell proliferation is occupied by chromaffin cells from mice. These cells have been known for some time to proliferate throughout life in vivo (Jurecka et al. 1978; Monkhouse 1986) and also exhibit some proliferation in vitro (Table 29). In vivo proliferation appears in several common mouse strains to be strain-dependent and in most instances to be less robust than in rats (A.S. Tischler and R.M. McClain, unpublished data). In contrast to the extreme rarity of pheochromocytomas in humans (Beard et al. 1983), various mouse strains have reported frequencies of pheochromocytomas that range from 0% to approximately 5% (Wright et al. 1990). It is not yet known whether the mouse strains with the highest rates of chromaffin cell proliferation also have the highest frequencies of pheochromocytomas.

Perspectives

Several investigations suggest that increased cell proliferation plays a role in the induction of neoplasia in a variety of target tissues by chemicals

Table 29. Species differences in mitogenic responses of adult chromaffin cells in vitro

	BrdU Incorporation In Vitro				
	Control	NGF	FGF	Forskolin	PMA
Rat	<1%	≤40%	≤40%	≤40%	≤10%
Human	<0.01%	<0.01%	<0.01%	<0.01%	<0.01%
Bovine	0	0	0	0	0
Mouse	<0.1%	0	≤5%	≤1%	≤1%

The table summarizes BrdU labeling indices in chromaffin cell cultures maintained for 2–5 days with BrdU and the indicated mitogens. Quantitative data for rat and human cells are in references by Tischler et al. (1993) and Tischler and Riseberg (1993), respectively. Data for bovine and mouse (12/SVJ × C57BL/6J) are unpublished data from A.S. Tischler and J. Riseberg. Forskolin is an activator of adenylate cyclase. Strains of animals supplying cells: rat (3- to 9-month-old male and female F344 Charles River Sprague-Dawley), bovine (adult female), mouse (12/SVJ × C57BL/6J; 3-month-old females). PMA, Phorbol myristate acetate, an activator of protein kinase C; NGF, nerve growth factor; FGF, fibroblast growth factor; BrdU, bromodeoxyuridine.

that have no apparent mutagenic or DNA-damaging activity (Ames and Gold 1990). In most such instances the mitogenic stimuli leading to secondary neoplasms are hormonal or are the result of cell death. Pheochromocytomas in rats appear to constitute a novel subset of secondary neoplasms in which the initial proliferative signals that provide the backdrop for neoplastic transformation are neurally mediated. It might be speculated that the events initiating neoplasia are mutations or other genetic alterations leading to constitutive activation or defective inhibition of portions of intracellular signaling pathways normally under neural control. This hypothesis is supported by studies showing that loss of innervation is one of the earliest changes in rat pheochromocytomas (Tischler and DeLellis 1988). Understanding of the pathogenesis of pheochromocytomas will ultimately require both identification of the genetic alterations that cause these tumors and elucidation of the consequences of those alterations on intracellular signaling. This information should also resolve the persisting question of why rat pheochromocytomas are almost always noradrenergic (Tischler and DeLellis 1988). One possible candidate gene is the *ret* proto-oncogene, a transmembrane tyrosine kinase that has recently been implicated in the pathogenesis of human familial multiple endocrine neoplasia type 2A (Mulligan et al. 1993).

Although the rarity of pheochromocytomas in humans might be sufficiently accounted for by a low turnover of human chromaffin cells, it is not yet clear whether the same is true for mice. Another possible explanation involves greater susceptibility of rats to particular mutations. Resolution of this issue will ultimately also require identification of the genetic abnormality in pheochromocytomas.

It might finally be asked *why* stimulation of chromaffin cell proliferation should lead to a high frequency of pheochromocytomas, while tumors may be less common in other tissues with higher rates of cell turnover. This question may be asked of any tissues with different frequencies of tumors and probably has many answers. In the adrenal medulla the answer may lie in unusual vulnerability to oxidative damage, both from nitric oxide released as a neurotransmitter from nerve endings that might regulate catecholamine secretion (Bredt et al. 1990) and as a by-product of oxidative reactions involved in catecholamine synthesis or degradation (Graham 1979).

Acknowledgements. Research discussed in this review was support by NIH grant CA 48017 and by a grant from the ILSI Risk Science Institute.

References

Ames BN, Gold LS (1990) Too many rodent carcinogens: mitogenesis increases mutagenesis. Science 249:970–971

Beard MC, Sheps SG, Kurland LT, Carney JA, Lei JT (1983) Occurrence of pheochromocytoma in Rochester, Minnesota, 1950–1979. Mayo Clin Proc 58:802–804

Bredt DS, Hwang PM, Snyder SH (1990) Localization of nitric oxide synthase indicating a neural role for nitric oxide. Nature 347:768–770

Claude P, Parada IM, Gordon KA, D'Amore PA, Wagner JA (1988) Acidic fibroblast growth factor stimulates adrenal chromaffin cells to proliferate and to extend neurites, but is not a long-term survival factor. Neuron 1:783–790

Diener RM (1988) Pheochromocytomas and reserpine: review of carcinogenicity bioassay. J Am Coll Toxicol 7:95–109

Frödin M, Hannibal J, Fahrenkrug J, Gammeltoft S (1993) Inhibition of rat chromaffin cell growth by pituitary adenylate cyclase-activating polypeptide 38. Abstracts of 7th international symposium on chromaffin cell biology and pharmacology, p 90

Gilad GM, McCarty R, Weise VK, Kopin IJ (1979) Strain differences in regulation of the sympatho-adrenal system. Brain Res 176:380–384

Graham DG (1979) On the origin and significance of neuromelanin. Arch Pathol Lab Med 103:359–362

Gratzner HG (1982) Monoclonal antibody to 5-bromo- and 5-iododeoxyuridine: a new reagent for detection of DNA replication. Science 218:474–475

Herman MA, Schulz CA, Claude PA (1991) Chronic exposure to an activator of protein kinase C mimics early effects of NGF in chromaffin cells. Dev Biol 146:558–568

Ito K, Sato A, Sato Y, Suzuki H (1986) Increase in adrenal catecholamine secretion and adrenal sympathetic nerve unitary activities with aging in rats. Neurosci Lett 69: 263–268

Jurecka W, Lassmann H, Horandner H (1978) The proliferation of adrenal medullary cells in newborn and adult mice. Cell Tissue Res 189:305–312

Lillien LE, Claude P (1985) Nerve growth factor is a mitogen for cultured chromaffin cells. Nature 317:632–634

Mahanthappa NK, Gage FH, Patterson PH (1990) Adrenal chromaffin cells as multipotential neurons for autografts. Prog Brain Res 82:33–39

Malhotra RK, Wakade TD, Wakade AR (1989) Cross-communication between acetylcholine and VIP in controlling catecholamine secretion by affecting cAMP, inositol, triphosphate, protein kinase C and calcium in rat adrenal medulla. J Neurosci 9:4150–4157

Malvaldi G, Mencacci P, Viola-Magni MP (1968) Mitoses in the adrenal medullary cells. Experientia 24:475–476

Maubert E, Tramu G, Croix D, Beauvillain JC, Dupouy JP (1990) Colocalization of vasoactive intestinal polypeptide and neuropeptide Y immunoreactivities in the nerve fibers of the rat adrenal gland. Neurosci Lett 113:121–126

McCarty R, Kopin IJ (1978) Sympatho-adrenal medullary activity and behavior during exposure to footshock stress:

comparison of seven rat strains. Physiol Behav 21:567–572
Monkhouse WS (1986) The effect of in vivo hydrocortisone administration on the labelling index and size of chromaffin tissue in the postnatal and adult mouse. J Anat 144:133–144
Mulligan LM, Kwok JB, Healey CS et al (1993) Germ-line mutations of the *ret* proto-oncogene in multiple endocrine neoplasia type 2A. Nature 363:458–460
Sietzen M, Schober M, Fischer-Colbrie R, Scherman D, Sperk G, Winkler H (1987) Rat adrenal medulla: levels of chromogranins, enkephalins, dopamine beta-hydroxylase and the amine transporter are changed by nervous activity and hypophysectomy. Neuroscience 22:131–139
Slotkin TA, Smith PG, Lau C, Barsis DL (1980) Functional aspects of development of catecholamine biosynthesis and release in the sympathetic nervous system. In: Parvez H, Parvez S (eds) Biogenic amines in development. Elsevier/ North Holland, Amsterdam, pp 29–48
Stemple DL, Mahanthappa NK, Anderson DJ (1988) Basic FGF induces neuronal differentiation, cell division and NGF dependence in chromaffin cells: a sequence of events in sympathetic development. Neuron 1:517–525
Tischler AS, Coupland RA (1994) Changes in the structure and function of the rat adrenal medulla. In: Mohr U, Dungworth DL, Capen CC (eds) Pathobiology of the aging rat. vol 2. ILSI, Washington DC, pp 245–268
Tischler AS, DeLellis RA (1988) The rat adrenal medulla. II. Proliferative lesions. J Am Coll Toxicol 7:23–44 (review)
Tischler AS, Riseberg J (1993) Different responses to mitogenic agents by adult rat and human chromaffin cells in vitro. Endocr Pathol 4:15–19
Tischler AS, Perlman RL, Costopoulos D, Horwitz J (1985) Vasoactive intestinal peptide increases tyrosine hydroxylase activity in normal and neoplastic rat chromaffin cell cultures. Neurosci Lett 61:141–146
Tischler AS, DeLellis RA, Nunnemacher G, Wolfe HJ (1988) Acute stimulation of chromaffin cell proliferation in the adult rat adrenal medulla. Lab Invest 58:733–735
Tischler AS, Ruzicka LA, Donahue SR, DeLellis RA (1989) Chromaffin cell proliferation in the adult rat adrenal medulla. Int J Devel Neurosci 7:439–448
Tischler AS, McClain RM, Childers H, Downing J (1991) Neurogenic signals regulate chromaffin cell proliferation and mediate the mitogenic effect of reserpine in the adult rat adrenal medulla. Lab Invest 65:374–376
Tischler AS, Ruzicka LA, Riseberg JC (1992) Immunocytochemical analysis of chromaffin cell proliferation in vitro. J Histochem Cytochem 40:1043–1045
Tischler AS, Riseberg JC, Hardenbrook MA, Cherington V (1993) Nerve growth factor is a potent inducer of proliferation and neuronal differentiation for adult rat chromaffin cells in vitro. J Neurosci 13:1533–1542
Tischler AS, Riseberg JC, Cherington V (1994) Multiple mitogenic signalling pathways in chromaffin cells: a model for cell cycle regulation in the nervous system. Neurosci Lett 168:181–184
Watanabe T, Masuo Y, Matsumoto H, Suzuki N, Ohtaki T, Masuda Y, Kitadu C, Fujino M (1992) Pituitary adenylate cyclase activating polypeptide provokes cultured rat chromaffin cells to secrete adrenaline. Biochem Biophys Res Commun 182:403–411
Wright JA, Wadsworth PF, Stewart MG (1990) Neuron-specific enolase immunoreactivity in rat and mouse phaeochromocytomas. J Comp Pathol 102:475–478

Hyperplasia and Pheochromocytoma, Adrenal Medulla, Rat

John D. Strandberg

Synonyms. Hyperplasia: nodular medullary hyperplasia, medullary hypertrophy, preneoplastic nodules, focal and diffuse hyperplasia; pheochromocytoma: medullary tumors, medullary nodules, medullary adenomas, medullary secretory cell tumors.

Gross Appearance

Adrenal medullary hyperplasia usually cannot be observed grossly, but on occasion the lesion can be seen as unilateral or, more often, bilateral enlargement of the glands. Medullary tumors may be too small to alter the gross appearance of the glands, or they may cause unilateral or bilateral enlargement. The cut surface of the medulla may have a nodular outline and may be fleshy white or reddish-brown due to an extensive vascular network in the tumor. Metastases of malignant pheochromocytomas occur rarely and are usually discovered only upon microscopic examination (Coleman et al. 1977; Anderson and Capen 1978; Goodman et al. 1979; Altman and Goodman 1979).

Microscopic Features

In formalin-fixed sections stained with hematoxylin and eosin (H&E) *diffuse hyperplasia* of the medulla is characterized by an increased number of medullary cells without the formation of nodules. Full cross-sections of the gland are necessary to detect diffuse medullary hyperplasia. In these cases the medullary cells are polygonal in shape and are arranged in nests and cords which are wider than those seen in the normal adrenal medulla. Although the number of cells in the medulla is increased, mitotic figures are rarely encountered. The adrenal cortex may be thinner than normal, but the cells at the inner margin are not compressed by the expanding medulla. Diffuse hyperplasia has been recognized by several authors and may be confirmed by morphometric techniques to assess medullary and cortical volumes (Tischler and DeLellis 1988a,b). It should be clearly differentiated from focal or nodular hyperplasia (Figs. 450, 451).

Pheochromocytomas in their earliest stages are found in the adrenal medulla and consist of cells that may resemble or differ from the normal medullary secretory cells. The large polyhedral cells with centrally placed spherical nuclei found in the normal medulla are replaced by similar cells with cytoplasm of less volume, but which is more basophilic in staining reaction and generally has larger hyperchromic nuclei. In the neoplastic state the normal packets of cells, surrounded by a delicate stroma, become larger, irregular in size, and more richly vascularized. In some tumors the cells may become individually isolated and quite pleomorphic, with giant bizarre nuclei; some contain abnormal mitotic figures. At times it is difficult in H&E stained sections to differentiate pheochromocytomas from adrenal cortical tumors. Zones of necrosis may be observed.

Replacement of cells of adjacent medulla and cortex is a feature of all pheochromocytomas. Compression is more often the hallmark of well-differentiated tumors. Invasion of cortical tissue, adrenal capsule, lymphatics, capillaries, vena cava, and periadrenal adipose tissue is a distinguishing feature of less differentiated or malignant pheochromocytoma. Metastasis to lymph nodes, lungs, or other organs is also characteristic of the malignant variety (Figs. 452–455).

Ultrastructure

Although by light microscopy all adrenal medullary cells appear similar, electron microscopy of adrenals from adult rats has revealed two major cell types (Eranko 1960) as well as one minor one (Tischler and DeLellis 1988). In preparations fixed with glutaraldehyde and postfixed with osmium tetroxide, norepinephrine is rendered insoluble and hence more electron dense. About 26% of the cells, type I, contain large, membrane-bound cytoplasmic granules measuring up to 0.3 µm in diameter and consisting of a highly electron-dense amorphous core, often eccentrically placed and separated from the unit membrane by a wide, electron-lucent space. These granules contain norepinephrine and are located in cells smaller than those secreting epinephrine. In the latter cells the granules containing epinephrine are somewhat smaller, measure up to 0.2 µm in diameter, and have a core which is more electron lucent. Thus, electron lucent granules indicate either epinephrine secretion or depleted norepinephrine granules. The secretory granules remain the major ultrastructural feature used to identify these cells and to separate them from tumors of the adrenal cortex. In addition, a third cell type representing about 1% of the cell population in the adrenal medulla has been termed small-granule containing cells (Tischler and DeLellis 1988). These have ultrastructural features intermediate between epinephrine and norepinephrine secreting cells and also possess synaptic vesicles. A clonal line of pheochromocytoma cells has been developed which respond to nerve growth factor in vitro by the development of neuritic processes (Tischler and Greene 1978).

Differential Diagnosis

Distinguishing features of proliferative lesions of the adrenal medulla of the rat may be described as follows.

Diffuse hyperplasia of the adrenal medulla (p. 411, this volume) involves all or most of the medullary secretory cells, which are increased in number and size and expand the volume of the medulla but do not form nodules. The cortex may appear thin but is not visibly compressed or invaded.

Focal or nodular hyperplasia (p. 412, this volume) is recognized by one or more focal accumulations of medullary cells, which are distinguished from preexisting cells by somewhat more basophilic cytoplasm and relatively larger nuclei. These cells do not invade or compress surrounding medulla or cortex. They tend to have uniform cytologic

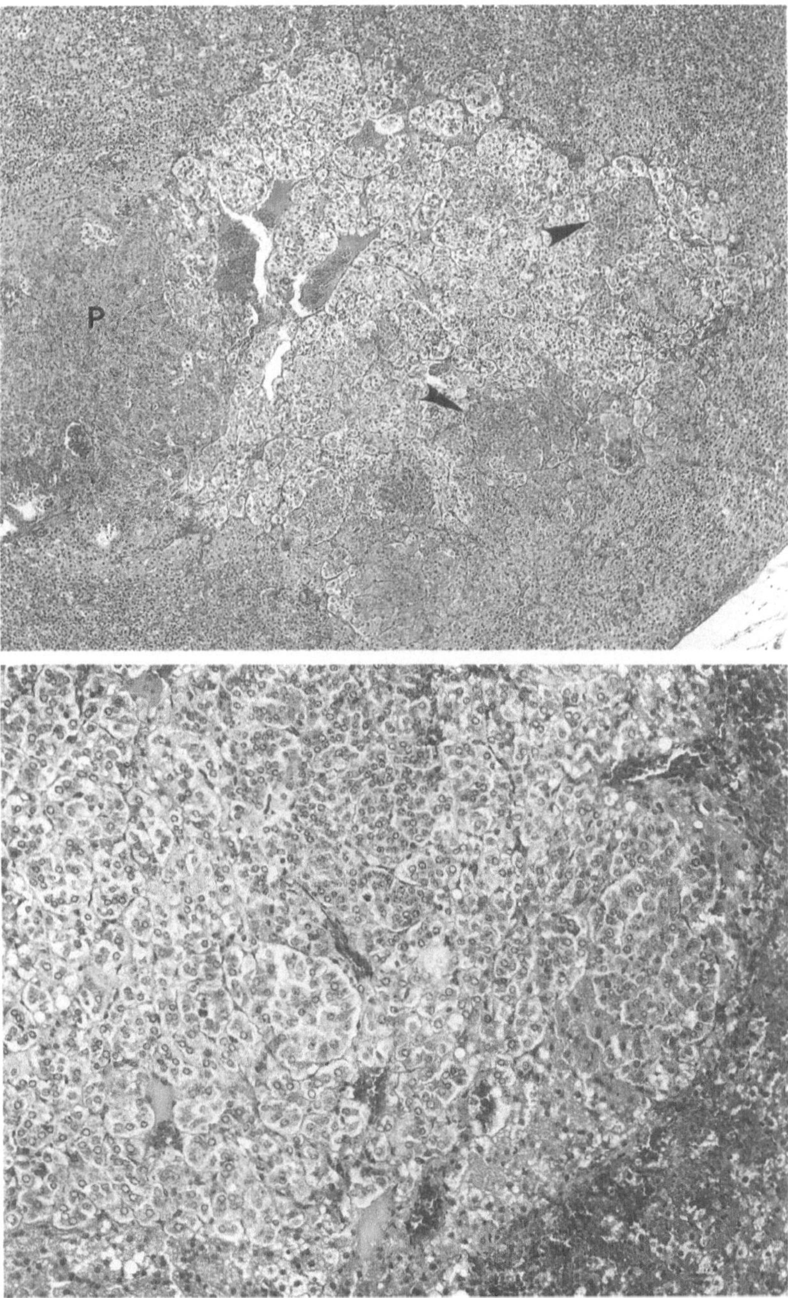

Fig. 450. (*above*) Focal hyperplasia, adrenal medulla, 24-month-old female Wistar rat. Note several foci of medullary hyperplasia (*arrows*), and a larger pheochromocytoma (*P*). Helley's fixative. H&E, ×50

Fig. 451. (*below*) Focal hyperplasia, adrenal medulla, aged Fischer 344 rat. Disorganized cords and nests of polygonal cells do not noticeably compress surrounding tissues. Formalin fixative. H&E, ×155

composition, with a high nuclear/cytoplasmic ratio.

Pheochromocytoma (benign, differentiated, or not otherwise specified) also arises in the adrenal medulla and is made up of neoplastic medullary secretory cells which grow and expand their total mass to compress and displace adjacent medulla or cortex.

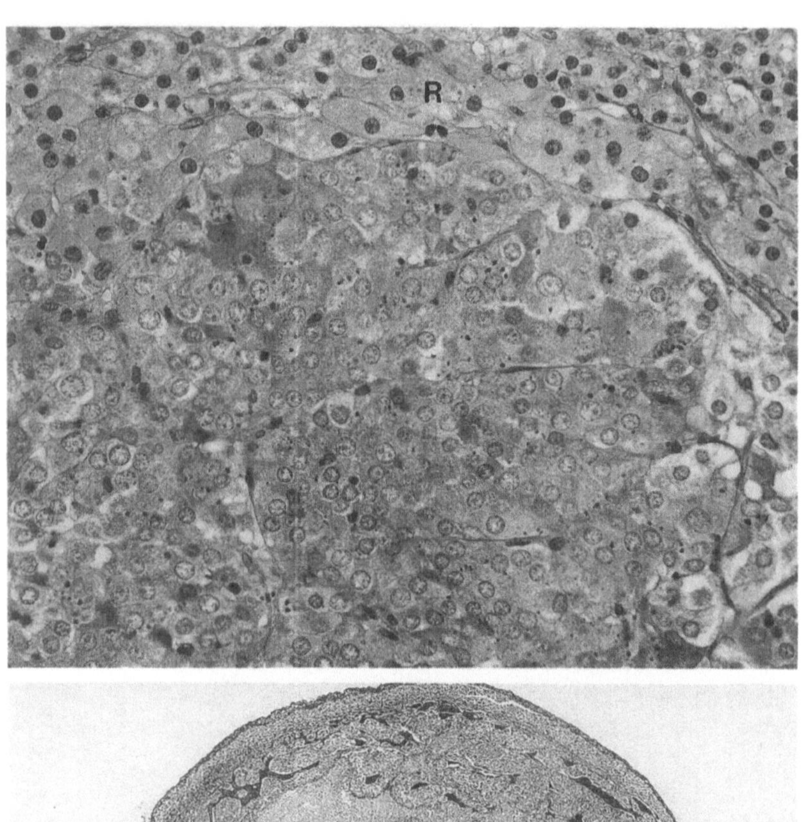

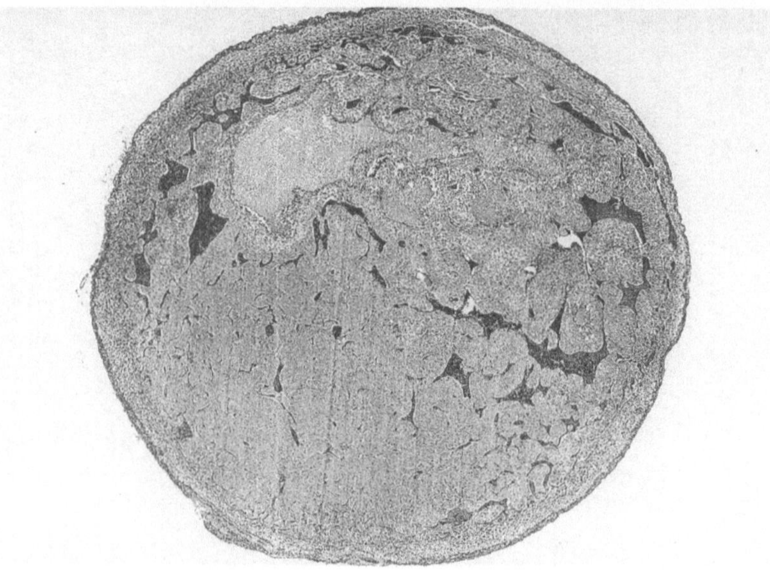

Fig. 452. (*above*) High magnification of pheochromocytoma in Fig. 450. Compression of zona reticularis (*R*). Adrenal medullary cells contain hematoxyphilic bodies as the result of use of Helley's fixative. H&E, ×340

Fig. 453. (*below*) A large pheochromocytoma distends the medulla of the adrenal from an aged Fischer 344 rat. The cortex is intact although compressed. Large vascular sinues are present within the tumor. Formalin. H&E, ×22

Malignant or undifferentiated pheochromocytomas are often cytologically similar to the differentiated type but grow by invading adjacent medulla, cortex, capsule, and blood, and lymph vessels. Some may extend into the adjacent adipose tissue or metastasize to lymph nodes, lungs or other organs.

It is obvious from the literature that not all authors agree with the above criteria. Considerable variation is found in terminology applied to cellular proliferations in the rat adrenal medulla. The difficulty in differentiating hyperplastic from benign and malignant lesions was further addressed by Tischler et al. (1990) in a study in

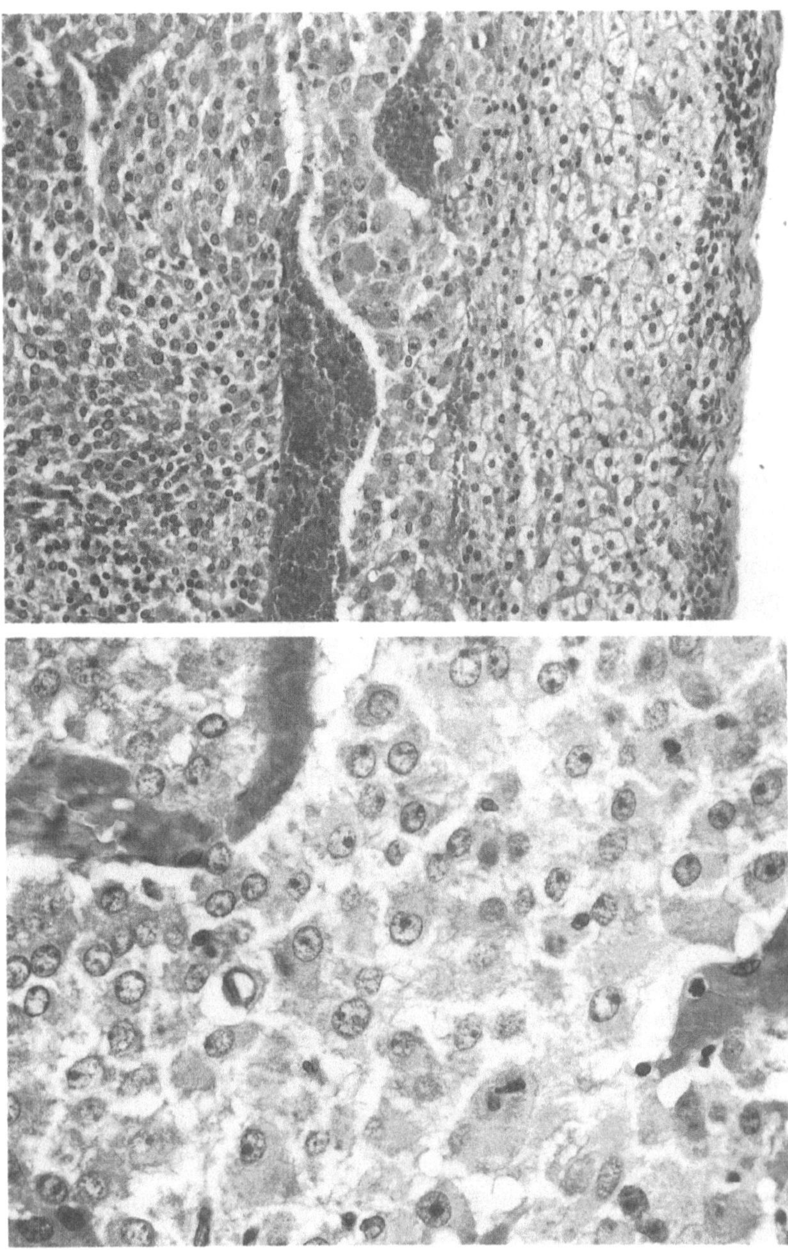

Fig. 454. (*above*) Higher magnification of Fig. 453; red cells fill sinusoidal spaces and large polygonal cells comprise the tumor. Formalin, H&E, ×22

Fig. 455. (*below*) Large pleomorphic cells of a pheochromocytoma lose special cytoplasmic staining following formalin fixation. Moderate pleomorphism of cells and nuclei may be observed. H&E, ×600

which lesions diagnosed as pheochromocytomas or nodular hyperplasias were assessed for the presence of norepinephrine production, a feature uniformly found in pheochromocytomas; they found it impossible to differentiate hyperplastic from neoplastic lesions on histologic grounds alone. A pragmatic descriptive approach to classification of proliferative medullary lesions has evolved (Tischler and Coupland 1994). Differentiation of medullary hyperplasia from pheochromocytoma is sometimes made on subjective grounds (Gilman et al. 1953; Yeakel 1947).

Hollander and Snell (1976) prefer to call all medullary cell proliferative lesions pheochromocytomas because they are unable to find any reliable histologic criteria to separate neoplastic from hyperplastic lesions. At the other extreme, Thompson et al. (1981) limit the diagnosis of pheochromocytoma to those proliferative lesions exhibiting excessive storage and synthesis of catecholamines.

It is evident that reports currently in the literature cannot be compared without careful consideration of the criteria used by each author for diagnosis of each entity. Future reports must continue to include precise criteria adhered to by the pathologist who conducted the study. Lesions of the adrenal medulla must be differentiated from infoldings or islands of normal cortical cells which may be encountered in a single section of the gland. Growth of neoplastic cells from the medulla into the cortex may produce a similar dilemma (Kovacs and Horvath 1973). Other neoplasms encountered in the adrenal medulla include ganglioneuromas (p. 427, this volume), neuroblastomas (p. 433), and neoplasms of the cortex (p. 438). Cortical neoplasms, especially those with a trabecular pattern, may resemble medullary proliferations, especially in H&E stained preparations. Pheochromoblastomas are also diagnosed by some investigators (Mohr et al. 1969). Interstitial cell tumors of the testis have been cited as neoplasms which may metastasize to the adrenal in some species and be mistaken for primary tumors (Thompson et al. 1981). However, this event has not been unequivocally demonstrated in the rat.

The terms *focal* or *nodular hyperplasia* should be reserved for those lesions which are characterized by aggregates of medullary cells which appear distinct and cytologically different from adjacent medullary cells. Cells comprising foci of nodular hyperplasia generally have relatively high nuclear/cytoplasmic ratios, with basophilic cytoplasm. Since hyperplastic medullary cells cannot be reliably distinguished from neoplastic medullary cells using standard morphological techniques, the distinction between hyperplastic and neoplastic nodules may be arbitrary. As a general rule, hyperplastic nodules are of smaller diameter and do not compress or invade adjacent medullary or cortical tissue (Figs. 450, 451). Most authors have relied on sections of formalin-fixed tissue stained with H&E to identify cells of the adrenal medulla. Others have depended on demonstration of chromaffin-positive material in the cytoplasm of the cells. Both major cell types, adrenaline-secreting and noradrenaline-secreting, in the rat adrenal medulla give a positive chromaffin reaction. Thus, this technique can be very helpful in identifying the cells as being of adrenal medullary origin. Staining intensity may vary in both normal and proliferative medullary cells. In a review of the rat adrenal Thompson et al. (1981) have summarized the other techniques which can be used to identify cellular subtypes in the medulla. These include the iodate reaction, the argentaffin reaction, and formalin-induced fluorescence, among others. These three reactions are used principally to differentiate noradrenaline-containing cells from those containing adrenaline or to demonstrate catecholamines.

Biologic Features

Natural History. In hyperplasia the adrenal medulla, as other endocrine organs, becomes hyperplastic in response to a variety of stimuli; these have included thiouracil, reserpine (Tischler et al. 1988), growth hormones (Russfield 1967), and nicotine (Eranko 1960; Staemmler 1935). Functional hyperplasia is often manifested uniformly throughout the medulla. However, in many of these hyperplastic states focal proliferations also can be recognized histologically. Because of the small size and irregular configuration of the gland complete cross-sections are necessary to recognize these lesions. Serial sectioning of glands gives even more information (Tischler and Greene 1978), but this technique is obviously not practicable in many instances. This author and others (Tischler 1989; Tischler and Coupland 1994; Hollander and Snell 1976; Staemmler 1935) feel that proliferative lesions of the adrenal medulla progress from hyperplasia to neoplasia, and that the neoplastic lesions can be properly termed pheochromocytomas. Progression of focal hyperplasia to pheochromocytoma is further suggested by increasing frequency in older animals. In some rat strains pheochromocytomas are found in well over 50% in animals over 2 years of age. There is a definite tendency for hyperplasia to appear prior to pheochromocytomas. However, these views are not universally held. In a discussion of the rat adrenal medulla Thompson et al. (1981) argued vehemently against both points, citing several sources dealing with both human and murine endocrine pathology. Adrenal medullary nodules have also been observed in aging male Long-Evans rats in association with proliferative lesions in other endocrine organs. These were viewed as a model of mixed multiple endocrine syndrome (Lee et al. 1982).

Secretory Activity. Only a few studies (Warren and Chute 1972; DeLellis et al. 1973; Cheng 1980) have been directed toward determining the secretory activity of hyperplasia or pheochromocytoma of the rat adrenal medulla; yet good evidence does exist of such activity. In the case of the transplantable pheochromocytoma in the NEDH rat, transplant-bearing animals have shown evidence of hypertension, elevated urinary catecholamine metabolites, renal arterial and arteriolar sclerosis, and focal myocardial degeneration (Warren and Chute 1972). These transplantable pheochromocytomas were demonstrated to contain high intracellular concentrations of primary catecholamines, indicated by the formaldehyde-vapor-induced fluorescence reaction (DeLellis et al. 1973).

Pathogenesis. Tischler and colleagues (1988) demonstrated that reserpine directly depletes catecholamine stores and increases neurogenic stimulation of chromaffin cells and proposed that prolongation of processes which increase proliferation of mature chromaffin cells may lead to pathologic proliferative states. This mitogenic effect was shown to be mediated by neurogenic signals and could be prevented by denervation of the gland (Tischler et al. 1991). Medullary cell proliferation may be induced by administration of xylitol and other polyols; an inhibitory effect on catecholamine synthesis coupled with stimulation of the medulla was postulated as the mechanism for hyperplasia (Boelsterli and Zbinden 1985). Dietary factors which increase absorption of calcium from the bowel have been noted to play a role in induction of this lesions; these factors include excessive food intake, excessive dietary calcium and phosphate and excessive intake of such food components as vitamin D and poorly absorbable carbohydrates leading to increased calcium absorption (Roe and Bar 1985). In these states the cellular proliferation is accompanied by an increased production of norepinephrine and a decrease in epinephrine/norepinephrine ratios (Tischler 1989). It has been noted that almost all adrenomedullary lesions in rats occur in animals with a high incidence of other endocrine tumors and thus might be analogous to multiple endocrine neoplasia syndromes seen in human populations (Tischler and DeLellis 1988). Control of cellular proliferation by neurogenic and hormonal signals are mechanisms which have been proposed to be of importance in hyperplasia and neoplasia of the adrenal medulla (Tischler et al. 1989, 1991a). Representatives of mechanisms by which this can be accomplished are outlined below.

Etiology. A variety of techniques and agents have been reported to induce adrenal medullary hyperplasia and neoplasia. Tischler et al. (1989) summarized these and grouped them into four major methods of action (Table 30). In all cases it appears that the neoplastic cells secrete norepinephrine. Tischler (1989) noted that the major difference between rat and human lesions is in their clinical context; human pheochromocytomas are solitary and sporadic and those in the rat are often multifocal and bilateral and associated with other proliferative endocrine lesions.

A substantial review of agents known to produce pheochromocytomas was published by Tischler and DeLellis (1988). It included those noted in Table 30 which groups these agents by the mechanism of action. Among those which affect the hypothalamic-endocrine axis is growth hormone; Russfield (1967) reported that growth

Table 30. Agents associated with proliferative changes in the rat adrenal medulla (based on Tischler et al. 1989)

Agents affecting hypothalamic-endocrine axis
Growth hormone
Estrogen
Antithyroid drugs
Alloxan
Neuroleptics
Agents affecting autonomic nervous system
Nicotine
Reserpine
Timolol
Dietary factors
Excess food
Excess Ca^{2+} intake or absorption
Miscellaneous
Gemfibrozil (hypolipidemic)
Zomepirone (anti-inflammatory)
Retinol Acetate
1,4-Dioxane
Diphenylamine
Ethylene glycol monoethyl ether
Bis(tri-*n*-butyltin)oxide (Wester et al. 1990)
Radiation

hormone administration to 40 Long-Evans rats resulted in adrenal medullary hyperplasia and pheochromocytomas. Similar results were reported by Moon et al. (1950).

The autonomic nervous system mediates the proliferative process for another group of chemicals reported to cause these lesions. These include nicotine (first studied by Staemmler (1935), thiouracil, and reserpine. Reserpine has been shown to increase the rate of proliferation of chromaffin cells in short-term experiments and also to induce adrenal medullary tumors in long-term experiments (Diener 1988). The action of reserpine in inducing mitosis in the medulla was shown to be neurologically mediated (Tischler et al. 1991a). The bioassay of reserpine with its conclusion that adrenal medullary hyperplasias and pheochromocytomas were produced was earlier the focus of voluminous rebuttals by Thompson and his coworkers (Bioassay of Reserpine 1980; Diener et al. 1980; Thompson et al. 1981).

As noted above, increased absorption of calcium from the bowel has been found to induce these lesions; this can result from excessive food intake or dietary calcium and phosphate and excessive vitamin D and poorly absorbable carbohydrates leading to increased calcium absorption (Roe and Bar 1985). In these states the cellular proliferation is accompanied by an increased production of norepinephrine and a decrease in epinephrine/norepinephrine ratios (Tischler 1989).

A miscellaneous group of agents with a range of possible actions have also been reported (Tischler et al. 1989) and are listed in Table 30. Several investigative groups have observed adrenal medullary tumors in irradiated animals (Rosen et al. 1961; Warren and Chute 1972). Castanera et al. (1968) reported adrenal medullary tumors in male Sprague-Dawley rats receiving whole-body X-ray or neutron irradiation. Of 121 tumors in 309 rats all but four were termed pheochromocytomas; three were pheochromoblastomas and one a myelolipoma.

An extensive literature has developed on a clonal line of rat pheochromocytoma cells (PC12 cells) both in vivo and in vitro. PC12 cells were first isolated by Greene and Tischler (1976) from a murine pheochromocytoma. These cells produce a range of normal products including norepinephrine and dopamine and resemble immature rat chromaffin cells. Neuronal differentiation of PC12 cells can be induced (Greene and Tischler 1976) and populations can be induced to produce neuropeptides as well (Tischler et al. 1991b).

Frequency. Adrenal medullary hyperplasia and pheochromocytoma are lesions frequently encountered in rats of several strains over 12 months of age (Crain 1958). Significant variability in incidence has been noted between laboratories, however, even when the same strain is considered (Tarone et al. 1981). They are often seen in Fischer and Wistar rats and are observed somewhat more frequently in male animals. Osborne-Mendel rats, which have a high incidence of cortical neoplasms, develop relatively few medullary tumors. In Table 31 the frequencies of natural and induced lesions are abstracted from the literature. Reviews of the frequency of these lesions have been conducted by Thompson et al. (1981) and more recently by Tischler and DeLellis (1988b).

Pheochromocytomas are frequently encountered in several strains of rats over 12 months of age (Crain 1958). However, significant variability occurs in the numbers found in the same strain in different laboratories (Tarone et al. 1981). Data on the reported frequency of medullary lesions in various strains of rats, from various laboratories, are presented in Table 31 (see also MacKenzie and Garner 1973 and Squire et al. 1978).

Comparison with Other Species

Hyperplasia of the adrenal medulla has been noted in the mouse (p. 421), although it appears less frequently than in the rat. Adrenal medullary hyperplasia and pheochromocytoma have been associated in human patients (Sipple's syndrome, type II multiple endocrine adenomatosis) with medullary thyroid carcinoma and parathyroid hyperplasia. This familial disease, inherited as an autosomal dominant trait, has some features of the adrenal lesions in the rat (DeLellis et al. 1973). Further studies are needed to ascertain whether other points of affinity result from any other comparable syndrome in rat and man.

Pheochromocytomas encountered in humans, cattle, mice, and dogs are histomorphologically similar to those observed in the rat. The variation in cell populations seen in the rat have been noted earlier. The incidence of familial pheochromocytomas in humans is comparable to the high prevalence of these lesions observed in certain rat

Table 31. Spontaneous tumors of the adrenal medulla, rat

Strain	Age	Lesion	Frequency (%)		Reference
			Male	Female	
Sprague-Dawley	–	Pheochromocytoma	2/82 (2.4)	5/43 (11.6)	Thompson et al. 1961
Sprague-Dawley	18 mo	Pheochromocytoma	2/181 (1.1)	2/179 (1.1)	Prejean et al. 1973
Sprague-Dawley	–	Pheochromocytoma	14/42 (33.3)	2/39 (5.1)	Suzuki et al. 1979
Sprague-Dawley (Holtzman)	1–18 mo	Pheochromocytoma	4/3387 (0.12)	3/1669 (0.18)	Schardein et al. 1968
Sprague-Dawley	18–31 mo	Pheochromocytoma	7/45 (15.6)	4/98 (4.1)	Thompson and Hunt 1963
Sprague-Dawley	29 mo	Pheochromocytoma	10/22 (45)		Ribelin et al. 1984
Sprague-Dawley	Life span	Proliferative lesions	(31)	(5)	Tischler and DeLellis 1988b
SD JCL	Life span	Proliferative lesions	(13)	(3)	Tischler and DeLellis 1988b
ACI	12–18 mo >18 mo	Pheochromocytoma	(0) (7)	(5) (4)	Hollander and Snell 1976
ACI	18–34 mo	Pheochromocytoma	7/55 (12.7)	10/209 (4.8)	Maekawa and Odashima 1975
Osborne-Mendel (OM)	12–18 mo >18 mo	Pheochromocytoma	0 0	0 0	Hollander and Snell 1976
Osborne-Mendel (OM)	Life span	Proliferative lesions	(2)	(1)	Tischler and DeLellis 1988b
F344	12–18 mo >18 mo	Pheochromocytoma	(5) (45)	(0) (5)	Hollander and Snell 1976
F344	Lifs span	Pheochromocytoma	7/160 (4.4)	1/192 (0.52)	Sass et al. 1975
F344	18–24 mo 24–30 mo 30–33 mo	Pheochromocytoma	1/40 (5.0) 2/47 (4.3) 1/15 (6.7)	– – –	Coleman et al. 1977
F344	24 mo	Pheochromocytoma (four with metastasis to lung) Medullary hyperplasia	158/1794 (8.8) 50/1794 (2.8)	55/1754 (3.1) 28/1754 (1.6)	Goodman et al. 1979
F344	29 mo	Pheochromocytoma	7/20 (35)	–	Ribelin et al. 1984
F344	Life span	Proliferative lesions	(30)	(15)	Tischler and DeLellis 1988b
CHbb	24–25 mo	Adenoma of adrenal medulla or pheochromocytoma	13/400 (3.3) (Male and female)		Tilov et al. 1976
CHbb:THOM	3/30 mo	Nodular hyperplasia of adrenal medulla	"Most"/380 (Male and female)		Von Seebach et al. 1975
GG (Wistar)	19–24 mo 25–30 mo	Pheochromocytoma	65/78 (83.3) 59/69 (85.5)	26/51 (51.0) 55/72 (76.4)	Gillman et al. 1953
GG	12–36 mo	Pheochromocytoma	137/218 (62.8)	127/268 (47.4)	Gilbert et al. 1958
Copenhagen	12–36 mo	Pheochromocytoma	35/44 (79.5)	25/32 (78.1)	Gilbert et al. 1958
BUF, F344, and WN	21 mo	Pheochromocytoma	(40)		Snell 1965
BN/Bi	27–39 mo	Pheochromocytoma	1/39 (2.6)	3/79 (3.8)	Hollander 1976
BN/Bi			6/74 (8.1)	16/236 (6.8)	
Long-Evans	Life span	Proliferative lesions	(38)		Tischler and DeLellis 1988b
NEDH	Life span	Proliferative lesions	(81)	–	Tischler and DeLellis 1988b
Rochester	18–24 mo	Medullary adenoma	5/279 (1.8)	5/368 (1.4)	Crain 1985
WAG/Rij	11–43 mo (average 33 mo)	Pheochromocytoma	–	7/290 (2.4)	Boorman and Hollander 1973
WAG/Rij	Life span	Pheochromocytoma	1/124 (0.8)	8/101 (7.9)	Burek 1978
(WAG × BN)F_1			8/67 (11.9)	2/68 (2.9)	
Wistar	19–30 mo	Hyperplasia	10/40 (25.0)	–	Jayne 1969
Wistar	Life span	Proliferative lesions	(86)	(74)	Tischler and DeLellis 1988b

strains. Similar, too, is the recognition of adrenal medullary hyperplasia, which is part of multiple endocrine adenomatosis and is considered the background in which both benign and malignant pheochromocytomas develop (Tischler and DeLellis 1988; Rosai 1981).

References

Altman NH, Goodman DG (1979) Neoplastic disease. In: Baker HJ, Lindsey JR, Weisbroth SH (eds) The laboratory rat, vol 1, chap 13. Academic, New York

Anderson MP, Capen CC (1978) The endocrine system. In: Benirschke K, Garner FM, Jones TC (eds) Pathology of laboratory animals, vol 1, chap 6. Springer, Berlin Heidelberg New York

Bioassay of reserpine for possible carcinogenicity (1980) National Cancer Institute carcinogenesis technical report series no 193, NTP no 80-16

Boelsterli UA, Zbinden G (1985) Early biochemical and morphological changes of the rat adrenal medullar induced by xylitol. Arch Toxicol 57:25–30

Boorman GA, Hollander CF (1973) Spontaneous lesion in the female WAG/Rij (Wistar) rat. J Gerontol 28:152–159

Burek JD (1978) Pathology of aging rats. CRC, Boca Raton

Castanera TJ, Jones DC, Kimeldorf DJ, Rosen VJ (1968) The influence of whole-body exposure to x-rays or neutrons on the life span distribution of tumors among male rats. Cancer Res 28:170–182

Cheng L (1980) Pheochromocytoma in rats. Incidence, etiology, morphology, and functional activity. J Environ Pathol Microbiol 4:219–228

Coleman GL, Barthold S, Osbaldiston GW, Foster S, Jonas AM (1977) Pathological changes during aging in barrier-reared Fischer 344 male rats. J Gerontol 32:258–278

Crain RC (1958) Spontaneous tumors in the Rochester strain of the Wistar rat. Am J Pathol 34:258–335

Delellis RA, Merk FB, Deckers P, Warren S, Balogh K (1973) Ultrastructure and in vitro growth characteristics of a transplantable rat pheochromocytoma. Cancer 32:227–235

Diener RM (1988) Pheochromocytomas and reserpine: review of carcinogenicity bioassay. J Am Col Toxicol 7:95–109

Diener RM, Rac VS, Thompson SW III, Spaet RH (1980) Review of the criticla findings contained withing DHHS publication N. NIH 80–1749: bioassay of reserpine for possible carcinogenicity. Toxicol Pathol 8:1–21

Eranko O (1960) Cell types of the adrenal medula. In: Vane JR, Wolstenholme GEW, O'Connor M (eds) Adrenergic mechanisms. Little, Boston, pp 103–110

Gilbert C, Gillman J, Loustalot P, Lutz W (1958) The modifying influence of diet and the physical environment on spontaneous tumour frequency in rats. Br J Cancer 12:565–593

Gillman J, Gilbert C, Spence (1953) Pheochromocytoma in the rat. Pathogenesis and collateral reactions and its relation to comparable tumours in man. Cancer 6:494–511

Goodman DG, Ward JM, Squire RA, Chu KC, Linhart MS (1979) Neoplastic and nonneoplastic lesion in aging F344 rats. Toxicol Appl Pharmacol 48:237–248

Greene LA, Tischler AS (1976) Establishment of a noradrenergic clonal line of rat adrenal pheochromocytoma cells which respond to nerve growth factor. Proc Natl Acad Sci USA 73:2424–2428

Hollander CF (1976) Current experience in using the laboratory rat in aging studies. Lab Anim Sci 26:320–328

Hollander CF, Snell KC (1976) Tumours of the adrenal gland. IARC Sci Publ 6:273–293

Jayne EP (1969) Atrophy and hyperplasia in the adrenal medulla. Geriatrics 24:115–119

Kovacs K, Horvath E (1973) Ultrastructural features of the corticomedullary cells in a human adrenocortical adenoma and in rat adrenal cortex. Anat Anz 134:387–393

Lee AK, DeLellis RA, Blount M, Nunnemacher G, Wolfe HJ (1982) Pituitary proliferative lesions in aging male Long-Evans rats. A model of mixed multiple endocrine neoplasia syndrome. Lab Invest 47:595–602

MacKenzie WF, Garner FM (1973) Comparison of neoplasms in six sources of rats. J Natl Cancer Inst 50:1243–1257

Maekawa A, Odashima S (1975) Spontaneous tumors in ACI/N rats. J Natl Cancer Inst 55:1437–1445

Mohr U, Altoff J, Kinzel V (1969) Geschwülste des Nebennierenmarkes bei der Ratte. Exp Pathol (Jena) 3:153–158

Moon HD, Simpson ME, Li CH, Evans H (1950) Neoplasms in rats treated with pituitary growth hormone. II. Adrenal glands. Cancer Res 10:364–370

Prejean JD, Peckham JC, Casey AE, Griswold DP, Weisburger EK, Weisburger JH (1973) Spontaneous tumors in Sprague-Dawley rats and Swiss mice. Cancer Res 33: 3768–2773

Ribelin WE, Roloff MV, Houser RM (1984) Minimally functional rat adrenal medullary pheochromocytomas. Vet Pathol 21:281–285

Roe FJ, Bar A (1985) Enzootic and epizootic adrenal medullary proliferative disease of rats: influence of dietary factors which affect calcium absorption. Hum Toxicol 4:27–52

Rosai J (1981) Ackerman's surgical pathology, 6th edn. Mosby, St Louis, pp 705–727

Rosen VJ, Castanera TJ, Jones DC, Kimeldorf DJ (1961) Islet cell tumors of the pancreas in the irradiated and non-irradiated rat. Lab Invest 10:608–616

Russfield AB (1967) Pathology of the endocrine glands, ovary and testis of rats and mice. In: Cotchin E, Roe FJC (eds) Pathology of laboratory rats and mice, chap 14. Blackwell Scientific, Oxford

Sass B, Rabstein LS, Madison R, Nims RM, Peters RL, Kelloff GJ (1975) Incidence of spontaneous neoplasms in F344 rats throughout the natural life span. J Natl Cancer Inst 54:1449–1456

Schardein JL, Fitzgerald JE, Kaump DH (1968) Spontaneous tumours in Holtzman-source rats of various ages. Vet Pathol 5:238–252

Snell KC (1965) Spontaneous lesions of the rat. In: Ribelin WE, McCoy JR (eds) Pathology of laboratory animals, chap 10. Thomas, Springfield

Squire RA, Goodman DG, Valerio MG, Fredrickson TN, Strandberg JD, Levitt MH, Lingeman CH, Harshbarger JC, Dawe CJ (1978) Tumors. In: Benirschke K, Garner FM, Jones TC (eds) Pathology of laboratory animals, vol II, chap 12. Springer, Berlin Heidelberg New York

Staemmler M (1935) Die chronische Vergiftung mit Nicotin. Ergebnisse experimenteller Untersuchungen an Ratten. Virchows Arch [Pathol Anat] 295:366–393

Suzuki H, Mohr U, Kimmerie G (1979) Spontaneous endocrine tumors in Sprague-Dawley rats. J Cancer Res Clin Oncol 95:187–196

Tarone RE, Chu KC, Ward JM (1981) Variability in the rates of some common naturally occurring tumors in Fischer 344 rats and (C57BL/6N × C3H/HeN) F_1 (B6C3F_1) mice. J Natl Cancer Inst 66:1175–1181

Thompson SW, Hunt RD (1963) Spontaneous tumors in the Spraue-Dawley rat: incidence rats of some types of neoplasms as determined by serial section versus single section technics. Ann N Y Acad Sci 108:832–848

Thompson SW, Huseby RA, Fox MA, Davis CL, Hunt RD (1961) Spontaneous tumors in the Sprague-Dawley rat. J Natl Cancer Inst 27:1037–1057

Thompson SW, Rac VS, Semoick DE, Antonchak B, Spaet RH, Schelhammer LE (1981) The adrenal medulla of rats. Thomas, Springfield

Tilov T, Köllmer H, Weisse I, Stötzer H (1976) Spontan auftretende Tumoren des Rattenstammes Chbb: THOM (SPF). Arzneimittelforschung 26:45–50

Tischler AS (1989) The rat adrenal medulla. Toxicol Pathol 17:330–332

Tischler AS, Coupland RE (1994) Changes in structure and funciton of the adrenal medulla. In: Mohr U, Dungworth DL, Capen CC (eds) Pathobiology of the aging rat, vol 2. ILSI, Washington DC, pp 245–268

Tischler AS, DeLellis RA (1988a) The rat adrenal medulla. I. The normal adrenal. J Am Coll Toxicol 7:1–21

Tischler AS, DeLellis RA (1988b) The rat adrenal medula. II. Proliferative lesions. J Am Coll Toxicol 7:23–44

Tischler AS, Greene LA (1978) Morphologic and cytochemical properties of a clonal line of rat adrenal pheochromocytoma cells which respond to nerve growth factor. Lab Invest 39:77–89

Tischler AS, DeLellis RA, Nunnemacher C, Wolfe HJ (1988) Acute stimulation of chromaffin cell proliferation in the adult rat adrenal medulla. Lab Invest 58:733–735

Tischler AS, Ruzicka LA, Donahue SR, DeLellis RA (1989) Chromaffin cell proliferation in the adult rat adrenal medulla. Dev Neurosci 7:439–448

Tischler AS, Ruzicka LA, Van Pelt CS, Sandusky GE (1990) Catecholamine-synthesizing enzymes and chromogranin proteins in drug-induced proliferative lesions of the rat adrenal medulla. Lab Invest 63:44–51

Tischler AS, Ruzicka LA, DeLellis RA (1991a) Regulation of neurotensin content in adrenal medullary cells: comparison of PC12 cells to normal rat chromaffin cells in vitro. Neuroscience 43:671–678

Tischler AS, McClain RM, Childers H, Downing J (1991b) Neurogenic signals regulate chromaffin cell proliferation and mediate the mitogenic effect of reserpine in the adult rat adrenal medulla. Lab Invest 65:374–376

Von Seebach HB, Lützen L, Kreiner E, Ueberberg H, Pappritz G, Dhom G (1975) Morphology of aging in rat adrenals. Verh Dtsch Ges Pathol 59:414–418

Warren S, Chute RN (1972) Pheochromocytoma. Cancer 29: 327–331

Wester PW, Krajnc EI, van Leeuwen FX, Loeber JG, van der Heijden CA, Vaessen HA, Helleman PW (1990) Chronic toxicity and carcinogenicity of bis (tri-n-butyltin) oxide (TBTO) in the rat. Food Chem Toxicol 28:179–196

Yeakel EH (1947) Medullary hyperplasia of the adrenal gland in aged Wistar albino and gray Norway rats. Arch Pathol 44:71–77

Adrenal Medullary Tumors, Mouse

Loic E. Longeart

Synonyms. Diffuse hyperplasia, focal hyperplasia, pheochromocytoma, ganglioneuroma, mixed adrenal medullary tumor, neuroblastoma.

Gross Appearance

While small medullary tumors are not visible grossly, large ones may result in a reddish-yellow, generalized enlargement of the affected adrenal gland (Smith et al. 1949). Medullary tumors cannot be distinguished grossly from adrenocortical tumors in the mouse (Dunn 1970).

Microscopic Features

Diffuse Hyperplasia. The medullary cells are diffusely increased in number and volume, resulting in expansion of the entire medulla. This puts pressure on the surrounding cortex and may result in its atrophy, but does not cause recognizable zones of compression. It should be emphasized that cortical atrophy is not uncommon in aging mice, particularly males (Faccini et al. 1990), and that the sole presence of such atrophy should not be mistaken for evidence of diffuse medullary hyperplasia. The normal medulla in mice, which has a pyriform shape, may reach the hilus and be incompletely surrounded by the cortex (Dunn 1970). In consequence, a practical indicator of diffuse medullary hyperplasia is a widening of the hilus (Fig. 456). In such instances medullary cells may extend into the periadrenal connective tissue but this should not be confused with invasion by malignant cells.

Focal Hyperplasia and Pheochromocytoma. Secretory cells of the adrenal medulla of the mouse give rise to a continuous spectrum of lesions ranging from focal hyperplasia to malignant pheochromocytoma. Focal proliferative changes in chromaffin cells are first recognized by increased basophilia of the cytoplasm of affected cells, distinguishing them from adjacent medullary secretory cells. These foci are otherwise composed of relatively uniform polyhedral cells, clearly resembling normal medullary secretory cells, with central nuclei and finely stippled cytoplasm. The packets of cells limited by the delicate stroma may appear larger in such foci, and the ratio of nucleus to cytoplasm may be increased. These foci may impinge upon cells of the adrenal cortex, but in the absence of compression of adjacent tissue, they are diagnosed as focal medullary hyperplasia," unless they are larger than 50% of a normal medulla, in which case they should always be called pheochromocytomas (Capen et al. 1994). More extensive growth and compression of adjacent tissue are generally accepted, although not necessarily biologically relevant, criteria for a diagnosis of pheochromocytoma. Pheochromocytomas are often sharply delineated from the adjacent medulla or cortex but are not usually encapsulated. They may replace the entire medulla. The proliferative cells are held in packets by a delicate stroma into which many capillaries extend. As the tumors become larger, the stroma tends to be less conspicuous, and the capillaries are distended with blood. Hemorrhage or necrosis may occur. The cytoplasm of the neoplastic cells, stained with H&E, is more basophilic than in normal medullary cells, but the tinctorial characteristics of the neoplastic cells vary a great deal. Bizarre nuclei may occur (Fig. 457). The mitotic index varies from one tumor to another and does not appear to be a particularly good indicator of malignancy (Frith and Ward 1988). A pheochromocytoma which penetrates the adrenal capsule and extends into the periadrenal adipose tissue and/or into the lumen of blood vessels is regarded as malignant. Metastases to the lungs may occur, and this is commonly correlated with tumor size (Figs. 458, 459).

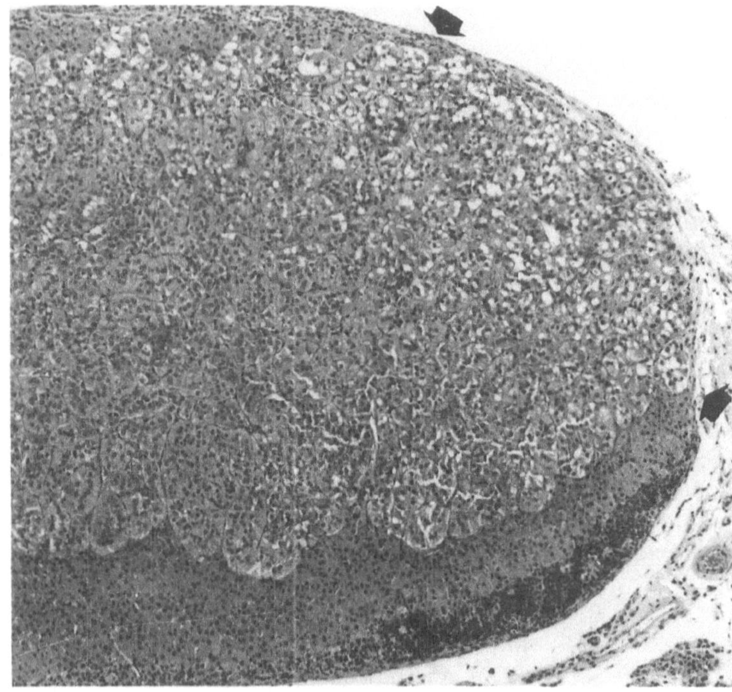

Fig. 456. Pheochromocytoma, adrenal medulla, mouse. Growth of the tumor has conspicuously widened the hilus (*between arrows*). H&E, ×80

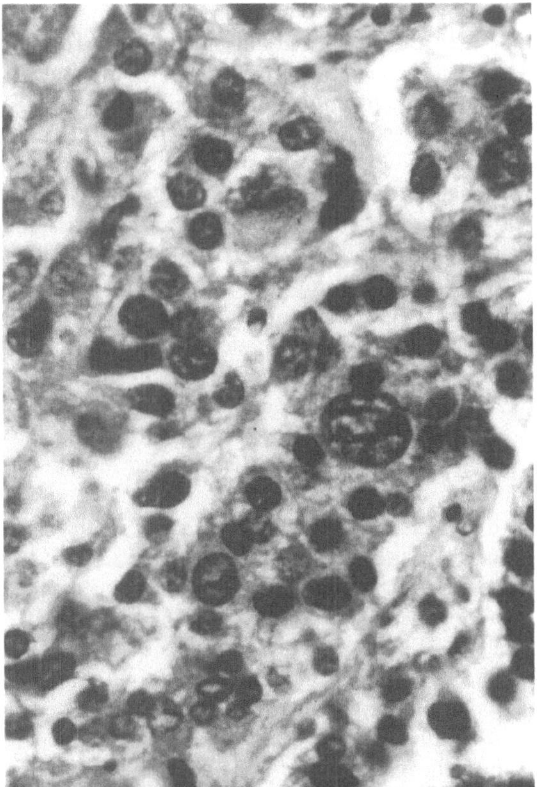

Fig. 457. Pheochromocytoma, adrenal medulla, mouse. Note enlarged and bizarre nuclei. H&E, ×500

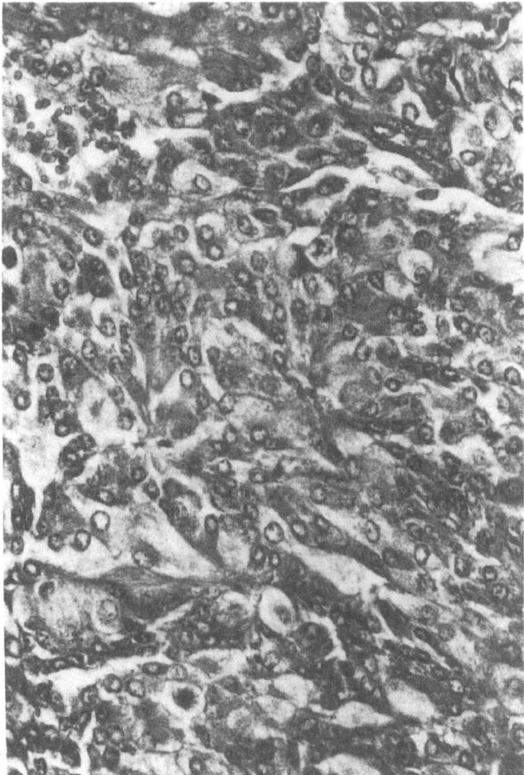

Fig. 458. Pheochromocytoma, adrenal medulla, mouse. Well-differentiated cells of malignant pheochromocytoma. H&E, ×300

Ganglioneuroma. These neoplasms are composed of large ganglion cells accompanied by supporting neural cells. The ganglion cells are characterized by the presence of an eccentric nucleus, with a prominent nucleolus and Nissl substance in the periphery of the abundant cytoplasm.

Mixed Adrenal Medullary Tumors. This term refers to neoplasms presenting features of both ganglioneuroma and pheochromocytoma, either intermingled or in separate areas. The occurrence of these peculiar neoplasms finds its explanation in the study of adrenal medullary cell lineages, which shows that primitive sympathetic cells (sympathogonia) develop either into neurons or chromaffin cells (Tischler and DeLellis 1988a).

Neuroblastoma. These neoplasms are composed of a dense sheet of small, hyperchromatic, tightly packed cells which occasionally form rosettes. In areas of decreased cellularity a fibrillary matrix resembling central nervous tissue is revealed. Occasional ganglion cells may be present. Metastases to the regional lymph nodes, liver, and bone may occur.

Ultrastructure

Ultrastructural studies of spontaneous medullary tumors have not been performed in the mouse, possibly owing to their rarity, the difficulty in recognizing them grossly, and the difficulty in distinguishing them grossly from adrenocortical tumors. The only ultrastructural study performed so far was on induced neuroblastomas (Aguzzi et al. 1990) and indicated that the matrix of the tumors is composed of a dense network of long axonic processes containing large numbers of membrane-bounded dense core vesicles, 80–100 nm in diameter, similar to those found in the cells of the adrenal medulla.

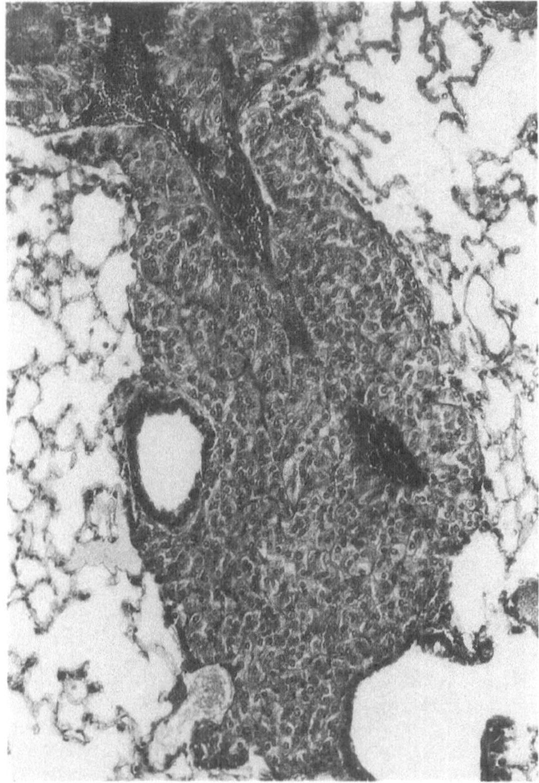

Fig. 459. Pheochromocytoma, adrenal medulla, mouse. Pulmonary metastasis of tumor depicted in Fig. 458. H&E, ×120

Differential Diagnosis

In the context of rodent bioassays diagnostic criteria for differentiation between focal hyperplasia and neoplasia, particularly in endocrine organs, have been established in a pragmatic approach for purposes of dealing with regulatory agencies. The boundaries between focal hyperplasia and pheochromocytoma are therefore arbitrary, and the question of their biologic relevance has been raised (Faccini et al. 1990). Nevertheless, the absence or presence of clear compression of adjacent tissue is usually accepted as the distinguishing factor between focal hyperplasia and pheochromocytoma. In addition, a size criterion, recently proposed by the European Registry of Industrial Toxicology Animal group (Capen et al. 1994), is that circumscribed lesions larger than 50% of the normal medulla should be called pheochromocytoma. This has proven usefül for these large lesions with no or only minimal compression.

The distinguishing features of malignancy for pheochromocytomas are also debatable. The only universally accepted criterion for malignancy of human pheochromocytoma is the presence of distant metastases in sites where chromaffin tissue is not normally expected, since capsular and even vascular invasion has been associated with benign clinical behavior (Ashley 1978). This is a somewhat controversial issue in rodents. Some authors, in view of the extrapolation of rodent bioassays to man, argue that distant metastasis remains the best and only reliable criterion of malignancy applicable to rodent pheochromocytomas (Greaves 1990; Tischler and DeLellis 1988b). A more commonly accepted viewpoint is that local evidence of invasive growth, i.e., invasion of the capsule, periadrenal fat, or vessels, warrants a diagnosis of malignancy (Capen et al. 1991; Faccini et al. 1990; Strandberg 1983). In the absence of published standardized criteria for proliferative lesions of mice it is useful to apply to mice the SOTP recommendations in rats (Brown et al. 1995), i.e., pheochromocytoma should be considered malignant if it invades the capsule and/or metastasises.

While the ganglioneuroma, neuroblastoma, and mixed medullary tumor are morphologically characteristic and discernable medullary tumors, it may sometimes be difficult in H&E preparations to distinguish pheochromocytoma from adrenocortical tumors. The chromaffin reaction, as well as the argentaffin or argyrophil reactions, are classical histochemical methods which possess a very low level of sensitivity and specificity and should not be used routinely (Capen et al. 1991). The demonstration of secretory granules under electron microscopy might prove useful in establishing the medullary nature of a tumor, providing that there is enough available tissue left after trimming for postfixation. Immunohistochemistry represents an alternative approach. Common markers, such as neuron-specific enolase (Fig. 460), chromogranin, or synaptophysin or more specific ones such as epinephrine and norepinephrine are easy to perform on formalin-fixed and paraffin-embedded material (Capen et al. 1991). In those cases where either ultrastructural or immunohistochemical results are equivocal, it should be borne in mind that there is ultrastructural evidence, at least in the rat, of the existence of corticochromaffin hybrid cells (Borstein et al. 1991; Kovacs and Horvath 1973), and that adrenocortical tumors with neuroendocrine differentia-

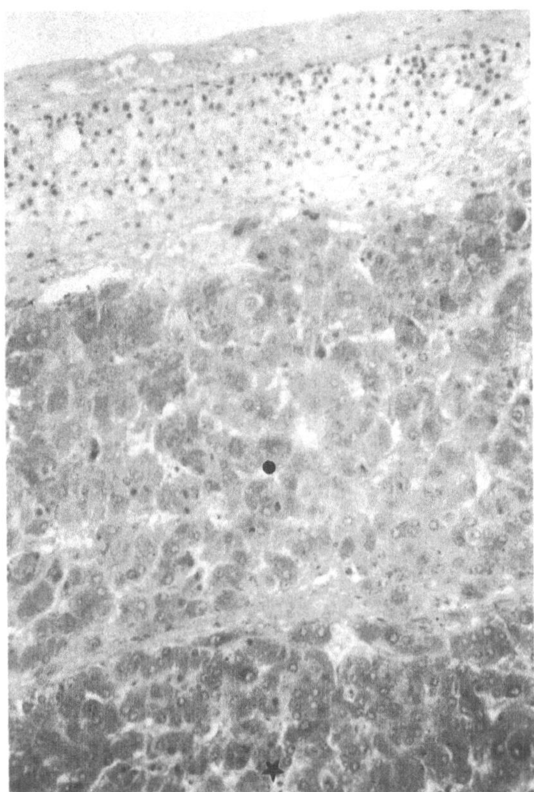

Fig. 460. Pheochromocytoma, adrenal medulla, mouse. Immunohistochemical staining for neuron-specific enolase, positive in tumor cells (*dot*) and in medulla (*star*). ×160

tion have been reported in humans (Miettinen 1992).

Biologic Features

Natural History. Medullary tumors have not been sufficiently studied in mice to draw firm conclusions as to whether they produce hormonal effects as they commonly do in rats and in humans. The only available report on the biologic features of pheochromocytomas in mice (Haran-Ghera et al. 1959) suggests that there might be some secretory activity of these tumors. In this experiment animals bearing a transplant of a pheochromocytoma exhibited, in early passages, severe respiratory distress presumably due to catecholamines. Unfortunately, the urine was not assayed for metabolites of adrenal hormones.

Etiology. A genetic factor has been suggested by Jones and Woodward (1954), who described an increased incidence of spontaneous tumors of the adrenal medulla in a cross between C3H females and stain-I males. This is further suggested by the high incidence of medullary hyperplasia, demonstrated by morphometric studies, in several substrains of mice such as the diabetic strain C57BL/KsJ db/db (Carson et al. 1982) and the AKR-derived senescence-accelerated murine model (Shino et al. 1987).

Some transgenic mice models for adrenal medullary tumors are now available. Helseth et al. (1992) generated a murine model for Cushing's disease in mice carrying the polyoma early region promoter linked to a cDNA encoding polyoma large T antigen. Quite unexpectedly these mice presented with nodular medullary hyperplasia. It is noteworthy that in this report "nodular medullary hyperplasia" on occasion referred to lesions featuring necrosis, compression of adjacent tissues, and numerous mitotic figures, all of which are generally accepted criteria by toxicologic pathologists as evidence for pheochromocytomas. Aguzzi et al. (1990) reported that transgenic mice carrying a cDNA to the polyoma virus middle T antigen linked to the thymidine kinase promoter developed multiple neuroblastoma, including in the adrenal, by 2–3 months of age. These tumors expressed the N-*myc* oncogene.

Very few chemicals have been reported to induce either medullary hyperplasia or neoplasia in mice, in contrast to rats. These include thiouracil and 1,1,2-trichloroethane (Ribelin 1984). In the older literature a variety of techniques were applied to increase the incidence of adrenal medullary tumors in mice, including irradiation (Haran-Ghera et al. 1959; Upton et al. 1960), castration (Smith et al. 1949), injection of polyoma virus (Stanton et al. 1959), and injection of parotid tumor or leukemia-producing viruses (Steward et al. 1958). These techniques induced only a slight increase in the incidence of medullary tumors.

Frequency. The incidence of spontaneous medullary tumors is generally low in common strains of laboratory mice. Since these tumors are sometimes quite small, they can be missed if only one section is studied. Multiple histologic sections may well increase the observed frequency of these tumors. Pheochromocytomas are rarely encountered in animals younger than 12 months of age (Frith 1983) and are still rarer in older animals. Selected data reported in the literature on the

Table 32. Incidence of pheochromocytoma in untreated mice (benign and malignant combined)

Strain	Males			Females			Reference
	n	Number	%	n	Number	%	
CD-1	99	2	2	102	0	0	Hamburger et al. (1975)
CD-1	891	5	0.56	890	4	0.45	Maita et al. (1988)
CD-1	405	1	0.24	407	4	0.98	Longeart, unpublished
CD-1	474	5	1.05	478	2	0.42	Lang (1987)
B6C3F1	2543	8	0.31	2522	7	0.27	Ward et al. (1979)
B6C3F1[a]	1716	20	1.2	1722	13	0.8	Haseman et al. (1985)
B6C3F1[b]	1051	23	2.2	1060	15	1.4	Haseman et al. (1985)
B6C3F1	244	3	1.2	246	1	0.4	Tamano et al. (1988)

[a] Untreated mice.
[b] Corn oil gavage.

incidence of pheochromocytomas in cohorts of aging mice from the most commonly used strains are presented in Table 32. Among these cohorts the highest incidence reported in a single control group is 6/50 (12%; Haseman et al. 1985). Ganglioneuromas are very uncommon in mice (Faccini et al. 1990). We have found only one brief account of a mixed medullary tumor (Frith and Ward 1988) and one of a neuroblastoma (Maita et al. 1988) in this species.

Comparison with Other Species

The morphologic features of medullary tumors are very similar across species. The occurrence of medullary tumors in mice is much less frequent than in most commonly used strains of laboratory rats. Moreover, the clinical context in mice and in rats is quite different. In mice, as in humans, medullary tumors are usually solitary and sporadic, whereas in rats they are frequently multifocal, bilateral, and associated with proliferative lesions in other endocrine glands, in that respect being reminiscent of the very rare mixed-type multiple endocrine neoplasia in humans (Tischler and DeLellis 1988b).

References

Aguzzi A, Wagner EF, Williams RL, Courtneidge SA (1990) Sympathetic hyperplasia and neuroblastomas in transgenic mice expressing polyoma middle T antigen. New Biol 2: 533–543

Ashley DJB (1978) Evan's histological appearances of tumours. Tumours of chromaffin tissue. Churchill Livingstone, Edinburgh, pp 311–327

Borstein SR, Ehrhart-Borstein M, Sherbaum WA (1991) Ultrastructural evidence for cortico-chromaffin hybrid cells in rat adrenals? Endocrinology 129:1113–1115

Brown WR, Gough A, Hamlin MH II, Hottendorf GH, Patterson DR (1995) Proliferative lesions of the adrenal in rats. In: Guides for toxicologic pathology. STP/ARP/AFIP, Washington (in press)

Capen CC, DeLellis RA, Yarrington JT (1991) Endocrine system. In: Haschek WM, Rousseaux CG (eds) Handbook of toxicologic pathology. Academic, San Diego, pp 675–760

Capen CC, DeLellis R, Deschl U, Hartig F, Karbe E, Konishi Y, Krinke GJ, Landes C, Mettler F, Rebel W, Riley MGI, Tuch K, Urwyler H (1994) Endocrine system. In: Mohr U (ed) International classification of rodent tumours, part I, vol 6. IARC, Lyon (IARC scientific publications no 122)

Carson KA, Hanker JS, Kirshner N (1982) The adrenal medulla of the diabetic mouse (C57BL/KsJ, db/db): biochemical and morphological changes. Comp Biochem Physiol 72:279–285

Dunn TB (1970) Normal and pathologic anatomy of the adrenal gland of the mouse, including neoplasms. J Natl Cancer Inst 44:1323–1389

Faccini JM, Abbott DP, Paulus GJJ (1990) Endocrine glands. In: Mouse histopathology: a glossary for use in toxicity and carcinogenicity studies. Elsevier, Amsterdam, pp 169–186

Frith CH (1983) Pheochromocytoma, adrenal medulla, mouse. In: Jones TC, Mohr U, Hunt RD (eds) ILSI monographs on pathology of laboratory animals, endocrine system, 1st edn. Springer, Berlin Heidelberg, pp 27–30

Frith CH, Ward JM (1988) Endocrine system. In: Frith CH, Ward JM (eds) Color atlas of neoplastic and non-neoplastic lesions in aging mice. Elsevier, Amsterdam, pp 33–48

Greaves P (1990) Endocrine glands. In: Histopathology of preclinical toxicity studies: interpretation and relevance in drug safety evaluation. Elsevier, Amsterdam, pp 677–755

Haran-Ghera N, Furth J, Buffett RF, Yokoro K (1959) Studies on the pathogenesis of neoplasms by ionizing radiation. II. Neoplasms of endocrine organs. Cancer Res 19:1181–1187

Haseman JK, Huff JE, Rao GN, Arnold JE, Boorman GA, McConnell EE (1985) Neoplasms observed in untreated and corn oil gavage control groups of F344/N and (C57BL/6N × C3H/HeN)Fl (B6C3Fl) mice. J Natl Cancer Inst 75: 975–984

Helseth A, Siegal GP, Haug E, Bautch VL (1992) Transgenic mice that develop pituitary tumors. A model for Cushing's disease. Am J Pathol 140:1071–1080

Homburger F, Russfield AB, Weisburger JH, Lim S, Chak SP, Weisburger EK (1975) Aging changes in CD-1 Ham/ICR mice reared under standard laboratory conditions. J Natl Cancer Inst 55:37–45

Jones EE, Woodward LJ (1954) Spontaneous adrenal medullary tumors in hybrid mice. J Natl Cancer Inst 15:449–461

Kovacs K, Horvath E (1973) Ultrastructural features of corticomedullary cells in a human adrenocortical adenoma and in rat adrenal cortex. Anat Anz 134:387–393

Lang PL (1987) Spontaneous neoplastic lesions in the Crl: CD-1 (ICR)BR mouse. Charles River technical report, 24-month studies, pp 7–13

Maita K, Hirano M, Harada T, Mitsumori K, Yoshida A, Takahashi K, Nakashima N, Kitasawa T, Enomoto A, Inui K, Shirasu Y (1988) Mortality, major cause of moribundity, and spontaneous tumors in CD-1 mice. Toxicol Pathol 16:340–349

Miettinen M (1992) Neuroendocrine differentiation in adrenocortical carcinoma. New immunohistochemical findings supported by electron microscopy. Lab Invest 66:169–174

Ribelin WE (1984) The effects of drugs and chemicals upon the structure of the adrenal gland. Fundam Appl Toxicol 4:105–119

Shino A, Tsukuda R, Omori Y, Matsuo T (1987) Histopathologic observations on the senescence-accelerated mice (SAM) reared under specific pathogen free conditions. Acta Pathol Jpn 37:1465–1475

Smith FW, Gardner WU, Li MH (1949) Adrenal medullary tumors (pheochromocytomas) in mice. Cancer Res 9: 193–198

Stanton MF, Steward SE, Eddy BE, Blackwell RH (1959) The oncogenic effect of tissue-culture preparations of polyoma virus on fetal mice. J Natl Cancer Inst 23:1441–1475

Steward SE, Eddy BE, Borgese N (1958) Neoplasms in mice inoculated with a tumor agent carried in tissue culture. J Natl Cancer Inst 20:1223–1243

Strandberg JD (1983) Pheochromocytoma, adrenal medulla, rat. In: Jones TC, Mohr U, Hunt RD (eds) Monographs on pathology of laboratory animals, endocrine system, 1st edn. Springer, Berlin Heidelberg New York, pp 22–27

Tamano S, Hagiwara A, Shibata MA, Kurata Y, Fukushima S, Ito N (1988) Spontaneous tumors in aging (C57BL/6N × C3H/HeN)Fl (B6C3Fl) mice. Toxicol Pathol 16:321–326

Tischler AS, DeLellis RA (1988a) The rat adrenal medulla. I. The normal adrenal. J Am Coll Toxicol 7:1–21

Tischler AS, DeLellis RA (1988b) The rat adrenal medulla. II. Proliferative lesions. J Am Coll Toxicol 7:23–44

Upton AC, Kimball AW, Furth J, Christenberry KW, Benedict WH (1960) Some delayed effects of atom-bomb radiations in mice. Cancer Res 20 [Suppl 8, 2]:1–59

Ward JM, Goodman DG, Squire RA, Chu KC, Linhart MS (1979) Neoplastic and nonneoplastic lesions in aging (C57BL/6N × C3H/HeN)Fl (B6C3Fl) mice. J Natl Cancer Inst 63:849–854

Ganglioneuroma, Adrenal, Rat

Gerd Reznik and Paul-Georg Germann

Synonyms. Tumor medullary benign, ganglioneuroma type (WHO)*; tumor medullary benign, complex type (WHO)*; complex pheochromocytoma.

Gross Appearance

The size of the neoplasms vary but are often as large as 20 mm in diameter (Fig. 461) and displace much of the affected adrenal. As a general rule, only one adrenal is involved.

Microscopic Features

In the presence of an expanded tumor mass in the medulla a small remnant of the adrenal gland can usually be found at one or both poles (Fig. 462). Smaller tumors are usually located within the adrenal medulla and are surrounded by pheochromocytes or by a thin compressed rim of adrenal cortex. In one series (Reznik et al. 1980) a ganglioneuroma infiltrated the capsule of the adrenal and invaded lymphatics; in another case tumor emboli of pheochromocytes were found in sections of the lung. Distant metastasis of the neural elements of ganglioneuromas has not been reported.

The main diagnostic feature of a ganglioneuroma is the presence of ganglion cells with supporting

* World Health Organization, International Classification of Rodent Tumors (Mohr 1992).

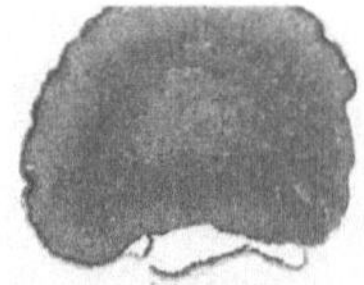

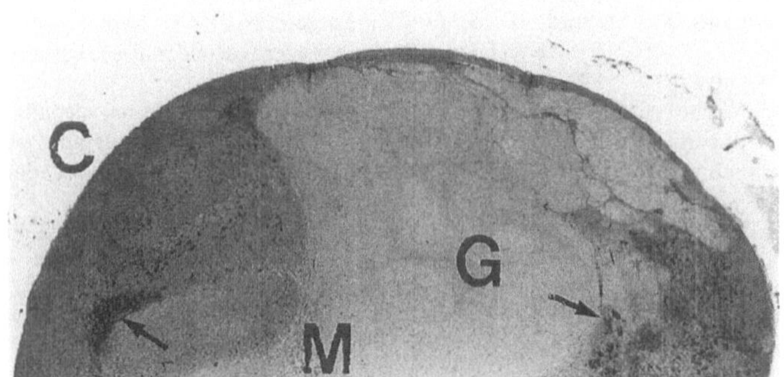

Fig. 461. Adrenal glands of a female F344 rat, 104 weeks old with a large ganglioneuroma (*G*). *C*, Cortex; M, medulla; *arrows*, hemorrhages. Note the size difference between the two adrenals. H&E, ×2.5

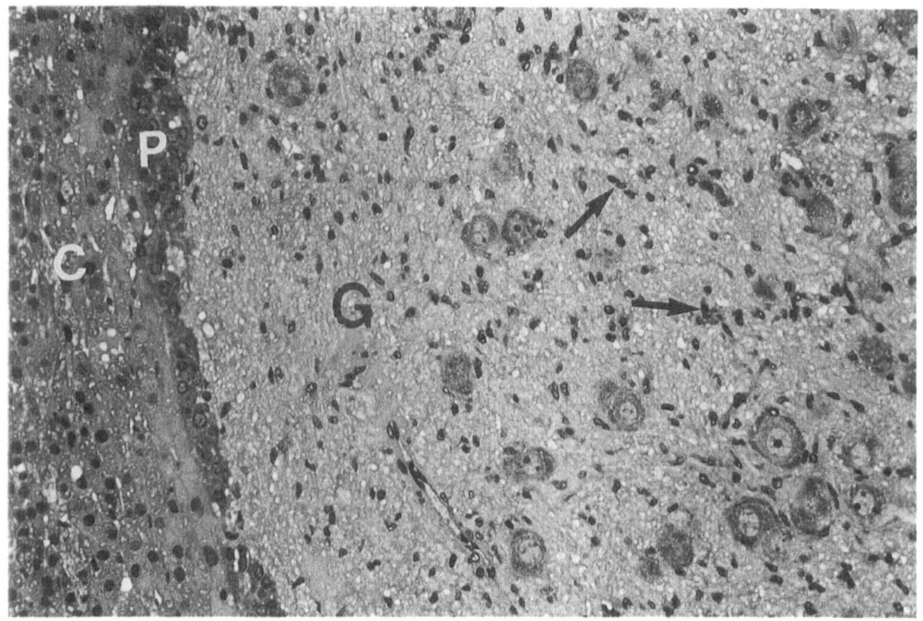

Fig. 462. Adrenal ganglioneuroma (*G*) of a female Sprague-Dawley rat, 99 weeks old. Cluster of ganglion cells in the S-100 positive Schwann's cell stroma (*arrows*). A small rim of pheochromocytes (*P*) demarcates the tumor from the cortex (*C*). *S*-100 PAP immunohistochemistry, hematoxylin, ×240

neural cells. The ganglion cells form small clusters (Figs. 462, 463) and are sometimes surrounded by large masses of supporting tissue. In other cases the ganglion cells displace the medulla and compress the adrenal cortex. The multipolar ganglion cells have large, pale nuclei with prominent, often eccentric nucleoli, and peripheral portions of the cytoplasm of the cells are positive with Nissl's stain after formaldehyde fixation (Fig. 463). Multiple nucleoli are commonly found, and the nuclear chromatin is often dispersed, resulting in a vesicular appearance of the nucleus.

The supporting cells, predominately of the Schwann's cell type, are small with little cyto-

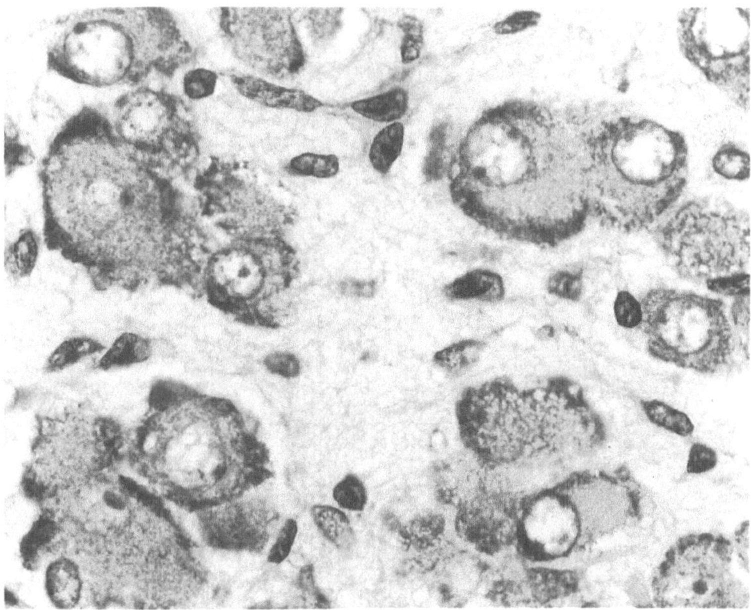

Fig. 463. Ganglioneuroma containing ganglion cells with nuclear chromatin mostly dispersed, which results in a vesicular appearance of the nucleus. Nissl stain, ×880

plasm. These Schwann's cell types frequently have a positive immunohistological reaction with S-100 protein, demonstrating a filamentous network, surrounding the individual ganglion cells (Figs. 464, 465). Sometimes the nuclei are elongated and form parallel bundles or are arranged in interlacing fascicles. In cross-sections the fascicles appear fibrous and resemble those found in schwannomas.

The proliferating pheochromocytes (chromaffin cells) which frequently occur with ganglioneuromas are mostly found in the outer portions of the ganglioneuroma, but a clearcut borderline between the two cell types is often difficult to detect. These pheochromocytoma cells are described on p. 411 (this volume). In certain areas of some tumors pheochromocytes appear to be differentiating into ganglion cells or arising from the same tumor stem cells as tumor ganglion cells. For this tumor type the synonym "tumor medullary benign, complex type" should be used, pointing out the coexistence of tumor areas with variable phenotypical differentiation.

Differential Diagnosis

A schwannoma as a second independent tumor can be found as a rare event coincidentally with a ganglioneuroma, as is demonstrated in Fig. 464. These composite tumors have to be separated from Schwann's cells belonging to the ganglioneuroma (Fig. 462).

Ultrastructure

Ganglioneuromas are made up of well-differentiated ganglion cells and stromal tissue consisting of Schwann's cells (Bolande 1979; Harkin and Reed 1969). The previously described morphologic features of the ganglion cells apparent under light microscopy may be confirmed using electron microscopy. Neurosecretory granules and axonal cytoplasmic reticulum (Nissl's substance) are characteristics of ganglion cells (Sandborn 1970; Reznik et al. 1980). Microtubules and neurofilaments are difficult to identify in formalin-fixed material. Schwann's cells are characterized by their tendency to surround the ganglion cells; they have long cytoplasmic extensions and possess a basement membrane (Weiss and Greep 1977; Boesel et al. 1978).

Biologic Features

The ganglioneuromas in one study (Reznik et al. 1980) were all located in the adrenal gland and were almost always associated with pheochromocytomas. About half of the ganglioneuromas in rats reported in the literature have been found

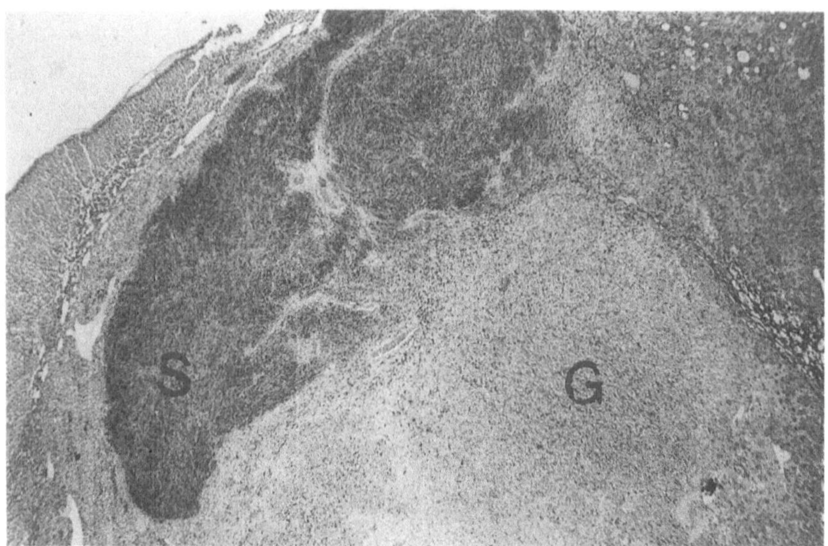

Fig. 464. Schwannoma (*S*) and a ganglioneuroma (*G*) in a female Wistar rat, 117 weeks old. S-100 strong positivity supports the clear distinction between these two tumors. *S*-100 PAP-immunohistochemistry, hematoxylin, ×24

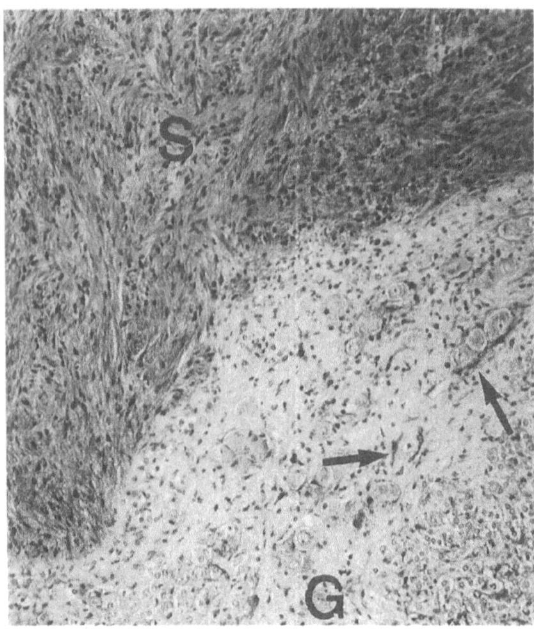

Fig. 465. Schwannoma (*S*) and a ganglioneuroma (*G*) in a female Wistar rat, 117 weeks old (larger magnification of the borderline of Fig. 464. S-100 positivity of Schwann's cell network is quite distinct (*arrows*). S-100 PAP-immunohistochemistry, hematoxylin, ×96

together with pheochromocytomas. This association of neoplastic growth of both ganglionic and medullary secretory cells has led some authors to refer to the lesion as mixed tumor, mixed neuroendocrine-neural tumor, or ganglioneuroma-pheochromocytoma, or more recently as tumor medullary benign, complex type or complex pheochromocytoma (Brown et al. in press; Hamlin and Banas 1990). Ganglion cells and pheochromocytes are both considered to differentiate from primitive sympathogonia arising in the neuroectoderm (Manger and Giffort 1977). Tumors which are a mixture of cells of neuroblast and pheochromocyte derivation have been reported in man and rats (Bolande 1979; Trump et al. 1977; Todd et al. 1970; Reznik et al. 1980). The close relationship in the development of these two tumor types may represent one of the possible differentiation patterns during the development of ganglioneuromas or may result from concomitant neoplastic changes in two cell types. It is also possible that sympathetic ganglion cells may develop from pheochromocytes, as demonstrated in tissue culture systems by the studies of Olson (1970) and DeLellis et al. (1973). Shafer and Atchison (1991) demonstrated the in vitro differentiation of cells from a rat pheochromocytoma cell line into ganglion cells after adding nerve growth factor to the culture medium.

Ganglioneuromas are rare in experimental animals (Barofsky et al. 1970; Fitzgerald et al. 1974; Glaister et al. 1977; Goodman et al. 1979; Hueper and Martin 1942; Reznik et al. 1980; Squire et al. 1978; Todd et al. 1970; MacKenzie and Garner 1973; Linhart et al. 1974), and only a few have been reported in other mammals (Capen 1978; Cimprich and Ardington 1975; Gupta and Singh 1978). The frequencies of ganglioneuromas found in F344, Sprague-Dawley, and Wistar rat strains are depicted in Fig. 466 (Morawietz et al. 1992; Reznik et al. 1980).

Comparison with Other Species

The association of ganglioneuromas with pheochromocytomas has been reported in the human adrenal gland (Trump et al. 1977). These have been referred to as mixed tumors or mixed neuroendocrine-neural tumors. Ganglioneuromas without coincident pheochromocytomas have been found in a number of human (Arseni et al. 1975) and animal organs including adrenal glands, cranium, spinal cord, and bulbar conjunctiva (Capen 1978; Gupta and Singh 1978; Nieberle and Cohrs 1967; Arseni et al. 1975; Cimprich and Ardington 1975).

Tumors of neurogenic origin (neuroblastoma, ganglioneuroblastoma, ganglioneuroma) are the most common solid abdominal neoplasms of children and arise in the adrenal medulla in 40% of the cases. Neuroblastoma, defined as a tumor composed of primitive neuroblasts derived from the neural crest, is described separately on p. 433 (this volume).

The occurrence of schwannoma with ganglioneuroma or pheochromocytoma is also described in humans (Chandrasoma et al. 1986; Min et al. 1988).

Ganglioneuroblastomas and ganglioneuromas are more mature neoplasms believed to develop from neuroblasts through cytodifferentiation (Bolande 1979). Pheochromocytoma, another adrenal tumor of neural crest origin, is believed to arise from mature pheochromocytes (medullary cells) of the adrenal medulla (Manger and Gifford 1977). This neoplasm in the rat and mouse is discussed, respectively, on pp. 411 and 421 (this volume).

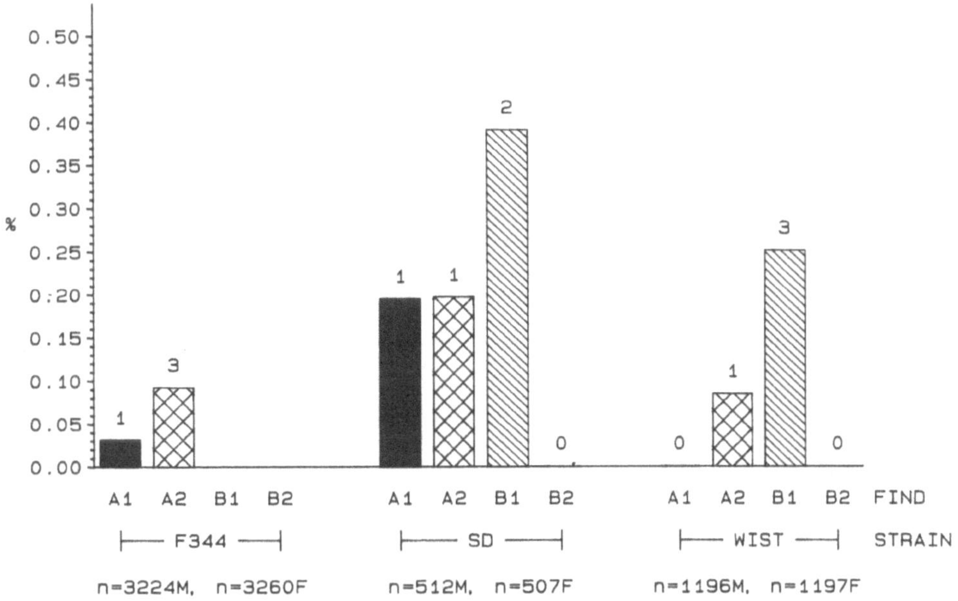

Fig. 466. Distribution of adrenal ganglioneuromas and tumors medullary, complex type in untreated control rats. Strains: F344, Sprague-Dawley (*SD*), and Wistar (*WIST*). *A1*, Ganglioneuroma, males; *A2*, ganglioneuroma, females; *B1*, tumor medullary, complex type, males; *B2*, tumor medullary, complex type, females

Acknowledgements. The authors wish to thank Dr. G.J. Krinke, Ciba Geigy (Switzerland), Dr. S.L. Eustis, NTP (USA), Dr. Barbara Lenz, Hoffman-La Roche (Switzerland), and Jerrold M. Ward, NCI (USA) for their supporting case material and Ms. Maureen Hall, EPL (USA) for her excellent photographs.

References

Arseni C, Horvath L, Carp N, Ciura V (1975) Intracranial ganglioneuromas in children. Acta Neurochir (Wien) 32: 270–286

Barofsky I, Matalka E, Russfield AB (1970) A ganglioneuroma in the adrenal medulla of a rat bearing a preoptic-anterior hypothalamic lesion. Cancer Res 30:2913–2916

Boesel CP, Suhan JP, Bradel EJ (1978) Ultrastructure of primitive neuroectodermal neoplasms of the central nervous system. Cancer 42:194–201

Bolande RP (1979) Developmental pathology. Am J Pathol 94:623–683

Brown WR, Gough A, Hamlin MH II, Hottendorf GH, Patterson DR (in press) Proliferative lesions of the adrenal glands of rats, pp 1–16 (In preparation by STP)

Capen CC (1978) Tumors of the endocrine glands. In: Moulton JE (ed) Tumors in domestic animals, 2nd edn. University of California Press, Berkeley, pp 388–392

Chandrasoma P, Shibata D, Radin R, Brown LP, Koss M (1986) Malignant peripheral nerve sheath tumor arising in an adrenal ganglioneuroma in an adult male homosexual. Cancer 57:2022–2025

Cimprich R, Ardington P (1975) Spinal ganglioneuroma in a steer. Vet Pathol 12:59–60

DeLellis RA, Merk FB, Deckers P, Warren S, Balogh K (1973) Ultrastructure and in vitro growth characteristics of a transplantable rat pheochromocytoma. Cancer 32:227–235

Fitzgerald JE, Schardein JL, Kurtz SM (1974) Spontaneous tumors of the nervous system in albino rats. J Natl Cancer Inst 52:265–273

Glaister JR, Samuels DM, Tucker MJ (1977) Ganglioneuroma-containing tumours of the adrenal medulla in Alderly Park rats. Lab Anim 11:35–37

Goodman DG, Ward JM, Squire RA, Chu KC, Linhart MS (1979) Neoplastic and non-neoplastic lesions in aging F344 rats. Toxicol Appl Pharmacol 48:237–248

Gupta PP, Singh B (1978) Ocular ganglioneuroma in Indian water buffaloes (Bubalus bubalis). Vet Pathol 15:138–139

Hamlin MH, Banas DA (1990) Adrenal Gland. In: Boorman GA, Eustis SL, Elwell MR, Montgomery CH Jr, Mackenzie WF (eds) Pathology of the Fischer rat: reference and atlas. Academic, San Diego, pp 501–518

Harkin JC, Reed RJ (1969) Tumors of the peripheral nervous system. In: Atlas of tumor pathology, 2nd series, fascicle 3. Armed Forces Institute of Pathology, Washington DC

Hueper WC, Martin GJ (1942) A tumor of the adrenal medulla in a castrated male rat. Cancer Res 2:294–295

Linhart MS, Cooper J, Martin RL, Page NP, Peters JA (1974) Carcinogenesis bioassay data system. Comput Biomed Res 7:230–248

MacKenzie WF, Garner FM (1973) Comparison of neoplasms in six sources of rats. J Natl Cancer Inst 50:1243–1257

Manger WM, Gifford RW (1977) Pheochromocytoma. Springer, Berlin Heidelberg New York

Min KW, Clemens A, Bell J, Dick H (1988) Malignant peripheral nerve sheath tumor and pheochromocytoma. Arch Pathol Lab Med 112:266–270

Mohr U (1992) International classification of rodent tumours. part 1. World Health Organization, Geneva (IARC science publication no 122)

Morawietz G, Rittinghausen S, Mohr U (1992) RITA – Registry of Industrial Toxicology Animal data – progress of the working group. Exp Toxicol Pathol 44:301–309

Nieberle K, Cohrs P (1967) Textbook of special pathological anatomy. Pergamon, Oxford

Olson L (1970) Fluorescence histochemical evidence for axonal growth and secretion from transplanted adrenal medullary tissue. Histochemistry 22:1–7

Reznik G, Ward JM, Reznik-Schüler H (1980) Ganglioneuromas in the adrenal medulla of F344 rats. Vet Pathol 17: 614–621

Sandborn EB (1970) Cells and tissues by light and electron microscopy, vol I. Academic, New York, pp 205–250

Shafer TJ, Atchison WD (1991) Transmitter, ion channel and receptor properties of pheochromocytoma (PC12) cells: a model for neurotoxicological studies. Neurotoxicology 12: 473–492

Squire RA, Goodman DG, Valerio MG, Fredrickson T, Strandberg JD, Levitt MH, Lingeman CH, Harshbarger JC, Dawe CJ (1978) Tumors. In: Benirschke K, Garner FM, Jones TC (eds) Pathology of laboratory animals, vol II. Springer, Berlin Heidelberg New York, pp 1052–1283

Todd GC, Pierce EC, Clevinger WG (1970) Ganglioneuroma of the adrenal medulla in rats. A report of three cases. Pathol Vet 7:139–144

Trump DL, Livingston JN, Baylin SB (1977) Watery diarrhea syndrome in an adult with ganglioneuroma-pheochromocytoma: identification of vasoactive intestinal peptide, calcitonin, and catecholamines and assessment of their biologic activity. Cancer 40:1526–1532

Weiss L, Greep RO (1977) Histology. McGraw-Hill, New York, pp 1111–1115

Neuroblastoma, Adrenal, Rat

Gerd Reznik and Paul-Georg Germann

Synonym. Sympathicoblastoma.

Gross Appearance

This neoplasm may be so small that it cannot be detected macroscopically.

Microscopic Features

With low magnification the adrenal medulla may be seen to be enlarged (Fig. 467). The histologic appearance of this neoplasm is quite distinctive. The tumor cells resemble the embryonic sympathogonia from which they are believed to arise and are generally small, each with a deeply stained elongated nucleus surrounded by inconspicuous cytoplasm. The nuclei are closely packed in parallel arrays and often form circular structures (rosettes, Fig. 468). The neoplasm is usually spherical, located in the adrenal medulla and surrounded by pheochromocytes. Neurofibrillary material is not clearly recognizable among the tumor cells. Distant metastases have not been reported.

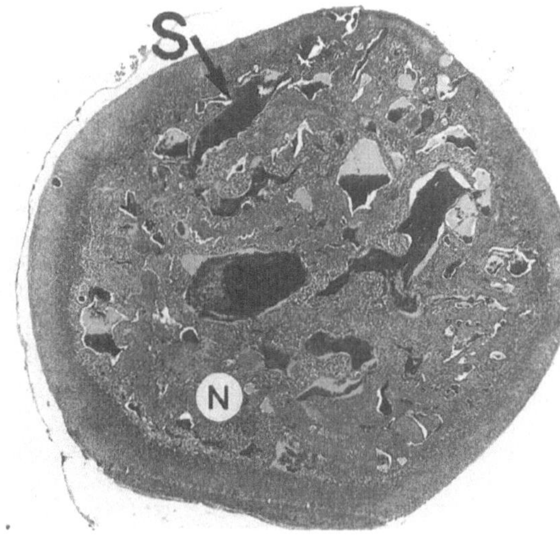

Fig. 467. Adrenal gland of a male F344 rat, 104 weeks old. Neuroblastoma (*N*) compressing the whole medulla. Severe vascular ectasia of sinusoids (*S*). H&E, ×3.3

Differential Diagnosis

Other medullary tumors of the adrenal gland, such as malignant pheochromocytomas, malignant complex pheochromocytomas, and malignant ganglioneuroblastomas occasionally contain areas of neuroblastic cells (Brown et al. in press; Hamlin and Banas 1990). Because the neuroblastic cell is not the dominating cell type, these tumors should be better diagnosed as medullary tumor, malignant, complex type (Krinke and Landes 1992). The diagnosis of neuroblastomas should be reserved for adrenal medullary neoplasms composed primarily (>80%) of neuroblasts (Fig. 468; Hamlin and Banas 1990).

Biologic Features

Only one other report of a neuroblastoma of the adrenal medulla in rats (Warren et al. 1966) was found in a search of the literature. In our study of 67 125 F344 male and female rats we found only one small neuroblastoma in the adrenal medulla of a 2-year-old untreated male (Reznik et al. 1980). The significance of this lesion is unknown.

Comparison with Other Species

Neuroblastomas are reported to occur in dogs, cattle, sheep, and chickens (Baumgartner 1931; Monlux et al. 1956; Trautwein 1958; Simon and Albert 1960; Sandersleben 1963; Jolly and Alley 1969; Frye and Clement 1970; Hollander and Snell 1976; Cordy 1978). Primary sites include the adrenal medulla and sympathetic ganglia. Although metastases are said to be common in peripheral neuroblastomas, few reports document this in the literature. In one case neuroblastoma of the cranial cervical ganglion in a 4-year-old springer spaniel was reported to metastasize to the kidney (Helman et al. 1980).

Neuroblastomas have been observed in human fetuses, in the newborn, and in infants only a few weeks old. Essentially this tumor is an embryonic neoplasm arising from still immature cells. In

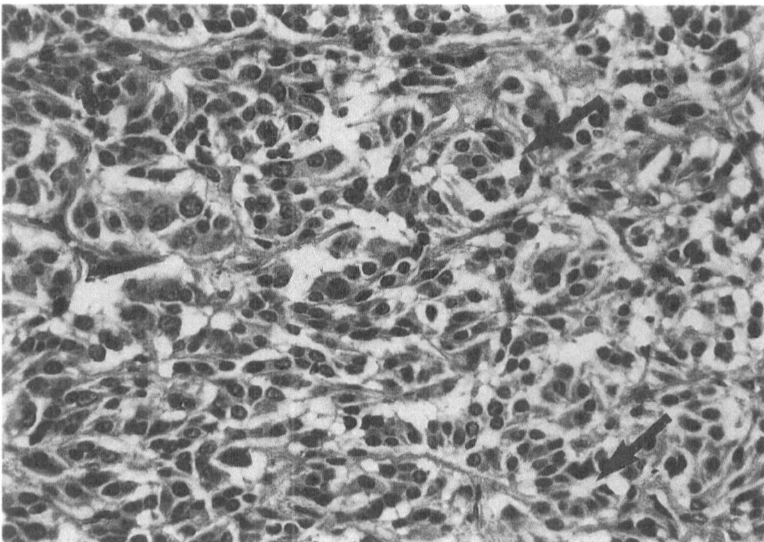

Fig. 468. Neuroblastoma in adrenal gland of a female Wistar rat, 140 weeks old. Note the rosettelike pattern (*arrows*). H&E, ×384

humans, the expression of markers for neuronal or neuroendocrine differentiation, for example, neurofilaments of different phosphorylation stages, chromogranin A, and synapthophysin, is variable in neuroblastomas, reflecting different molecular maturation stages of these embryonic precursor cells (Trojanowski et al. 1991). Additionally, a coexpression of other immunohistological markers as a sign of their variable histogenic differentiation has been observed, for example, rhabdomyogenous markers such as muscle-specific actin, desmin or myoglobin, and neuromelanin (Layfield and Glasgow 1991; Gonzalez-Crussi and Hsueh 1988).

Neuroblastomas of the brain may be found at autopsy in children under 3 months of age who have died of other causes. Although a rare form of malignant disease in adults, neuroblastoma is one of the most common tumors of childhood, occurring in children under 10 years of age, and is most frequent during the first 2 years of life. Infrequently, neuroblastoma develops in adolescents, but very rarely in adults or elderly people (Koop and Hernandez 1964; Williams and Donaldson 1973). In about two-thirds of cases neuroblastomas in adults arise in the abdomen, originating most frequently from the adrenal gland and neighboring sympathetic ganglia. Other sites of origin include the sympathetic ganglia in the pelvis, the posterior mediastinum, and less commonly the ganglia of the cervical sympathetic chain. Rarely, a neuroblastoma develops in the kidney or from small peripheral ganglia in the viscera (Azarelli et al. 1977).

Acknowledgements. The authors wish to thank Dr. S.L. Eustis, NTP (USA), and Jerrold M. Ward, National Cancer Institute (USA), for their supporting case material and Ms. Maureen Hall, Experimental Pathology Laboratories (USA) for her excellent photographs.

References

Azarelli F, Richards DE, Anton AH, Roessmann U (1977) Central neuroblastoma. Electron microscopic observations and catecholamine determinations. J Neuropathol Exp Neurol 36:384–397

Baumgartner H (1931) Ein Fall von bösartigem Neuroblastom beim Rind. Z Krebsforsch 34:174–184

Brown WR, Gough A, Hamlin MH II, Hottendorf GH, Patterson DR (in press) Proliferative lesions of the adrenal glands of rats, pp 1–16 (In preparation by STP)

Cordy DR (1978) Tumors of the nervous system and eye. In: Moulton JE (ed) Tumors in domestic animals, 2nd edn. University of California Press, Berkeley, pp 437–439

Frye FL, Clement ED (1970) Sympathicoblastoma in a dog. J Am Vet Med Assoc 156:900–901

Gonzalez-crussi F, Hsueh W (1988) Bilateral adrenal ganglioneuroblastoma with neuromelanin. Cancer 61:1159–1166

Hamlin MH, Banas DA (1990) Adrenal gland. In: Boorman GA, Eustis SL, Elwell MR, Montgomery CA Jr, MacKenzie WF (eds) Pathology of the Fischer rat, reference and atlas. Academic, San Diego, pp 501–518

Helman RG, Adams LG, Hall CL, Read WK (1980) Metastatic neuroblastoma in a dog. Vet Pathol 17:769–773

Hollander CR, Snell KC (1976) Tumours of the adrenal gland. IARC Sci Publ 6:273–294

Jolly RD, Alley MR (1969) Medulloblastoma in calves. Vet Pathol 6:463–468
Krinke GJ, Landes C (1992) Toxicologic pathology of the rodent adrenal medulla. In: ILSI handout of histopathology seminar on the endocrine system of laboratory animals 1992, session C
Koop CE, Hernandez JR (1964) Neuroblastoma: experience with 100 cases in children. Surgery 56:726–733
Layfield LI, Glasgow BJ (1991) Rhabdomyosarcomatous differentiation in a neuroblastoma. Diagn Cytopathol 7:193–197
Monlux AW, Anderson WA, Davis CL (1956) A Survey of tumors occurring in cattle, sheep and swine. Am J Vet Res 17:646–677
Reznik G, Ward JM, Reznik-Schüler H (1980) Ganglioneuromas in the adrenal medulla of F344 rats. Vet Pathol 17:614–621
Sandersleben J (1963) Blastome der Spinalnervenwurzeln und der Rückenmarkshäute als Ursache von Lähmungen beim Fleischfresser. Berl Munch Tieraerztl Wochenschr 76:129–133
Simon J, Albert LT (1960) Two cases of neuroblastomas in dogs. J Am Vet Med Assoc 136:210–214
Trautwein G (1958) Über ein Sympathoblastom des Haushuhnes. DTW Dtsch Tierarztl Wochenschr 65: 353–356
Trojanowski JQ, Molenaar WM, Baker DL, Pleasure D, Lee VMY (1991) Neural and neuroendocrine phenotype of neuroblastomas, ganglioblastomas, ganglioneuromas and mature versus embryonic adrenal medullary cells. Advances in neuroblastoma research 3:335–341
Warren S, Grozdev L, Gates O, Chute RN (1966) Radiation induced adrenal medullary tumors in the rat. Arch Pathol 82:115–118
Williams TE, Donaldson MH (1973) Neuroblastoma in clinical pediatric oncology. In: Sutow WW, Vietti TY, Fernback DY (eds) Clinical pediatric oncology. Mosby, St Louis, pp 384–410

Focal Hyperplasia, Adrenal Cortex; Rat

John D. Strandberg

Synonyms. Foci of cellular alteration, nodular hyperplasia, hyperplastic nodules.

Gross Appearance

The smallest and earliest lesions are inapparent on gross examination. Larger areas of hyperplasia and adenomas appear as discrete nodular swellings within the adrenal cortex, resulting in its enlargement. The nodules may be of the same color as the adjacent cortex or contrast with it by being either paler yellow or darker.

Microscopic Features

For the purposes of this review, focal hyperplasia is described as a separate entity. It is rather arbitrarily separated from cortical adenoma even though the two lesions are often part of a continuous spectrum of disease. Histologic features do not necessarily predict behavior. Several criteria, summarized by Hamlin and Banas (1990) must be considered in their diagnosis.

The foci of cellular alteration are most commonly found in the zona fasciculata and the zona reticularis. They are roughly spherical collections of adrenal cortical cells which do not compress the surrounding cortical parenchyma (Figs. 469, 470). The cells themselves may be of several types and are indistinguishable from those found in cortical adenomas. Hyperplastic cells may closely resemble those of the surrounding cortex and possess round vesicular nuclei and pale eosinophilic cytoplasm which is often slightly vacuolated. Some foci may be formed of cells with highly vacuolated cytoplasm, while others are populated by smaller cells with denser, more basophilic cytoplasm. Foci with mixtures of these cell populations also occur (Hamlin and Banas 1990). Mitotic activity tends to be low in all these lesions. At times there are also large blood-filled spaces or sinusoids located within the areas. Thrombosis and necrosis are often a part of the process as well. In addition, the author has noted foci of altered cells in the zona glomerulosa of Brown Norway rats. These subcapsular foci are composed of cells with pale cytoplasm and have discrete margins. They show no evidence of progression to form adenomas or carcinomas.

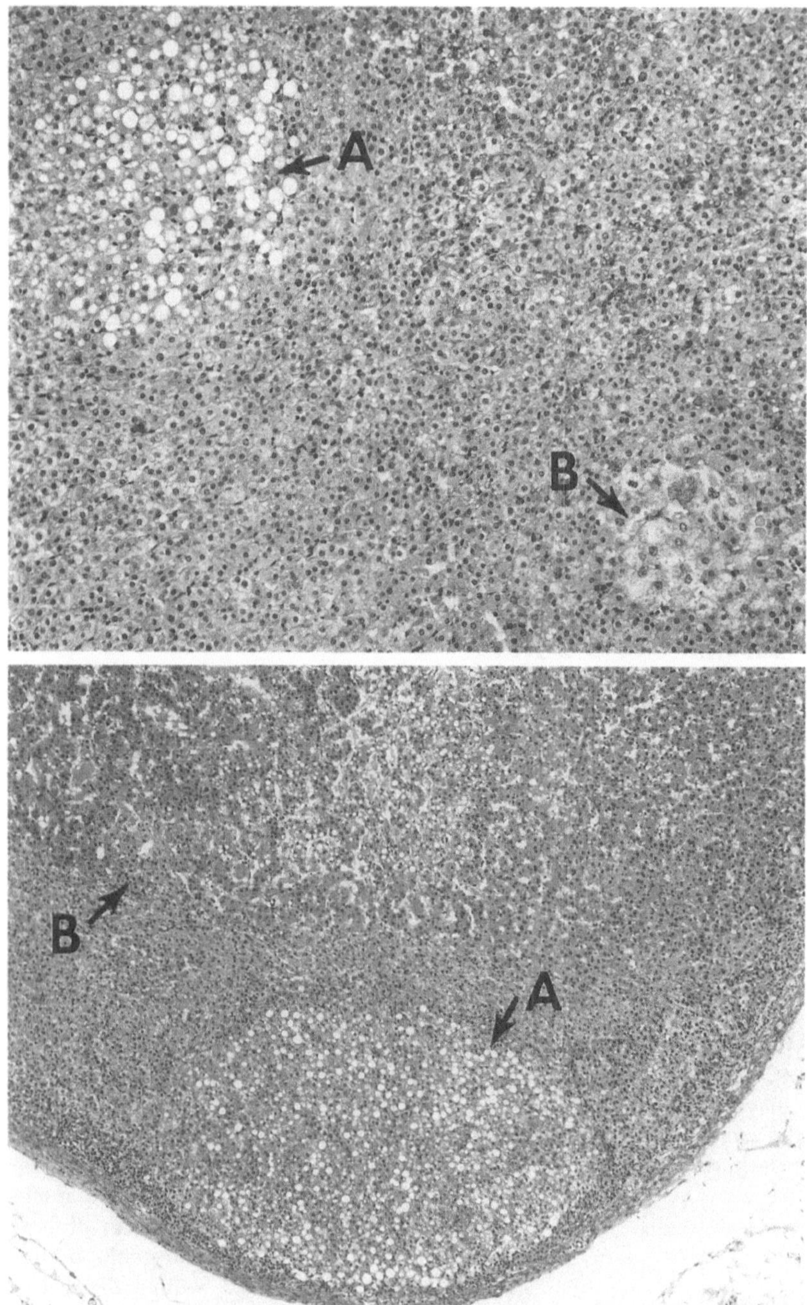

Fig. 469. (*above*) Two foci of hyperplasia in the adrenal cortex of a 21-month-old female OM rat. The larger (*A*) is composed of cells filled with large lipid droplets. The smaller focus (*B*) has cells with broad, palely eosinophilic cytoplasm. Helley's fixative. H&E, ×220

Fig. 470. (*below*) Adrenal from a 21-month-old female OM rat containing a small focus of hyperplasia (*A*) of lipid-laden cells in the outer zona fasciculata. A larger cortical adenoma (*B*) occupies much of the inner cortex and is composed of cords of well-differentiated cortical cells. Helley's fixative. H&E, ×70

Ultrastructure

Ultrastructural studies have been performed on several types of adrenal lesions. Aniline induces adrenal cortical lipid hyperplasia in which the hyperplastic cells accumulate lipid and cholesterol. The changes include degeneration of mitochondria, hypertrophy of smooth endoplasmic reticulum, and dilatation of the Golgi. These changes are more pronounced in the inner cortex and resemble congenital adrenal hyperplasia as seen in humans (Kovacs et al. 1971). Sugihara et al. (1973) reported nodules in the zona fasciculata of male Wistar rats 12–24 months of age. Two-thirds of these animals had nodules that could be divided into three types on the basis of their cytologic features. These were termed: (a) hyperplastic small-cell type with many elongated mitochondria and high levels of alkaline phosphatase, (b) hyperplastic large-cell type with abundant smooth endoplasmic reticulum and increased levels of steroid 3 β-ol-dehydrogenase, and (c) lipid droplet type in which the cells contained many round mitochondria with lamellar or whorling cristae, intramitochondrial deposits, and increased levels of secondary alcohol dehydrogenase. Six of these lesions were termed large adenomatous nodules, but the authors did not address the question of whether they were neoplasms.

Differential Diagnosis

The principal differential diagnostic problem is in separating various adrenal lesions from one another. The terminology (hyperplasia vs. neoplasia) is often of practical importance particularly in those cases in which these lesions are found in bioassay studies. One somewhat arbitrary criterion is the absence of compression of adjacent cortical tissue in hyperplasia. Other lesions which must be differentiated include hyperplasia and neoplasms of the adrenal medulla which may resemble these lesions histologically at times. In this case the demonstration of chromaffin granules is decisive. Also those instances in which there is extensive vascular dilatation must be separated from hemangiomatous lesions. Adrenal cortical cells in this instance are not intermingled with vasculature. In all cases diagnosis is facilitated if multiple sections of the gland are examined, and a full cross-section including the medulla is essential. Serial sectioning has been recommended as a way to diminish the number of small lesions that are overlooked in single-sectioning techniques (Thompson and Hunt 1963).

As noted above, criteria used to categorize proliferative lesions of the rat adrenal cortex on morphologic grounds have been somewhat subjective resulting in considerable variation in terminology encountered in published reports. Some individuals are reluctant to designate as neoplasms any but the largest or most obviously invasive or metastatic lesions, resulting in the term nodular hyperplasia being employed for many proliferative lesions. Others note that since one cannot on histopathologic grounds reliably differentiate hyperplastic lesions from benign tumors, all nodular growths should be considered potentially neoplastic and termed adenomas or, if they invade or metastasize, carcinomas. A recently presented discussion of adrenal cortical lesions in Fischer 344 rats nicely summarizes criteria which are helpful in differentiating hyperplasia from neoplasia (Hamlin and Banas 1990). However, the variance in nomenclature and criteria used in diagnosis makes it difficult to compare historical data derived from different studies (see "Adenoma, Adrenal Cortex, Rat," this volume).

Biologic Features

Focal adrenal cortical hyperplasia, cortical adenomas, and adenocarcinomas are seen with increasing frequency in older animals of several strains of rats (Boorman and Hollander 1973). Very high numbers have been encountered in the Osborne-Mendel (OM) strain, while and Sprague-Dawley rats tend to have fewer lesions (Tables 33, 34). With the exception of the OM rats, most of these lesions are seen in animals older than 18 months. There is also a difference between sexes, although this varies somewhat from strain to strain and from laboratory to laboratory. In general, these lesions occur somewhat more commonly in female animals, which normally tend to have larger glands. Age and sex differences in incidence are noted in induced lesions as well as in those occurring spontaneously (Korenchevsky and Paris 1950; Iglesias and Mardones 1958; Goldman 1967; Russfield 1967; Schardein et al. 1968; Noble 1977; Squire et al.

Table 33. Spontaneous lesions of adrenal cortex

Strain	Age	Lesion	Frequency (%)		Reference
			Male	Female	
Sprague-Dawley	–	Cortical adenocarcinoma	1/43 (2.3)	0/82	Thompson et al. 1961
Sprague-Dawley	18 mo	Cortical adenoma	11/179 (6.1)	16/181 (8.8)	Prejean et al. 1973
		Cortical carcinoma	1/179 (0.56)	0/181	
Sprague-Dawley	–	Cortical adenoma	3/42 (7)	4/39 (10)	Suzuki et al. 1979
ACI	12–18 mo	Cortical tumors	0	0	Hollander and Snell 1976
	>18 mo		0	0	
ACI	18–34 mo	Cortical adenoma	1/55 (1.8)	1/209 (0.5)	Maekawa and Odashima 1975
		Cortical carcinoma	1/55 (1.8)	1/209 (0.5)	
Osborne-Mendel	12–18 mo	Cortical tumors	(50)	(65)	Hollander and Snell 1976
(OM)	>18 mo		(73)	(95)	
OM	>18 mo	Adenomas or adenocarcinomas	53/59 (90)		Snell and Stewart 1959
	12–17 mo	Hyperplastic nodules or small adenomas	17/26 (65)		
BUF	12–18 mo	Cortical tumors	(13)	(5)	Hollander and Snell 1976
	>18 mo		(33)	(62)	
WAG/Rij	Life span	Adrenal cortical adenoma	7/124 (6)	40/101 (40)	Burek 1978
	Life span	Carcinoma	2/124 (2)	2/101 (2)	
WAG/Rij	8–11 mo	Adrenal cortical adenoma		0/1	Boorman and Hollander 1973
	12–15 mo			0/4	
	16–19 mo			0/9	
	20–23 mo			3/7 (42.9)	
	24–27 mo			10/44 (22.7)	
	28–31 mo			26/84 (31.0)	
	32–35 mo			25/81 (30.9)	
	36–39 mo			16/54 (29.6)	
	40–43 mo			3/6 (50.0)	
	Total			83/290 (28.6)	
WAG/Rij	Life span	Adrenal cortical tumors	7/106 (7)	91/301 (31)	Hollander 1976
BN/Bi	Life span	Adrenal cortical adenoma	5/39 (13)	17/79 (22)	Hollander 1976
		Adrenal cortical carcinoma	0/39	4/79 (5)	
BN/Bi	Life span	Adenoma	9/74 (12)	45/236 (19)	Burek 1978
		Carcinoma	1/74 (1)	22/236 (9)	
F_1	Life span	Adenoma	21/67 (31)	15/68 (22)	Burek 1978
		Carcinoma	2/67 (3)	5/68 (7)	
F344	12–18 mo	Cortical tumors	0	0	Hollander and Snell 1976
	>18 mo		(6)	0	
F344	Life span	Adrenal cortical tumors (three carcinomas with pulmonary metastasis)	17/160 (11)	11/192 (6)	Sass et al. 1975
Sprague-Dawley	–	Cortical carcinoma	1/63 (1.6)	0/114	Thompson and Hunt 1963
F344	4–33 mo	Cortical adenoma	2/144 (1.4)	–	Coleman et al. 1977
F344	Life span	Adenoma	4/1794 (0.22)	1/1754 (0.05)	Goodman et al. 1979
F344	Life span	Cortical adenoma	13/1794 (0.72)	19/1754 (1.10)	Goodman et al. 1979
		Cortical carcinoma	3/1794 (0.16)	3/1754 (0.17)	
		Cortical hyperplasia	22/1794 (1.2)	39/1754 (2.2)	
Sprague-Dawley (Holtzman-source)	1½–18 mo	Cortical adenoma	38/3387 (1.1)	53/1699 (3.1)	Schardein et al. 1968
Wistar	–	Adenoma-like nodules	11/60 (18.3)	–	Jayne 1957
Wistar	12–24 mo	Intracortical nodules	60/90 (67)	–	Sugihara et al. 1973
WN	12–18 mo	Cortical tumors	0	10	Hollander and Snell 1976
	>18 mo		(8)	(12)	
M520	12–18 mo	Cortical tumors	0	0	Hollander and Snell 1976
	>18 mo		(20)	(40)	

Table 34. Induced adrenal cortical lesions

Strain: Treatment	Age	Diagnosis	Frequency (%)		Reference
			Males	Females	
Sprague-Dawley Control	–	Adrenal tumors	2/80 (2.5)	3/80 (3.8)	Berdjis 1967
Irradiation			10/78 (12.8)	11/76 (13.2)	
Sprague-Dawley Control	–	Adenomas	5/129 (3.8)	–	Castanera et al. 1968
		Carcinomas	1/129 (0.7)	–	
Whole-body irradiation	–	Adenomas	49/309 (15.9)	–	
		Carcinomas	7/309 (2.3)	–	

1978; Goodman et al. 1979; Yarrington and Johnston 1994).

The lesions outlined above are distinct from cellular proliferations of specific zones of the adrenal cortex which have been induced by hormonal stimuli directed at certain populations. Marked generalized adrenal cortical hyperplasia has been seen in rats implanted with tumor cells which secreted corticotropin-releasing hormone (Hammer et al. 1992). They are also quite different from the generalized hypertrophy of the zona fasciculata and zona reticularis which occur with advancing age and attributed to high levels of circulating ACTH (Rebuffat et al. 1992).

References

Boorman GA, Hollander CF (1973) Spontaneous lesions in the female WAG/Rij (Wistar) rat. J Gerontol 28:152–159

Goldman AS (1967) Experimental model of congenital adrenal cortical hyperplasia produced in utero with an inhibitor of 11-beta-steroid hydroxylase. J Clin Endocrinol Metab 27: 1390–1394

Goodman DG, Ward JM, Squire RA, Chu KC, Linhart MS (1979) Neoplastic and nonneoplastic lesions in aging F344 rats. Toxicol Appl Pharmacol 48:237–248

Hamlin MH II, Banas DA (1990) Adrenal gland. In: Boorman GA, Eustis SL, Elwell MR, Montgomery CL Jr, McKenzie WF (eds) Pathology of the Fischer rat. Academic, San Diego, pp 501–518

Hammer GD, Mueller G, Liu B, Petrides JS, Roos BA, Low MJ (1992) Ectopic corticotropin-releasing hormone produced by a transfected cell line chronically activates the pituitary-adrenal axis in transkaryotic rats. Endocrinology 130:1975–1985

Iglesias R, Mardones E (1958) Spontaneous and transplantable functional tumor of the adrenal cortex in the A × C rat. Br J Cancer 12:20–27

Korenchevsky V, Paris SK (1950) Cooperative effects of endocrinological factors and processes of aging in producing adenoma-like structures in rats. Cancer 3:903–922

Kovacs K, Blascheck JA, Yeghiayan E, Hatakeyama S, Gardell C (1971) Adrenocortical lipid hyperplasia induced in rats by aniline. A histologic and electron microscopic study. Am J Pathol 62:17–34

Noble RL (1977) Hormonal control of growth and progression in tumors of Nb rats and a theory of action. Cancer Res 37:82–94

Rebuffat P, Belloni AS, Rocco S, Andreis PG, Neri G, Malendowicz LK, Gottardo G, Mazzocchi G, Nussdorfer GG (1992) The effects of aging on the morphology and function of the zonae fasciculata and reticularis of the rat adrenal cortex. Cell Tissue Res 270:265–272

Russfield AB (1967) Pathology of the endocrine glands, ovary and testis of rats and mice. In: Cotchin E, Roe FJC (eds) Pathology of laboratory rats and mice, chap 14. Blackwell Scientific, Oxford

Schardein JL, Fitzgerald JE, Kaump DH (1968) Spontaneous tumors in Holtzman-Source rats of various ages. Vet Pathol 5:238–252

Squire RA, Goodman DG, Valerio MG, Fredrickson TN, Strandberg JD, Levitt MH, Lingeman CH, Harshbarger JC, Dawe CJ (1978) Tumors. In: Benirschke K, Garner FM, Jones TC (eds) Pathology of laboratory animals, vol II, chap 12. Springer, Berlin Heidelberg New York

Sugihara H, Kawai K, Tsuchiyama H (1973) Pathology of intracortical nodules in rat adrenal glands, especially on their fine-structure. Acta Pathol Jpn 23:253–260

Thompson SW, Hunt RD (1963) Spontaneous tumors in the Sprague-Dawley rat: incidence rates of some types of neoplasms as determined by serial section versus single section technics. Ann NY Acad Sci 108:832–848

Yarrington JT, Johnston JO (1994) Aging in the adrenal cortex. In: Mohr U, Dungworth, DL, Capen CC (eds) Pathobiology of the aging rat, vol 2. ILSI, Washington DC, pp 227–244

Adenoma, Adrenal Cortex, Rat

John D. Strandberg

Synonyms. Nodular hyperplasia, nodules, hyperplastic nodules, foci of cellular alteration (often used erroneously).

Gross Appearance

The smallest and earliest lesions are not seen on gross examination. Large foci of hyperplasia and adenomas, indistinguishable grossly, occur as discrete nodular swellings within and often compressing the cortex. The focal enlargement may be the same color, paler yellow, or darker than the surrounding cortex.

Microscopic Features

The cells which make up adenoma of the adrenal cortex clearly resemble those of the zona reticulata or zona fasciculata from which they arise. These cells may vary somewhat in appearance (Duprat et al. 1990), are large polygonal cells with eosinophilic cytoplasm containing clear lipid droplets which may vary considerably in size from adenoma to adenoma or within a single tumor. In other cases the cells are of normal size or even smaller with slightly basophilic cytoplasm (Hamlin and Banas 1990). The cells lack normal orientation and are sometimes arranged in irregular cords but clearly grow by expansion and compress the adjacent cortex (Fig. 471). Their nuclei are usually densely stained; only occasionally is the nucleolus conspicuous (Fig. 472). Dilated sinusoids, filled with blood, often constitute a large part of the tumor mass (Fig. 473).

Differential Diagnosis

Hamlin and Banas (1990) and Yarrington and Johnson (1994) have clearly summarized criteria useful in differential diagnosis of proliferative lesions of the rat adrenal cortex. The general basis for differentiating adrenal cortical adenomas from areas of focal cortical hyperplasia is the concept that adenomas are expansive lesions as evidenced by compression of surrounding cortex. These neoplasms may have delicate connective tissue capsules. In other respects the cell populations which are encountered are those described for focal cortical hyperplasia. Blood-filled lakes or sinusoids are more commonly seen in adenomas than in foci of hyperplasia. Mitotic figures and cellular atypia are rarely encountered. The occasional difficulty in differentiating adenomas from focal hyperplasia is discussed further on p. 437 (this volume).

Biologic Features

Adrenal cortical tumors and hyperplasias may be functional (Iglesias and Mardones 1958). This is often indicated by atrophy of the gland surrounding a lesion or lipid depletion and atrophy of the contralateral adrenal; similar atrophy is observed in the adrenals of rats with transplanted carcinomas (Snell and Stewart 1959). Cells from the transplantable adrenal carcinoma have been shown to be capable of synthesis and metabolism comparable to those derived from normal cortex (Mason et al. 1983). Assay of cells for biochemical and hormonal activity has principally used transplantable carcinomas because of the volume of tissue that is available for use and the reproducibility of the system. Such tumors have been shown to produce a variety of hormones, among them erythropoietin (Cohen et al. 1957; Meineke 1969). Adrenal cortical tumors induced by estrogens respond to hormonal stimuli, and isolated cells in vitro show altered function as compared with cells of the normal rat cortex (McMillan et al. 1971; Sharma 1973; see Table 3).

Pathogenesis. Study of the pathogenesis of adrenal tumors has used experimental settings in which the lesions have been induced by castration, administration of hormones, and irradiation. In these situations there is a progression of lesions which mimic those seen in spontaneous neoplasms. This spectrum begins with foci of hyperplasia, which most commonly occur in the zona fasciculata; these may be multiple and have the morphology described above. Depending on the rat strain and experimental protocol, they are

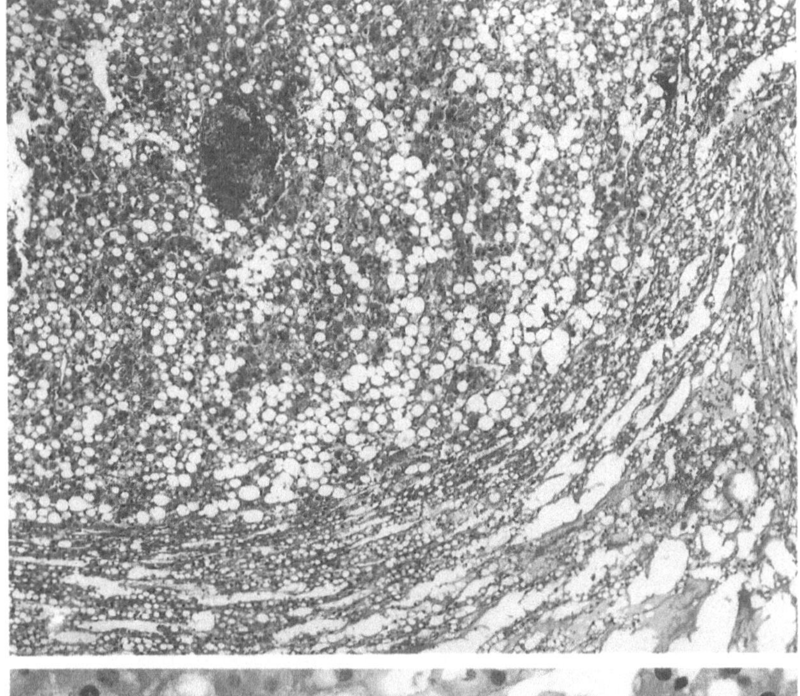

Fig. 471. A segment of a large cortical adenoma compressing surrounding adrenal tissue, 26-month-old female OM rat. Both the tumor and the cortex contain abundant lipid in the form of clear cytoplasmic droplets. Helley's fixative. H&E, ×70

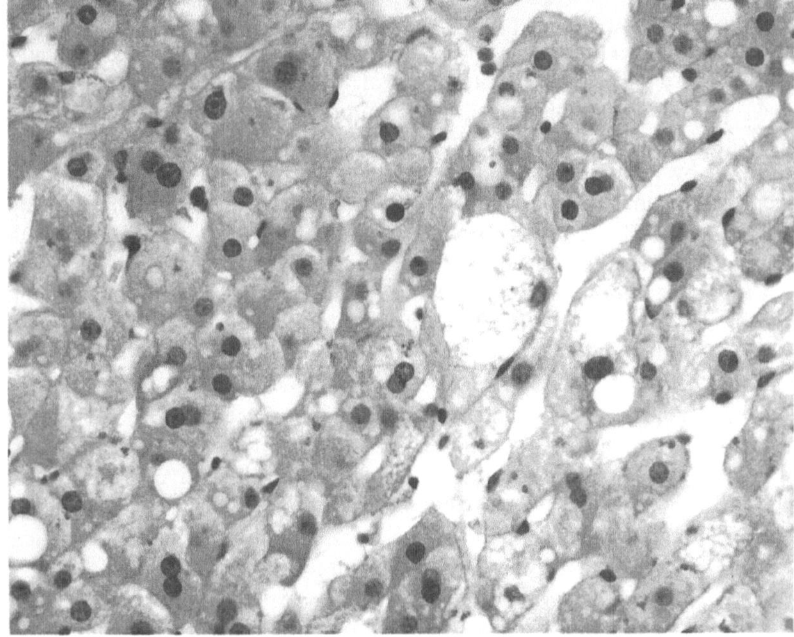

Fig. 472. Higher magnification of cells from the adenoma illustrated in Fig. 471. There is some cellular pleomorphism. The amount of cytoplasmic lipd varies from cell to cell. Helley's fixative. H&E, ×430

followed in time, usually after 18 months of age, by the appearance of cortical adenomas. These tend to be present in smaller numbers than the hyperplasias. There is usually a single adenoma per adrenal. To some extent the various morphological types of lesions reflect the amount of lipid secretion stored within the cells. The distended vascular channels may represent distortion of sinusoidal channels previously existing in the gland or may be the result of degeneration and necrosis of tumor cells with subsequent angiectasis.

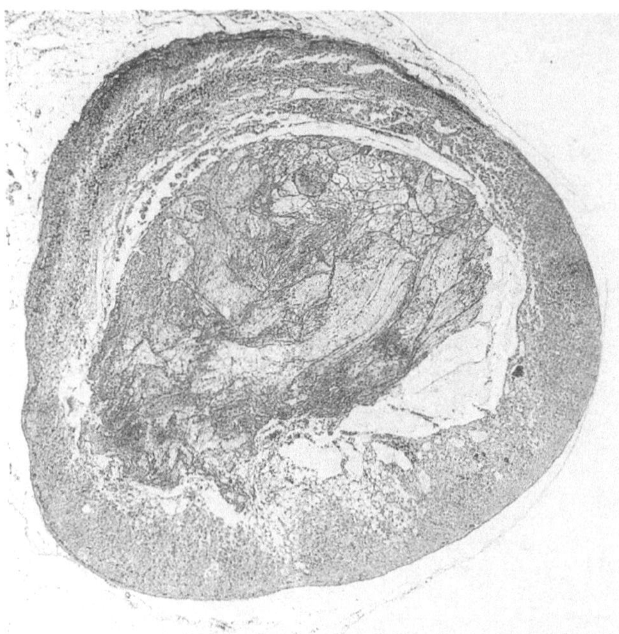

Fig. 473. The central area of a large cortical adenoma is occupied by clotted blood and some necrotic debris. Most of the gland is occupied by tumor. Tissue was obtained from a 24-month-old female OM rat. Helley's fixative. H&E, ×16

Etiology. Hormonal manipulations can be used to induce these lesions (Cohen et al. 1957; Korenchevsky and Paris 1950). Houssay et al. (1955) observed that castration caused a focal modification of the cortex after 1–4 months. This was followed by nodular hyperplasia in 2–8 months and by adenomas in 6–12 months. These occurred in 25%–55% of the rats. None of these tumors ever metastasized despite the histologic features of carcinoma in some of them. Administration of estrogen in several forms was found to cause both benign and malignant neoplasms (Dunning et al. 1953).

Estrogen-induced lesions may be capable of metastasis and often show hormonal dependence, requiring estrogen for continued growth and spread. This hormonal dependence is not a uniform characteristic; some carcinomas are capable of autonomous growth following transplantation (Nichols 1971; Noble 1977).

Fission neutron irradiation has also been found to lead to the production of cortical adenocarcinomas in male Buffalo rats (Vogel and Zaldivar 1970). Other investigators using ionizing radiation also reported adrenal tumors (Castanera et al. 1968; Rosen et al. 1961). In Sprague-Dawley rats the initial response was degeneration of the cortex followed by development of proliferative centers (Berdjis 1967). Pollard and Sharon (1971) noted no cortical tumors following irradiation of Wistar and Fischer rats but found instead adenomas of the medulla.

Adrenal tumors have been reported to result from chronic administration of certain chlorinated hydrocarbons. An association of chlorobenzilate with cortical adenomas was found in low-dose male and high-dose female rats, although the Osborne-Mendel (OM) strain used in the study has a high background incidence (Bioassay 1978). Kepone and hexachlorobenzene were found to produce hyperplasia of the cortex in Sherman strain rats (Kimbrough 1979). Carcinomas and sarcomas of the adrenal cortex have been reported in OM rats ingesting endrin (Reuber 1978); the NCI bioassay of this compound, however, was negative for induction of cortical tumors.

Other carcinogens which have been reported to cause adrenal cortical tumors include *N,N'*-2,7-fluorenylene bis-2,2,2-trifluoroacetamide (2,7-FAA-F6) as well as 2,7-FAA (Morris et al. 1963). Several adenomas and carcinomas were also found in OM rats fed *p*-dimethylaminoazobenzene (Mulay and Eyestone 1955). The statistical significance of the difference from controls may be questioned, and the natural high frequency of this strain must be pointed out. Administration of aniline (aminobenzene) causes lipid hyperplasia of the cortex. The mechanism is postulated to be the lowering of blood corticosterone with resulting increase in ACTH secretion and subsequent hyperplasia. The cells in the hyperplastic cortex are laden with lipid and cholesterol. This lesion resembles congenital adrenal hyperplasia of humans and hyperplasia following treatment with aminoglutethimide (Kovacs et al. 1971). A similar hyperplastic lesion has been produced in animals treated in utero with metyrapone, an inhibitor of 11β-steroid hydroxylase (Goldman 1967; see Table 34).

In another study transformed cell lines obtained by Kirsten murine sarcoma virus infection of adrenal cells from young rats were found to produce tumors with a variety of histologic patterns upon being inoculated into animals. These included pleomorphic carcinomas and sarcomas as well as mixed and anaplastic tumors (Auersperg et al. 1981).

Comparison with Other Species

Focal adrenal cortical hyperplasia, cortical adenoma, and cortical adenocarcinomas of rats resemble in morphology and behavior the same lesion observed in mice. Morphological similarities can be seen in others of the more common domestic species, as well as in humans. In all these the major problem has been in the differentiation of hyperplasias from benign tumors and of adenomas from adenocarcinomas (Russfield 1967; Anderson and Capen 1978; Squire et al. 1978; Altman and Goodman 1979; Goodman et al. 1979, Duprat et al. 1990, Hamlin and Banas 1990).

References

Altman NH, Goodman DG (1979) Neoplastic diseases. In: Baker HJ, Lindsey JR, Weisbroth SH (eds) The laboratory rat, vol I, chap 13. Academic, New York

Anderson MP, Capen CC (1978) The endocrine system. In: Benirschke K, Garner FM, Jones TC (eds) Pathology of laboratory animals, vol I, chap 6. Springer, Berlin Heidelberg New York

Auersperg N, Wan MW, Sanderson RA, Wong KS, Mauldin D (1981) Morphologic and functional differentiation of Kirsten murine sarcoma virus-transformed rat adrenocortical cell lines. Cancer Res 41:1763–1771

Berdjis CC (1967) Pathogenesis of radiation-induced endocrine tumors. Oncology 21:49–60

Bioassay of chlorobenzilate for possible carcinogenicity (1978). CAS no 510-15-6. DHEW/PUB/NIH-78-1325, NCI-CG-TR-75. US Government Printing Office, Washington DC

Boorman GA, Hollander CF (1973) Spontaneous lesions in the female WAG/Rij (Wistar) rat. J Gerontol 28:152–159

Burek JD (1978) Pathology of aging rats. CRC, Boca Raton

Castanera TJ, Jones DC, Kimeldorf DJ, Rosen VJ (1968) The influence of whole body exposure to X-rays or neutrons on the life span distribution of tumors among male rats. Cancer Res 28:170–182

Cohen AI, Furth J, Buffett RF (1957) Histologic and physiologic characteristics of hormone-secreting transplantable adrenal tumors in mice and rats. Am J Pathol 33:631–651

Coleman GL, Barthold S, Osbaldiston GW, Foster S, Jonas AM (1977) Pathological changes during aging in barrier-reared Fischer 344 male rats. J Gerontol 32:258–278

Dunning WF, Curtis MR, Segaloff A (1953) Strain differences in response to estrone and the induction of mammary gland, adrenal, and bladder cancer in rats. Cancer Res 13:147–152

Duprat P, Snell KC, Hollander CF (1990) Tumours of the adrenal gland. In: Turusov V, Mohr U (eds) Pathology of tumours in laboratory animals, vol. 1, 2nd edn. IARC Sci Publ 99:573–596

Goldman AS (1967) Experimental model of congenital adrenal cortical hyperplasia produced in utero with an inhibitor of 11-beta-steroid hydroxylase. J Clin Endocrinol Metab 27:1390–1394

Goodman DG, Ward JM, Squire RA, Chu KC, Linhart MS (1979) Neoplastic and nonneoplastic lesions in aging F344 rats. Toxicol Appl Pharmacol 48:237–248

Hamlin MH II, Banas DA (1990) Adrenal gland. In: Boorman GA, Eustis SL, Elwell MR, Montgomery CL Jr, McKenzie WF (eds) Pathology of the Fischer rat. Academic, San Diego, pp 501–518

Hollander CF (1976) Current experience in using the laboratory rat in aging studies. Lab Anim Sci 26:320–328

Hollander CF, Snell KC (1976) Tumours of the adrenal gland. IARC Sci Publ 6:273–294

Houssay BA, Houssay AB, Cardeza AF, Pinto RM (1955) Tumeurs surrénales oestrogéniques et tumeurs hypophysaires chez les animaux castrés. Schweiz Med Wochenschr 85:291–296

Iglesias R, Mardones E (1958) Spontaneous and transplantable functional tumor of the adrenal cortex in the A × C rat. Br J Cancer 12:20–27

Jayne EP (1957) Histochemical and degenerative changes in the adrenal cortex of the rat with age. J Gerontol 12:2–8

Kimbrough RD (1979) The carcinogenic and other chronic effects of persistent halogenated organic compounds. Ann NY Acad Sci 320:415–418

Korenchevsky V, Paris SK (1950) Cooperative effects of endocrinological factors and processes of aging in producing adenoma-like structures in rats. Cancer 3:903–922

Kovacs K, Blascheck JA, Yeghiayan E, Hatakeyama S, Gardell C (1971) Adrenocortical lipid hyperplasia induced in rats by aniline. A histologic and electron microscopic study. Am J Pathol 62:17–34

Maekawa S, Odashima S (1975) Spontaneous tumors in ACI/N rats. J Natl Cancer Inst 55:1437–1445

Mason JI, Murry BA, Aberhart DJ (1983) The synthesis and metabolism of [6-3H]-25-hydroxycholesterol in rat adrenal tumor cells. J Steroid Biochem 18:765–769

McMillan BH, Ney RL, Schorr I (1971) Guanyl cyclase activity in normal adrenals and a corticosterone producing adrenal cancer of the rat. Endocrinology 89:281–283

Meineke HA (1969) The origin of erythropoietin in rats with transplants of an adrenal cortical carcinoma. Proc Soc Exp Biol Med 132:651–655

Morris HP, Wagner BP, Ray FE, Stewart HL, Snell KC (1963) Carcinogenic effects of N, N′-2,7-fluorenylenebis-2,2,2-trifluoroacetamide (2,7-FAA-F6) administered orally to Buffalo strain rats. J Natl Cancer Inst 30:143–161

Mulay AS, Eyestone WH (1955) Transplantable adrenocortical adenocarcinomas in Osborne-Mendel rats fed a carcinogenic diet. J Natl Cancer Inst 16:723–739

Nichols TM (1971) The morphological effects of estrogen removal on an estrogen-dependent adrenocortical carcinoma in rats. Cancer Res 31:1042–1050

Noble RL (1977) Hormonal control of growth and progression in tumors of Nb rats and a theory of action. Cancer Res 37:82–94

Pollard M, Sharon N (1971) Irradiation-induced lesions in germfree rats. J Natl Cancer Inst 47:229–234

Prejean JD, Peckham JC, Casey AE, Griswold DP, Weisburger EK, Weisburger JH (1973) Spontaneous tumors in Sprague-Dawley rats and Swiss mice. Cancer Res 33:2768–2773

Reuber MD (1978) Carcinomas, sarcomas and other lesions in Osborne-Mendel rats ingesting endrin. Exp Cell Biol 46:129–145

Rosen VJ, Castanera TJ, Jones DC, Kimeldorf DJ (1961) Islet-cell tumors of the pancreas in the irradiated and non-irradiated rat. Lab Invest 10:608–616

Russfield AB (1967) Pathology of the endocrine glands, ovary and testis of rats and mice. In: Cotchin E, Roe FJC (eds) Pathology of laboratory rats and mice, chap 14. Blackwell Scientific, Oxford

Sass B, Rabstein LS, Madison R, Nims RM, Peters RL, Kelloff GJ (1975) Incidence of spontaneous neoplasms in F344 rats throughout the natural life-span. J Natl Cancer Inst 54:1449–1456

Schardein JL, Fitzgerald JE, Kaump DH (1968) Spontaneous tumors in Holtzman-source rats of various ages. Vet Pathol 5:238–252

Sharma RK (1973) Metabolic regulation of steroidogenesis in adrenocortical carcinoma cells of rat. Effect of adrenocorticotropin and adenosine cyclic 3′:5′-monophosphate on corticosteroidogenesis. Eur J Biochem 32:506–512

Snell KC, Stewart HL (1959) Variations in histologic pattern and functional effects of a transplantable adrenal cortical carcinoma in intact, hypophysectomized, and newborn rats. J Natl Cancer Inst 22:1119–1155

Squire RA, Goodman DG, Valerio MG, Fredrickson TN, Strandberg JD, Levitt MH, Lingeman CH, Harshbarger JC, Dawe CJ (1978) Tumors. In: Benirschke K, Garner FM, Jones TC (eds) Pathology of laboratory animals, vol II, chap 12. Springer, Berlin Heidelberg New York

Sugihara H, Kawai K, Tsuchiyama H (1973) Pathology of intracortical nodules in rat adrenal glands, especially on their fine-structure. Acta Pathol Jpn 23:253–260

Suzuki H, Mohr U, Kimmerle G (1979) Spontaneous endocrine tumors in Sprague-Dawley rats. J Cancer Res Clin Oncol 95:187–196

Thompson SW, Hunt RD (1963) Spontaneous tumors in the Sprague-Dawley rat: incidence rates of some types of neoplasms as determined by serial section versus single section technics. Ann N Y Acad Sci 108:832–848

Thompson SW, Huseby RA, Fox MA, Davis CL, Hunt RD (1961) Spontaneous tumors in the Sprague-Dawley rat. J Natl Cancer Inst 27:1037–1057

Vogel HH Jr, Zaldivar R (1970) Malignant tumours of the rat adrenal gland induced by fission neutron irradiation. Int J Radiat Biol 18:267–270

Yarrington JT, Johnston JO (1994) Aging in the adrenal cortex. In: Mohr U, Dungworth, DL, Capen CC (eds) Pathobiology of the aging rat, vol 2. ILSI, Washington DC, pp 227–244

Adenocarcinoma, Adrenal Cortex, Rat

John D. Strandberg

Synonyms. Adrenal cortical carcinoma, adenocarcinoma, cortical (M) adrenal gland (WHO).*

Gross Appearance

Adenocarcinomas of the adrenal cortex often distort the gland and may extend through the capsule into the surrounding tissues. When metastatic lesions occur they are usually small and on occasion may be found in the liver or the lungs. These tumors tend to be soft, containing little connective tissue. Areas of thrombosis, hemorrhage, and necrosis may make the tissue friable.

Microscopic Features

In contrast to adenomas which are characteristically circumscribed and well-differentiated,

* World Health Organization, International Classification of Rodent Tumors (Mohr 1992)

adenocarcinomas tend to occupy large areas of the cortex and to have poorly defined boundaries. They may invade the capsule and extend into surrounding tissues (Figs. 474, 475). Such regional invasion as well as distant metastasis are the factors most helpful in arriving at a diagnosis of malignancy (Fig. 476). Varying cellular differentiation is encountered ranging from cells which closely resemble normal cells of the zona fasciculata to anaplastic, poorly differentiated epithelial cells with irregular, variable-sized nuclei. The cells of adenocarcinomas are often found in disorganized trabecular patterns with large areas of hemorrhage and necrosis. Mitotic activity may be high. Carcinomas and other adrenal proliferative lesions may be accompanied by atrophic cortical tissue in the contralateral gland. The cellular morphology within lesions reflects the amount of lipid secretion stored within the cells. Distended vascular channels may represent distortion of sinusoidal channels previously existing in the gland or may be the result of degeneration and necrosis of tumor cells with subsequent angiectasis.

Ultrastructure

Kovacs and Horvath (1973) described cells in the rat adrenal cortex containing granules typical of catecholamine secretion. These were found in the inner layers of the zona fasciculata or zona reticularis. The cells also contained mitochondria similar to those of medullary cells, rod-shaped with lamellar cristae, and presumably arose from the adrenal medulla. The presence of these cells, previously noted by French workers, adds further to the confusion surrounding classification of the rat adrenal medullary tumors. The presence of catecholamine granules should identify cells of the medulla which appear to be in the cortex. Electron microscopy has shown transplantable cortical adenocarcinomas to have a decrease in intracellular lipid and a 2.5-fold increase in nuclear size. The mitochondria are elongated but are of decreased volume compared to normal cells of the zona fasciculata (Moore et al. 1978). In estrogen-dependent carcinomas similar changes are seen. In regressive carcinomas a dramatic infiltration of the tumor by eosinophils has been noted (Nichols 1971).

Differential Diagnosis

As noted above, the main differential diagnostic problem is in separating proliferative adrenal cortical lesions from one another. The terminology employed by pathologists to designate lesions, i.e., hyperplasia vs. neoplasia, is often of practical importance, particularly in those cases in which these lesions are found in bioassays. Other lesions which must be differentiated include hyperplasias and neoplasias of the adrenal medulla which

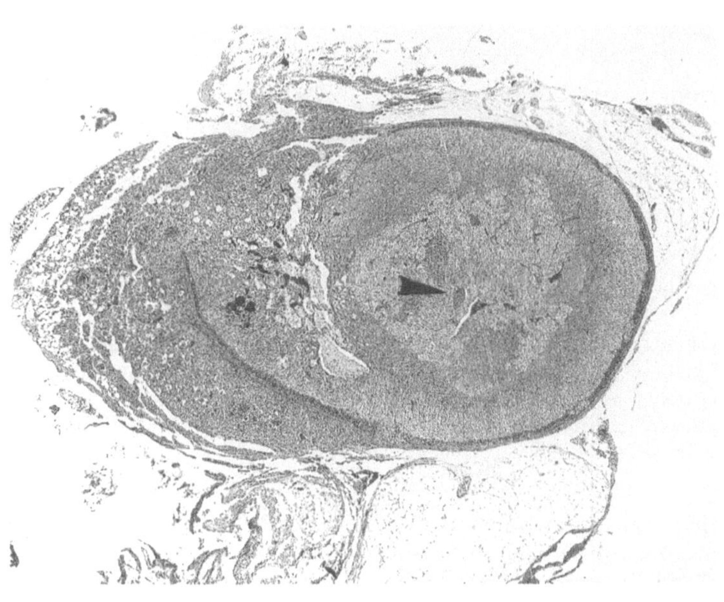

Fig. 474. An adrenal gland from a 24-month-old female OM rat contains a large cortical carcinoma which has broken through the capsule and extends into the surrounding tissues. Nests of tumor cells are present in veins in the medulla (*arrow head*) and there are co-existing proliferative lesions of the medulla. Helley's fixative. H&E, ×22

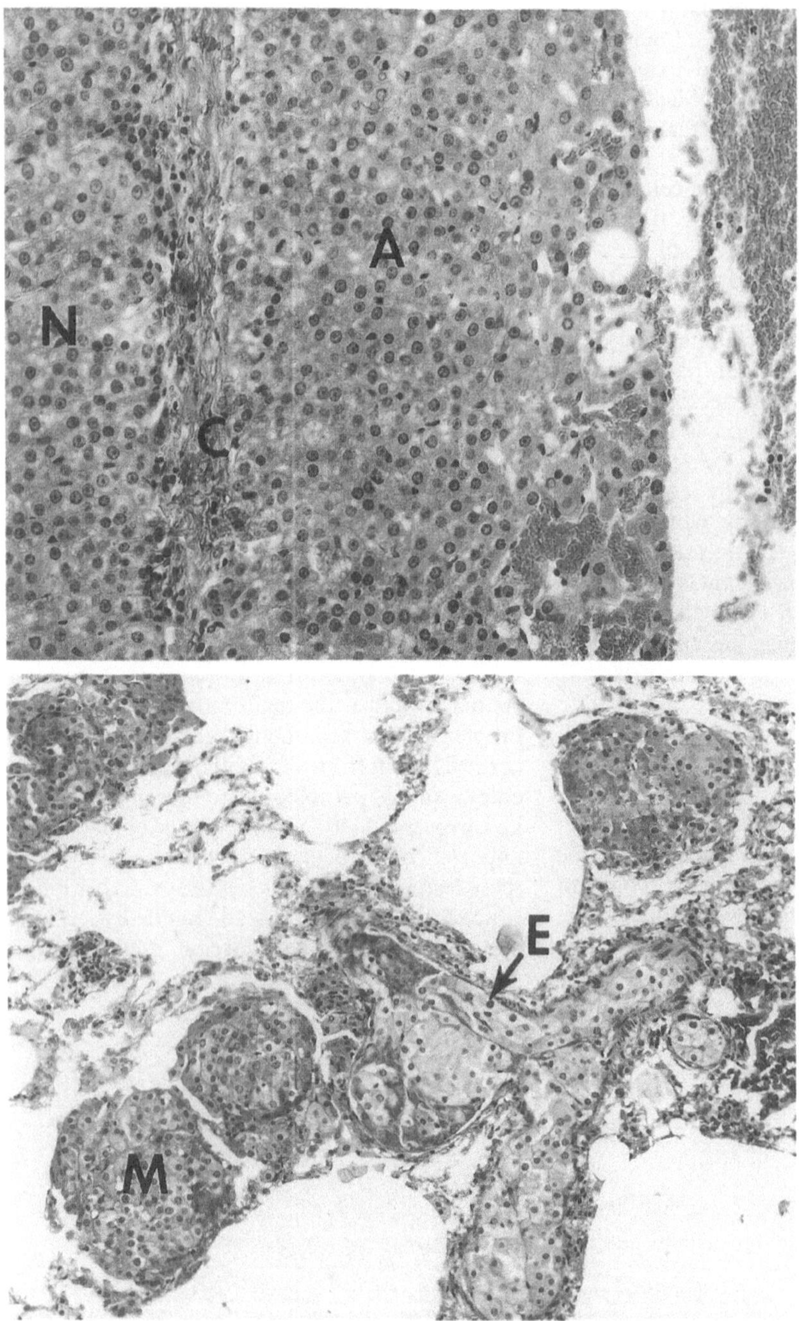

Fig. 475. (*above*) Extracapsular invasion of a cortical adenocarcinoma (*A*) from a 21-month-old female OM rat. The neoplastic cells closely resemble those of the normal cortical tissue (*N*) underlying the capsule (*C*). Helley's fixative. H&E, ×275

Fig. 476. (*below*) Pulmonary metastasis of a cortical adenocarcinoma in a 24-month-old female OM rat. Note tumor emboli (*E*) in vessels and metastatic foci (*M*) in alveolar spaces. Helley's fixative. H&E, ×160

share the same small organ, and which may histologically resemble cortical lesions at times. Those instances in which there is extensive vascular dilatation must be separated from hemangiomatous lesions. In all cases diagnosis is facilitated if multiple sections of the gland are examined, and a full cross-section including the medulla is essential. The essential differentiating feature of carcinomas of the adrenal cortex is their tendency to invade adjacent tissues or blood and lymph vessels and to metastasize.

Biologic Features

Natural History. Adrenal cortical hyperplasia, cortical adenomas, and adenocarcinomas are seen with increasing frequency in older animals of several strains of rats (Boorman and Hollander 1973; Hamlin and Banas 1990; Duprat et al. 1990; Yarrington and Johnston 1994). Very high numbers have been encountered in the Osborne-Mendel (OM) strain, while Fischer 344 and Sprague-Dawley rats tend to have fewer lesions (see Tables 33, 34). With the exception of the OM rats, most of the lesions are seen in animals older than 18 months. In general, these lesions occur somewhat more commonly in females, which normally tend to have larger adrenals, although this varies with different strains and laboratories. Age and sex differences in frequency are noted in induced as well as spontaneous lesions. Dunning et al. (1953) reported the induction of adenomas and adenocarcinomas in rats of the August strain by administration of estrone. The tumors were produced in 36% of the male animals but in only two of the females surviving for 150 days. One of the neoplasms metastasized to the lungs. The number of tumors induced by this treatment was considerably less in the three other rat strains employed in the study.

Adrenal cortical tumors and hyperplasias may be functional. This is often indicated by atrophy of the gland surrounding a lesion or lipid depletion and atrophy of the contralateral adrenal; similar atrophy is observed in the adrenals of rats with transplanted carcinomas (Iglesias and Mardones 1958; Snell and Stewart 1959). Assays of cells of biochemical and hormonal activity have been performed principally on transplantable carcinomas because of the volume of available tissue and reproducibility of the system. Such tumors have been shown to produce a variety of hormones including erythropoietin (Cohen et al. 1957; Meineke 1969). Adrenal cortical tumors induced by estrogens respond to hormonal stimuli, and isolated cells in vitro have altered function as compared with cells of the normal rat cortex (McMillan et al. 1971; Sharma 1973). Iglesias and Mardones (1958) reported that following transplant of a functional adrenal cortical tumor to A × C rats more metastatic lesions were found in the males.

Pathogenesis. The pathogenesis of adrenal tumors is covered on p. 440 (this volume). The occurrence of cortical adenocarcinomas is also an event of later life. Cortical adenocarcinomas are usually unilateral, although at times both glands may be involved. There is usually good correlation among the numbers of all three types of proliferative cortical lesions in situations in which carcinomas are found.

Etiology. The experimental induction of adrenal cortical hyperplasias, adenomas, and adenocarcinomas is discussed in connection with adenomas, on p. 442 (this volume).

Frequency. See Tables 33 and 34.

Comparison with Other Species

Focal adrenal cortical hyperplasia, cortical adenoma and cortical adenocarcinomas of rats resemble in morphology and behavior the same lesions observed in mice. Morphologic similarities can be seen in other of the more common domestic species, as well as in humans.

References

Boorman GA, Hollander CF (1973) Spontaneous lesions in the female WAG/Rij (Wistar) rat. J Gerontol 28:152–159

Cohen AI, Furth J, Buffett RF (1957) Histologic and physiologic characteristics of hormone-secreting transplantable adrenal tumors in mice and rats. Am J Pathol 33:631–651

Dunning WF, Curtis MR, Segaloff A (1953) Strain differences in response to estrone and the induction of mammary gland, adrenal and bladder cancer in rats. Cancer Res 13:147–152

Duprat P, Snell KC, Hollander CF (1990) Tumours of the adrenal gland. In: Turusov V, Mohr U (eds) Pathology of tumours in laboratory animals, vol 1, 2nd edn. IARC Sci Publ 99:573–596

Hamlin MH II, Banas DA (1990) Adrenal gland. In: Boorman GA, Eustis SL, Elwell MR, Montgomery CL Jr, McKenzie WF (eds) Pathology of the Fischer rat. Academic, San Diego, pp 501–518

Iglesias R, Mardones E (1958) Spontaneous and transplantable functional tumor of the adrenal cortex in the A × C rat. Br J Cancer 12:20–27K, Horvath E (1973) Ultrastructural features of corticomedullary cells in a human adrenocortical adenoma and in rat adrenal cortex. Anat Anz 134:387–393

McMillan BH, Ney RL, Schorr I (1971) Guanyl cyclase activity in normal adrenals and a corticosterone producing adrenal cancer of the rat. Endocrinology 89:281–283

Meineke HA (1969) The origin of erythropoietin in rats with transplants of an adrenal cortical carcinoma. Proc Soc Exp Biol Med 132:651–655

Mohr U (1992) International classification of rodent tumors. World Health Organization, IARC Science Publication no 122

Moore RN, Penney DP, Averill KA (1978) Rat adrenocortical carcinoma 494: an integrated structural stereological and biochemical analysis. Anat Rec 190:703–717

Nichols TM (1971) The morphological effects of estrogen removal on an estrogen-dependent adrenocortical carcinoma in rats. Cancer Res 31:1042–1050

Sharma RK (1973) Metabolic regulation of steroidogenesis in adrenocortical carcinoma cells of rat. Effect of adrenocorticotropin and adenosine cyclic 3′ : 5′-monophosphate on corticosteroidogenesis. Eur J Biochem 32:506–512

Snell KC, Stewart HL (1959) Variations in histologic pattern and functional effects of a transplantable adrenal cortical carcinoma in intact, hypophysectomized, and newborn rats. J Natl Cancer Inst 22:1119–1155

Yarrington JT, Johnston JO (1994) Aging in the adrenal cortex. In: Mohr U, Dungworth DL, Capen CC (eds) Pathobiology of the aging rat, vol 2. ILSI, Washington DC, pp 227–244

Adenoma and Carcinoma, Adrenal Cortex, Mouse

James E. Heath

Synonyms. Adrenocortical adenoma, adrenocortical carcinoma, adrenocortical adenocarcinoma.

Gross Appearance

Adenomas of the adrenal cortex in mice are often not visible grossly but may appear as a slightly enlarged adrenal gland when compared to the contralateral organ. Carcinomas often appear as enlarged adrenal glands of up to 5 mm or more in diameter. The affected adrenal is usually spherical or lobulated and may vary from flesh colored to dark red or brown.

Microscopic Features

Proliferative lesions of the mouse adrenal cortex usually arise in the zona glomerulosa (subcapsular area) and may involve type A and/or type B cells. Type A cells are elongated, fibroblastic cells with fusiform nuclei and scant cytoplasm. Type B cells are rounded or polyhedral with comparatively abundant amphophilic and often vacuolated cytoplasm. Less frequently hyperplasia and neoplasia appear to originate in the zona fasciculata.

Adenomas of the adrenal cortex are believed to be preceded by subcapsular cell hyperplasia (p. 464, this volume) which consists of focal aggregations of type A and type B cells (Fig. 477). The hyperplasia usually consists of an elliptical or wedge-shaped band of spindle-shaped cells contiguous with the capsule and extending into the zona fasciculata. Smaller numbers of plump, type B cells may be interspersed among the more prominent type A cells. There is little compression or displacement of the normal cortex nor protrusion beyond the capsular surface.

Adenomas are composed of varying combinations of type A and type B cells. They appear typically as nodular masses containing either or both cell types which compress or displace the underlying zona fasciculata and occasionally the medulla and usually protrude above the capsular surface (Figs. 478, 479). Individual cells are morphologically and tinctorially similar to those seen with focal hyperplasia except that mild cytomegaly, especially of type B cells, may be evident. The tumor cells are frequently arranged in cords and packets of two to several cells thickness which are separated by fibrovascular septa. There is usually a clear line of demarcation between the adenoma and the adjacent adrenal tissue.

Carcinomas are typically larger than adenomas and they may attain such size that little or no remaining adrenal cortex is visible in the section. Individual cells may favor the A or the B type although the cell type distinction in carcinomas is usually less apparent than in focal hyperplasia and adenoma. Carcinomas frequently consist of solid sheets of closely arranged, relatively small cells with ovoid to fusiform nuclei and scant cytoplasm (Figs. 480–482). The plump, round type

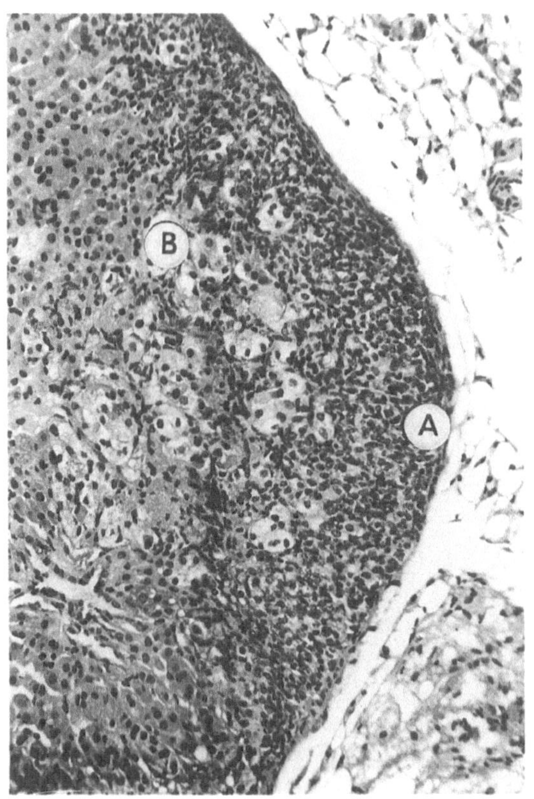

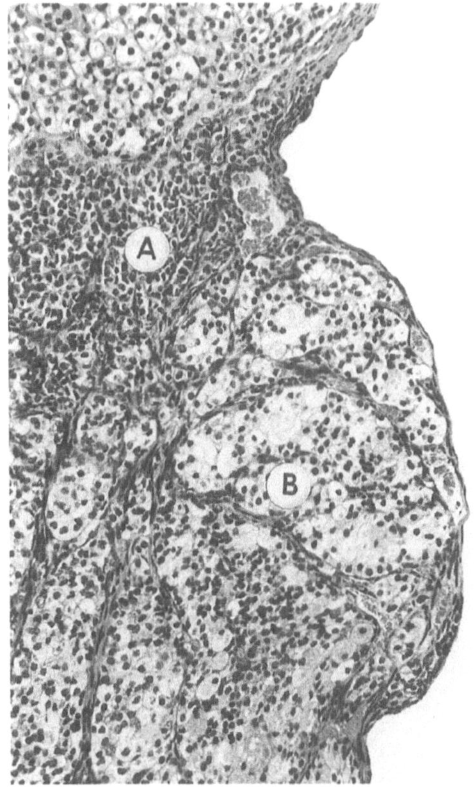

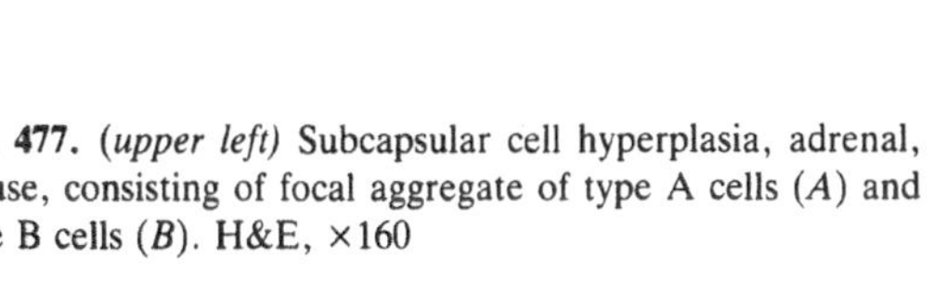

Fig. 477. (*upper left*) Subcapsular cell hyperplasia, adrenal, mouse, consisting of focal aggregate of type A cells (*A*) and type B cells (*B*). H&E, ×160

Fig. 478. (*lower right*) Subcapsular cortical adenoma, adrenal, mouse, protruding above capsular surface of adrenal gland. H&E, ×40

Fig. 479. (*upper right*) Cortical adenoma, adrenal, mouse, composed of well differentiated type A (*A*) and type B cells (*B*). H&E, ×160

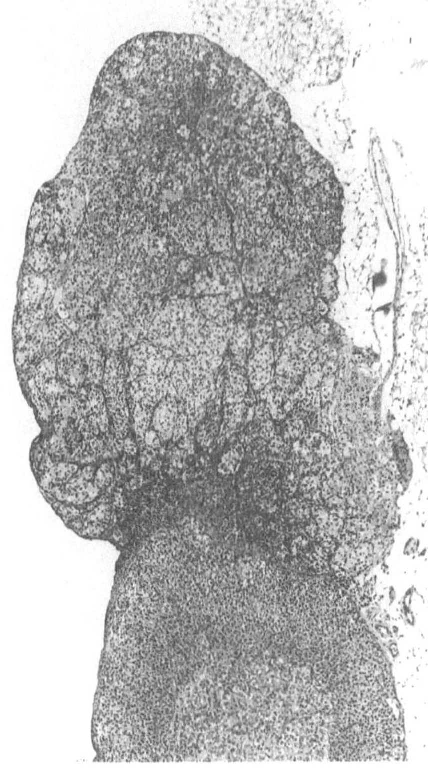

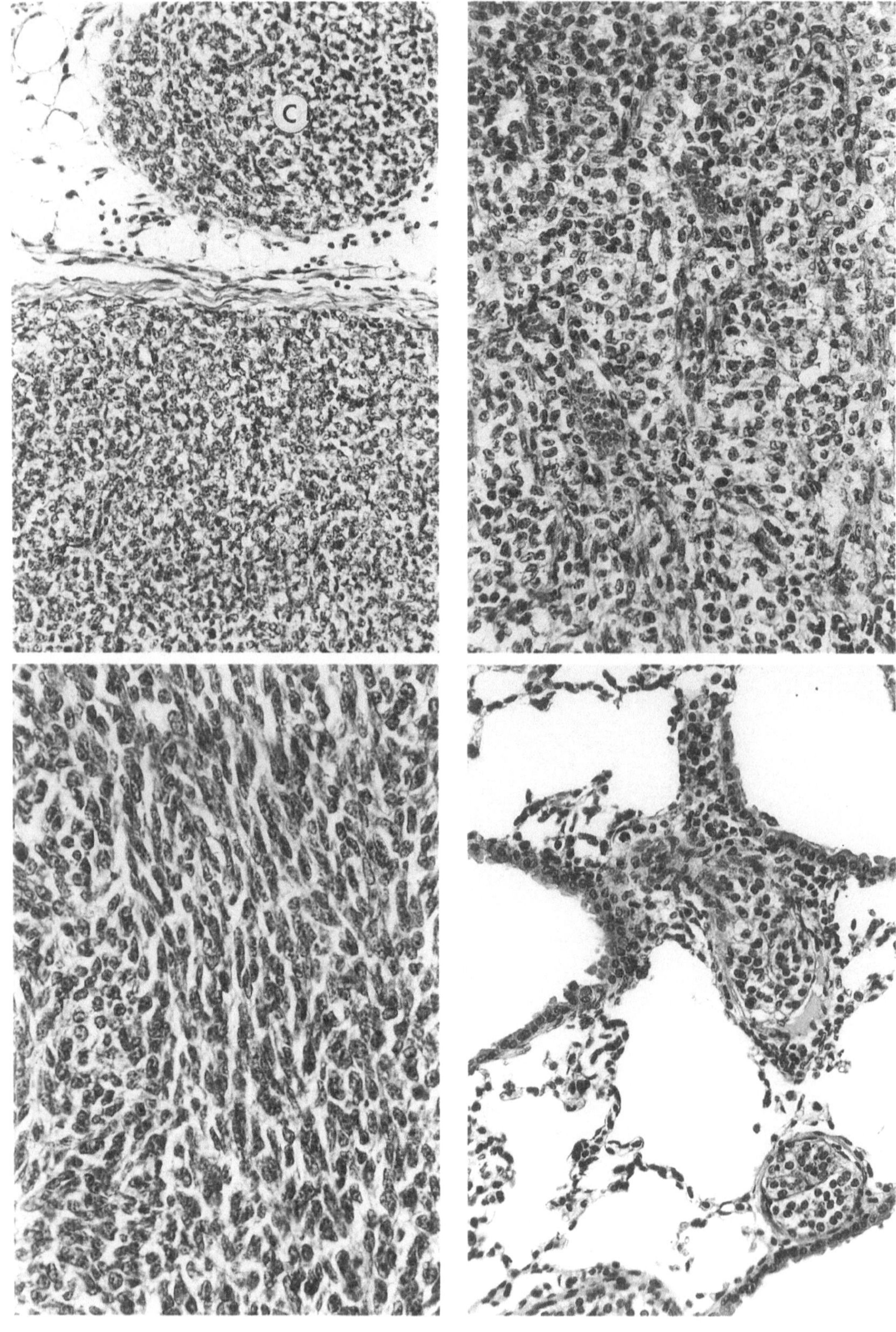
C

B cells typically seen in adenomas and focal hyperplasia are less seen frequently in carcinomas. Tumors composed mainly of type A cells may present a whorled or herringbone pattern suggestive of fibrosarcoma. Mitotic activity is usually moderate to marked. Metastasis to the lung is observed occasionally (Fig. 483).
Hyperplasia and neoplasia originating in the zona fasciculata is occasionally seen in mice. Unlike the proliferative changes that arise in the subcapsular zone, the lesions occurring in the zona fasciculata are composed of plump, round cells with strongly eosinophilic, often vacuolated cytoplasm. Focal hyperplasia in this region consists of a poorly to well demarcated focus of cortical cells which may compress the surrounding parenchyma, but in which the normal cellular structure is retained (Fig. 484). The cells within the hyperplastic focus generally maintain the normal perpendicular arrangement relative to the adrenal capsule. Varying degrees of cortical cell hypertrophy usually accompany the focal hyperplasia, but nuclear atypia or mitosis are usually not evident. Adenomas which occur in the zona fasciculata resemble focal hyperplasia except that they are generally larger, result in greater parenchymal compression, and usually show some degree of cellular atypia (Figs. 485, 486). In contrast to focal hyperplasia, the normal perpendicular arrangement of cells relative to the capsule is usually lost, resulting in an absence of normal architectural relationships. Carcinomas arising in the zona fasciculata are rarely observed in mice.

Ultrastructure

Ultrastructural studies on adrenal cortical neoplasms in mice are limited. One type A carcinoma from a 562-day-old BALB/c mouse was evaluated using transmission electron microscopy (Frith 1983). The presence of large cytoplasmic lipid droplets and desmosomes suggested that the neoplastic cells were epithelial and adrenocortical in origin.

◀

Fig. 480. (*upper left*) Cortical carcinoma, adrenal, mouse, with invasion of pericapsular fat (*C*). H&E, ×200

Fig. 481. (*lower left*) Adrenal cortical carcinoma, mouse, composed largely of cells with type A morphology. H&E, ×400

Fig. 482. (*upper right*) Cortical carcinoma, adrenal, mouse, composed of densely packed cells primarily of type B morphology. H&E, ×250

Fig. 483. (*lower right*) Metastasis to lung of adrenal cortical carcinoma, mouse. The neoplastic cells have type B characteristics. H&E, ×200

Differential Diagnosis

Adrenal cortical adenomas must be distinguished from cortical hyperplasia and cortical carcinomas, and criteria for each of these are presented above (see "Microscopic Features"). Cortical carcinomas could be confused with pheochromocytomas. Cortical carcinomas usually contain areas of spindle cells, even in those made up principally of type B cells. The diagnosis of pheochromocytoma can be aided by the use of immunohistochemical staining or electron microscopy to demonstrate the neurosecretory granules characteristic of this tumor.

Biologic Features

Natural History and Pathogenesis. Proliferative lesions of the mouse adrenal cortex consist of a spectrum of changes which begin with focal hyperplasia. Hyperplastic foci may progress to adenomas, and adenomas may progress to carcinomas, although hyperplasia or adenoma in any given animal is not necessarily destined to progress to the next classification. Because of the morphological continuum from one category to the next, classification is somewhat arbitrary, and a predetermined set of criteria for each classification is necessary for compiling meaningful data in safety and carcinogenicity assays. Fusiform, type A cells are usually observed initially in hyperplastic foci. Although hyperplastic foci and tumors of the adrenal cortex may contain predominately type A or type B cells, in most instances they are composed of a combination of both cell types. Type A cells, under hormonal influence, may undergo transformation to plump, lipid-containing type B cells, which are capable of secreting sex hormones (Woolley 1950). Transplantation studies have shown tumors composed of type B cells to have estrogenic activity, resulting in mammary gland hyperplasia in the host animal (Dunn 1970). Other cell lines of type A morphology appeared hormonally inactive.

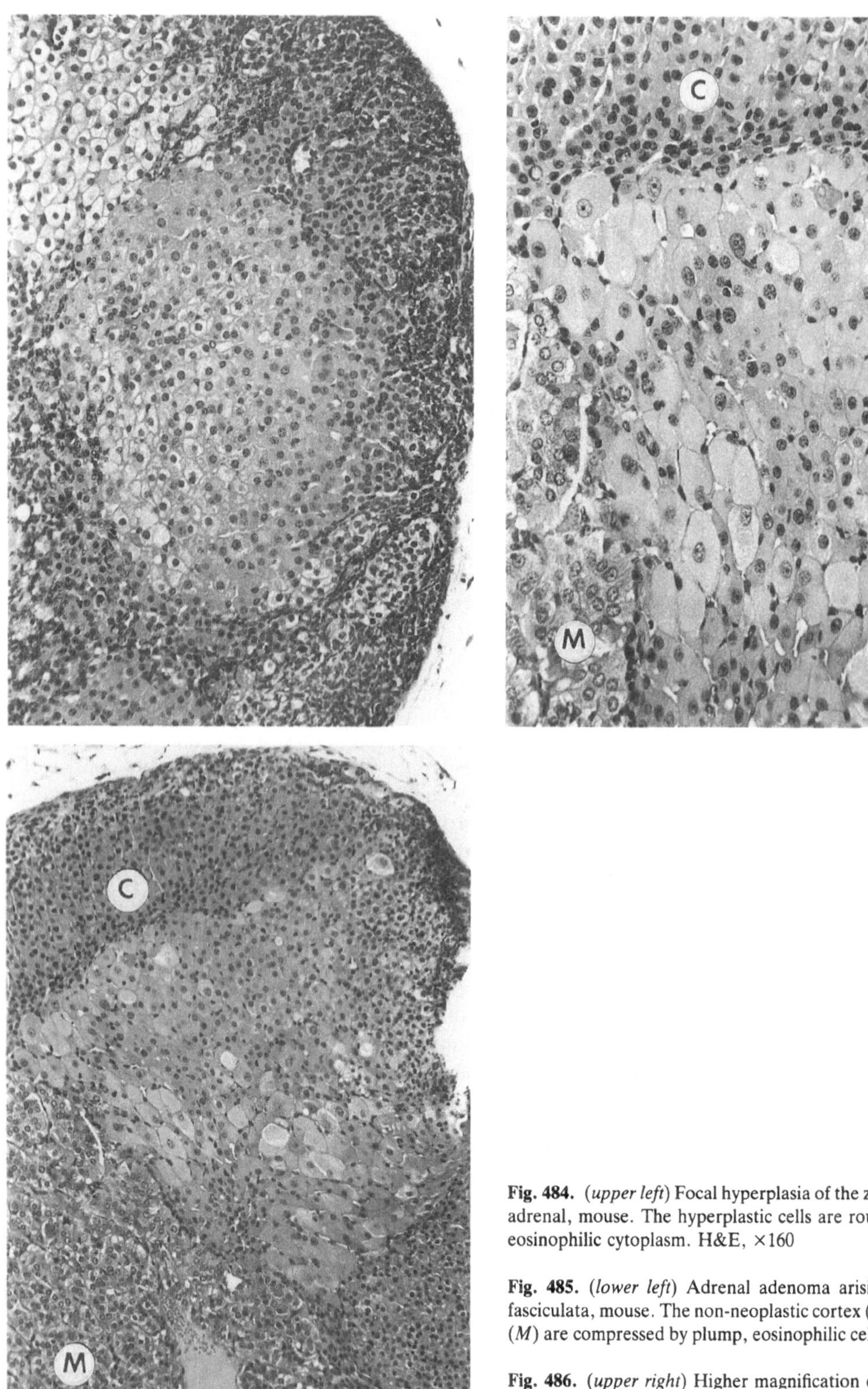

Fig. 484. (*upper left*) Focal hyperplasia of the zona fasciculata, adrenal, mouse. The hyperplastic cells are rounded and have eosinophilic cytoplasm. H&E, ×160

Fig. 485. (*lower left*) Adrenal adenoma arising in the zona fasciculata, mouse. The non-neoplastic cortex (*C*) and medulla (*M*) are compressed by plump, eosinophilic cells. H&E, ×100

Fig. 486. (*upper right*) Higher magnification of Fig. 485 with plump cells of adenoma arising in zona fasciculata with encroachment on non-neoplastic cortex (*C*) and medulla (*M*). H&E, ×200

Etiology. It has long been recognized that adrenal subcapsular cell proliferation can be induced in both males and females of certain mouse strains by gonadectomy (Fekete and Little 1945; Woolley 1950). This change appears to be mediated through the pituitary gland by accelerated release of gonadotrophic hormone. Increased gonadotropin secretion results in proliferation of type A cells which subsequently undergo transformation to type B cells. Depending on the mouse strain, gonadectomy may result in hyperplastic nodules, adenomas, or carcinomas (Woolley and Bittner 1952; Martinez and Bittner 1955). Carcinogenicity assays of xenobiotics have not often resulted in adrenal cortical tumors in mice. However, cortical neoplasms have been induced by administration of the chemical carcinogen 7,12-dimethylbenz(a)anthracene (DMBA) and by ionizing radiation (Marchant 1967; Mody 1969; Haran-Ghera et al. 1959). Tumor induction by both DMBA exposure and irradiation was enhanced by gonadectomy.

Frequency. The frequency of spontaneous adrenal cortical tumors is low in most strains of mice although the incidence in the NH and BALB/c lines is considered higher than in most other strains (Table 35). Adenomas occur more frequently than carcinomas in all strains for which data are available. The incidence of adrenal cortical tumors increases with age in male and female mice and is especially increased in aging females of the NH and BALB/c strains, probably due to reduced ovarian function.

Comparison with Other Species

Unlike adrenal cortex tumors in mice, those in rats most often arise in the zona fasciculata and are reported to secrete primarily glucocorticoid hormones. Spontaneous tumor incidence is considered relatively low for most rat strains although it often increases markedly after 18 months of age. Frequency is reported to be high in the Osborne-Mendel line, in which the majority of rats of both sexes have cortical tumors by 18 months of age (Snell and Stewart 1959), and also in aging WAG/Rij and BN/Bi rats (Burek 1978). Adrenocortical tumors occur fairly frequently in old dogs and are usually encountered as incidental findings at necropsy (Capen 1993). They are occasionally implicated in a Cushing's-type syndrome in dogs due to excessive glucocorticoid secretion (Siegel et al. 1967). Adenomas, carcinomas, and hyperplasias of the adrenal cortex are reported to be relatively common in some hamster strains, most often in old males, and may originate in the zona glomerulosa or zona fasciculata (Strandberg 1987). Cortical tumors are considered to be infrequent in nonhuman primates, guinea pigs, rabbits, and cats. Among domestic animal species they are seen most frequently in ruminants and are reported to occur with a high incidence in castrated male goats (Capen 1993; Richter 1958).

Adrenocortical tumors in human beings are relatively rare, with adenomas occurring in about 2%–8% of adult autopsies and carcinomas occurring even more infrequently (Sommers 1985).

Table 35. Incidence of spontaneous adrenal cortical neoplasms in various mouse strains

Strain	Sex	Experimental period (weeks)	Incidence (%)		Reference
			Adenoma	Carcinoma	
CD-1	Male	0–104	8/891 (0.9)	0/891 (0.0)	Maita et al. 1988
	Female	0–104	4/890 (0.5)	3/890 (0.3)	
$B6C3F_1$	Male	0–110	14/2543 (0.5)	3/2543 (0.1)	Ward et al. 1979
	Female	0–110	9/2522 (0.3)	0/2522 (0.0)	
BALB/c	Male	46–98	11/338 (3.6)	0/338 (0.0)	Frith et al. 1983
	Female	46–98	18/419 (4.3)	0/419 (0.0)	
C57BL/6	Male	46–98	1/348 (0.3)	0/348 (0.0)	Frith et al. 1983
	Female	46–98	0/416 (0.0)	0/416 (0.0)	
NH	Male	>52	1/8 (12.5)	0/8 (0.0)	Kirschbaum et al. 1946
	Female	>52	13/14 (92.9)	0/14 (0.0)	

There is no sex predilection and the tumors may occur in individuals of any age, although they are seen most often in adults. Unlike the murine tumors, which are virtually nonexistent in young animals, a substantial portion of human adrenocortical tumors occur in children. Most cortical adenomas in man are nonfunctional, although up to 50% of carcinomas are believed to be hormonally active (Ritchie 1990). The most common clinical manifestation of functional cortical tumors is Cushing's syndrome due to hypersecretion of cortisol, while virilization or feminization syndromes from androgen or estrogen excess are seen less frequently. Functional neoplasms are twice as likely to occur in women as in men.

References

Burek JD (1978) Pathology of aging rats. CRC, West Palm Beach, pp 42–46

Capen CC (1993) The endocrine glands. In: Jubb KV, Kennedy PC, Palmer N (eds) Pathology of domestic animals, vol III. Academic, San Diego, pp 267–347

Dunn TB (1970) Normal and pathologic anatomy of the adrenal gland of the mouse, including neoplasms. J Natl Cancer Inst 44:1323–1389

Fekete E, Little CC (1945) Histological study of adrenal cortical tumors in gonadectomized mice of the cc strain. Cancer Res 5:220–226

Frith CH (1983) Adenoma and carcinoma, adrenal cortex, mouse. In: Jones TC, Mohr U, Hunt RD (eds) Monographs on pathology of laboratory animals, endocrine system. Springer, Berlin Heidelberg New York, pp 49–56

Frith CH, Highman B, Burger G, Sheldon WD (1983) Spontaneous lesions in virgin and retired breeder BALB/c and C57BL/6 mice. Lab Anim Sci 33(3):273–286

Haran-Ghera N, Furth J, Buffett RF, Yokorok (1959) Studies on the pathogenesis of neoplasms by ionizing radiation. II. Neoplasms of endocrine organs. Cancer Res 19:1181–1187

Kirschbaum A, Frantz M, Williams WL (1946) Neoplasms of the adrenal cortex in non-castrate mice. Cancer Res 6: 707–711

Maita K, Hirano M, Harada T, Mitsumori K, Yoshida A, et al. (1988) Mortality, major cause of moribundity, and spontaneous tumors in CD-1 mice. Toxicol Pathol 16(3): 340–349

Marchant J (1967) Development of adrenal cortical carcinoma in C3H mice following castration and the administration of 7,12-dimethylbenz(a)anthracene. Br J Cancer 21:750–754

Martinez C, Bittner JJ (1955) Postcastrational adrenal tumors in unilaterally adrenalectomized C3H mice. Cancer Res 15:612–613

Mody JK (1969) A new type of transplantable adrenal tumor and its comparative histopathology. Cancer Res 29: 1254–1261

Richter WR (1958) Adrenal cortical adenomata in the goat. Am J Vet Res 19:895–901

Ritchie AC (1990) Adrenal glands. In: Richie AC (ed) Boyd's textbook of pathology, vol II, 9th edn. Lea and Febiger, Philadelphia, pp 1458–1481

Siegel ET, O'Brien JB, Pyle L, Schryver HF (1967) Functional adrenocortical carcinoma in a dog. J Am Vet Med Assoc 150:760–766

Snell KC, Stewart HL (1959) Variations in histologic pattern and functional effects of transplantable adrenal cortical carcinoma in intact, hypophysectomized and new-born rats. J Natl Cancer Inst 22:1119–1132

Sommers SC (1985) Adrenal glands. In: Kissane JM, Anderson WA (eds) Anderson's pathology, vol II, 8th edn. Mosby, St Louis, pp 1429–1450

Strandberg JD (1987) Neoplastic diseases. In: Van Hoosier GL, McPherson CW (eds) Laboratory hamsters. Academic, Orlando, pp 157–168

Ward JM, Goodman DG, Squire RA, Chu KC, Linhart MS (1979) Neoplastic and nonneoplastic lesions in aging (C57BL/6N × C3H/HeN)F, (B6C3F$_1$) mice. J Natl Cancer Inst 63(3):849–854

Woolley GW (1950) Effect of hormonal substances on adrenal cortical tumor formation. Cancer Res 10:250 (abstract)

Woolley GW, Dickie MM, Little CC (1952) Adrenal tumors and other pathological changes in reciprocal crosses in mice. I Strain DBA × strain CE and the reciprocal. Cancer Res 12:142–152

Amyloidosis, Adrenal, Mouse

Bernard Sass

Synonyms. Amyloid degeneration, hyalin degeneration, amyloid infiltration.

Gross Appearance

The gross appearance of the lesion has not been described in the mouse.

Microscopic Features

The zona reticularis, the histologically nondistinct inner part of the cortex of the adrenal gland, is usually the first site for the intercellular deposition of amyloid. As the deposits increase, they form a linear pattern in the zona fasciculata (Dunn 1967; Figs. 487, 488), but the zona glomerulosa is usually spared. In adrenals that are mildly affected there are amyloid deposits in the connective tissues. In H&E preparations these deposits take the eosin stain and are translucent and acidophilic (Dunn 1967). Inflammatory cells are not found in the amyloidotic mouse adrenal. Amyloid may sometimes be associated with ceroid pigment in the zona reticulata.

Ultrastructure

Naeser and Westermark (1977) described the structure of amyloid in renal glomeruli of strain *Ob/ob* mice, examined by transmission electron microscopy, as consisting of 100-Å-wide, rigid, nonbranching strands, twisted into two filaments.

Differential Diagnosis

Amyloid may be distinguished from ceroid and from other hyalines by the Congo red, crystal violet, Sirius red, and methyl violet stains, and by the thioflavine T method which requires a source of ultraviolet light. Newer methods include immunoperoxidase and potassium permanganate (Luna 1968; van Rijswijk and van Heusden 1979; Fujihara et al. 1980). Amyloid stained with Congo red gives a bright green birefringence with polarized light, and even pinpoint areas of amyloid are revealed by the technique (Figs. 489, 490). Amyloid is also commonly found in the spleen, liver, and intestine of mice with adrenal amyloidosis.

Biologic Behavior

Pathogenesis. The pathogenesis of amyloidosis has not yet been elucidated. Several mechanisms for its formation have been postulated (Scarpelli and Chiga 1977). One of these is that amyloid deposits may arise from cells of the reticuloendothelial system, such as plasma cells or macrophages, which infiltrate the tissues and produce immunoglobulin amyloid; this is then deposited locally. Another possibility is that a circulating precursor substance that is rendered insoluble is deposited by some as yet unknown mechanism. Jakob and Hilgenfeld (1972) reviewed work on a factor that accelerates the induction of amyloidosis by casein. They demonstrated that the onset of amyloidosis was accelerated in isogenic mice of the Decin strain and in allogenic mice of strains AB and Strong A, casein-treated by intravenous injection of spleen cells or various derivatives of spleen cells, such as homogenates and filtrates. These preparations hastened the onset of amyloidosis when they were obtained from casein-treated isogenic donors, but not when they were obtained from untreated donors. Cells obtained from amyloidotic bovine kidney accelerated the onset of casein-induced amyloidosis in recipient mice of the Decin strain.

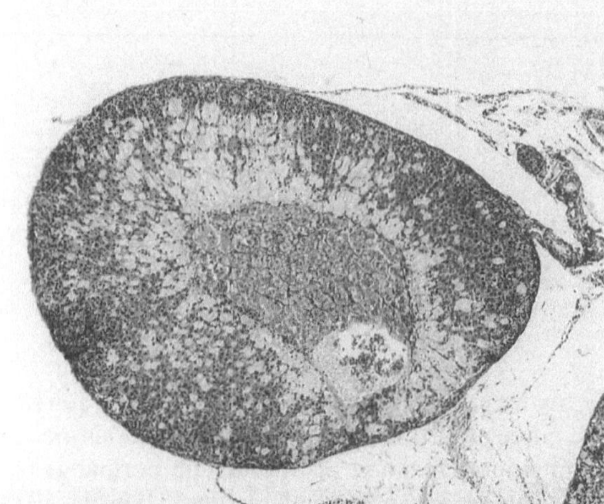

Fig. 487. Amyloidosis adrenal mouse. Zona reticularis is largely replaced by amyloid which extends into the zona fasciculata. H&E, ×54

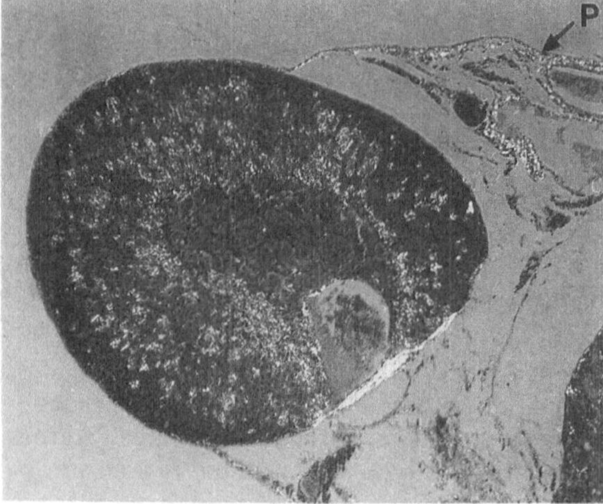

Fig. 488. Amyloidosis adrenal mouse. Birefringence in the adrenal cotex. Birefringence also in the capsule and adjacent peritoneum (*P*). Congo red stain, illuminated with polarized light, ×54

Etiology. Primary amyloidosis, as defined by Dunn (1965), is directly related to a genetic factor or factors in a given inbred mouse strain. Secondary amyloidosis is produced by the administration of chemicals such as casein (Dunn 1967), methylcholanthrene and Freund's adjuvant. Tulaney (1978) postulated that thymic influence may be an etiologic factor, inasmuch as thymectomy hastens the onset of casein-induced amyloidosis. He also found that pregnancy did not affect the time of onset or frequency of amyloidosis in outbred Swiss mice that received a 5.0% solution of sodium caseinate five times weekly. Other influences cited by Dunn (1967) which promote the increased deposition of amyloid include adrenal cortical hormone secretion and thyroidectomy. Dunn (1967) and Galton (1963) also mention ectoparasites and repeated needle punctures as probable causes of amyloidosis. In addition, Page and Glenner (1972) concluded from their studies that social interaction, especially fighting among males, was an important factor that increased amyloidosis.

Frequency. Primary amyloidosis occurs most frequently in inbred mice of the A, Y, BL, and NH strains (Dunn 1967). Of these strains, NH also has the hightest percentage of renal amyloidosis. A high degree of susceptibility to amyloidosis of the adrenal gland does not necessarily coincide with a high frequency of generalized amyloidosis. Strains most frequently affected with amyloidosis of the adrenal gland are, in decreasing order, A, L, C3H, C57 and CBA. Naeser and Westermark (1977) found amyloid deposition in 60% of mice of strain *ob*/*ob*. Of 13 obese *ob*/*ob* animals, 12 had adrenal deposits, as did 10 of 15 lean *Ob*/*ob* controls. Andervont and

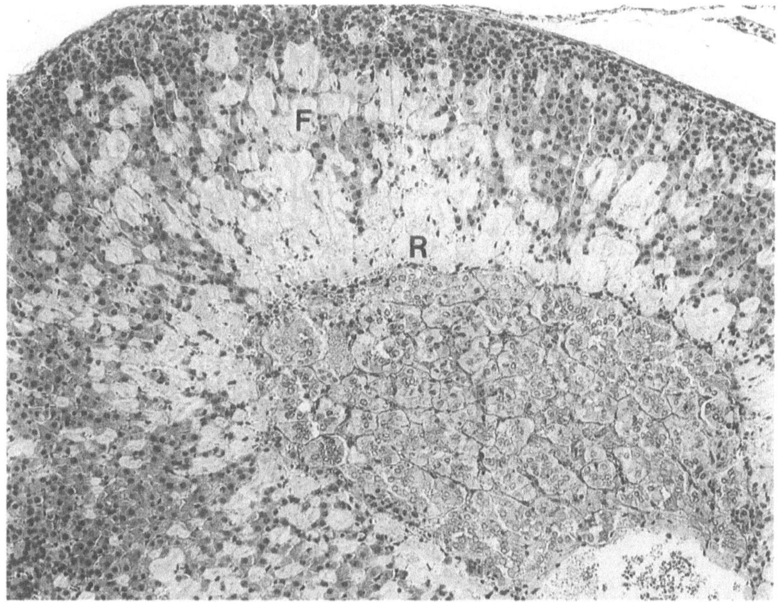

Fig. 489. Amyloidosis mouse adrenal. Higher magnification of Fig. 487. The amyloid is principally in the zonae reticularis (*R*) and fasciculata (*F*). H&E, ×130

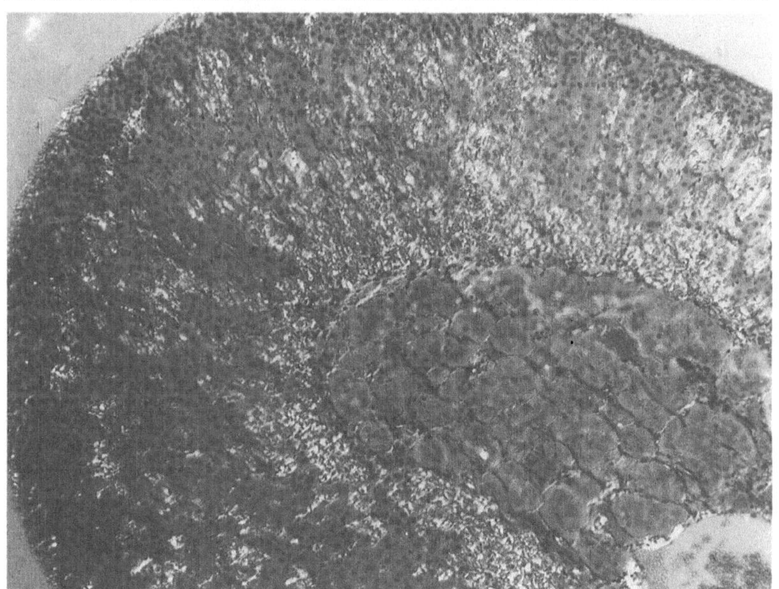

Fig. 490. Amyloidosis mouse adrenal. Birefringent amyloid in zonae reticularis and fasciculata. Congo red stain with polarized illumination, ×130

Dunn (1970) studied the frequency of severe amyloidosis in wild mice and hydrids. All of 34 inbred wild mice, but only four of 25 outbred controls developed amyloidosis. Hybrid offspring of a wild inbred male and strain A females all developed amyloidosis, while off-spring of a wild outbred male and strain A females did not. Thus genetic homogeneity appears to increase the frequency of primary amyloidosis.

References

Andervont HB, Dunn TB (1970) Amyloidosis in wild house mice during inbreeding and in hybrids derived from inbred strains and wild mice. J Natl Cancer Inst 44:719–727

Dunn TB (1965) Spontaneous lesions of mice. In: Ribelin WE, McCoy JR (eds) Pathology of laboratory animals. Thomas, Springfield, chapter 11

Dunn TB (1967) Amyloidosis in mice. In: Cotchin E, Roe FJC (eds) Pathology of laboratory rats and mice. Blackwell Scientific, Oxford, chapter 7

Fujihara S, Balow JE, costa JC, Glenner GG (1980) Identification and classification of amyloid in formalin-fixed,

paraffin-embeded tissue sections by the unlabeled immunoperoxidase method. Lab Invest 43:358–365
Galton M (1963) Myobic mange in the mouse leading to skin ulceration and amyloidosis. Am J Pathol 43:855–865
Jakob W, Hilgenfeld M (1972) Beschleunigte Amyloidbidung bei Mäusen durch Organmaterial von Tieren mit Spontnamyloid. Zentrabl Allg Pathol 116:94–97
Luna L (1968) Methods for carbohydrates and mucoproteins. In: Manual of histologic staining methods of the Armed Forces Institute of Pathology. McGraw-Hill, New York, chapter 10
Naeser P, Westermark P (1977) Amyloidosis in ageing obese hypergly cemic mice and their lean litter-mates. A morphological study. Acta Pathol Microbiol Scand [A] 85:761–767
Page DL, Glenner GG (1972) Social interaction and wounding in the genesis of "spontaneous" murine amyloidosis. Am J Pathol 67:555–570
Scarpelli DG, Chiga M (1977) Cell injury and errors in metabolism. In: Anderson WAD, Kissane JM (eds) Pathology. Mosby, St Louis, chapter 3
Tulaney O (1978) Experimental amyloidosis in mice of different ages: effect of neonatal thymectomy and pregnancy. Isr J Med Sci 14:459–465
van Rijswijk MH, van Heusden CWGJ (1979) The potassium permanaganate method: a reliable method for differentiating amyloid AA from other forms of amyloid in routine laboratory practice. Am J Pathol 97:43–58

Lipogenic Pigmentation, Adrenal Cortex, Mouse

Charles H. Frith

Synonyms. Ceroid deposition, "brown degeneration," ceroidogenesis, ceroid degeneration, aging pigment, lipofuscin.

Gross Appearance

Lipogenic pigmentation in the mouse adrenal is not visible grossly.

Microscopic Features

The deposition of ceroid or lipogenic pigment in the adrenal initially occurs in cortical cells near the corticomedullary junction and eventually encircles the medulla (Fig. 491). Small amounts of the pigment appear as granular to amophous, yellowish–brown material in the cytoplasm of the epithelial cells. When the amount of pigment increases in each cell the cytoplasm becomes distended, brown, and foamy in appearance. Nuclei may become pyknotic and the cells resemble macrophages. Sometimes they fuse to form multinucleated giant cells. Occasionally, cells containing the pigment extend into the medulla. The pigment is positive following periodic acid Schiff reaction (PAS; Fig. 492) and is acid-fast when appropriately stained (Dunn 1970).

Ultrastructure

An examination of the ultrastructural aspects of the pigment (Samorajski and Ordy 1967) revealed cytoplasmic particles of various sizes and electron densities. This suggested that the pigment originated in cells of the inner cortex and that it was endogenous.
Samorajski and Ordy (1967) also reported that the quantity of pigment increased with age and that many of the cells coalesced to form multinucleated cells with unusually large pigment inclusions. Reactions specific for lipid pigment included positive staining for sulfatides, peroxidases, and vicinal polyhydroxyl groups. Figures 493 and 494 demonstrate clumps of ceroid pigment in the cytoplasm of adrenal cortical epithelial cells.

Differential Diagnosis

Hemosiderin-laden macrophages may appear in the adrenal cortex and may superficially resemble cortical epithelial cells distended with ceroid. Stains for iron, such as Prussian blue, will identify the iron content of hemosiderin, but ceroid should be distinguished by its positive reaction to PAS and its acid-fast properties. The existence of so many approximate synonyms illustrates well the

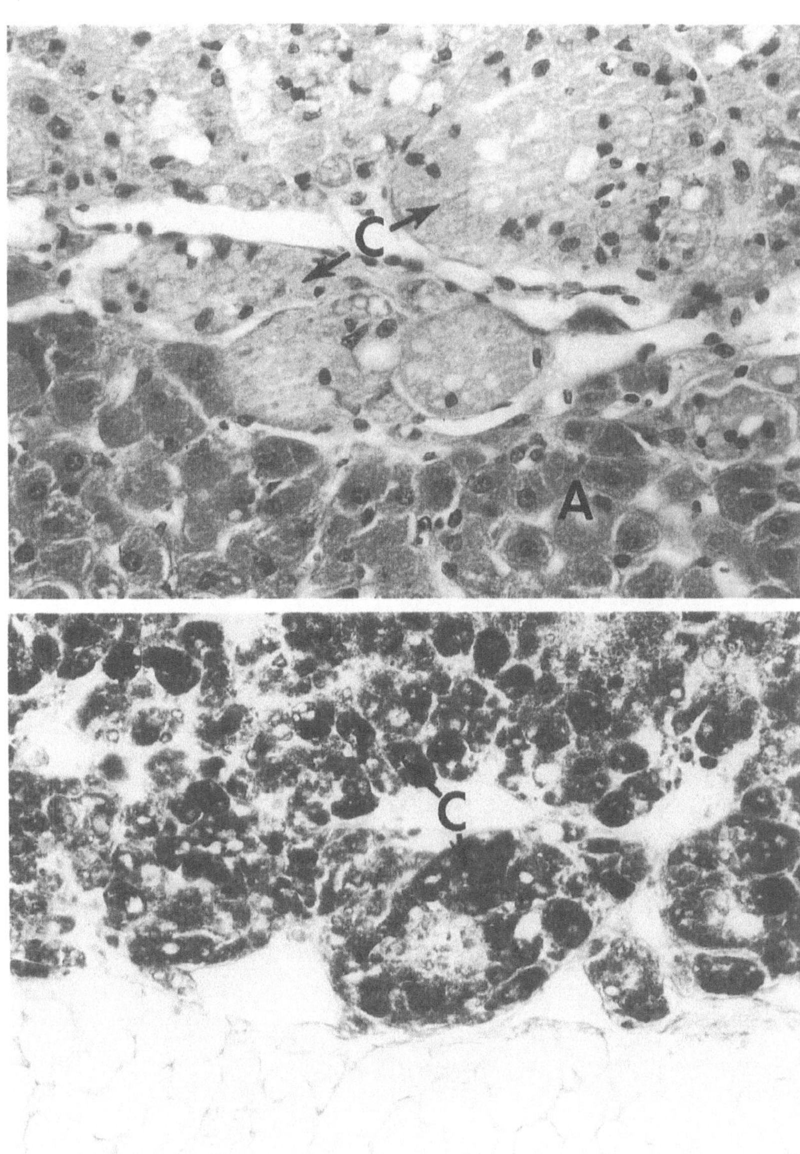

Fig. 491. Ceroid (*C*) in mouse adrenal cortical cells as compared with normal adrenocortical cells (*A*). H&E, ×300

Fig. 492. Ceroid (*C*) in mouse adrenal cortical cells. PAS, ×300

confusion concerning the exact nature of lipogenic pigments.

Biologic Features

Cramer (1939) reported a positive correlation between the incidence of ceroid deposition and mammary tumors in mice, but other investigators have since refuted that correlation. Schardein et al. (1967) confirmed that the brown pigment was histochemically identical to ceroid, and interpreted the deposition as lipid products resulting from altered fat metabolism. They consistently induced ceroid pigment in the adrenal gland of mice by administration of ethinylestradiol. Ultrastructurally, ceroid formation progressed from small pigment granules morphologically similar to lysosomes, to large composite pleomorphic pigment bodies composed of granular and membranous components.

Firminger (1952) compared the adrenal ceroid to pigment found in the interstitium of the testes of mice given diethylstilbestrol. Studies at the

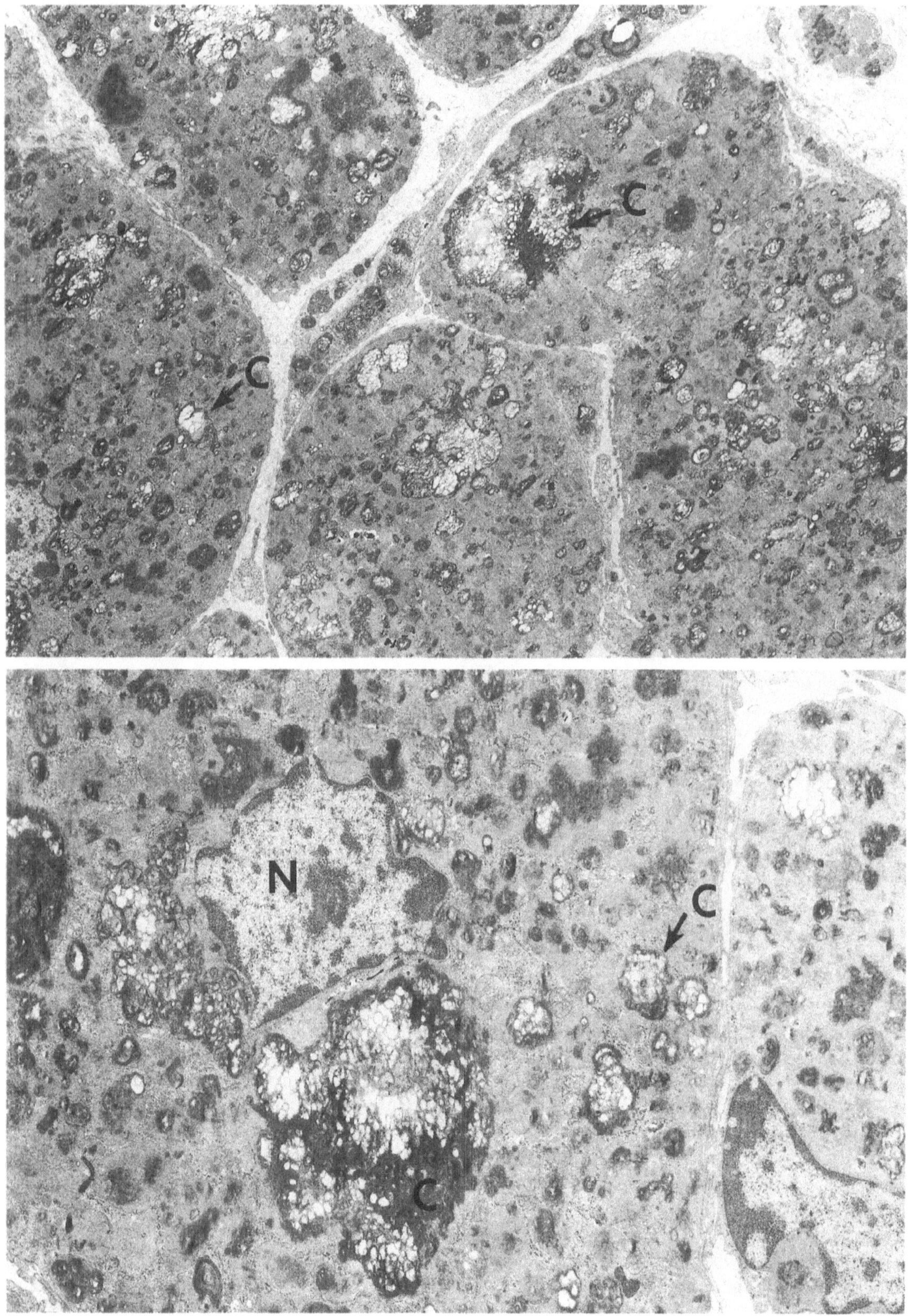

Fig. 493. (*above*) Ceroid pigment (*C*) in cytoplasm. Electron micrograph, uranyl acetate–lead citrate, ×3900

Fig. 494. (*below*) Ceroid pigment (*C*) in cytoplasm. *N* Nucleus. Electron micrograph, uranyl acetate–lead citrate, ×8775

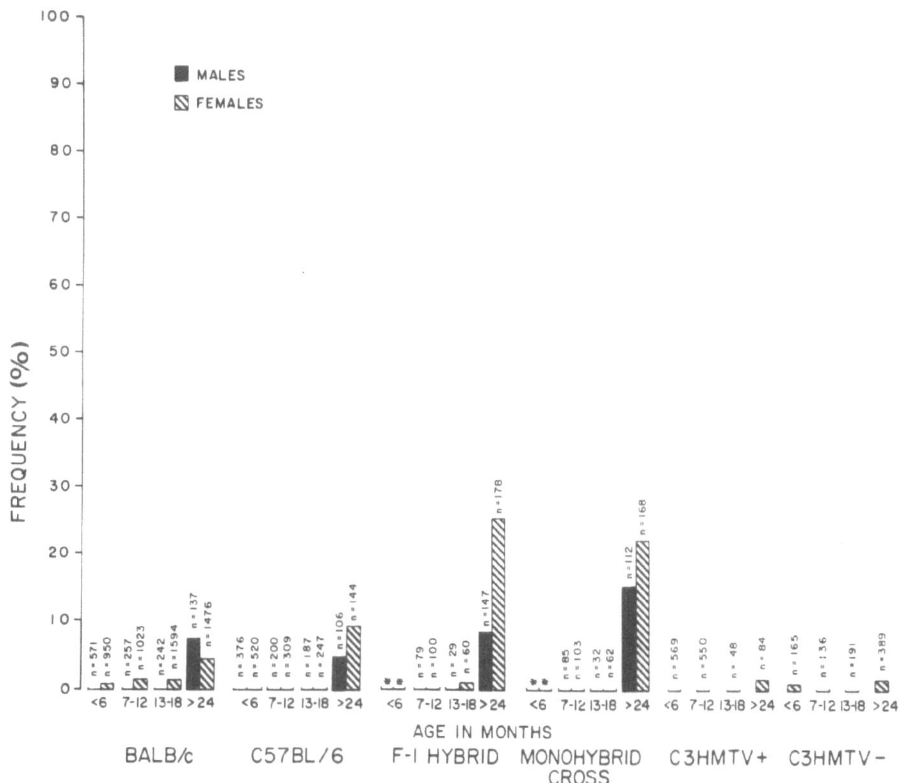

Fig. 495. Adrenal ceroid in untreated mice. *Asterisk*, no data; *F-1 hybrid*, C57BL/6 females × BALB/c males; *Monohybrid*, F-1 females × F-1 males; *n*, total number of animals examined

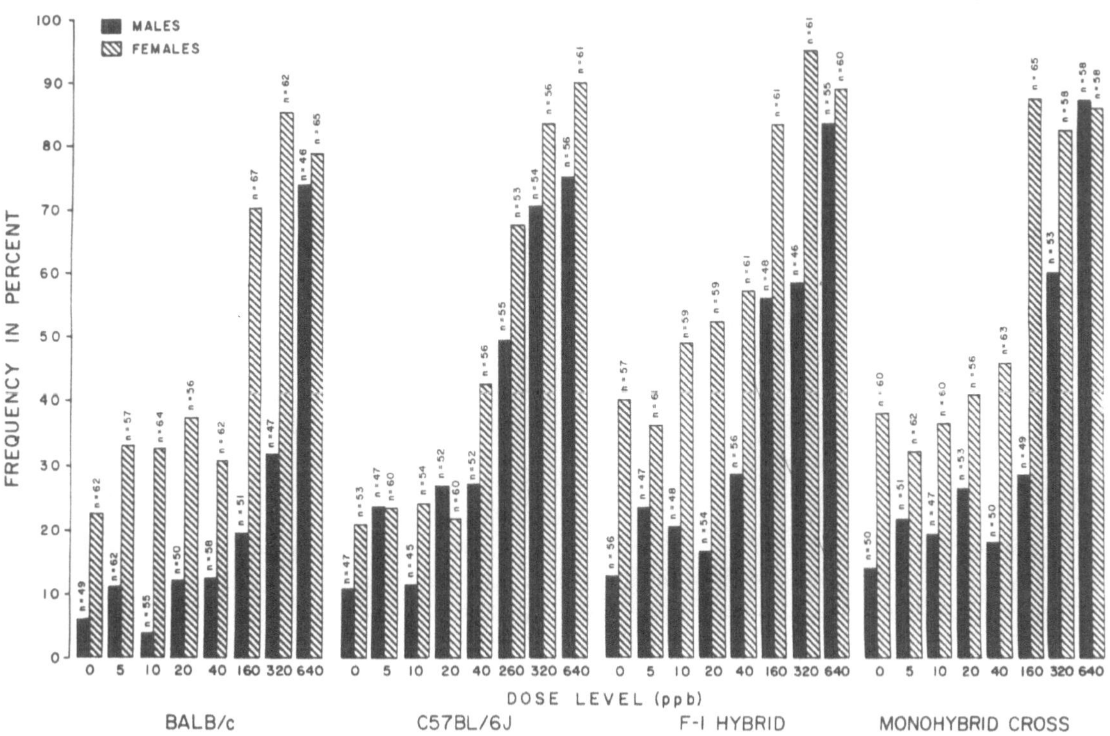

Fig. 496. Ceroid in the adrenal glands of mice treated with diethylstilbestrol. *F-1 hybrid*, C57BL/6J females × BALB/c males; *Monohybrid*, F-1 females × F-1 males; *n*, total number of animals examined

National Center for Toxicological Research have shown that ceroid is rare in untreated mice until after 24 months of age (Fig. 495), and that diethylstilbestrol increases the incidence of the deposition of ceroid in the adrenals of mice (Fig. 496).

Comparison with Other Species

Lipogenic pigment, similar if not identical to lipofuscin or ceroid, may be found in adrenal cortical cells in the rat (see p. 462, this volume). The accumulation of such pigment is more extensive in older animals. Other organs of several species have been reported to accumulate similar pigment. The production and storage of this pigment are enhanced by dietary deficiency of antioxidants such as vitamin E (Smith et al. 1972).

References

Cramer W (1939) On the association between brown degeneration of the adrenals and the incidence of mammary cancer in two inbred strains of mice. Am J Cancer 37:342–354

Dunn TB (1970) Normal and pathologic anatomy of the adrenal gland of the mouse, including neoplasms. J Natl Cancer Inst 44:1323–1389

Firminger HI (1952) Apparent identity of pigmented lipoid in cells in adrenal gland and interstitium of testis of mice following administration of stilbestrol. J Natl Cancer Inst 13:225–227

Samorajski T, Ordy JM (1967) The histochemistry and ultrastructure of lipid pigment in the adrenal glands of aging mice. J Gerontol 22:253–367

Schardein JL, Patton GR, Lucas JA (1967) The microscopy of "brown degeneration" in the adrenal gland of the mouse. Anat Rec 159:291–309

Smith HA, Jones TC, Hunt RD (1972) Mineral deposits, pigments. In: Jones TC, Hunt RD (eds) Veterinary pathology, 4th edn. Lea and Febiger, Philadelphia, chapter 3

Lipogenic Pigmentation, Adrenal Cortex, Rat

George A. Parker and Marion G. Valerio

Synonyms. Lipofuscin, ceroid, ceroid-like pigment, abnutzungs pigment, wear-and-tear pigment, pigment of brown atrophy, chromolipoid, hemofuscin, cytolipochrome, acid-fast pigment, aging pigment, pigment of vitamin E deficiency.

Gross Appearance

Lipogenic pigmentation of the adrenal cortex usually is not severe enough to be seen grossly in rats.

Microscopic Features

Lipogenic pigment in the adrenal gland of the rat is usually seen in adrenocortical cells of the inner layers (zona reticularis) of the cortex. With mild involvement the amorphous to granular, yellowish brown pigment is present typically in randomly scattered cells. With more severe involvement the pigment is present in greater quantity in nearly all adrenocortical cells in the inner cortex and may involve a lesser number of cells in the outer cortex. Some of the lipogenic pigment exhibits a brown autofluorescence. It is usually PAS-positive, sudanophilic even in paraffin-embedded sections, and may be acid-fast (Ward and Reznik-Schuller 1980).

Ultrastructure

Differences in nomenclature hinder the interpretation of reports on the ultrastructural appearance of lipogenic pigments, and no such published information with regard to the rat adrenal gland is available. Lipofuscin in man is known to consist of highly electron-dense granules that often include membranous structures and usually are in a perinuclear location (Cotran et al. 1989). They may exist as small spherical globules or as very large irregular masses (Cheville 1976; see Figs. 493, 494).

Differential Diagnosis

Severely affected adrenocortical epithelial cells may be so distended with lipogenic pigment that they resemble pigment-laden macrophages. These cells must be distinguished from hemosiderin-laden macrophages, which are also quite common along the sinusoids of the inner adrenal cortex of aged rats. Nuclear position within the cell and chromatin distribution are helpful in this differentiation. Where definitive differentiation is required, iron stains can be used to distinguish the iron-positive hemosiderin from the iron-negative lipochrome pigments. Positive staining with PAS and variable acid fastness also help to identify lipogenic pigments.

Biologic Features

Heterophagocytosis of extracellular particles and autophagocytosis of intracellular structures both result in ingested material in phagosomes, which acquire digestive hydrolases by fusion with pre-existing digestive vacuoles or enzyme-laden granules. Material in the digestive vacuoles is hydrolyzed to undigestible debris or soluble intermediates which can be reutilized or released from the cell. Some debris, largely lipid, remains in effete digestive vacuoles called residual bodies. In some cells the debris-filled residual bodies are known to fuse with the plasma membrane by reverse esotropy and discharge their debris to the extracellular milieu. In other cells this apparently cannot occur, and debris-filled residual bodies accumulate for the lifetime of the cell (LaVia and Hill 1975).

Lipogenic pigments result from peroxidation of lipids in heterophagocytized or autophagocytized subcellular organelles, resulting in aldehydes and lipoperoxides which undergo polymerization to yield insoluble residues. Deficiencies of antioxidants such as vitamin E are associated with formation of an increased amount of these residues. Chemical analysis of lipofuscin reveals approximately 50% lipid residues, 30% protein residues, and 20% nonextractable, unidentifiable material (Robbins and Cotran 1974).

There is some difference of opinion on the nomenclature that should be applied to lipogenic pigments, particularly the terms lipofuscin and ceroid. The commonly occurring "wear-and-tear" pigment, the development of which is described above, is generally considered to be lipofuscin. There is less concurrence on the criteria used to differentiate ceroid. Ceroid was first described in the liver of rats with experimentally induced cirrhosis (Lillie et al. 1941) and has since been produced in a number of species (Jones and Hunt 1983). A histochemically similar pigment occurs in a number of animal species with vitamin E deficiency (Jones and Hunt 1983). Most disagreements in terminology center around the histochemical features used to distinguish ceroid from lipofuscin, particularly the acid fastness and autofluorescence of the pigments. One pathology textbook describes ceroid as a variant of lipofuscin that has become acid-fast and autofluorescent, but not different from lipofuscin in any significant way (Robbins and Cotran 1974). Another author describes ceroid as a variant of lipofuscin which is associated with disturbances of vitamin E and fatty acid metabolism but points out the ultrastructural resemblance of ceroid to lipofuscin and states that ceroid may also be encountered with no indication of how it evolved (Cheville 1976). In the latter description both lipofuscin and ceroid are autofluorescent, but ceroid possesses the additional quality of acid fastness. A third text refers to lipofuscin and ceroid as histochemically indistinguishable, but suggests continued use of the different terms to be justified by the different circumstances involved in formation of the pigments (Jones and Hunt 1983).

To summarize, it appears that lipogenic pigments are formed continually in a variety of cells from lipid-containing precursors of intracellular or extracellular origin. Their production and accumulation are enhanced by deficiencies in antioxidants such as vitamin E. Some forms of the pigments may be subclassified by histochemical means, but the subclassification probably has little biologic significance in the context of diagnostic histopathology. (See also "Lipogenic Pigmentation, Adrenal Cortex, Mouse," this volume.)

Data are not presently available on the precise frequency of occurrence of lipogenic pigmentation in the adrenals of rats. It was observed in some aged rats in a gerontology study but was not specifically studied (Burek 1978). In our experience, some degree of lipogenic pigmentation is a very common, perhaps routine finding in the adrenals of aged F344 rats, and Sprague-Dawley rats. Accumulation in young animals usually indicates excessive turnover of cellular organelles or a disorder in cell metabolism (Hamlin and Banas 1990).

Comparison with Other Species

Lipogenic pigmentation of the adrenals, commonly referred to as brown degeneration, is a very common finding in some strains of laboratory mice (Russfield 1967; Dunn 1970) (see also "Lipogenic Pigmentation, Adrenal Corex, Mouse," this volume). Usually only the zona reticularis is involved, but in severe cases the major part of the cortex may be populated by pigment-laden cells. The pigment is chemically compatible with ceroid (Russfield 1967). Diets high in unsaturated fat result in lipogenic pigmentation of the adrenals in strains of mice that normally do not have the pigment. Its development is inhibited by feeding vitamin E or use of a diet that contains only saturated fatty acids (Tobin and Birnbaum 1947).

References

Burek JD (1978) Pathology of aging rats. CRC, West Palm Beach, p 42

Cheville NF (1976) Cell pathology. Iowa State University Press, Ames, p 70

Cotran RS, Kumar V, Robbins SL (1989) Robbins pathologic basis of disease. Saunders, Philadelphia

Dunn TB (1970) Normal and pathologic anatomy of the adrenal gland of the mouse, including neoplasms. J Natl Cancer Inst 44:1323–1389

Hamlin MH, Banas DA (1990) Adrenal gland. In: Boorman GA, Eustis SL, Elwell MR, Montgomery CA, MacKenzie WF (eds) Pathology of the Fischer rat. Academic, New York, p 506

Jones TC, Hunt RD (1983) Veterinary pathology, 5th edn. Lea and Febiger, Philadelphia, pp 98–101

LaVia MF, Hill RB Jr (1975) Principles of pathobiology, 2nd edn. Oxford University Press, New York, p 53

Lillie RD, Daft FS, Sebrell WH (1941) Cirrhosis of the liver in rats on a deficient diet and the effect of alcohol. Public Health Rep 56:1255–1258

Robbins SL, Cotran RS (1974) Pathologic basis of disease. Saunders, Philadelphia, p 47

Russfield AB (1967) Pathology of the endocrine glands, ovary and testis of rats and mice. In: Cotchin E, Roe FJC (eds) Pathology of laboratory rats and mice. chap 14. Blackwell Scientific, Philadelphia

Tobin CE, Eirnbaum ıP (1947) Some factors influencing brown degeneration of the adrenal gland in the Swiss albino mouse. Arch Pathol 44:269–281

Ward JM, Reznik-Schuller H (1980) Morphological and histochemical characteristics of pigments in aging F344 rats. Vet Pathol 17:678–685

Subcapsular-Cell Hyperplasia, Adrenal, Mouse

Dawn G. Goodman

Synonyms. Subcapsular-cell reaction; spindle-cell hyperplasia of the adrenal cortex; type A cell hyperplasia; fibrous degeneration of the zona glomerulosa; cortical scars.

Gross Appearance

Generally, this lesion is not observed grossly. In older mice, the capsular surface of the adrenal may be slightly irregular. Occasionally, nodules may be present if the lesion has become focally extensive or developed into a neoplasm (p. 448, this volume).

Microscopic Features

In older mice of many strains proliferation of spindle cells, either focally or diffuse, occurs beneath the capsule of the adrenal gland (Fig. 497). This change may involve the zona glomerulosa and extend downward into the cortex between the cords of the zona fasciculata, often having a wedge shape. It may be so extensive as to replace large portions of the cortex. Occasionally, the proliferation may be nodular and may progress to neoplasms.

Microscopically, the cells are oval to fusiform with eilliptical nuclei and scant, basophilic cytoplasm (Fig. 498); mitotic figures are rare. These cells have been referred to as type A cells and are the predominant cell type seen. Type B cells are occasionally observed, usually when the lesion is

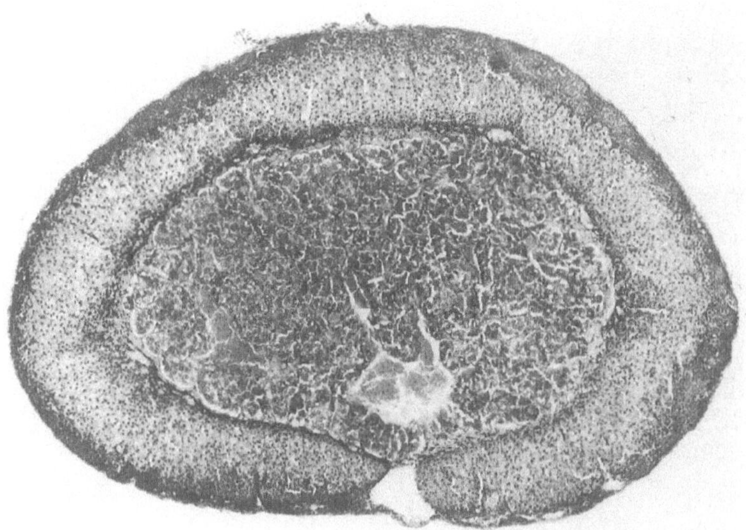

Fig. 497. Diffuse subcapsular-cell hyperplasia of the mouse adrenal gland with foci extending downward into the cortex. H&E, ×65

extensive. However, they are most commonly found in neoplasms. They are large, round to polygonal cells with abundant eosinophilic or vacuolated cytoplasm and round, vesicular nuclei. They may occur as single cells scattered among the spindle cells or in small nests surrounded by the spindle cells (Fig. 499; Jayne 1963).

Ultrastructure

Sato (1967) studied the fine structure of the mouse adrenal cortex at various ages. He described thickening of the capsule with age, associated with an increased number of cell layers. With electron microscopy an increase in collagen fibrils and in the number of capsular cells was seen. Particularly in older animals capsular cells contained few organelles, consisting primarily of polygonal mitochondria, occasional lipid droplets, and membrane-bound dense bodies. Desmosomes were observed attaching adjacent capsular cells and membranes surrounding groups of capsular cells resembled basement membranes. In Sato's opinion, these cells may represent reserve cells of the zona glomerulosa.

Differential Diagnosis

This lesion is quite characteristic microscopically. In the past it has been thought to represent scarring (Löwenthal 1931; Whitehead 1932) or "fibrous degeneration" of the zona glomerulosa (Delost et al. 1958). The primary problem in diagnosis arises with extensive focal lesions i.e., whether the lesion is a focal hyperplasia or has progressed to neoplasia. When the proliferation is large, nodular, and compresses adjacent tissue, it is generally considered to be neoplastic (p. 448, this volume).

Biological Features

Subcapsular-cell hyperplasia is commonly observed in older mice of many strains. The incidence of the lesion in various strains is not well documented. It is rarely observed in young mice, but is more frequent and more severe with age. In some strains, the lesion tends to be more extensive in females than in males. The severity of the lesion also varies greatly between individuals of the same strain, sex and age.
Gonadectomy usually enhances its development in both male and female mice. The lesion develops at an early age following castration, becoming quite severe, and adrenal cortical tumors usually arise from the lesion in such animals (Dunn 1970, 1979; Woolley 1950).

Comparison with Other Species

Subcapsular-cell hyperplasia is rarely seen spontaneously in other species. Nodular subcapsular

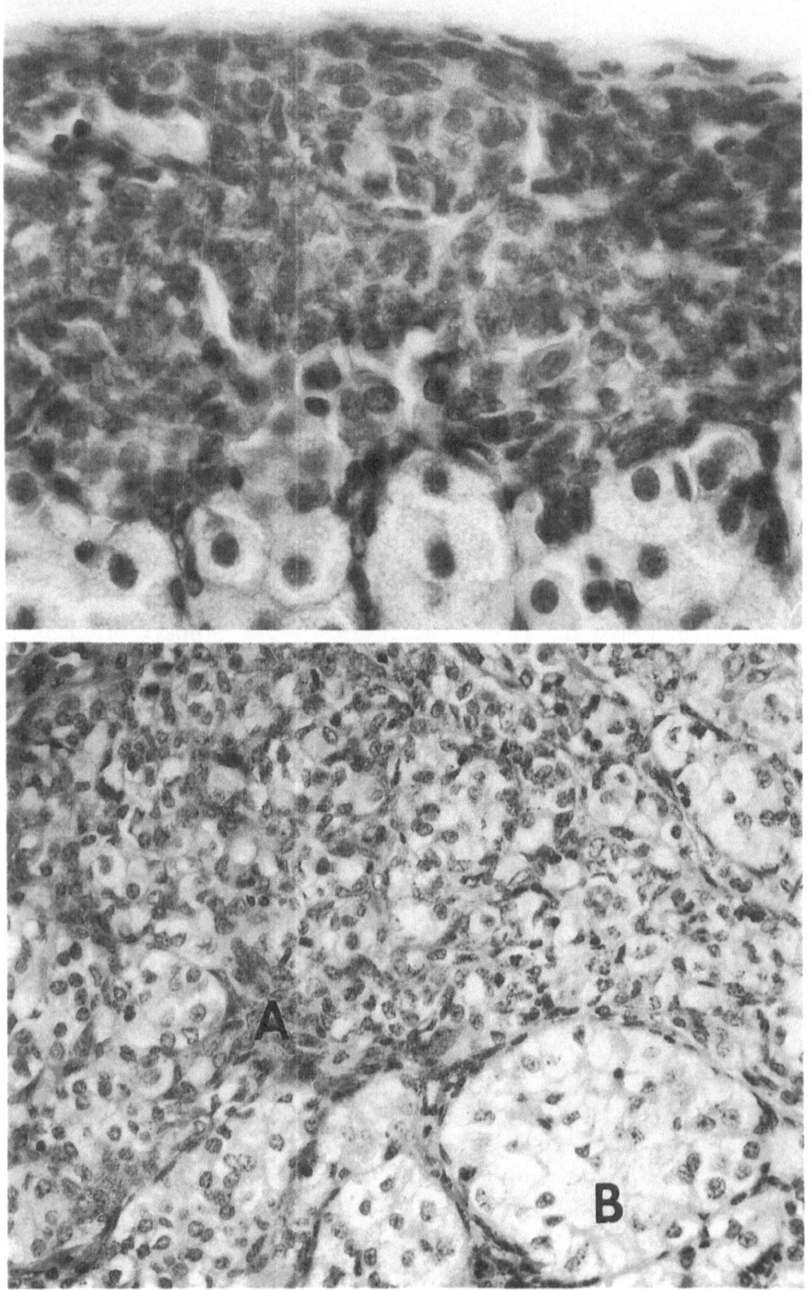

Fig. 498. (*above*) Subcapsular-cell hyperplasia, composed of oval to fusiform type A cells. H&E, ×900

Fig. 499. (*below*) Subcapsular-cell hyperplasia, composed primarily of nests of large, polygonal type B cells (*B*) intermixed with fusiform type A cells (*A*). H&E, ×330

spindle-cell proliferations, including neoplasms, have been described as occurring spontaneously in hamsters (Pour et al. 1976), increasing in size after castration (Cantin 1971; Murthy and Russfield 1966; Russfield 1966). Subcapsular-cell proliferations in rats (Cardeza 1956) and nodular spindle-cell lesions in goats (Richter 1958) have been described as observed following gonadectomy.

References

Cantin M (1971) Adrenocortical structure and function in ovariectomized hamsters. Rev Can Biol 30:125–134

Cardeza AF (1956) Histology of adrenal tumors in castrated rats. Acta Unio Int Contra Cancrum 12:149–152

Delost P, Delost H, Vincent AM (1958) Etude pondérale morphologique et histochimique de la surrénale chez la souris âgée multipare. CR Soc Biol (Paris) 152:1059–1062

Dunn TB (1970) Normal and pathologic anatomy of the adrenal gland of the mouse, including neoplasms. J Natl Cancer Inst 44:1323–1389

Dunn TB (1979) Tumours of the adrenal gland. IARC Sci Publ 23:475–485

Jayne EP (1963) A histo-cytologic study of the splenic cortex in mice as influenced by strain, sex and age. J Gerontol 18:227–234

Löwenthal K (1931) Nebennieren: In: Jaffe R (ed) Anatomie und Pathologie der Spontanerkrankungen der kleinen Laboratoriumstiere. Springer, Berlin Heidelberg New York

Murthy ASK, Russfied AB (1966) Evidence for three types of benign adrenal tumors in Syrian hamsters. Arch Pathol Lab Med 81:140–145

Pour P, Mohr U, Althoff J, Cardesa A, Kmoch N (1976) Spontaneous tumors and common diseases in two colonies of Syrian hamsters. III. Urogenital system and endocrine glands. J Natl Cancer Inst 56:949–961

Richter WR (1958) Adrenal cortical adenomata in the goat. Am J Vet Res 19:895–901

Russfield AB (1966) Tumors of the endocrine glands and secondary sex organs. Public Health Service Publication no 1332. US Government Printing Office, Washington DC, chapter IV

Sato T (1967) Age and sex differences in the fine structure the mouse adrenal cortex. Nagoya J Med Sci 30:225–251

Whitehead R (1932) Abnormalities of the mouse suprarenal. J Pathol 35:415–418

Woolley GW (1950) Experimental endocrine tumors with special reference to the adrenal cortex. Recent Prog Horm Res 5:382–405

Chemically Induced Adrenocortical Degenerative Lesions

John T. Yarrington and James F. Reindel

Synonyms. Chemically induced adrenocorticolysis, adrenocortical necrosis, adrenal cortical degeneration.

Introduction

Adrenocortical degenerative lesions can be induced by a wide range of structurally dissimilar and functionally unrelated compounds. A review of the literature indicates that the adrenal gland, particularly the cortex, is the endocrine organ most frequently affected by chemical injury (Ribelin 1984; Colby 1988). Examples of prototypic adrenotoxicants associated with adrenocortical degeneration include glucocorticoids (Sasano et al. 1966; Purjesz et al. 1964), 7,12-dimethylbenzanthracene (Murad et al. 1973), aminoglutethimide (Camacho et al. 1967; Malendowicz 1972), spironolactone (Fischer and Horvat 1971), 2,2-bis (parachlorophenyl)-1,1 dichlorethane (*o,p′*-DDD; Nelson and Woodward 1949; Hennigar et al. 1964), α-(1,4-dioxido-3-methyl-quinoxalin-2-yl)-*N*-methylnitrone (DMNM; Yarrington et al. 1981, 1985; Capen et al. 1991), amphenone (Hertz et al. 1955), and 1,1′ thiodiethylidene-ferrocene (MDL 80,478; Capen et al. 1991; Yarrington et al. 1983). With many of these compounds degenerative changes in the adrenal cortex occur, in conjunction with functional alterations in steroidogenesis.

The adrenal cortex is predisposed to chemical insult because of at least two major factors. Adrenocortical cells of most animal species contain large stores of membrane-bound lipids used primarily as substrate for steroidogenesis. Many adrenotoxicants are lipophilic and can therefore accumulate in these lipid-rich cells (Mohammed et al. 1985; Hallberg 1990). In addition, cortical cells are richly endowed with enzymes capable of xenobiotic metabolism, including many enzymes of the cytochrome P-450 family (Hornsby 1989; Colby 1988). Many of these enzymes function in the biosynthesis of endogenous steroids and are localized in membranes of the endoplasmic reticulum and mitochondria. A number of toxic xenobiotics can serve as (pseudo)substrates for these enzymes and can be metabolized to reactive toxic species. These reactive species elicit toxic effects either by direct covalent interactions with cellular macromolecules or through oxygen activation with the generation of various free radicals (Colby 1988).

Examples of chemicals that are bioactivated by enzymes of the adrenal cortex to toxic reactive species include spironolactone, 7,12-dimethylbenz(a)anthracene, carbon tetrachloride, 4-chlorobiphenyl, 3-methylsulfonyl-1,1-dichloro-2,2-dicholorphenylethylene, Nifurtimox, and *o,p'*-DDD. For spironolactone the 17-hydroxylase enzymes of steroid metabolism may be involved in generation of toxic species since coincubation with the 17-hydroxylase inhibitor SU-10 603 has been shown to protect guinea pig adrenal cortical tissue from corticolysis induced by spironolactone alone (Colby 1988). The effects of 7,12-dimethylbenz(a)anthracene may also be related to enzyme specific bioactivation of the toxicant since the administration of 11β-hydroxylase inhibitors such as metyrapone and SU-9055 prevent compound-induced necrosis in rats (Currie et al. 1962; Szabo and Lippe 1989). Carbon tetrachloride, on the other hand, can be bioactivated by a number of cytochrome P-450 enzymes to toxic species (Brogan et al. 1984; Colby 1988).

Species Considerations

Animal species can differ in susceptability and sensitivity to the adrenotoxic effects of certain compounds. Some adrenotoxic chemicals such as DMNM and 1,1' thioethylidene-ferrocene cause adrenal cortical lesions in numerous species, including dogs, rats, and monkeys (Yarrington et al. 1981, 1983, 1985; Capen et al. 1991). The susceptibility and sensitivity of other compounds to adrenotoxicants differ among animal species. The compound PD 132301-2 elicits adrenotoxicity in certain species including dogs, guinea pigs, rabbits, and monkeys; other species such as rats and hamsters are resistant to adrenocortical necrosis even at high doses (Reindel et al. 1992). Still other compounds are associated with limited species-specific toxicity such as *o,p'*-DDD in the dog and humans and 7,12-dimethylbenzanthracene in the rat (Nelson and Woodward 1949; Murad et al. 1973). The causes of species differences in susceptibility and sensitivity to adrenotoxicants are not entirely clear, but differences in pathways of metabolism in the adrenal cortex, pharmacokinetic factors, or ancillary metabolism in other tissues such as the liver may be involved.

The specific cortical zone affected by an adrenotoxicant and the nature of histologic changes induced by a compound may also vary between animal species. In monkeys PD 132301-2 induces a narrow band of cytotoxic cortical cell degeneration restricted to the middle to outer zona fasciculata and a reduction of the fine vacuolation or vesciculation of remaining cortical cells (Reindel et al. 1992; Fig. 500). In dogs this compound causes widespread degeneration and necrosis of the zona fasciculata/reticularis and lesser portions of the zona glomerulosa (Dominick et al. 1993b). The zona fasciculata is the principal target of PD 130301-2 in guinea pigs; the zona reticularis is largely spared (Reindel et al. 1992; Dominick et al. 1993a). With aminoglutethimide there are species differences in the nature of induced histologic responses (Malendowicz 1972). This compound causes cortical cell lipid vacuolation in the zona fasciculata of rats but not in hamsters. Adrenal gland enlargement occurs in

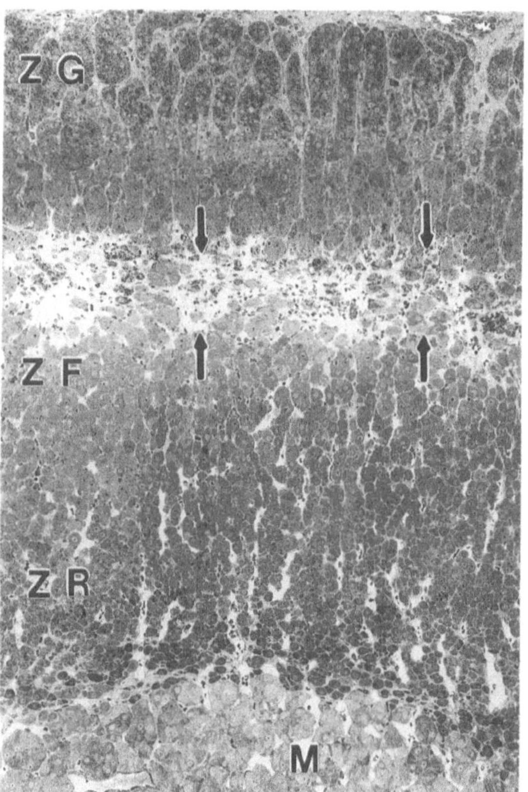

Fig. 500. A thin band-like zone of cortical cell necrosis (*arrows*) is present in the mid to outer zona fasciculata (*ZF*) of monkeys given 50 mg/kg per day and greater of PD 132301-2 for 2 weeks. Depletion of fine lipid vacuoles is evident in the remaining cells of the zona fasciculata and reticularis (*ZR*). The zona glomerulosa (*ZG*) and medulla (*M*) are illustrated. H&E, ×100

both hamsters and rats. However, in hamsters this is attributed to an increased size of the zona reticularis while in rats it is caused by hyperplasia of the zona glomerulosa and fasciculata cortical cells. There may be several reasons for the zone selective alterations in certain species. The distribution of certain drug and steroid-metabolizing enzymes differ amongst cortical zones (Eacho and Colby 1983; Colby et al. 1987) and may account for some zone selectivity of the toxic insult encountered with certain xenobiotics. In addition, animal species differ in principal steroid products generated by the adrenal cortex. Thus, they presumably differ in amount and nature of specific steroid synthesizing enzymes that are capable of xenotiotic metabolism.

Gross Appearance

The gross appearance of adrenal glands following chemical insult depends on the nature of the degenerative change. Adrenotoxicants which cause vacuolar degeneration of cortical cells

Table 36. Examples of chemically induced microscopic and ultrastructural degeneration of the adrenal cortex

Compound	Histology	Ultrastructure	References
Aminoglutethimide	Cortical vacuolar degeneration	Mitochondrial hypertrophy and cavitation	Camacho et al. 1967; Malendowicz 1972; Racela et al. 1969
o,p'-DDD	Cortical vacuolar degeneration	Mitochondrial vacuolation and SER dilatation	Nelson and Woodward 1949; Hennigar et al. 1964; Powers et al. 1974
a-(1,4-Dioxido-3-methyl-quinoxalin-2-yl)-*N*-methylnitrone	Cortical granular and vacuolar degeneration	Mitochondrial vacuolation and SER dilatation	Yarrington et al. 1981; Yarrington et al. 1985; Capen et al. 1991
1,1' Thio-diethylidene-ferrocene (MDL 80,478)	Cortical granular and vacuolar degeneration	Mitochondrial vacuolation and increased lipid droplets	Yarrington et al. 1983; Capen et al. 1991
Triparanol (MER 29)	Cortical eosinophilic degeneration and inclusions	Decreased lipid droplets; mitochondrial alterations; SER hypertophy; lysosomal formation	Volk and Scarpelli 1964; Dietert and Scallen 1969
Amphenone	Cortical fatty degeneration	Mitochondrial alterations	Hertz et al. 1955; Luse 1967
7,12 Dimethylbenzan-thracene	Cortical necrosis	Mitochondrial alterations	Murad et al. 1973
Corticosteroids (e.g., prednisolone, dexamethasone)	Cortical atrophy	Increased lipid droplets surrounded by membranous "whorls"; increased myelin figures and lysosomes	Sasano et al. 1966; Purjesz et al. 1964; Rhodin 1971
Propylthiouracil	Ceroid degeneration of zona reticularis	Liposomal and mitochondrial degeneration	Moore and Callas 1975
Spironolactone	Inclusions and hypertrophy of zona glomerulosa	Lipid droplets surrounded by whorls of SER ("spirono-lactone bodies") and mitochondrial alterations	Fisher and Horvat 1971
Hexadimethrine bromide	Necrosis of zona glomerulosa and infarction of zona fasciculata and zona reticularis	Protein-containing vacuoles and hyalin bodies; microthrombi	Marek and Peifer 1971; Marek et al. 1973
R01-8307, a sulfated mucopolysaccharide	Condensation of the zona glomerulosa		Abbott et al. 1966
PD 132301-2	Cortical cell coarse vacuolation and zonal necrosis	SER aggregation, mitochondrial changes; autophagosome formation	Dominick et al. 1993a Domimick et al. 1993b Reindel et al. 1992

SER, Smooth endoplasmic reticulum.

without appreciable corticolysis may cause no grossly apparent alterations or can induce adrenal enlargement. Compounds which cause corticolysis may cause a range of responses, depending in part on the duration and severity of the injury.

Representative of the macroscopic adrenal effects caused by corticolytic chemicals is the toxicity due to DMNM. Adrenals of rats treated with 100 mg/kg DMNM per day for 7 weeks were small and the cortex substantially thinned relative to the medulla. Mean adrenal weight of treated rat adrenals (0.041 ± 0.004 g) were approximately two-thirds of controls (0.064 ± 0.003 g; Yarrington et al. 1981). Small adrenals with thin cortices were also identified in dogs administered PD 132301-2 at 6 mg/kg per day and greater for 2 weeks (Dominick et al. 1993b). Dogs sacrificed moribund prior to the end of the dosing period had adrenal enlargement and hemorrhage. Reparative responses may occur following zonal necrosis and may restore the adrenal cortex to normal thickness and contour, or they can result in an irregular and nodular appearence of the cortex due to irregular hyperplasia of scattered foci of residual cortical cells.

Microscopic Features

Table 36 presents examples of chemically induced microscopic degeneration of the adrenal cortex of laboratory animals. Degenerative changes induced by most adrenotoxicants consist of vacuolar degeneration (coarse vacuolation, lipid accumulation, fatty change) of adrenocortical cells and/or cortical cell necrosis (granular degeneration, adrenocorticolysis, cortical necrosis, cortical atrophy) in selective zones of the adrenal cortex. Infiltrates of mixed or mononuclear inflammatory cells are commonly present during

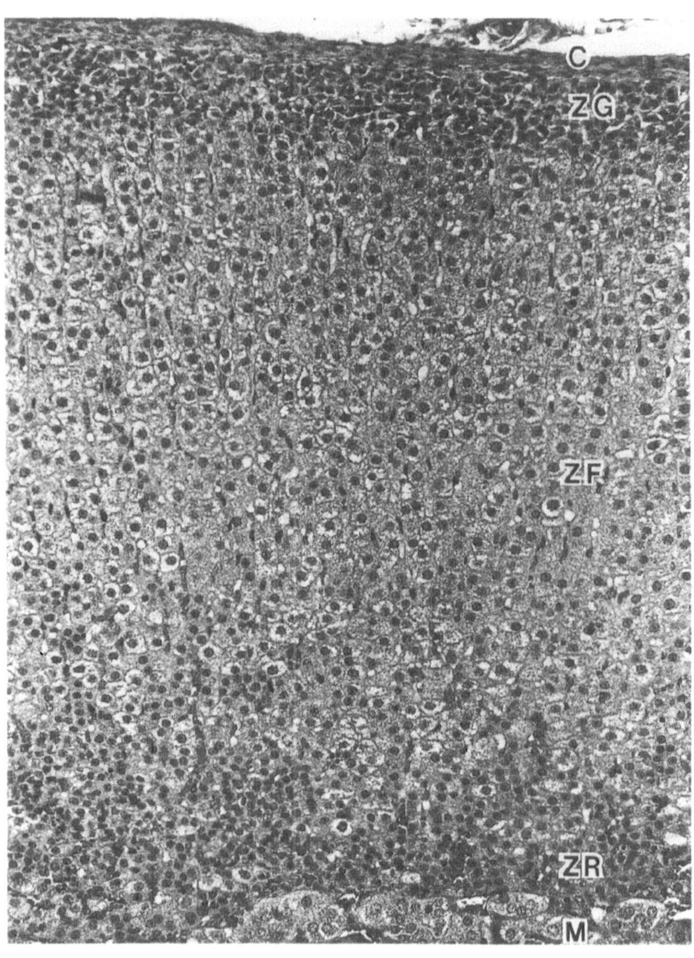

Fig. 501. The normal adrenal cortex of a rat contains a distinct zona glomerulosa (*ZG*), zona fasciculata (*ZF*), and zona reticularis (*ZR*). An adjacent area of medulla (*M*) and the capsule (*C*) are illustrated in the figure. H&E, ×100

various stages of the degenerative process; hemorrhage may or may not be present. Dystrophic mineralization occasionally occurs secondary to tissue necrosis. Other cellular changes that may be chemically related but are not clearly degenerative include: cortical cell hypertrophy or hyperplasia, depletion of fine lipid vacuoles (reduced vesiculation), increased cytoplasmic eosinophilia, and intracytoplasmic inclusions.

Compared to a normal adrenal cortex (Fig. 501), diffuse adrenocortical degeneration caused by the potent adrenocortical toxic chemical DMNM begins in the zona reticularis. The earliest lesions, which may initially result in cortical enlargement, consist of granular and vacuolar degeneration of cortical cells. Increasing the treatment duration or dose results in vacuolation spreading to the other zones. With time, the entire cortex including the zona glomerulosa is involved (Fig. 502). Condensation or collapse of these areas with or without hemorrhage may follow cellular necrosis. In addition, a mixed population of inflammatory cells including neutrophils, macrophages, and lymphocytes may be present in the adrenal cortex of dogs treated with DMNM (≥15 mg/kg per day), 1,1′ thiodiethylidene-ferrocene (75 mg/kg per day) or *o,p′*-DDD (50 mg/kg per day). Acute degenerative lesions caused by 7,12 dimethylbenzanthracene in rats can best be described as frank necrosis of the cortex with hemorrhage and secondary mineralization (Murad et al. 1973). The examples of microscopic changes listed above reflect acute to subacute injury. Zonal atrophy with stromal collapse and fibrosis in association with focal hyperplastic areas of cortical remnants (Fig. 503) are subacute to chronic histological changes resulting in small adrenals of rats treated with 50 mg/kg per day of DMNM for 90 days Fig. 504). Atrophy and fibrosis have also been chronic lesions associated with *o,p′*-DDD treatment of

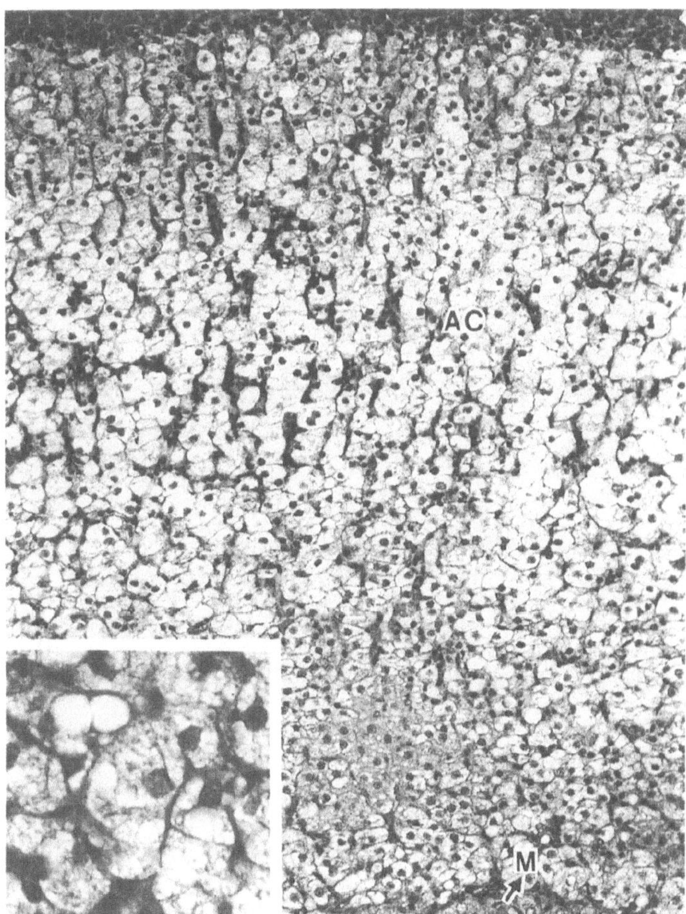

Fig. 502. Vacuolar and granular degeneration of the adrenal cortex (*AC*) of a rat treated with 100 mg/kg per day α-(1,4-dioxido-3-methylquinoxalin-2-yl)-*N*-methylnitrone for 35 days. A portion of the medulla (*M*) can also be observed. ×100. *Insert*, higher magnification of degenerative changes, H&E, ×250

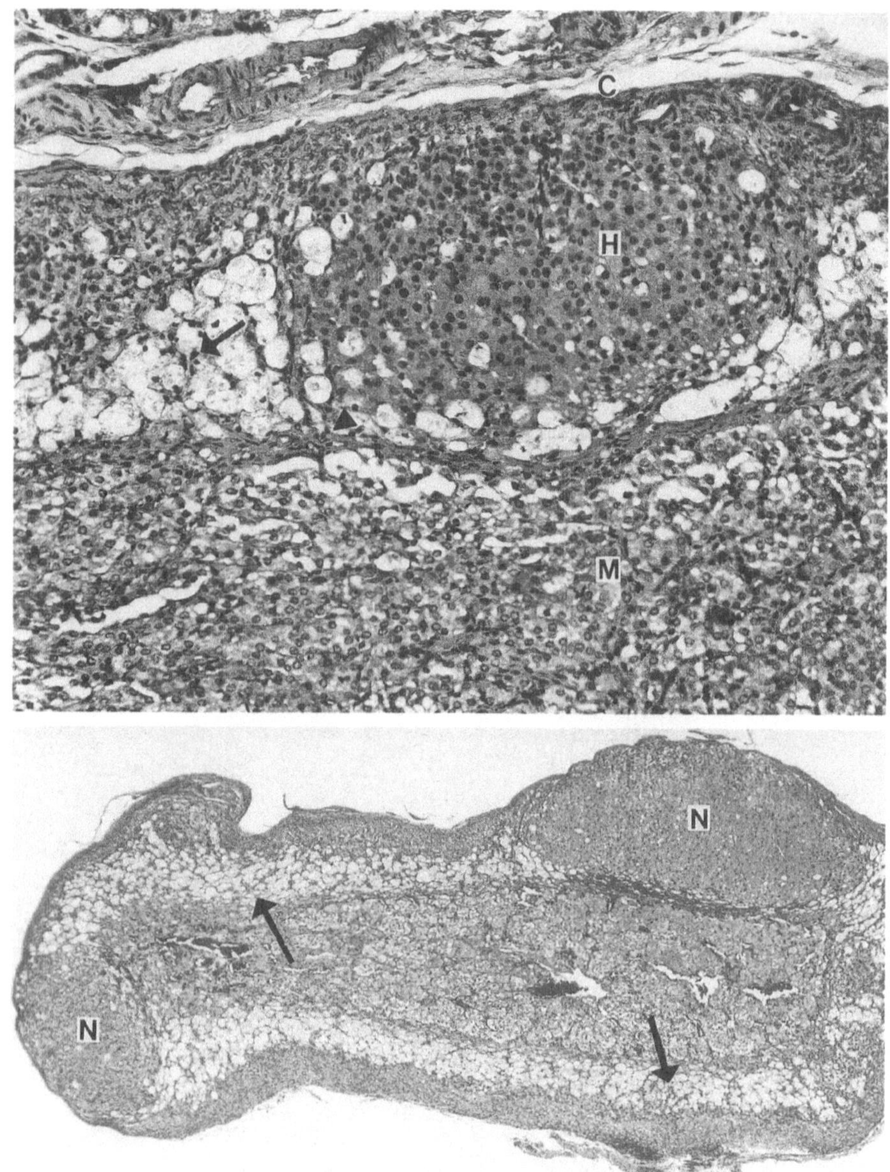

Fig. 503. (*above*) Narrow cortex, vacuolar atrophy (*arrow*) and mild fibrosis (*arrowhead*) in association with focal hyperplasia (*H*) of cortical remnants are prominent findings in the adrenal of a rat treated with 50 mg/kg per day α-(1,4-dioxido-3-methylquinoxalin-2-yl)-N-methylnitrone for 90 days. The capsule (*C*) and medulla (*M*) are also present. H&E, ×100

Fig. 504. (*below*) A small adrenal with areas of cortical vacuolar atrophy (*arrows*) and nodular hyperplasia (*N*) frequently resulted when rats were treated with 50 mg/kg per day α-(1,4-dioxido-3-methylquinoxalin-2-yl)-*N*-methylnitrone for 90 days. H&E, ×25

dogs (Nelson and Woodward 1949; Kaminsky et al. 1962).

Repair responses occur in the damaged adrenal cortex following withdrawal of toxicants and can be relatively complete even when the extent of cortical injury has been substantial. Repair of the adrenal cortex following administration of corticolytic doses of DDD to dogs occurs largely within 10–12 weeks of drug withdrawal (Powers et al. 1974). During repair severely damaged cells and cell fragments are consumed by macrophages. Mildly affected cells are moved centripetally toward the medulla by regenerating cortical cells that originate from the outer cortex. Minor residual changes detected 36 weeks after drug withdrawal consisted of the persistence of some macrophages and lipofuscin-rich reticularis cells at the mildly fibrotic reticularis-medullary junction. In PD 132301-2 treated guinea pigs, near complete reversal of zona fasciculata effacement occurred within 2 weeks of drug withdrawal (Dominick et al. 1993a). Minor mononuclear infiltrates and foci of mineralization persisted in the restored region.

Ultrastructure

Ultrastructural changes caused by the action of some adrenocortical toxic compounds are listed in Table 36. Typically the zona reticularis and zona fasciculata are most severely affected by these compounds, although all layers may eventually become involved. The type of injury is frequently related to dose and duration of chemical exposure. Dose-related differences in cellular responses can be seen in fasciculata cells of monkeys treated with PD 132301-2 for 2 weeks. At low doses cortical cells had proliferation of endoplasmic reticulam, depletion of small lipid vacuoles, and an increase in myelin figures, autophagosomes, and residual bodies in cortical cells (Reindel et al. 1993). At higher doses there was cortical cell lysis, disruption of trabeculae, and the presence of increased numbers of phagolysosome-laden tissue macrophages.

The profound cytoplasmic granular and vacuolar degeneration noted microscopically in rat adrenal cortices as a result of treatment with DMNM appears ultrastructurally as severe mitochondrial damage and lipid accumulation (Fig. 505). Disruption of mitochondria and smooth endoplasmic reticulum caused by adrenocortical toxic chemicals is not surprising since during adrenal steroidogenesis cytochrome P450-associated 11β- and 18-hydroxylation occurs in mitochondrial membranes while 17α- and 21-hydroxylation occurs in microsomal fractions (endoplasmic reticulum;

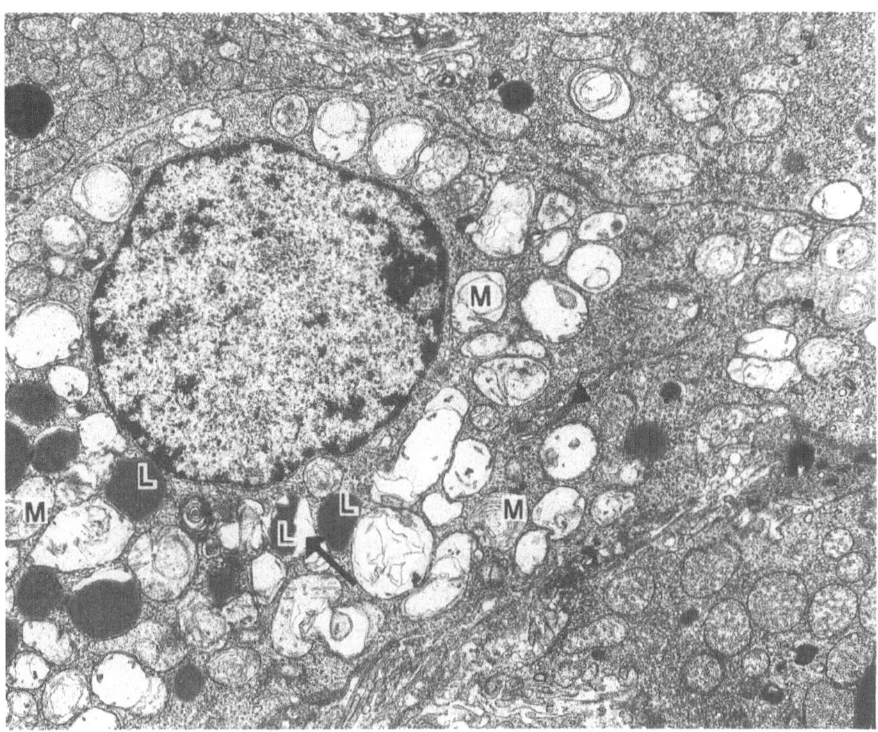

Fig. 505. Cell of the zona fasciculata of the adrenal cortex of a rat treated with 100 mg/kg per day α-(1,4-dioxido-3-methylquinoxalin-2-yl)-*N*-methylnitrone for 21 days. Vacuolated mitochondria (*M*) and increased lipid droplets (*L*), some undergoing lipolysis (*arrow*), are distinct features. Areas of moderate dilation of smooth endoplasmic reticulum (*arrowhead*) can also be observed. TEM, ×8000

Mitani 1979). Furthermore, mitochondria of steroidogenic tissues are intimately associated with the endoplasmic reticulum. More severe ultrastructural injury due to the potent adrenocorticolytic chemicals can cause cortical cells to have dense-appearing cytoplasm, chromolysis, and disruption of their plasma membrane, all of which are features of necrosis. Macrophages containing cholesterol clefts, numerous lipid droplets, and membranous debris are frequently observed among these necrotic cells. As a result of necrosis and possibly inhibition of steroidogenesis considerable amounts of lipid material may coalesce into larger, poorly defined extracellular masses in the adrenal cortex of DMNM-treated rats (Yarrington et al. 1985). In contrast to the potent adrenocortical toxic compounds, spironolactone, which promotes sodium diuresis by competitively antagonizing aldosterone at peripheral receptor sites, causes ultrastructural findings of so-called spironolactone bodies in the zona glomerulosa. These bodies are foci of hypertrophic smooth endoplasmic reticulum surrounding a core of lipid. They may result from the impaired production of aldosterone, although stimulation and the resultant hypertrophy of the zona gomerulosa due to the activation of the renin-angiotensin system is the more likely cause (Fisher and Horvat 1971).

Biologic Features

Chemically induced adrenocortical degeneration frequently results in functional alterations in

Table 37. Pharmacologic inhibition of adrenal steroid biosynthesis or effects

Compound	Steroid or conversion site inhibited	Mechanism of action	References
Aminoglutethimide	Cholesterol to pregnenolone	Competitive inhibition of 20 α-hydroxylase	Cohen 1968
o,p'-DDD	Cholesterol to pregnenolone 11-Deoxycortisol to cortisol	Decreased production or availability of TPNH (NADPH) 11β-Hydroxylase	Hart et al. 1971
DMNM	Cholesterol to pregnenolone?	Unknown	Yarrington et al. 1985; Capen et al. 1991
Triparanol	Desmosterol (24-dehydrocholesterol) to cholesterol	Inhibited reduction of 24, 25 bond	Steinberg and Avigan 1960
Cyanoketone	Δ^5-3β-ol Steroids to Δ^4-3-oxo steroids	3β-Hydroxysteroid dehydrogenase inhibited	Liddle 1974
SU-9055	Cortisol Aldosterone	Inhibition of 17 α-hydroxylase Interference of oxidation at the carbon-18	Liddle 1974
SU-8000	Cortisol Aldosterone	Inhibition of 17 α-hydroxylase Interference of oxidation at the carbon-18	Liddle 1974
Metyrapone	11-Deoxycortisol to cortisol DOC to corticosterone	Inhibition of 11β-hydroxylase	Liddle 1974
SKF 12185	11-Deoxycortisol to cortisol DOC to corticosterone	Inhibition of 11β-hydroxylase	Liddle 1974
RO1-8307/ Heparinoids	Aldosterone	Inhibition of aldosterone; mechanism unknown	Abbott et al. 1966
Spironolactone	Aldosterone	Competitive inhibition of peripheral receptor sites, resulting in sodium diuresis	Fisher and Horvat 1971; Liddle 1974
Amphenone	Non-specific inhibition	Inhibition of 20α-hydroxylase? 11β-, 17α-, and 21-hydroxylases	Temple and Liddle 1970
PD 132301-2	Esterification of cholesterol	Inhibition of acyl-CoA: cholesterol acyltransferase (ACAT)	Dominick et al. 1993a

steroidogenesis or secretion of corticosteroids that can be assessed by various in vivo parameters. Reductions in serum and plasma levels of corticosteroids have been reported following treatment with compounds that ablate the zona fasciculata and reticularis (Vilar and Tullner 1959; Holloszy and Eisenstein 1961; Dexter et al. 1967). Basal levels of blood corticosteroids are not, however, a sensitive marker for compromised adrenal steroidogenesis. ACTH stimulation tests are a more sensitive measure of adrenal cortical reserves following cortical injury. Suppressed adrenal responsiveness in the form of decreased blood corticosteroids following ACTH stimulation has been documented in animals treated with a number of toxicants (Yarrington et al. 1985; Hertz et al. 1955; Dexter et al. 1967; Hennigar et al. 1964). Alterations in serum electrolytes secondary to adrenocortical insufficiency can also occur as a result of adrenocortical necrosis. Serum aldosterone concentrations have not been used routinely as an index of adrenal cortical reserves but may be useful in assessing altered function associated with hypertrophy of the zona glomerulosa.

In vitro studies to assess the specific cellular consequences of toxicant exposure have been useful in determining specific drug-related alterations in pathways of steroidogenesis. The development of adrenocortical degeneration caused by adrenocortical toxic chemicals is frequently correlated with their ability to inhibit steroidogenesis (Table 37). In general, the potent adrenocortical toxic compounds primarily inhibit the intramitochondrial conversion of cholesterol to pregnenolone, which correlates with ultrastructural findings of increased numbers of lipid droplets and cholesterol clefts and prominent effects on mitochondria and endoplasmic reticulum. Aminoglutethimide, for example, appears to cause these effects by the competitive inhibition of 20α-hydroxylase (Cohen 1968). The action of *o,p'*-DDD on adrenal steroidogenesis is less well defined. Although *o,p'*-DDD has been shown partially to inhibit 11β-hydroxylation, its principal effect appears to be its ability to inhibit the conversion of cholesterol to pregnenolone by reducing within the adrenal cortical cell the production or availability of reduced triphosphopyridine nucleotide (NADPH), an essential cofactor for steroid hydroxylation (Hart et al. 1971). Little is known at present about the effects of potent adrenocortical toxic drugs DMNM and 1,1' thiodiethylidene-ferrocene on adrenal steroidogenesis. Some adrenocortical toxic compounds frequently inhibit specific enzyme systems or affect the metabolism of one class of steroids. For example, the heparinoid compound R01-8307, a sulfated mucopolysaccharide with low anticoagulant activity, selectively inhibits aldosterone secretion while at the same time causing distinct selective condensation of the zona glomerulosa of the adrenal cortex (Abbott et al. 1966).

References

Abbott EC, Monkhouse FC, Steiner JW, Laidlaw JC (1966) Effect of a sulfated mucopolysaccharide (R01-8307) on the zona glomerulosa of the rat adrenal gland. Endocrinology 78:651–654

Brogan WC, Eacho PI, Hinton DE, Colby HD (1984) Effects of carbon tetrachloride on adrenocortical structure and function in guinea pigs. Toxicol Appl Pharmacol 75:118–127

Camacho AM, Cash R, Brough AJ, Wilroy RS (1967) Inhibition of adrenal steroidogenesis by amino-glutethimide and the mechanism of action. JAMA 202:114–120

Capen CC, DeLellis RA, Yarrington JT (1991) Endocrine system. In: Haschek-Hock WM, Rousseaux CG (eds) Handbook of toxicologic pathology. Academic, Orlando, pp 675–759

Cohen MP (1968) Aminoglutethimide inhibition of adrenal desmolase activity. Proc Soc Exp Biol Med 127:1086–1090

Colby HD (1988) Adrenal gland toxicity: chemically induced dysfunction. J Am Coll Toxicol 7:45–69

Colby HD, Pope MR, Johnson PB, Sherry JH (1987) Effects of cadmium in vitro on microsomal steroid metabolism in the inner and outer zones of the guinea pig adrenal cortex. J Biochem Toxicol 2:1–11

Currie AR, Helfenstein JE, Young S (1962) Massive adrenal necrosis in rats caused by 9,10-dimethyl-1,2-benzanthracene and its inhibition by metyrapone. Lancet ii:1199–1200

Dexter RN, Fishman LM, Ney RL, Liddle GW (1967) Inhibition of adrenal corticosteroid synthesis by aminoglutethimide: Studies of the mechanism of action. J Clin Endocrinol Metab 27:473–480

Dietert SE, Scallen TJ (1969) An ultrastructural and biochemical study of the effects of three inhibitors of cholesterol biosynthesis upon murine adrenal gland and testis. J Cell Biol 40:44–60

Dominick MA, Bobrowski WA, MacDonald JR, Gough AW (1993a) Morphogenesis of a zone-specific adrenocortical cytotoxicity in guinea pigs administered PD 132301-2, an inhibitor of acyl-CoA: cholesterol acyltransferase. Toxicol Pathol 21:54–62

Dominick MA, McGuire EJ, Reindel JF, Bobrowski WF, Bocan TMA, Gough AW (1993b) Subacute toxicity of a novel inhibitor of acyl-CoA: cholesterol acyltransferase in beagle dogs. Fundam Appl Toxicol 20:217–224

Eacho I, Colby HD (1983) Regional distribution of microsomal drug and steroid metabolism in the guinea pig adrenal cortex. Life Sci 32:1119–1127

Fisher ER, Horvat B (1971) Experimental production of so-called spironolactone bodies. Arch Pathol 91:471–478

Hallberg E (1990) Metabolism and toxicity of xenobiotics in the adrenal cortex with particular reference to 7,12-dimethylbenz(a)anthracene. J Biochem Toxicol 5:71–90

Hart MM, Swackhamer ES, Straw JA (1971) Studies on the site of action of *o,p'*-DDD in the dog adrenal cortex. II. TPNH- and corticosteroid precursor-stimulation of *o,p'*-DDD-inhibited steroidogenesis. Steroids 17:575–586

Hennigar GR, Fleckner RA, Golding MR (1964) Degeneration and regeneration of the adrenal cortex following administration of DDD (2,2-bis (parachlorophenyl)-1,1 dichlorethane. Bull N Y Acad Med 40:161–166

Hertz R, Tullner WW, Schricker JA, Dhyse FG, Hallman LF (1955) Studies on amphenone and related compounds. Recent Prog Horm Res 11:119–147

Holloszy J, Eisenstein AB (1961) Effect of triparanol (MER/29) on corticosterone secretion by rat adrenals. Proc Soc Exp Biol Med 107:347–349

Hornsby PJ (1989) Steroid and xenobiotic effects on the adrenal cortex: mediation by oxidative and other mechanisms. Free Radic Biol Med 6:103–115

Kaminsky N, Luse S, Hartroft P (1962) Ultrastructure of adrenal cortex of the dog during treatment with DDD. J Natl Cancer Inst 29:127–159

Liddle GW (1974) The adrenal cortex. In: Williams RH (ed) Textbook of endocrinology. Saunders, Philadelphia, pp 233–283

Luse S (1967) Fine structure of the adrenal cortex. In: Eisenstein AB (ed) The adrenal cortex. Little Brown, Boston, pp 1–69

Malendowicz LK (1972) Steatotic degeneration of rat adrenocortical cells after treatment with aminoglutethimide. Acta Histochem (Jena) 43:350–360

Marek J, Pfeifer U (1971) Microthrombi as a partial cause of adrenal damage due to hexadimethrine bromide (Polybrene). Verh Dtsch Ges Pathol 55:706–709

Marek J, Pfeifer U, Motlik K (1973) Ultrastructure of the protein-containing vacuoles and hyaline droplets in rat adrenocortical cells following Polybrene. Virchows Arch B Cell Pathol 14:273–283

Mitani F (1979) Cytochrome P450 in adrenocortical mitochondria. Mol Cell Biochem 24:21–44

Mohammed A, Hallberg E, Rydstrom J, Slanina P (1985) Toxaphene: accumulation in the adrenal cortex and effect on ACTH-stimulated corticosteroid synthesis in the rat. Toxicol Lett 24:137–143

Moore NA, Callas G (1975) Observations on the fine structure of propylthiouracil-induced "brown degeneration" in the zona reticularis of mouse adrenal cortex. Anat Rec 183: 293–302

Murad TM, Leibach J, Von Hamm E (1973) Latent effect of DMBA on adrenal glands of Sprague-Dawley rats: an ultrastructural study. Exp Mol Pathol 18:305–315

Nelson AA, Woodward G (1949) Severe adrenal cortical atrophy (cytotoxic) and hepatic damage produced in dogs by feeding 2,2-bis (parachlorophenyl)-1,1-dichlorethane (DDD or TDE). Arch Pathol 48:387–394

Powers JM, Hennigar GR, Grooms G, Nichols J (1974) Adrenal cortical degeneration and regeneration following administration of DDD. Am J Pathol 75:181–194

Purjesz I, Sturcz J, Huttner I (1964) The effect of chronic prolonged water loading on prednisolone induced adrenocortical atrophy. Experimentia 20:688–689

Racela A Jr, Azarnoff D, Svoboda D (1969) Mitochondrial cavitation and hypertrophy in rat adrenal cortex due to aminoglutethimide. Lab Invest 21:52–60

Reindel JF, Dominick MA, Krause B (1992) Comparative adrenotoxicity of a novel acyl-CoA: cholesterol acyltransferase (ACAT) inhibitor (PD 132301-2) in laboratory animals. Toxicol Pathol 20:A642

Reindel JF, Dominick MA, Bocan TM, Gough AW, McGuire EJ (1994) Toxicologic effects of a novel acyl-CoA: cholesterol acyltransferase (ACAT) inhibitor in cynomolgus monkeys. Toxicol Pathol 22:510–518

Rhodin JA (1971) The ultrastructure of the adrenal cortex of the rat under normal and experimental conditions. J Ultrastruct Res 34:23–71

Ribelin WE (1984) The effects of drugs and chemicals upon the structure of the adrenal gland. Fundam Appl Toxicol 4:105–109

Sasano N, Ichinoe F, Hirano K (1966) Histological and enzyme histochemical studies on adrenocortical atrophy induced by hydrocortisone, dexamethasone and paramethasone. Nippon Naibunpi Gakkai Zasshi 41:1432–1437

Steinberg D, Avigan J (1960) Studies of cholesterol biosynthesis. II. The role of desmosterol in the biosynthesis of cholesterol. J Biol Chem 235:3127–3129

Szabo S, Lippe IT (1989) Adrenal gland: chemically induced structural and functional changes in the cortex. Toxicol Pathol 17:317–329

Temple TE, Liddle GW (1970) Inhibitors of adrenal steroid biosynthesis. Annu Rev Pharmacol 10:199–218

Vilar O, Tullner WW (1959) Effects of *o,p'*-DDD on histology and 17-hydroxycorticosteroid output of the dog adrenal cortex. Endocrinology 65:80–86

Volk TL, Scarpelli DG (1964) Alterations of fine structure of the rat adrenal cortex after the administration of triparanol. Lab Invest 13:1205–1214

Yarrington JT, Huffman KW, Gibson JP (1981) Adrenocortical degeneration in dogs, monkeys and rats treated with α-(1,4-dioxido-3-methylquinoxalin-2-yl)-*N*-methylnitrone. Toxicol Lett 8:229–234

Yarrington JT, Huffman KW, Leeson GA, Sprinkle DJ, Loudy DE, Gibson JP (1983) Comparative toxicity of the hematinic MDL 80,478 – effects on the liver and adrenal cortex of the dog, rat and monkey. Fundam Appl Toxicol 3:86–94

Yarrington JT, Loudy DE, Sprinkle DJ, Gibson JP, Wright GL, Johnston JO (1985) Degeneration of the rat and canine adrenal cortex caused by α-(1,4-dioxido-3-methylquinoxalin-2-yl)-*N*-methylnitrone (DMNM). Fundam Appl Toxicol 5:370–381

Nodular Cortical Hyperplasia, Adrenal, Thymectomized Mouse*

Frantisek Zak

Synonyms. Adrenocortical nodules, adrenocortical lipid hyperplasia, nodular hyperplasia, "B" cell hyperplasia, hyperplastic clear cell nodule.

Gross Appearance

Occasional minute rounded yellow nodules may be seen within the adrenal cortex. The brown patches of ceroid may also be seen grossly.

Microscopic Features

In about 40% of aged thymectomized mice, single or multiple adrenocortical nodules of varying size may be seen with the light microscope (Fig. 506). Generally, these hyperplastic nodules consist of clear, lipid-laden cells which are sometimes larger than those of the normal zona fasciculata and vary in size and shape (Fig. 507). These cells of the zona fasciculata correspond to the so-called type B cells of Woolley and Little (1945) and Dunn (1970, 1979) and are arranged in cords and clusters (Fig. 508). The nodules, if multiple, are separated by fibrovascular stroma and are situated wholly within the cortex toward its periphery, or, occasionally, near the center of the gland in relation to the main vein. The larger nodules distort the architecture of the adrenal cortex and may elevate the capsule.

Clusters of these hyperplastic cortical cells sometimes protrude through gaps in the fibrous capsule, usually around blood vessels, into the periadrenal fat tissue (Fig. 509). Although these extrusions commonly arise from underlying nodules, they may also be encountered in areas where the cortex appears normal. Histologic evidence of malignant degeneration of these hyperplastic nodular lesions has not been observed in our material.

In sham-operated and untreated control mice all these changes occurred less frequently and usually at a more advanced age (20 or more months).

Differential Diagnosis

Adenoma of the adrenal cortex may be distinguished from nodular cortical hyperplasia by the compression of normal tissues adjacent to the adenoma. Compression and invasion of adjacent tissues, and metastases to other sites, are features which distinguish carcinomas of the adrental cortex.

Biologic Features

Natural History. Although in the adult animal removal of the thymus is not associated with a significant depression of the immune response (Comsa et al. 1977; Hess 1968; Pierpaoli and Sorkin 1972; Walter and Israel 1979), thymectomy performed shortly (up to 48 h) after birth can produce severe effects in some species (Hess et al. 1963; McIntire et al. 1964). Mice, for instance, thymectomized at birth and maintained under conventional conditions, grow normally for a time but then develop a syndrome characterized by marked wasting, lethargy, ruffled fur, hunched posture, sometimes diarrhea, and eventually death (McIntire et al. 1964). The earlier in life thymectomy is performed, the higher the frequency of the wasting syndrome. However, thymectomy after 1 week of age is not associated with any significant incidence of this syndrome (Pierpaoli and Besedovsky 1975), and wasting does not occur in neonatally thymectomized mice maintained under SPF or germ-free conditions (McIntire et al. 1964; Pierpaoli and Besedovsky 1975; Walter and Israel 1979). The primary factor in the pathogenesis of the postneonatal thymectomy wasting syndrome thus appears to be an environmental one, presumably an infectious agent (mouse hepatitis virus is one) to which only neonatally thymectomized mice, because of their diminished immunological capacity, are susceptible. Athymic hairless (nude) mice have a pro-

* The lesions found in the adrenals of mice that are thymectomized at birth and kept under specific pathogen-free (SPF) or germ-free conditions to old age consist of (a) ceroid deposits in the cortex, (b) subcapsular spindle-cell hyperplasia, and (c) nodular cortical hyperplasia. The first two are described elsewhere in this volume (pp. 458, 464); Nodular cortical hyperplasia is described in this section.

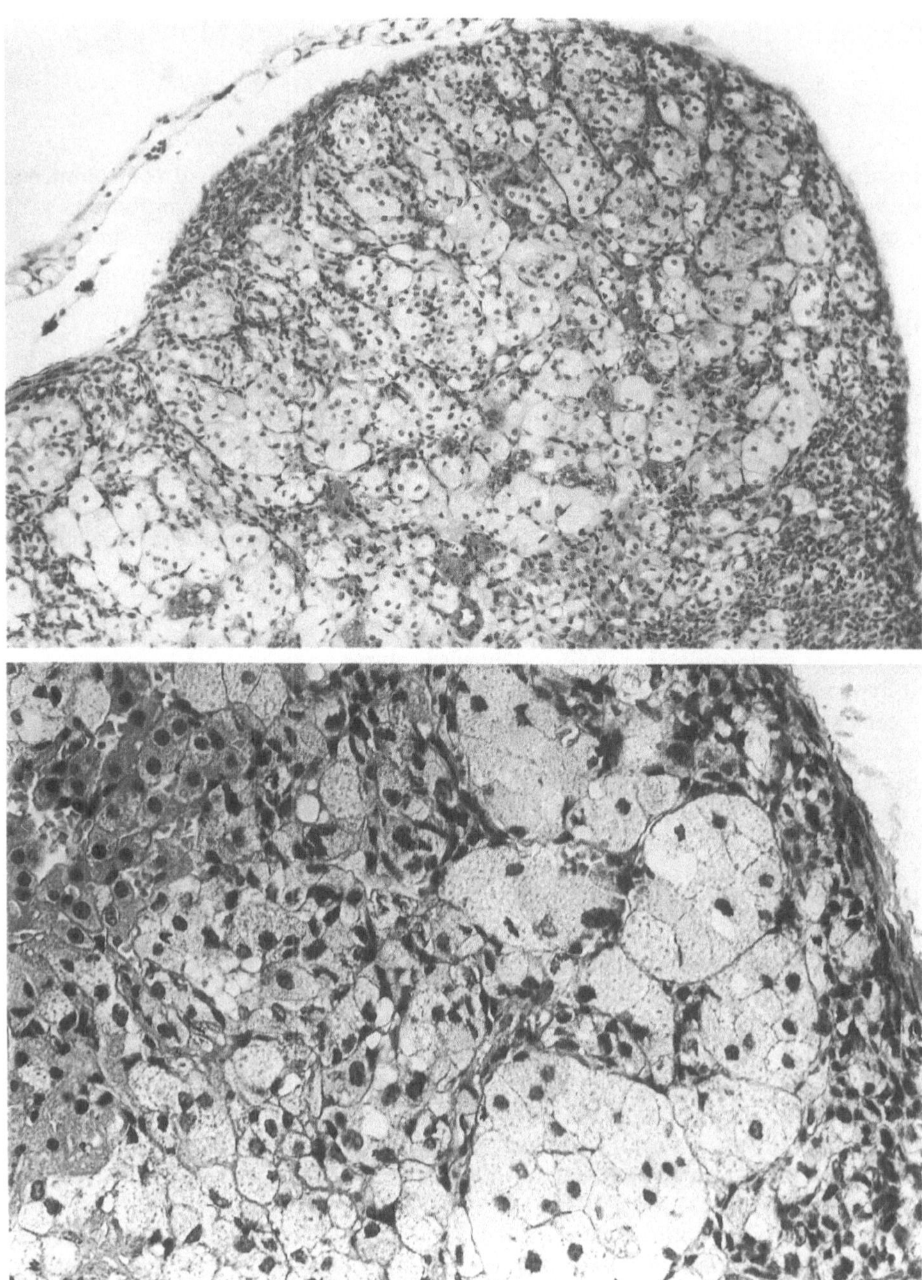

Fig. 506. (*above*) Adrenal of a male MAG mouse 64 weeks after thymectomy. Hyperplastic and hypertrophied adrenal cortical type B cells in noducle which elevates adrenal capsule. H&E, ×100

Fig. 507. (*below*) Adrenal of a male MAG mouse 64 weeks after thymectomy. Large lipid-laden pleomorphic B-cells in adrenal cortex. H&E, ×250

gressive wasting syndrome that reduces their life span to 2–4 months in conventional breeding conditions, but in an SPF environment they survive for 10 months or longer (Pierpaoli and Sorkin 1972).

However, in mice with congenital absence of the thymus, as well as in neonatally thymectomized mice, there is marked deficiency of small lymphocytes throughout the body, mainly in the paracortical zones of lymph nodes, in the splenic white

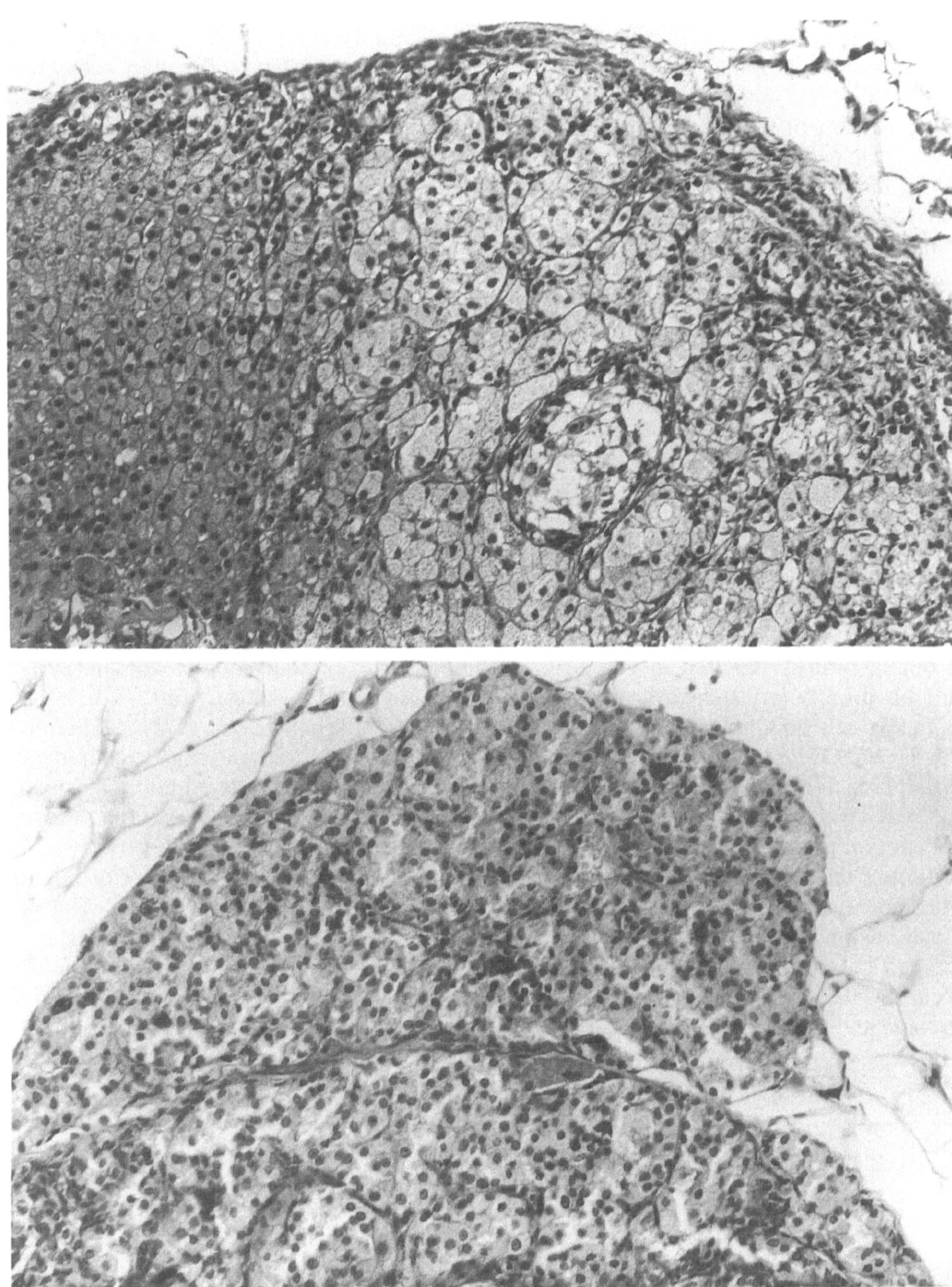

Fig. 508. (*above*) Adrenal of a female MAG mouse 67 weeks after thymectomy. Clusters of hyperplastic cortical type B cells in adrenal cortex. H&E, ×130

Fig. 509. (*below*) Adrenal of a female MAG mouse 62 weeks after thymctomy. Extrusion of hyperplastic cortical type B cells through the adrenal capsule. H&E, ×130

pulp, and in the circulating blood (Hess 1968; McIntire et al. 1964; Pierpaoli and Sorkin 1972; Walter and Israel 1979). The animals exhibit an impaired ability to develop delayed-type hypersensitivity, and are tolerant of homografts, and sometimes even of heterografts (Hess et al. 1963). The production of immunoglobulins to some antigens is normal but to others, e.g., sheep red cells or egg white, it is impaired (Comsa et al. 1977). Specific derangements of thyroid and gonadal functions were observed in neonatally thymectomized mice (Pierpaoli and Besedovsky 1975). Although severe degenerative changes in the adrenal cortex of wasted thymectomized animals have been described (Comsa et al. 1977; Hess 1968), in surviving "noninfected" animals or in animals held under SPF conditions, only transitory stimulation of the adrenal cortex was noted in subacute experiments (Comsa et al. 1977; Deschaux et al. 1974, 1979; Pierpaoli and Besedovsky 1975).

Pathogenesis. Hyperplastic clear cell nodules in mice correspond to the so-called type B cell adenomas or microadenomas of Woolley and Little (1945; Dunn 1970, 1979). Present evidence indicates that they are not neoplastic. They may occur infrequently in old, untreated mice of various strains (Cotchin and Roe 1967; Dunn 1970); however, in young mice their spontaneous occurrence has not been described. The frequency of occurrence of this lesion in MAG and CFI mice in our laboratory is noted in Fig. 510. Succinic and β-hydroxybutyric dehydrogenases remain low in the B cell nodules (Cotchin and Roe 1967; Neville and O'Hare 1982). B cell hypertrophy and hyperplasia are dependent on ACTH secretion and may be prevented by hypophysectomy.
Stimulation with ACTH or stress causes transformation of the foamy cells in the zona fasciculata to compact cells, from which cholesterol can be rapidly depleted. Under continuous influence of the corticotropic stimulus, lipoid repletion may occur in the cortex after the initial depletion (Neville and O'Hare 1982). As a sequel to persistent increase in corticotropic stimulation, focal hyperplasia may take place, sometimes with discontinuous proliferation of adrenocortical cells, along the vessels and nerves, through the capsule, even into the periadrenal fat tissue (Dobbie 1969).

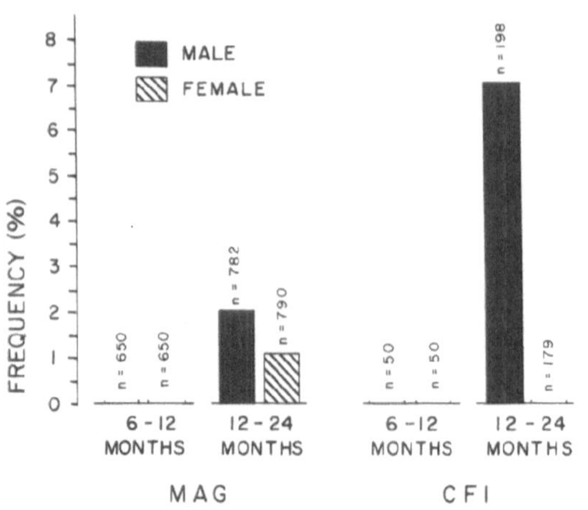

Fig. 510. Cortical (B cell) hyperplasia in mice. *n*. total number of animals examined

Etiology. A few adrenocortical hyperplastic nodules appear to have been induced experimentally in mice by various forms of irradiation (Cotchin and Roe 1967; Dunn 1970), and by dimethylbenzanthracene, a chemical which induces necrosis, but no tumors in rats. A markedly increased incidence of these adrenocortical hyperplastic nodules has been described in castrated male and ovariectomized female mice (Dunn 1970; Woolley and Little 1945).

Comparison with Other Species

Nodular hyperplasia is common in the adrenal cortex of adult rabbits, golden (Syrian) hamsters, rats, mice, dogs, cats, horses and baboons (Benirschke et al. 1978). Sometimes it may be present in both adrenals, generally as small, multiple, unencapsulated foci. Diagnostic terms such as adenomatous hyperplasia, microadenoma or cortical adenoma have been used to describe these lesions (Jayne 1953, 1963; Cotchin and Roe 1967; Dobbie 1969; Nelson 1980). The literature concerning adenomas and hyperplastic nodules in the adrenal cortex of rodents is confusing; the differentiation of one from the other is subjective and often equivocal. Adrenocortical nodules of similar histologic appearance are very common in man (Dobbie 1969; Nelson 1980; Neville and O'Hare 1982), but despite numerous recent advances there is still no convincing explanation of their functional properties. According to Neville and O'Hare (1982) the nodules in man are localized overgrowths of adrenocortical cells and not true neoplasms. Extrusions of cortical cells through the fibrous capsule and intracapsular or extracapsular adrenal nodules are surely not histologic signs of malignant growth; they may frequently be observed during detailed histologic examination of adult adrenal glands in man (Dobbie 1969), dog (Hullinger 1978), and rat (Jayne 1953). We have also observed adrenocortical extrusions in old mice. These changes are regarded as sequelae of tropic stimuli to the adrenal cortex and have been seen in increasing frequency with age in man (Dobbie 1969).

References

Benirschke K, Garner FM, Jones TC (1978) Pathology of laboratory animals. Springer, Berlin Heidelberg New York

Comsa J, Philipp EM, Leonhardt H (1977) Effects of thymectomy on the endocrine glands of the rat. Isr J Med Sci 13:354-362

Cotchin E, Roe FJC (1967) Pathology of laboratory rats and mice. Blackwell, Oxford

Deschaux P, Flores JL, Fontanges R (1974) Influence de la thymectomie sur les glandes surrénales. Arch Int Physiol Biochim 82:115-121

Deschaux P, Massengo B, Fontanges R (1979) Edocrine interaction of the thymus with the hypophysis, adrenals and testes. Thymus 1:95-108

Dobbie JW (1969) Adrenocortical nodular hyperplasia: the ageing adrenal. J Pathol 99:1-18

Dunn TB (1970) Normal and pathologic anatomy of the adrenal gland of the mouse, including neoplasms. JNCI 44:1323-1389

Dunn TB (1979) Tumours of the adrenal gland. In: Turusov VS (ed) Pathology of tumours in laboratory animals, vol II: tumours of the mouse. IARC, Lyon (IARC scientific publications no 23)

Hess MW (1968) Experimental thymectomy: possibilities and limitations. Springer, Berlin Heidelberg New York

Hess MW, Cottier H, Stoner RD (1963) Primary and secondary antitoxin responses in thymectomized mice. J Immunol 91:425-430

Hullinger RL (1978) Adrenal cortex of the dog (Canis familiaiaris). I. Histomorphologic changes during growth, maturity and aging. Anat Histol Embryol 7:1-27

Jayne EP (1953) Cytology of the adrenal gland of the rat at different ages. Anat Rec 115:459-483

Jayne EP (1963) A histo-cytologic study of the adrenal cortex in mice as influenced by strain, sex, and age. J Gerontol 18:227-234

McIntire KR, Sell S, Miller JF (1964) Pathogenesis of the postneonatal thymectomy wasting syndrome. Nature 204: 151-155

Nelson DH (1980) The adrenal cortex: physiological function and disease, vol XVII: major problems in internal medicine. Saunders, Philadelphia

Neville AM, O'Hare MJ (1982) The human adrenal cortex. Springer, Berlin Heidelberg New York

Pierpaoli W, Besedovsky HO (1975) Role of the thymus in programming of neuroendocrine functions. Clin Exp Immunol 20:323-328

Pierpaoli W, Sorkin E (1972) Alterations of adrenal cortex and thyroid in mice with congenital absence of the thymus. Nature 238:282-285

Walter JB, Israel MS (1979) General pathology, 5th edn. Churchill-Livingstone, Edinburgh

Woolley GW, Little CC (1945) The incidence of adrenal cortical carcinoma in gonadectomized female mice of the extreme dilution strain. I. Observations on the adrenal cortex. Cancer Res 5:193-202

Lipid Hyperplasia, Adrenal Cortex, Rat

Christian Landes, Georg Krinke, and Frantisek Zak

Synonyms. Lipid adrenal hyperplasia, adrenocortical lipid hyperplasia, adrenocortical lipid transformation, adrenal change due to adrenostatic drugs, congenital lipoid adrenal hyperplasia in man.

Gross Appearance

The adrenals are enlarged, the gland surface is smooth; on cross-section the cortex appears to be markedly widened, showing diffuse, pale yellow or ivory white discoloration. A two- to fourfold increase in adrenal weight was observed in subchronic studies (Malendowicz 1972a). In a chronic (24-month) carcinogenicity study with aminoglutethimide, lipid hyperplasia progressed to neoplastic lesions, manifested by the macroscopic presence of nodules and masses in the adrenal gland, and adrenal weight increase amounted to eight times the control values.

Microscopic Features

Enlargement of the hyperplastic adrenal gland is due to diffuse increase in number and size of adrenal cortical cells; the medulla remains intact (Fig. 511). Most of the cortical cells accumulate large amounts of cytoplasmic lipids, acquiring a finely alveolate to coarsely vacuolate appearance (Fig. 512). Accumulation of lipid is apparent through the full width of the cortex, with loss of cortical zonation especially between the zonae glomerulosa and fasciculata. Extensive accumulation of lipids may result in occurrence of large

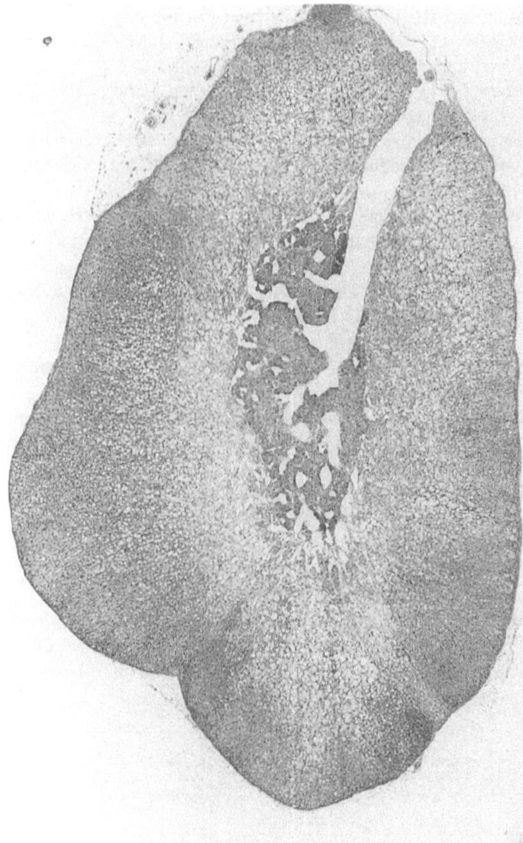

Fig. 511. Diffuse lipid hyperplasia of the adrenal cortex, rat treated with aminoglutethimide. The cortex is devoid of clear zonation and unusually large in proportion to the medulla. H&E ×20

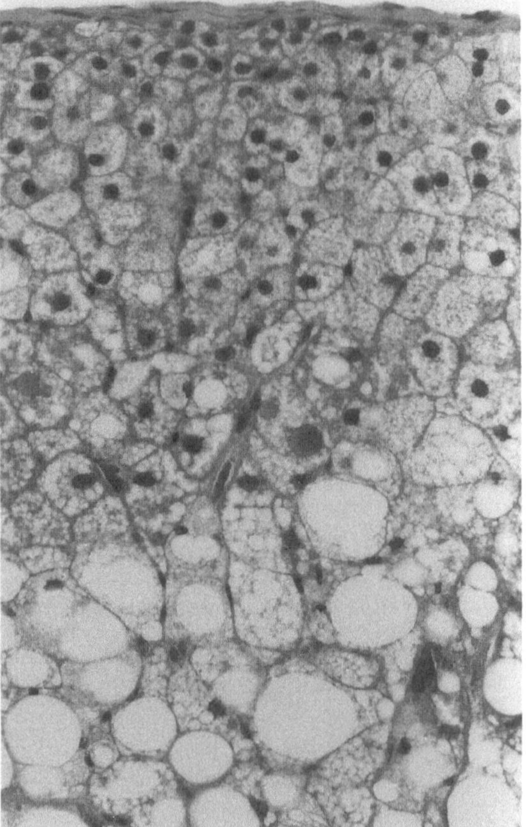

Fig. 512. Lipid hyperplasia, adrenal cortex, rat treated with aminoglutethimide. Lipid-laden cells, partly finely alveolate, partly coarsely vacuolated. H&E, ×400

ballooned cells and occasional formation of needle-shaped or rhombic crystals within the cytoplasm, believed to be cholesterol or cholesterol esters depending on their morphology and lipid solubility (Marek et al. 1970; Motlik et al. 1973; Starka and Motlik 1971). The altered cells, especially in the outer third of the adrenal cortex, undergo histochemical changes evidenced by an increase in acid hydrolases, particularly acid phosphatase, and by a depression or even loss of activity of lactate, malate, succinic acid, 3β-hydroxysteroid, isopropanol, and glucose-6-phosphate dehydrogenases (Malendowicz 1972b; Motlik et al. 1973) and $NADH_2$ tetrazolium reductase. PAS-positive droplets may be found in some altered cells (Marek and Motlik 1978).

When lipid hyperplasia progresses to neoplasia, some neoplastic cells have compact, eosinophilic cytoplasm, but in others features of lipid hyperplasia are seen. The presence of occasional mitotic figures in such cells (Fig. 513) indicates active cell division of cells affected by lipid hyperplasia which may lead to neoplasia. Figure 514 presents

▶

Fig. 513. (*upper left*) Lipid-laden adrenocortical cells, one undergoing mitotic division, rat treated with aminoglutethimide. H&E, ×1000

Fig. 514. (*lower left*) Adrenocortical adenoma, rat treated with aminoglutethimide. The circumscribed neoplastic lesion compresses adrenal cortex affected by lipid hyperplasia, H&E, ×20

Fig. 515. (*upper right*) Adrenocortical adenoma (same as in Fig. 514) is composed of both lipid-laden and compact, eosinophilic cells. H&E, ×200

Fig. 516. (*lower right*) Adrenocortical carcinoma, rat treated with aminoglutethimide. The tumor contains both lipid-laden and compact, eosinophilic cells, growing in trabecular pattern. H&E, ×200

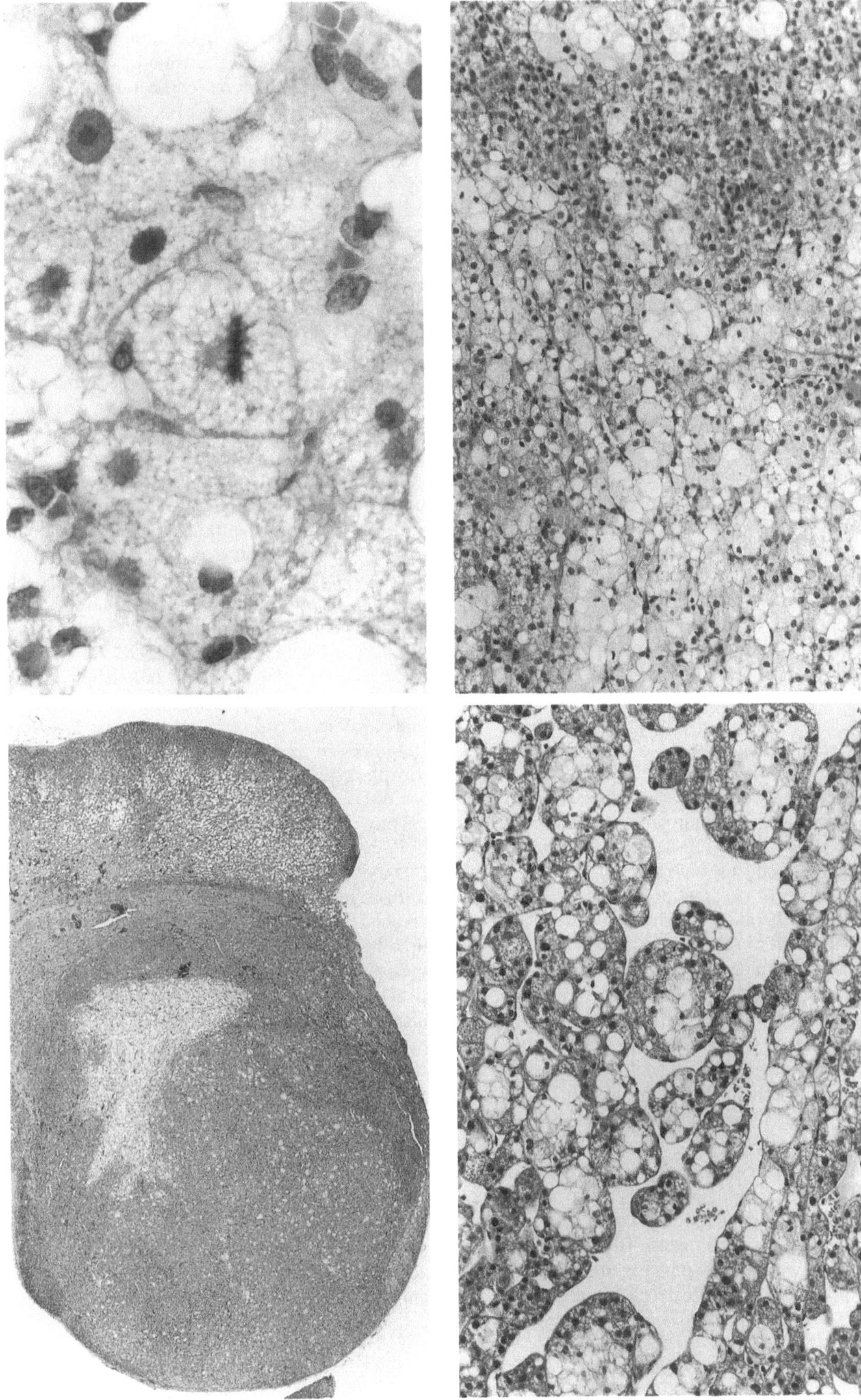

an example of cortical adenoma; this tumor is composed predominantly of lipid-laden cells but also contains compact, eosinophilic cells (Fig. 515). In Fig. 516 a trabecular growth pattern is evident in the cortical carcinoma.

Ultrastructure

Apart from hypertrophy of the smooth endoplasmic reticulum (Marek et al. 1971) the most striking changes in the adrenocortical cells of aminoglutethimide-treated rats (20–40 mg/kg per day) are the intramitochondrial membrane-bound cavities of differing size (up to 6 µm) which are regarded as pathologic equivalents of mitochondrial vesicles (Marek and Motlik 1978; Marek et al. 1970; Racela et al. 1969). The cavities are either empty or contain fine fibrillar or homogeneous lipid material of moderate electron density. For these changes the term "lipoid transformation of the adrenocortical mitochondria" has been introduced. At the periphery of this intramitochondrial lipid material myelinlike structures are often found. After the dissolution of the membranous component of mitochondria affected by lipid accumulation, free cytoplasmic lipids aggregate and large lipid droplets form.

Differential Diagnosis

Conditions associated with increased adrenocortical size/weight include prolonged stress reaction (Uno et al. 1989), effects of adrenocorticotropic hormone, and Cushing's disease. Adrenal pathology of acute stress is poorly documented, and there are therefore no clearly defined histologic features that can be used to identify characteristic stress morphology in the adrenal cortex. Depletion of lipids and hypertrophy of compact, eosinophilic cells have been attributed to stress (Neville and O'Hare 1982; Russfield 1967). Since the adrenal cortex of young healthy rats is composed of cells with compact, eosinophilic cytoplasm, lipid depletion and transformation of lipid-laden to this type of cell may be difficult to discern.

Likewise, increased levels of plasma ACTH (of exogenous or endogenous, "ectopic" origin) have been associated with hypertrophy of compact, eosinophilic cortical cells. In lipid hyperplasia induced with adrenostatic agents the cytoplasm of proliferating cortical cells is alveolated and vacuolated rather than compact, due to intracellular accumulation of lipids, although the proliferative stimulation is attributed to increased ACTH levels. Bilateral cortical hyperplasia in Cushing's disease consists of both lipid-laden and compact cells. In contrast to cortical hypofunction occurring in adrenostatic agent induced lipid hyperplasia, in Cushing's disease the proliferating adrenal cortex is hyperfunctional. We are not aware of naturally occurring Cushing's disease in rats, although adrenocortical hyperplasia coinciding with pituitary adenomas is frequent in aging rats. There is good evidence for stimulation of ACTH-producing pituitary cells in aminoglutethimide-treated rats (Zak 1983). This, however, is in reaction to inhibited adrenal steroidogenesis, so that the order of events is reversed in chemically induced lipid hyperplasia in comparison to Cushing's disease.

Adrenocortical vacuolar (fatty) degeneration may be induced with a number of agents interfering with corticosteroid synthesis, including aminoglutethimide. The lesion may progress into cortical necrosis and loss of zonation and fibrosis with resulting atrophy manifested by decreased adrenal size and weight (Yarrington 1983). The apparently opposite effects of adrenostatic agents – cortical hyperplasia, on the one hand, and atrophy, on the other – can obviously be explained by differences in conditions of exposure, such as dose levels and frequency or duration of treatment.

Morphologic features provide insufficient basis for discrimination of induced from naturally occurring proliferative adrenocortical lesions, as lipid-laden cells may occur in both situations (Strandberg 1983a–c). The presence of bilateral, diffuse hyperplasia with cells exhibiting finely alveolate cytoplasm, however, is suggestive of lipid hyperplasia. It is of interest that despite the mesodermal origin of adrenal cortex, adrenocortical tumors are classified as adenomas or carcinomas even if they are composed predominantly of cells containing fat, comparable to those encountered in lipomas.

Biologic Features

Pathogenesis and Sequelae of the Aminoglutethimide-Induced Adrenocortical Lesions. Aminoglutethimide, an amino derivative of the hypnotic agent glutethimide, was initially introduced as an anticonvulsant in 1958 (Santen and Henderson

1981). The observation of adrenal insufficiency in patients receiving this drug (Camacho et al. 1967; Cash et al. 1967; Givens et al. 1968; Hughes and Burley 1970) led to restriction of its use to an investigational drug in 1966. Since that time data from numerous studies have been published, focusing on the experimental pathology and pathophysiology, as well as on biochemical investigations on the mechanisms and sites of action of this compound as an inhibitor of steroidogenesis (Cohen 1968; Dexter et al. 1967; Malendowicz 1972a). It has been shown that aminoglutethimide inhibits the enzymatic conversion of cholesterol to pregnenolone by suppressing 20α-hydroxylation of the cholesterol side chain, the initial step for side-chain cleavage. This blocking action is primarily responsible for the adrenocortical changes. The intracellular accumulation of lipids is due to storage of nonutilized natural steroid precursors. Under such conditions the negative feedback mechanism results in an increase in ACTH secretion, leading to diffuse adrenocortical hyperplasia (Goldman 1967, 1970a,b).

Treatment. Aminoglutethimide has been found useful (a) in the palliation of Cushing's syndrome, particularly the malignant variety, by suppressing adrenocortical secretion, (b) in the relief of bone pain in some patients with metastatic carcinoma of the breast or prostate, and (c) in reducing the blood pressure of patients with low renin hypertension (Liddle et al. 1976; Bentley 1981; Neville and O'Hare 1982; Santen et al. 1974; Smilo et al. 1967). Aminoglutethimide is a nonsteroidal agent inhibiting a number of cytochrome P-450 dependent enzymes. Therefore the aminoglutethimide-induced aromatase inhibition, representing an effect desirable for estrogen deprivation in treatment of estrogen-dependent breast cancer, is not quite specific. Recently, novel nonsteroidal aromatase inhibitors have been developed, with highly specific effects on estrogen biosynthesis and minimal or absent inhibition of adrenal steroidogenesis (Bhatnagar et al. 1990).

Frequency. In a chronic (24-month) carcinogenicity study with aminoglutethimide in rats, lipid hyperplasia occurred frequently and affected about 30% of animals treated with 30 mg/kg and about 85% of those treated with 60 mg/kg. The number of male and female rats bearing adrenocortical adenomas or carcinomas was increased to about 9% in males and 26% in females treated with 60 mg/kg per os, compared to about 7% expected in untreated control animals of both sexes of same strain and comparable age (Morawietz et al. 1992), indicating a probable progression of hyperplasia to neoplasia, especially in females.

Comparison with Other Species

Lipid hyperplasia is a term used for a peculiar diffuse hyperplasia of the adrenal cortex, described originally in man as an adrenocortical disorder based on a congenital deficiency of enzyme systems involved in the early stages of steroid biosynthesis (Prader and Gurtner 1955; Siebenmann 1957). A morphologically similar adrenocortical lesion has been produced experimentally in rats by administration of several adrenostatic drugs, especially aminoglutethimide. In contrast to animals, mitochondrial changes in adrenocortical cells of human patients treated with aminoglutethimide (1–2 g daily for varying periods of time) are not a prominent feature. The only mitochondrial changes observed are focal loss of the vesicular cristae and concomitant fibrillary loosening of the mitochondrial matrix (Marek and Motlik 1975). The most striking ultrastructural finding described in adrenocortical cells of man is the intracytoplasmic accumulation of lipids, mostly as rounded liposomes of variable size. In some of the cortical cells focal cytoplasmic degradation may be observed, culminating in coagulative necrosis or, in others, cytolysis. In some areas of the adrenal cortex, activated lipophagic histiocytes are the prevalent cells.

References

Bentley PJ (1981) Endocrine pharmacology: physiological basis and therapeutic applications. Cambridge University Press, Cambridge

Bhatnagar AS, Häusler A, Schieweck K, Lang M, Bowman R (1990) Highly selective inhibition of estrogen biosynthesis by CGS 20267, a new nonsteroidal aromatase inhibitor. J Steroid Biochem Mol Biol 37:1021–1027

Camacho AM, Cash R, Brough AJ, Wilroy RS (1967) Inhibition of adrenal steroidogenesis by aminoglutethimide and the mechanism of action. JAMA 202:114–120

Cash R, Brough AJ, Cohen MNP, Satoh PS (1967) Aminoglutethimide (Elipten-Ciba) as an inhibitor of adrenal steroidogenesis: mechanism of action and therapeutic trial. J Clin Endocrinol Metab 27:1239–1248

Cohen MP (1968) Aminoglutethimide inhibition of adrenal desmolase activity. Proc Soc Exp Biol Med 127:1086–1090

Dexter RN, Fishman LM, Ney RL, Liddle GW (1967) Inhibition of adrenal corticosteroid synthesis by aminoglutethimide: studies of the mechanism of action. J Clin Endocrinol Metab 27:473–480

Givens JR, Coleman S, Britt L (1968) Anatomical changes produced in the human adrenal cortex by aminoglutethimide. Clin Res 16:441

Goldman AS (1967) Experimental congenital adrenocortical hyperplasia: persistent postnatal deficiency in activity of 3 beta-hydroxysteroid dehydrogenase produced in utero. J Clin Endocrinol Metab 27:1041–1049

Goldman AS (1970a) Production of congenital lipoid adrenal hyperplasia in rats and inhibition of cholesterol side-chain cleavage. Endocrinology 86:1245–1251

Goldman AS (1970b) Experimental congenital lipoid adrenal hyperplasia: prevention of anatomic defects produced by aminoglutethimide. Endocrinology 87:889–893

Hughes SW, Burley DM (1970) Aminoglutethimide: a "side effect" turned to therapeutic advantage. Postgrad Med J 46:409–416

Liddle GW, Hollifield JW, Slaton PE, Wilson HM (1976) Effects of various adrenal inhibitors in low-renin essential hypertension. J Steroid Biochem 7:937–940

Malendowicz LK (1972a) Karyometrical and histochemical studies of adult male rat adrenal cortex after treatment with aminoglutethimide. Endokrinologie 60:60–74

Malendowicz LK (1972b) Comparative studies of the effects of aminoglutethimide, metopirone, ACTH and hydrocortisone on the adrenal cortex of adult male rats. I. Karyometric studies. Virchows Arch [B] 11:55–65

Marek J, Thoenes W, Motlik K (1970) Lipoide Transformation der Mitochondrien in Nebennierenrindenzellen nach Aminoglutethimid (Elipten Ciba). Virchows Arch [B] 6: 116–131

Marek J, Motlik K (1975) Ultrastructural changes of the adrenal cortex in Cushing's syndrome treated with aminoglutethimide (Elipten Ciba). Virchows Arch [B] 18:145–156

Marek J, Motlik K (1978) Ultrastructure of acute adrenocortical damage due to aminoglutethimide (Elipten Ciba). Virchows Arch [B] 27:173–187

Marek J, Pfeifer U, Motlik K (1971) Hypertrophie des glatten endoplasmatischen Reticulum in Nebennierenrinden-Zellen nach Aminoglutäthimid. Virchows Arch [B] 8:36–41

Morawietz G, Rittinghausen S, Mohr U (1992) RITA – Registry of Industrial Toxicology Animal data – progress of the working group. Exp Toxicol Pathol 44:301–309

Motlik K, Pinsker P, Starka L, Hradec E (1973) Effects of aminoglutethimide (Elipten Ciba), a steroid biosynthesis blocking agent, on adrenal glands in Cushing's syndrome. Virchows Arch [A] 360:11–26

Neville AM, O'Hare MJ (1982) The human adrenal cortex. Springer, Berlin Heidelberg New York

Prader A, Gurtner HP (1955) Das Syndrom des Pseudohermaphroditismus masculinus bei kongenitaler Nebennierenrinden-Hyperplasie ohne Androgenilberproduktion (adrenaler Pseudohermaphroditismus masculinus). Helv Pediatr Acta 10:397–412

Racela A Jr, Azarnoff D, Svoboda D (1969) Mitochondrial cavitation and hypertrophy in rat adrenal cortex due to aminoglutethimide. Lab Invest 21:52–60

Russfield AB (1967) Pathology of the endocrine glands, ovary and testis of rats and mice. In: Cotchin E, Roe FJC (eds) Pathology of laboratory rats and mice, Blackwell Scientific, Oxford

Santen RJ, Henderson IC (1981) A comprehensive guide to the therapeutic use of aminoglutethimide. Pharmanual 2. Karger, Basel

Santen RJ, Lipton A, Kendall J (1974) Successful medical adrenalectomy with aminoglutethimide. Role of altered drug metabolism. JAMA 230:1661–1665

Siebenmann RE (1957) Die kongenitale Lipoidhyperplasie der Nebennierenrinde mit Nebennierenrinde-Insuffizienz. Schweiz Z Allg Pathol (Basel) 20:77–84

Smilo RP, Earl JM, Forsham PH (1967) Suppression of tumorous adrenal hyperfunction by aminoglutethimide. Metabolism 16:374–377

Starka L, Motlik K (1971) The influence of injected aminoglutethimide on the morphology of rat adrenal cortex and adrenal metabolism of progesterone. Endokrinologie 58: 75–86

Strandberg JD (1983a) Focal hyperplasia, adrenal cortex, rat. In: Jones TC, Mohr U, Hunt RD (eds) Monographs on pathology of laboratory animals, endocrine system. Springer, Berlin Heidelberg New York, pp 37–41

Strandberg JD (1983b) Adenoma, adrenal cortex, rat. In: Jones TC, Mohr U, Hunt RD (eds) Monographs on pathology of laboratory animals, endocrine system. Springer, Berlin Heidelberg New York, pp 41–45

Strandberg JD (1983c) Adenocarcinoma, adrenal cortex, rat. In: Jones TC, Mohr U, Hunt RD (eds) Monographs on pathology of laboratory animals, endocrine system. Springer, Berlin Heidelberg New York, pp 46–49

Uno H, Tarara R, Else JG, Suleman MA, Sapolsky RM (1989) Hippocampal damage associated with prolonged and fatal stress in primates. J Neurosci 9:1705–1711

Yarrington JT (1983) Chemically induced adrenocortical lesions. In: Jones TC, Mohr U, Hunt RD (eds) Monographs on pathology of laboratory animals, endocrine system. Springer, Berlin Heidelberg New York, pp 69–75

Zak F (1983) Lipid Hyperplasia, adrenal cortex, rat. In: Jones TC, Mohr U, Hunt RD (eds) Monographs on pathology of laboratory animals, endocrine system. Springer-Verlag, Heidelberg, Berlin, New York, pp 80–84

Zak M, Kovacs K, McComb DJ, Heitz PU (1985) Aminoglutethimide-stimulated corticotrophs. An immunocytologic, ultrastructural and immunoelectron microscopic study of the rat adenohypophysis. Virchows Arch [B] 49:93–106

Mouse Hepatitis Viral Infection, Adrenal, Mouse

Stephen W. Barthold

Synonyms. Hepatoencephalitis virus, murine hepatitis viral infection.

Gross Appearance

Mice that are ill or dying from mouse hepatitis virus (MHV) infection may have gross lesions in a number of organs, depending upon the infecting virus strain and a number of host factors. Livers may be diffusely pale, have random depressed white spots and petechiae, or be roughly nodular with depression of intervening parenchyma. Hepatitis may be accompanied by small amounts of peritoneal exudate. Mice infected with enterotropic strains may have dilated, fluid- and gas-filled intestines with thin, translucent walls. The spleen may be enlarged and the thymus reduced. The majority of infections in adult, immunocompetent mice are asymptomatic, with no gross lesions (Barthold 1987; Barthold et al. 1982, 1985; Biggers et al. 1964; Hierholzer et al. 1979; Piazza 1969). Depending upon infecting virus strain, athymic nude mice may develop wasting syndrome with neurological signs, hepatic lesions and splenomegaly (Hirano et al. 1975; Sebesteny and Hill 1974; Tamura et al. 1977). Nude mice infected with enterotropic strains of virus may have no overt disease or segmental thickening of the bowel wall, particularly the cecum and ascending colon, and mesenteric lymph node enlargement without hepatitis (Barthold et al. 1985).

Microscopic Appearance

Depending on virus and host factors, focal necrosis, leukocytic infiltration, and syncytium formation may be found in a variety of organs including liver, brain, spinal cord, olfactory mucosa, lung, lymphoid organs, pancreas, small intestine, cecum, and colon. Syncytia may arise from mesothelium, lymphoreticular cells, endothelium, glia, neurons, enterocytes, and parenchymal cells (Barthold 1987, 1988; Barthold and Smith 1987; Barthold et al. 1982, 1985, 1993; Biggers et al. 1964; Piazza 1969). Adrenal cortical or medullary cells may form syncytia in multisystemic viral infections (unpublished). Vacuolization of adrenal parenchyma, especially the zonae glomerulosa and fasciculate, and medullary edema and hyperemia have been reported in experimental MHV-3 infection (Piazza 1969).

Ultrastructure

Lytically infected cells develop a number of nonspecific degenerative changes. Viral particles are seen in dilated cisternae of endoplasmic reticulum and to a lesser extent within cytoplasm and cytoplasmic vesicles. Virions have a nonhomogeneous central nucleoid surrounded by a less dense peripheral ring and an envelope with spikes. The envelope is acquired by budding through internal cytoplasmic membranes. Virus leaves the cell by exocytosis or cytolysis. Tissue culture cells infected with MHV strain A59 develop round or oval reticular inclusions and tubular bodies measuring approximately 1–2 nm. Reticular inclusions are composed of 250–400 Å threads in a dense matrix of 35 Å granules. Tubular bodies are composed of tubular structures 160–250 Å in diameter which may be continuous with the cytoplasmic tubular system. Ribosomes are in the cytoplasmic matrix between tubules. Viral particles bud into the cisternae of the tubules (David-Ferreira and Manaker 1965). Tubular bodies also have been found in hepatocytes of MHV A59 infected mice and enterocytes of mice infected with MHV-Y (Barthold et al. 1982; Piazza 1969).

Differential Diagnosis

When they can be found, syncytia are characteristic of MHV in many organs. Adrenal syncytia must be differentiated from clusters of hematopoietic elements or leukocytes. Adrenal lesions are likely to occur only in disseminated infections of susceptible hosts. Thus, evaluation of other more commonly affected tissues for MHV lesions is confirmatory.

Biologic Features

Natural History. The majority of natural MHV strains are only mildly pathogenic, and infections are likely to be subclinical. MHV infections may be manifest in a number of ways, depending on route of exposure, virus strain, dose, mouse strain, immunocompetency, age, and coinfection with other agents (Barthold 1987). Some strains are weakly pathogenic, even in athymic nude mice (Hirano et al. 1975), while others are highly virulent in adult mice (LePrevost et al. 1975). A common sign of infection is perturbed immune responsiveness of mice (Barthold 1987). MHV infections in immunocompetent mice are generally acute, with no persistence of the virus (Barthold and Smith 1987, 1990; Barthold et al. 1993). Misunderstanding about MHV persistence in mice has been perpetuated by observations of exacerbation of acute disease with immunosuppressive agents in subclinically infected mice (Barthold and Smith 1990; Piazza 1969). Exacerbation of disease can occur only in the early phase of infection, not after mice have recovered (Barthold and Smith 1990). Host immunity to MHV is virus strain specific, with immune mice susceptible to repeated subclinical reinfections with different strains of the virus (Barthold and Smith 1989; Homberger et al. 1992), thus suggesting persistence of virus when mice are immunosuppressed during active reinfection. Although mouse pups are most susceptible to disease, outbreaks of MHV in breeding populations are rapidly attenuated by maternal antibody, which protects young mice through their age-related susceptibility. Maternally derived immunity is short-lived, but once it has waned, mice are at an age when clinical signs are not apparent when they become infected (Barthold et al. 1988; Homberger et al. 1992). MHV is not likely to be vertically transmitted from dam to fetus (Barthold et al. 1988).

MHV strains, as coronaviruses of other species, have primary tropism for either respiratory or enteric mucosa. Respiratory MHV strains initially replicate in nasal mucosa, then readily disseminate in susceptible hosts to other organs. Enterotropic MHV strains tend to be much more selective in their tissue tropism, with infections restricted largely to the intestine. Thus, these two basic types of infection result in markedly different disease manifestations (Barthold 1987; Barthold and Smith 1987; Barthold et al. 1993). Enterotropic MHV strains tend to be highly contagious, causing severe disease in neonatal mice, with explosive outbreaks with high mortality when first introduced to a naive population. Neonates may die within 24–48 h of exposure (Barthold et al. 1982, 1993; Biggers et al. 1964; Hierholzer et al. 1979). Respiratory strains of MHV tend to be less contagious, but young mice are also most susceptible to disease manifestations, which include hepatitis and encephalitis (Barthold 1987; Barthold and Smith 1987). Neurotropism is an experimentally emphasized attribute of certain MHV strains and is usually a feature of the polytropic, respiratory types of virus, with development of encephalitis and demyelination upon intracerebral inoculation (Barthold 1987; Piazza 1969). Neurotropic strains of MHV can also infect brain directly via olfactory neural pathways or through viremia (Barthold 1988; Barthold and Smith 1987). Athymic nude mice and other immunologically compromised mice are prone to severe manifestations when infected with respiratory strains of MHV (Barthold et al. 1985; Hirano et al. 1975; Taguchi et al. 1979; Sebesteny and Hill 1974) but less so with enterotropic strains of MHV (Barthold et al. 1985).

Transplantable tumors, particularly leukemia lines, may become contaminated with MHV. The virus can be carried for many passages with no adverse effect but may break out following immunosuppression, chemotherapeutic regimens, or introduction into a susceptible host, resulting in acute disease or abnormal host tumor biology (Barthold 1987; Braunsteiner and Friend 1954).

Pathogenesis. MHV strains vary considerably in their virulence and relative organotropism but can be divided into respiratory and enteric biotypes (Barthold 1987). Respiratory strains of the virus infect nasal epithelium (but not the lower respiratory epithelium), then disseminate in susceptible hosts to multiple organs. These viruses are pantropic, infecting and causing disease in many organs, of which the liver and brain are prominent because of their clinical effects. Brain infection can take place along olfactory neural pathways or via viremia. Lymphoid tissues are also a very common target, even in subclinically infected mice, resulting in immunological aberrations.

When respiratory viruses infect neonatal, athymic or other immunologically compromised strains of mice, their full disease manifestations become evident (Barthold and Smith 1987, 1990; Hirano et al. 1975). Immunocompetent mice vary in their susceptibility to MHV infection but recover from infection with no carrier state, although they can be reinfected with other strains of the virus (Barthold and Smith 1987, 1989). In contrast, enterotropic MHV strains are much more restrictive in their tissue tropism, targeting enterocytes and to a much lesser extent other tissues. Although mice of all ages are susceptible to infection, disease is highly age associated due to kinetics of intestinal epithelium. Infection of adult immunologically compromised mice, such as athymic nude mice, results in chronic infection, but clinical signs may be mild or absent (Barthold et al. 1982, 1985; Barthold and Smith 1990; Biggers et al. 1964; Hierholzer et al. 1979). Outcome of infection with MHV is highly dependent upon infecting virus strain, dose, route of inoculation, host age, genotype, and immune status (Barthold 1987).

Etiology. MHV is a coronavirus with numerous strains that vary widely in their biologic effects. MHV strains share extensive cross-reactive antigens, but host immunity to infection is virus strain specific (Barthold and Smith 1989; Homberger et al. 1992). To date there is no means of defining the biologic behavior or specific strain identity with genetic or antigenic means. This is irrelevant, as MHV is highly mutable and prone to recombination. Although the mouse is the natural host for MHV, rats can support experimental infections (Barthold and Smith 1989; Taguchi et al. 1979).

Frequency. MHV is very frequent in colonies of laboratory mice. The frequency of adrenal lesions in MHV-infected mice is low, as most infections are very mild without dissemination to organs such as the adrenal. They are most apt to be seen in immunologically compromised mice, such as nude mice, or in experimentally inoculated infant mice or mice infected with atypically virulent strains of MHV.

Comparison with Other Species

Coronaviruses are generally species specific, infect a number of host species, and have a wide spectrum of lesions, including peritonitis in cats, bronchitis in chickens, and enteritis in many species, especially in neonates. Like MHV, different strains of a particular species of coronavirus have either primary respiratory or enteric tropism. Human coronaviruses are generally associated with upper respiratory infections, and, as with mice, humans are subject to repeated infections with different strains of coronavirus (Barthold 1987).

References

Barthold SW (1987) Mouse hepatitis virus biology and epizootiology. In: Bhatt PN, Jacoby RO, Morse HC III, New AE (eds) Viral and mycoplasmal infections of laboratory rodents. Effects on biomedical research. Academic, New York, pp 571–601

Barthold SW (1988) Olfactory neural pathway in mouse hepatitis virus nasoencephalitis. Acta Neuropathol (Berl) 76:502–506

Barthold SW, Smith AL (1987) Response of genetically susceptible and resistant mice to intranasal inoculation with mouse hepatitis virus JHM. Virus Res 7:225–239

Barthold SW, Smith AL (1989) Virus strain specificity to challenge immunity to coronavirus. Arch Virol 104:187–196

Barthold SW, Smith AL (1990) Duration of mouse hepatitis virus infection: studies in immunocompetent and chemically immunosuppressed mice. Lab Anim Sci 40:133–137

Barthold SW, Smith AL, Lord PFS, Bhatt PN, Jacoby RO (1982) Epizootic coronaviral typhlocolitis in sucking mice. Lab Anim Sci 32:376–383

Barthold SW, Smith AL, Povar ML (1985) Enterotropic mouse hepatitis virus infection in nude mice. Lab Anim Sci 35:613–618

Barthold SW, Beck DS, Smith AL (1988) Mouse hepatitis virus and host determinants of vertical transmission and maternally-derived passive immunity in mice. Arch Virol 100:171–183

Barthold SW, Beck DS, Smith AL (1993) Enterotropic coronavirus (mouse hepatitis virus) in mice: influence of host age and strain on infection and disease. Lab Anim Sci 43:276–284

Biggers DC, Kraft LM, Sprinz H (1964) Lethal intestinal virus infection of mice (LIVIM). An important new model for study of the response of the intestinal mucosa to injury. Am J Pathol 45:413–422

Braunsteiner H, Friend C (1954) Viral hepatitis associated with transplantable mouse leukemia. I. Acute hepatic manifestations following treatment with urethane or methylformamide. J Exp Med 100:665–677

David-Ferreira JF, Manaker RA (1965) An electron microscope study of the development of a mouse hepatitis virus in tissue culture cells. J Cell Biol 24:57–78

Hierholzer JC, Broderson JR, Murphy FA (1979) New strain of mouse hepatitis virus as the cause of lethal enteritis in infant mice. Infect Immun 24:508–522

Hirano N, Tamura T, Taguchi F, Ueda K, Fujiwara K (1975) Isolation of low-virulent mouse hepatitis virus from nude mice with wasting syndrome and hepatitis. Jpn J Exp Med 45:429–432

Homberger FR, Barthold SW, Smith AL (1992) Duration and strain-specificity of immunity to enterotropic mouse hepatitis virus. Lab Anim Sci 42:347–351

LePrevost C, Levy-Leblond E, Virelizier JL, Dupuy JM (1975) Immunopathology of mouse hepatitis virus type 3 infection. I. Role of humoral and cell-mediated immunity in resistance mechanisms. J Immunol 114:221–225

Piazza M (1969) Hepatitis in mice. In: Piazza M (ed) Experimental viral hepatitis, chap II. Thomas, Springfield

Sebesteny A, Hill AC (1974) Hepatitis and brain lesions due to mouse hepatitis virus accompanied by wasting in nude mice. Lab Anim 8:317–326

Taguchi F, Yamada A, Fujiwara F (1979) Asymptomatic infection of mouse hepatitis virus in the rat. Arch Virol 59:275–279

Tamura T, Taguchi F, Ueda K, Fujiwara F (1977) Persistent infection with mouse hepatitis virus of low virulence in nude mice. Microbiol Immunol 21:683–691

Adenovirus Infection, Adrenal, Mouse

Stephen W. Barthold

Gross Appearance

No lesion in the adrenal is visible to the naked eye in this infection.

Microscopic Appearance

Microscopic changes associated with this agent include inclusion body formation, necrosis, and inflammation in multiple organs (Heck et al. 1972). Adrenal changes occur primarily in all zones of cortical epithelium, but medullary cells and, less often, endothelium may be involved. Virus-induced inclusions are common and may be present in 80% of cortical epithelial cells in severe case (Figs. 517, 518). Inclusions vary in morphology depending upon stage of development. Inclusions appear first as slightly phloxinophilic single or paired ring forms or small spherules. Ring forms have sharply delineated, hematoxylinophilic outer and inner rims. Spherules are strongly phloxinophilic and vary in size up to the full capacity of the nucleus. Some spherules are surrounded by numerous tiny granules. Spherules later become dense and stain intensely with both pholxine and hematoxylin. Flower forms are very dense and are surrounded by radiating strands which divide the peripheral nucleus into septae. The cytoplasm of infected cells becomes eosinophilic and shrunken. Cellular disintegration intermixed with includion-bearing cells is usually seen. Leukocytic infiltration is frequent and most conspicuous in the late infection (Hoenig et al. 1974; Margolis et al. 1974).

Ultrastructure

Sequential changes in adrenal epithelium reflect a continuum of virus-host interaction, although cellular changes in a single specimen are always asynchronous with many stages occurring in different cells in the same area. The earliest change is an increase in the size and number of nucleoli, with the adjacent formation of round masses of finely punctate or fibrillar electron-dense material. These rounded masses detach and enlarge (E inclusion), some taking ring forms with electronlucent centers. E inclusions contain three components: (a) a finely fibrillar matrix of intermediate electron density (E_1); (b) a coarsely punctate component of high electron density, 150 Å granules (E_2); (c) highly electron-dense, finely granular material in irregular condensations throughout the matrix (E_3). Some E_3 material

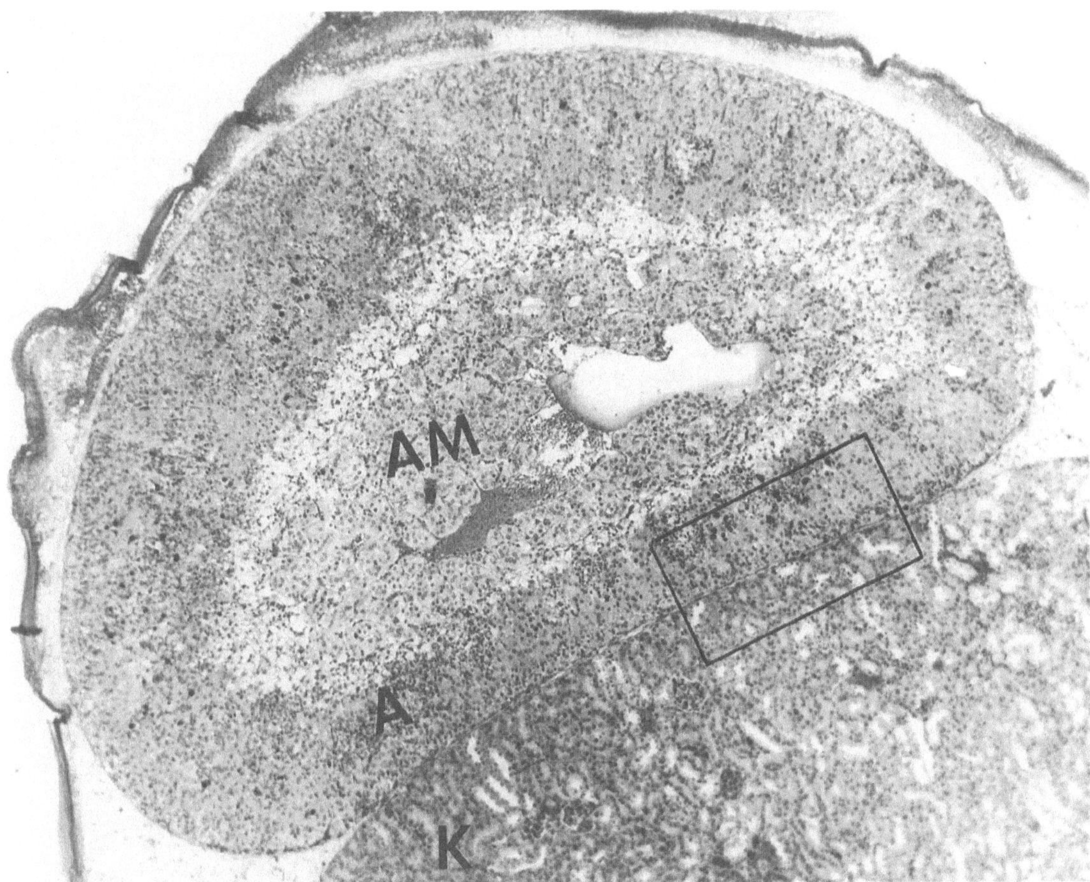

Fig. 517. Severe necrosis and clusters of inclusion bodies in adrenal cortex (*A*) following experimental inoculation with mouse adenovirus, FL strain. The adjacent kidney (*K*) is not involved. *Field marked* is magnified in Fig. 518. (*AM*) medulla; H&E, ×250. (Courtesy of George Margolis, MD, and American Journal of Pathology)

becomes peripheral in inclusions and disperses throughout the nucleoplasm. Remaining E_3 increases in volume until it becomes the main mass of a large central body in the nucleus (L inclusion). The L inclusion develops electron-lucent holes and edges which enlarge and coalesce. Electron-dense 80–100 Å particles form in these spaces, giving rise to 670–700 Å hexagonal virus particles with or without dense cores. Virions increase and form aggregates and crystals as the mass of the L inclusion decreases. Flower forms seen with light microscopy are not seen with electron microscopy, since they represent L inclusions with virus at their periphery, modified by histological artifact. As virions increase the nuclear membrane disrupts, followed by rapid degenerative changes in the cytoplasm, then by dissolution of the cell membrane. Phagocytosomes of neutrophils and monocytes contain viral aggregates, and free virus may be seen in their cytoplasm. L inclusions are also found in endothelial cells and monocytes, but virion formation is absent (Hoenig et al. 1974).

Differential Diagnosis

Mouse adenovirus adrenal changes must be differentiated from other changes such as intranuclear inclusion bodies, necrosis and inflammation induced by other viral agents, including murine cytomegalovirus and polyoma virus.

Biologic Features

Natural History. At least two serotypes of mouse adenovirus have been identified in naturally

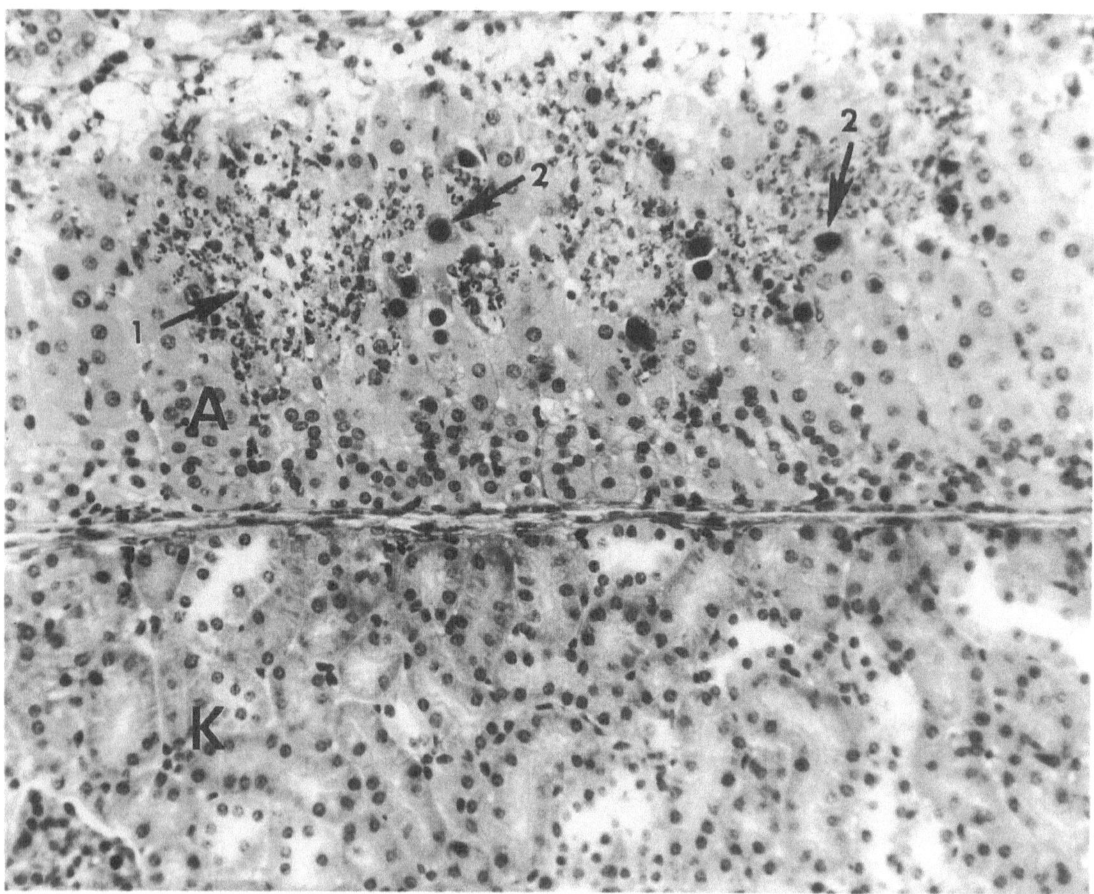

Fig. 518. Enlargement of filed in Fig. 517, demonstrating necrosis, inflammation (*1*), and intranuclear inclusions (2) in adrenal cortex (*A*), with sparing of adjacent kidney (*K*). H&E, ×600. (Courtesy of George Margolis, MD, and American Journal of Pathology)

infected mice with distinctly different disease spectra (van der Veen and Mes 1974). Strain FL causes a subclinical multisystemic infection with prolonged viruria in adult mice and is the only strain that infects the adrenal. Infection is transmitted by direct contact and the virus has been isolated from urine and nasal tissue of experimentally infected mice, but not from saliva or feces (Hartley and Rowe 1960; van der Veen and Mes 1973). Strain K87 also causes subclinical infection, which appears, however, to be limited to the intestine. Virus is transiently shed from feces, but cannot be detected in nasal tissue or urine (Sugiyama et al. 1967).

Pathogenesis. The FL strain produces a fatal infection in suckling mice within 10 days of intraperitoneal, intracerebral, or intranasal inoculation (Hartley and Rowe 1960; Heck et al. 1972). The virus also produces a generalized infection, with occasional deaths in weanling and adult mice (Hartley and Rowe 1960; van der Veen and Mes 1973). Mice develop a viremia within 1–4 days following inoculation, with disseminated lesions and virus replication in brown fat, myocardium, adrenal gland, spleen, brain, pancreas, liver, intestine, salivary glands, and kidney appearing between 3 and 5 days. Characteristic lesions include type A intranuclear inclusions in areas of necrosis and inflammation (Hartley and Rowe 1960; Heck et al. 1972; Margolis et al. 1974). There is strong adrenotropism, with qualitatively more severe lesions occurring in the adrenal in contrast to other organs (Margolis et al. 1974). Virus can be shed in urine for at least 2 years after infection of adult mice (van der Veen and Mes 1973).

Etiology. Adenoviruses occur in many species, but are generally species specific. Mouse adenovirus is naturally restricted to the mouse, but rat sera have been found to contain antibodies to mouse adenovirus (Smith et al. 1986). Clinical disease or lesions in the rat have not been found, virus has not been isolated, and rats cannot be experimentally infected with mouse adenovirus FL or K87 (Smith and Barthold 1987). One report describes adenovirus-type inclusions in the intestines of rats. Viral particles were seen but the agent was not isolated (Ward and Young 1976).

Frequency. Serologic evidence of natural infection with mouse adenovirus (FL strain) was found in 11% of mouse colonies tested in one study (Parker et al. 1966). Seroconversion to the FL strain of mouse adenovirus has rarely been seen in recent years. This agent may be a contaminant of transplantable tumors. The K87 strain of mouse adenovirus appears to be more common in laboratory mouse colonies, but its prevalence tends to be low, possibly because of its inefficient transmission among older mice, which are resistant to infection (Smith and Barthold 1987). Strains FL and K87 are two distinct, unrelated serotypes. FL antigen has been generally used in serological surveys, but use of this antigen in seroassays fails to detect antibody to the K87 strain (Smith et al. 1986; Lussier 1987).

Comparison with Other Species

Adrenal disease occurs in man in a variety of systemic virus infections, including herpes simplex, cytomegalovirus, Coxsackie B, varicella, vaccinia and Dengue hemorrhagic fever. Adenovirus has been isolated from the adrenal in a case of fatal illness in a child. Because of its high degree of adrenotropism (Margolis et al. 1974), mouse adenovirus provides a model system to study the effect of virus damage on the adrenal cortex.

References

Hartley JW, Rowe WP (1960) A new mouse virus apparently related to the adenovirus group. Virology 11:645–647

Heck FC Jr, Sheldon WG, Gleiser CA (1972) Pathogenesis of experimentally produced mouse adenovirus infection in mice. Am J Vet Res 33:841–846

Hoenig EM, Margolis G, Kilham L (1974) Experimental adenovirus infection of the mouse adrenal gland. II. Electron microscopic observations. Am J Pathol 75:375–394

Lussier G (1987) Serological relationship between mouse adenovirus strains FL and K87. Lab Anim Sci 37:55–57

Margolis G, Kilham L, Hoenig EM (1974) Experimental adenovirus infection of the mouse adrenal gland. I. Light microscopic observations. Am J Pathol 75:363–374

Parker JC, Tennant RW, Ward TG (1966) Prevalence of viruses in mouse colonies. Natl Cancer Inst Monogr 20: 25–36

Smith AL, Barthold SW (1987) Factors influencing susceptibility of laboratory rodents to infection with mouse adenovirus strains K87 and FL. Arch Viral 95:143–148

Smith AL, Winograd DF, Burrage TG (1986) Comparative biological characterization of mouse adenovirus strains FL and K87 and seroprevalence in laboratory rodents. Arch Virol 91:233–246

Sugiyama T, Hashimoto K, Sasaki S (1967) An adenovirus isolated from the feces of mice. II. Experimental infection. Jpn J Microbiol 11:33–42

van der Veen J, Mes A (1973) Experimental infection with mouse adenovirus in adult mice. Arch Virol 42:235–241

van der Veen J, Mes A (1974) Serological classification of two mouse adenoiruses. Arch Virol 45:386–387

Ward JM, Young DM (1976) Laten adenoviral infection of rats: Intranuclear inclusions induced by treatment with a cancer chemotherapeutic agent. J Am Vet Med Assoc 169:952–953

Murine Cytomegalovirus Infection, Adrenal, Mouse

Stephen W. Barthold

Synonyms. Salivary gland virus infection, cytomegalic inclusion disease virus infection.

Gross Appearance

In acute generalized murine cytomegalovirus infections, foci of necrosis may be seen as small areas of discoloration in multiple organs, especially the liver. Gross lesions are not associated with other forms of infection.

Microscopic Appearance

Adrenal lesions occur concomitantly with generalized visceral infection. Focal necrosis with cytomegaly and intranuclear inclusion bodies occur in salivary glands, meninges, brain, liver, spleen, adrenals, lymph nodes, peritoneal connective and adipose tissue, lungs, kidneys, gut, pancreas, skeletal and cardiac muscle, and brown fat (Lussier 1975; McCordock and Smith 1936). Adrenal lesions range from a few cortical cells with intranuclear inclusions, mild necrosis, and neutrophilic leukocytic infiltration to extensive hemorrhagic necrosis of cortical tissue with an abundance of intranuclear inclusions. Inclusion-bearing cells have greatly enlarged nuclei and increased cell volume (cytomegaly). Characteristic Cowdry-type A intranuclear inclusions are surrounded by a clear halo and marginated chromatin. Inclusions are Feulgen-positive and PAS-negative. Halo formation is probably an artifact of shrinkage, since it is not present in material fixed in and embedded in osmic acid Araldite (Ruebner et al. 1964). Mice that survive the acute disease may have focal cortical degenerative changes and mononuclear leukocyte infiltration (McCordock and Smith 1936; Lussier 1975).

Ultrastructure

Cells infected with murine cytomegalovirus develop a number of nonspecific degenerative changes. These changes include initial nuclear swelling with peripheral aggregation of chromatin. Dense bodies are found in the nucleolus and less often in the nucleoplasm. Early viral particles appear in the nucleus within 2–3 days of infection. These particles possess an inner, often incomplete ring surrounded by a capsid, which forms from hollow fibrillar material in the nucleolus. The inner ring condenses to form a spherical nucleoid. Particles acquire a second membrane as they traverse the inner nuclear membrane which may become tortuous and multiple. A relatively small proportion of complete viral particles are present in the cytoplasm, either as free particles or in membrane-bound vesicles (Ruebner et al. 1964; Henson and Strano 1972).

Differential Diagnosis

Differential diagnosis must include consideration of other agents which cause adrenal cortical necrosis. Intranuclear inclusion bodies are readily visualized with murine cytomegalovirus infection, narrowing the alternatives primarily to mouse adenovirus, which produces similar cortical changes, or polyoma virus, which involves the medulla. Focal leukocytic infiltrates are seen in the adrenal under a variety of circumstances, including infections by polyoma and lymphocytic choriomeningitis viruses.

Biologic Features

Natural History. Murine cytomegalovirus is generally of low virulence and in most instances produces no clinical signs. Natural infections are localized to the salivary glands. Infection is very common in wild mice, but rare in laboratory mice. Transmission occurs via inhalation or ingestion of the virus, which is shed in saliva, tears, and urine. Acute generalized infection is followed by chronic persistent infection, with localized viral replication in some tissues for up to 4 months after experimental inoculation. Latency, in which the virus is harbored in a nonreplicative state, occurs frequently in mice. In utero infection does not typically occur (Lussier 1975; Brodsky and Rowe 1958).

Pathogenesis. Within 7 days of experimental inoculation, young mice develop generalized viral infection, including leukocyte-associated viremia. Acutely ill mice have multifocal necrotizing lesions with cytomegaly and inclusion bodies in multiple organs. Inclusions are always present in the adrenals under these circumstances. Following recovery from the acute disease, there is chronic persistent infection of salivary glands, kidneys, lacrimal glands, and lymphoid tissues, with replication and shedding of the virus and the continued presence of intranuclear inclusions (Lussier 1975; McCordock and Smith 1936). The course of experimental infection depends upon route of inoculation, age and strain of mouse, virulence of the virus strain, and the immune status of the host. Salivary glands are preferentially infected, regardless of these factors, and natural infections are localized to the salivary gland (Lussier 1975). Immunosuppression of latently infected animals results in exacerbation of generalized disease (Gardner et al. 1974; Jordan et al. 1977; Lussier 1975). Disseminated disease has been observed rarely in naturally infected, aging laboratory mice (Chen and Cover 1988). During acute sublethal infection, the virus induces transient immunosuppression and suppression of interferon response, and may modify host response to other murine-infectious agents (Lussier 1975).

Etiology. Murine cytomegalovirus belongs to the cytomegalovirus subgenus of the herpesvirus group. Several strains have been obtained from laboratory and wild mice. Cytomegaloviruses are generally species-specific, and different viruses have been described in mice, guinea pigs, hamsters, various other rodents, man, nonhuman primates, moles, pigs, dogs, sheep, and horses (Lussier 1975; Plotkin and Furukawa 1978).

Frequency. Infection is not common in laboratory mice under natural conditions, but occurs frequently in wild mice (Lussier 1975). The potential for transmission from wild to laboratory mice is therefore always present. Adrenal lesions are usually present in acute, generalized disease, but rarely under other circumstances.

Comparison with Other Species

Generalized human cytomegalovirus infection is a common complication following immunosuppressive regimens. It causes a fatal pneumonia and disseminated cytomegalic inclusion disease. The natural history of the murine disease closely resembles that of man (Jordan et al. 1977; Lussier 1975).

References

Brodsky I, Rowe WP (1958) Chronic subclinical infection with mouse salivary gland virus. Proc Soc Exp Biol Med 99: 654–655

Chen HC, Cover CE (1988) Spontaneous disseminated cytomegalic inclusion disease in an aging laboratory mouse. J Comp Pathol 98:489–493

Gardner MB, Officer JE, Parker J, Estes JD, Rongey RW (1974) Induction of disseminated virulent cytomegalovirus infection by immunosuppression of naturally chronically infected wild mice. Infect Immun 10:966–969

Henson D, Strano AJ (1972) Mouse cytomegalovirus. Necrosis of infected and morphologically normal submaxillary gland acinar cells during termination of chronic infection. Am J Pathol 68:183–202

Jordan MC, Shanley JD, Stevens JG (1977) Immunosuppression reactivates and disseminates latent murine cytomegalovirus. J Gen Virol 37:419–423

Lussier G (1975) Murine cytomegalovirus (MCMV). Adv Vet Sci Comp Med 19:223–247

McCordock HA, Smith MG (1936) The visceral lesions produced in mice by the salivary gland virus of mice. J Exp Med 63:303–310 (+ 3 plates)

Plotkin SA, Furukawa T (1978) Herpesviridae: Cytomegalovirus. In: Hsiung G-D, Green RH (eds) CRC handbook series in clinical laboratory science, Section H: Virology and rickettsiology, vol I, part 2. CRC Press, West Palm Beach, pp 93–112

Ruebner BH, Miyai K, Slusser RJ, Wedemeyer P, Medearis DN Jr (1964) Mouse cytomegalovirus infection. An electron microscopic study of hepatic parenchymal cells. Am J Pathol 44:799–821

Polyoma Virus Infection, Adrenal, Mouse

Stephen W. Barthold

Synonyms. SE (Stewart-Eddy) polyoma virus, parotid tumor virus infection.

Gross Appearance

This agent induces tumors in a variety of organs, most commonly the parotid salivary glands. Adrenal tumors are unilateral or bilateral. They are very soft, fleshy, and pale pink with foci of internal hemorrhage. Their surfaces are smooth and glistening. Large tumors may be multinodular and reach 2.5 cm in diameter. Metastases are often widespread to liver, lungs, ovary, pancreas, and peripheral lymph nodes (Stewart 1955, 1960).

Microscopic Appearance

The polyoma virus produces a wide variety of tumors (Stanton et al. 1959; Stewart 1955, 1960). Both degenerative and neoplastic lesions occur in the adrenal medulla but not in the cortex of susceptible mice. During the acute infection, epithelial cells enlarge, nuclei swell, and intranuclear inclusion bodies develop. Adjacent cells, not involved in replicative viral infection, are mitotically active. Focal perivascular lymphocytic infiltrates may be seen. Medullary neoplasms are composed of chromaffin-negative, deeply basophilic, round to ovoid cells with relatively scant cytoplasm and slightly oval, hyperchromatic nuclei. Cells grow in clumps separated by thin bands of connective tissue. Early tumors contain many enlarged cells as in the acute infection. As tumors enlarge, they invade and compress cortical tissue, and necrosis is frequent. Some tumors become anaplastic with fusiform cell types (Buffett and Levinthal 1962; Stewart 1955, 1960; Stewart et al. 1958).

Ultrastructure

Cells in replicative infection develop arrays of closely packed viral particles in their nuclei. Crystalloids may form and completely fill the nucleus, or the particles may be less regularly arranged. Phagocytes may contain phagosomes with aggregates of virus derived from adjacent lytic cells. Tumors may have rare cells with small aggregates of viral particles, but virus is present only in small quantities (Eddy 1960; Howatson et al. 1960; Stewart 1960).

Differential Diagnosis

Acute polyoma viral infection of the adrenal must be differentiated from infections by other agents which induce the formation of intranuclear inclusion bodies, including murine cytomegalovirus and adenovirus. The latter agents produce changes in the adrenal cortex. Perivascular lymphocytic infiltrates are found in the adrenal under a variety of circumstances, but specific agents include lymphocytic choriomeningitis virus and murine cytomegalovirus. Spontaneous medullary tumors possess chromaffin-positive columnar cells bordering vascular channels with polarization of nuclei along the arterial poles of the cells (Jones and Woodward 1954). Tumor cells induced by polyoma virus are chromaffin-negative, lack polarization, and are more basophilic (Stewart 1955).

Biologic Features

Natural History. Polyoma virus generally occurs as a subclinical infection of laboratory and wild mice. The virus is excreted from urine, saliva and, to a lesser extent, feces for at least 120 days. Mice are infected most readily by intranasal installation of virus. Excretion of virus is most efficient from newborn mice, but infection does not spread readily among weanling or adult mice. In wild populations, infection is probably maintained in contaminated nesting areas, since the agent is highly stable. Laboratory colonies may be infected by accidental exposure to experimental virus or to contaminated transplantable tumor lines. Infection is maintained best in laboratory mice when conditions allow close contact among weanling mice with excrete virus relatively inefficiently. Newborn mice may avoid infection because the statistical chance of acquiring infection in the first few days of life is small and they may be protected by maternal antibody. Transplacental infection does not occur, but virus can be reactivated with renewal of virus shedding in persistently infected pregnant mice that were infected as neonates (McCance and Mims 1979).

Infection with polyoma virus usually does not result in spontaneous tumor development under natural conditions. This apparently is due to the rapid development of resistance to the oncogenic effect with age, to the low statistical probability of a neonate acquiring infection during the critical age period, to the presence of maternal antibody and to the amount of virus produced; finally, natural routes of exposure are relatively ineffective for tumor induction. Nevertheless, characteristic polyoma viral tumors have been observed in several colonies under natural conditions. These events followed shortly after the colonies were exposed to virus for the first time (Rowe 1961).

Pathogenesis. Polyoma virus in vitro can follow three different courses upon infection of a susceptible cell: (a) lytic infection, in which a permissive cell is destroyed by viral replication; (b) transformation, in which the viral genome is incorporated permanently into the genome of the cell; or (c) abortive infection, in which transformed cells lose the virus after several cell divisions. In the process of infection and transformation, polyoma virus induces several virus-directed antigens, including small, middle, and large T antigens and tumor-specific transplantation antigens (TSTA). In addition, viral structural antigens also are produced in lytic infections. These events play a critical role in the pathogenesis of polyoma virus in vivo.

The outcome of infection largely depends upon the host's immune response to the virus or to viral-induced tumor neoantigens, particularly TSTA. Adult mice which are fully immunocompetent mount an efficient and rapid immune response to both the virus and the tumor, preventing both generalized infection and tumor development. Neonatal mice have an ineffective, delayed immune response, allowing generalized viral infection, excretion of virus, and growth of transformed cells to the point that neoplastic growth can no longer be controlled (Allison 1980). Susceptibility to the oncogenic effects of polyoma virus is most pronounced during the first 24 h of life, after which it rapidly declines (Barthold and Olson 1974).

Neonates have a high mortality 2–4 weeks after subcutaneous inoculation of the virus. There is marked retardation of growth rate and severe thymic atrophy. About 1 week after infection, renal tubular epithelial cells swell, vacuolate, and develop intranuclear inclusions. With the development of an immune response to the virus at about 2 weeks, lymphocytes and plasmacytes infiltrate perivascular tissue in involved areas. Within the next 2 weeks, similar changes are common throughout many organs. At about 2 months, multicentric foci of undifferentiated, mitotically active cells evolve in multiple organs. Grossly visible tumors develop in up to 100% of mice surviving between 2 and 4 months (Buffet and Levinthal 1962). Most of the tumors that develop are types that do not occur spontaneously (Stewart 1960). The most frequent tumors are parotid gland tumors, but a wide variety of epithelial and mesenchymal tumors evolve from many organs, including adrenal medulla (Stanton et al. 1959; Stewart 1955, 1960). Natural routes of infection have a similar outcome, with fewer tumors. Oronasal inoculation of neonates results in virus replication in nasal mucosa, submaxillary salivary glands and lungs, followed by viremic dissemination to multiple organs, including kidney. By day 12 virus is cleared from most sites but persists in lung and kidney for months (Dubensky et al. 1984). Natural infection of athymic nude mice has resulted in posterior paralysis due to development of vertebral tumors and central nervous system lesions reminiscent of progressive multifocal leukoencephalopathy (McCance et al. 1983; Sebesteny et al. 1980).

Etiology. Polyoma virus belongs to and is the type species of the polyomavirus subgroup of the papovavirus group. The virus measures 40–45 nm in diameter and contains double stranded, circular DNA. All strains of mice are susceptible to infection with polyoma virus and some strains are highly susceptible to tumor induction (Barthold and Olson 1974; Stewart 1960). Polyoma virus is also capable of producing sarcomas in experimentally inoculated hamsters, rats, ferrets, guinea pigs, rabbits, and Mastomys. In contrast to mice, hamsters readily develop tumors after intranasal installation of virus and there is no sharp development of resistance with age (Barthold and Olson 1974; Rowe 1961).

Frequency. Polyoma virus was at one time a common agent in both laboratory and wild mice (Rowe 1961), but the virus is not commonly found at present in laboratory mouse colonies. It may be found as a permanent contaminant of transplantable tumor lines. Although polyoma virus can induce spontaneous development of tumors under natural conditions, this event is rare, apparently due to complex epizootiological factors. Adrenal medullary tumors have been noted in up to 36% of polyoma-virus-inoculated mice when exposed 8 h after birth. Low doses of virus result in development of parotid tumors only (Stewart 1955, 1960). Thus, the likelihood of spontaneous adrenal tumors induced by this agent under natural conditions is very low.

Comparison with Other Species

Polyoma virus of mice is the type species for the polyomavirus subgroup of Papoviridae. Members of this subgroup tend to be species specific, but infect a wide range of hosts, including humans. Human infections are usually asymptomatic, with urinary excretion of virus, except in immunocompromized hosts, which may develop clinical signs. Humans and nonhuman primates with acquired immunodeficiency can develop central nervous system disease, progressive multifocal leukoencephalopathy (King et al. 1983) as is seen in athymic nude mice (Sebesteny et al. 1980). Hamsters are host to another polyomavirus. Unlike mice, hamsters of all ages develop persistent infections with natural exposure. Hamster papovavirus can cause epizootics of transmissible lymphomas when introduced to a naive hamster population (Barthold et al. 1987).

References

Allison AC (1980) Immune responses to polyoma virus and polyoma virus-induced tumors. In: Klein G (ed) Viral oncology. Raven, New York

Barthold SW, Olson C (1974) Papovavirus-induced neoplasia. In: Melby EC Jr, Altman NH (eds) Handbook of laboratory animal science, vol II, CRC, Cleveland, chapter 9

Barthold SW, Bhatt PN, Johnson EA (1987) Further evidence for papovavirus as the probable etiology of transmissible lymphoma of Syrian hamsters. Lab Anim Sci 37:283–288

Buffet RF, Levinthal JD (1962) Polyoma virus infection in mice. Arch Pathol 74:513–526

Dubensky TW, Murphy FA, Villarreal LP (1984) Detection of DNA and RNA virus genomes in organ systems of whole mice: patterns of mouse organ infection by polyomavirus. J Virol 50:779–783

Eddy BE (1960) The polyoma virus. Adv Virus Res 7:91–102

Howatson AF, McCulloch EA, Almeida JD, Siminovitch L, Axelrad AA, Ham AW (1960) Studies in vitro, in vivo and by electron microscope of a virus recovered from a C3H mouse mammary tumor: relationship to polyoma virus. JNCI 24:1131–1151

Jones EE, Woodward LJ (1954) Spontaneous adrenal medullary tumors in hybrid mice. JNCI 15:449–461

King NW, Hunt RD, Letvin NL (1983) Histopathologic changes in macaques with an acquired immunodeficiency syndrome (AIDS). Am J Pathol 113:382–388

McCance DJ, Mims CA (1979) Reactivation of polyoma virus in kidneys of persistently infected mice during pregnancy. Infect Immuno 25:998–1002

McCance DJ, Sebesteny A, Griffin BE, Balkwill F, Tilly R, Gregson NA (1983) A paralytic disease in nude mice associated with polyoma virus infection. J Gen Virol 64: 57–67

Rowe WP (1961) The epidemiology of mouse polyoma virus infection. Bacteriol Rev 25:18–31

Sebesteny A, Tilly R, Balkwill F, Trevan D (1980) Demyelination and wasting associated with polyomavirus infection in nude (nu/nu) mice. Lab Anim 14:337–345

Stanton MF, Stewart SE, Eddy BE, Blackwell RH (1959) Oncogenic effect of tissue-culture preparations of polyoma virus on fetal mice. JNCI 23:1441–1475

Stewart SE (1955) Neoplasms in mice inoculated with cell-free extracts or filtrates of leukemic mouse tissues. I. Neoplasms of the parotid and adrenal glands. JNCI 15:1391–1415

Stewart SE (1960) The polyoma virus. Adv Virus Res 7:61–90

Stewart SE, Eddy BE, Borgese N (1958) Neoplasms in mice inoculated with a tumor agent carried in tissue culture. JNCI 20:1223–1243

Lymphocytic Choriomeningitis Virus Infection, Adrenal, Mouse

Stephen W. Barthold

Gross Appearance

Gross changes are usually absent, but mice may have splenomegaly, pale liver, and pleural exudate. Adrenal glands are unremarkable (Lillie and Armstrong 1945; Maurer 1964).

Microscopic Appearance

Adrenal changes occur as a component of generalized lymphocytic choriomeningitis virus (LCMV) infection. Chronically infected mice develop nonsuppurative inflammatory lesions and lymphoreticular proliferation in virtually every tissue, especially lung and liver. Neonatally infected mice with persistent infections develop renal glomerular endothelial and mesangial proliferation, basement membrane thickening, intracapillary hyalinization, and capillary occlusion. Brain lesions are mild unless mice are inoculated intracerebrally. Splenomegaly is due to lymphoreticular proliferation. Adrenal glands, like other organs, may have focal or diffuse lymphocytic infiltrates in the cortex, medulla, or periglandular adipose tissue. In acutely ill mice, foci of adrenal cortical necrosis may be seen. Necrosis of lymphocytes also occurs in thymus and lymph nodes in the acute disease (Findlay and Stern 1936; Lillie and Armstrong 1945; Maurer 1964; Oldstone and Dixon 1969).

Ultrastructure

Lymphocytic choriomeningitis viral antigen is ubiquitous in cells throughout the body in persistent infections, but only a very small proportion of cells contain visible virus particles. In cell culture, less than 5% of infected cells manufacture discernible virus. Thus, the likelihood of visualizing virus in infected tissues is remote. Viral particles are pleomorphic, ranging from 50 to 300 nm in diameter. They bud from the cell membrane, have small spikes on their envelope and contain 1–8 electron-dense internal granules. Infectious particles have a diameter of 106 ± 14 nm (Blechschmidt and Thomssen 1976; Dalton et al. 1968). Since the virus seldom produces lytic changes in infected cells, other ultrastructural findings are rare.

Differential Diagnosis

The nonspecific lymphocytic infiltrates in the adrenal and other organs of mice infected with the virus mimic the effects of other viruses such as murine cytomegalovirus and polyoma virus. In contrast to LCMV, these latter agents induce intranuclear inclusion bodies. Focal lymphocytic infiltrates may also occur in the adrenal in the absence of an infectious agent.

Biologic Features

Natural History. Lymphocytic choriomeningitis virus is very prevalent in wild mice, which are the reservoir host. Laboratory rodents may acquire the infection from wild rodents or, more commonly, via contamination of transplantable tumors. When immunocompetent, adult mice are infected with the virus, virus is effectively eliminated with minimal or no disease. On the other hand mice infected in utero or as neonates experience chronic persistent infections which are usually subclinical, but eventually result in a chronic wasting syndrome (Oldstone and Dixon 1969, 1970). These carrier mice chronically excrete virus and readily transmit it to their offspring or cohorts. A small proportion of mice that naturally acquire infection after weaning may exhibit clinical signs which include rough hair coats, drowsiness, emaciation, weakness, photophobia, and conjunctivitis. Their movement is slow, stiff, and creeping (Maurer 1964). Acute disease can be induced in mice between 5 and 7 days after intracerebral or intraperitoneal inoculation of virus. Death occurs at 6–8 days while mice are convulsing in a typical, extended posture. Intranasal or subcutaneous inoculation of virus results in an acute infection with subclinical or transient illness (Hotchin 1971). Naturally infected mice with subclinical infections may manifest convulsions due to activation of virus following intracerebral injection of sterile foreign material (Maurer 1964). Infection is transmitted by the airborne route or by contamination of the environment with infected urine. Various bloodsucking arthropods have been shown experimentally to transmit the agent (Hotchin 1971). Contact infection through nasal secretions is the most important means of transmission in a naive mouse population. Once infection is enzootic, the intrauterine route becomes the primary means of transmission within a colony (Traub 1936).

Pathogenesis. The pathogenic mechanisms of LCMV infection in the mouse have been extensively studied. The virus itself is considered to be basically harmless to mice, since infected cells continue to function normally although the virus induces a host-homograft response to virus-induced neoantigens on infected cells, resulting in illness and death (Hotchin 1971). This hypothesis is not absolutely true, since the virus itself is lethal in some mouse strains, causing direct viral damage. In other strains, the immune response is the harmful component, while in still others, neither virus nor immune response is harmful (Volkert and Lundstedt 1971). Generally, when mice are infected in utero or as neonates, they develop a tolerance which allows a persistent infection with high titers of virus in many tissues of the body. The mechanism of this tolerant state has not been completely defined, but one feature is profound depression of cell-mediated immunity to the virus. Disease can be precipitated in these mice by injection of virus-sensitized T cells. Persistent infection can be induced in adult mice by immunosuppression or in nude mice without such manipulation (Christoffersen et al. 1976; Oldstone and Dixon 1969; Volkert and Lundstedt 1971). Mice persistently infected with nonpathogenic strains of the virus can develop signs of organ dysfunction, such as endocrinopathies, as a result of virus infection of target cells without cytolysis (Oldstone et al. 1982). Depending largely upon the genetic strain, neonatally infected mice eventually develop glomerulonephritis as the result of antigen excess immune complex deposition, focal hepatic necrosis, and extensive lymphoid proliferations and interstitial mononuclear leukocyte infiltrates throughout the body (Lillie and Armstrong 1945; Oldstone and Dixon 1969, 1970). Disease development depends on the amount of virus, the extent of antibody response, and the interaction between virus and antibody. Mouse strains that allow high virus and antibody titers develop the earliest and most severe disease (Oldstone and Dixon 1969, 1970). When conditions favor an effective immune response, for example, low virus dose, neurotropism, route of exposure and age, mice develop both a humoral and cell-mediated immune response with elimination of the virus. Cell-mediated immunity appears to be most crucial in freeing mice of virus (Oldstone and Dixon 1969, 1970; Volkert and Lundstedt 1971). A thymic nude mice have persistent infections (Dykewicz et al. 1992).

Etiology. Lymphocytic choriomeningitis virus is an enveloped RNA virus of the arenavirus group. Virus strains vary in pathogenicity but cannot be differentiated serologically. Strains that have been passaged to develop viscerotropic properties tend to induce persistent infection, while brain-passaged strains develop neurotropic properties and are lethal to newborn mice. Lethal strains are termed "aggressive" and nonlethal strains, "docile." Wild virus strains are docile, viscerotropic types (Hotchin 1971). The agent occurs naturally in mice, hamsters, guinea pigs, chinchillas, cotton rats, foxes, dogs, nonhuman primates and man. Numerous other species are experimentally susceptible. Hamsters develop persistent infection with excretion of high titers of virus. Guinea pigs are highly susceptible, even through intact skin, and develop pneumonia, pulmonary edema, and meningitis (Maurer 1964).

Frequency. This viral infection is commonplace in wild and rare in laboratory mice, but prevalence depends largely upon their source and husbandry. Transplantable tumors are frequently contaminated with the virus and are the most common source of infection in laboratory mice (Bhatt et al. 1986; Dykewicz et al. 1992). Natural infections are usually subclinical. Lesions, under these circumstances, are not well developed in the brain and are rather nonspecific in other organs. Thus, a diagnosis cannot be made by morphology alone. Adrenal lesions are common in the experimental chronic disease.

Comparison with Other Species

Lymphocytic choriomeningitis virus infection is largely innocuous in the mouse, its natural host, with lesions related to the host's immune response to the agent. In other species, injury related to the virus itself appears to be the primary mechanism of disease, and the immune response does not play a decisive role in the pathogenesis (Volkert and Lundstedt 1971). Adrenal lesions are constantly present in the infected rat and guinea pig (Lillie and Armstrong 1945).

In man LCMV produces disease ranging in severity from inapparent infection to a rare, fatal disease. It usually results in a mild, influenza-like illness. Lesions may include meningitis, encephalitis, myocarditis, parotitis, orchitis, and pneumonia. Multisystemic disease is seen in fatal cases. Infections in the laboratory are easily contracted (Hotchin 1971).

References

Bhatt PN, Jacoby RO, Barthold SW (1986) Contamination of transplantable murine tumors with lymphocytic choriomeningitis virus. Lab Anim Sci 36:136–139

Blechschmidt M, Thomssen R (1976) Electron-microscopic identification of infectious particles of lymphocytic choriomeningitis. Med Microbiol Immunol (Berl) 162:193–199

Christoffersen PJ, Volkert M, Rygaard J (1976) Immunological unresponsiveness of nude mice to LCM virus infection. Acta Pathol Microbiol Scand [C] 84:520–523

Dalton AJ, Rowe WP, Smith GH, Wilsnack RE, Pugh WE (1968) Morphological and cytochemical studies on lymphocytic choriomeningitis virus. J Virol 2:1465–1478

Dykewicz CA, Dato M, Fisher-Hoch SP, Howarth MV, Perez-Oronoz GI, Ostroff SM, Gary H Jr, Schonberger LB, McCormick JB (1992) Lymphocytic choriomeningitis outbreak associated with nude mice in a research institute. JAMA 267:1349–1353

Findlay GM, Stern RO (1936) Pathological changes due to infection with the virus of lymphocytic choriomeningitis. J Pathol Bacteriol 43:327–338

Hotchin J (1971) The contamination of laboratory animals with lymphocytic choriomeningitis virus. Am J Pathol 64: 747–769

Lillie RD, Armstrong C (1945) Pathology of lymphocytic choriomeningitis in mice. Arch Pathol 40:141–152

Maurer FD (1964) Lymphocytic choriomeningitis. Lab Anim Care 14:415–419

Oldstone MBA, Dixon FJ (1969) Pathogenesis of chronic disease associated with persistent lymphocytic choriomeningitis viral infection. I. Relationship of antibody production to disease in neonatally infected mice. J Exp Med 129:483–505

Oldstone MBA, Dixon FJ (1970) Pathogenesis of chronic disease associated with persistent lymphocytic choriomeningitis viral infection. II. Relationship of the anti-lymphocytic choriomeningitis immune response to tissue injury in chronic lymphocytic choriomeningitis disease. J Exp Med 131:1–19

Oldstone MBA, Sinha YN, Blount P, Tishon A, Rodriguez M, von Wedel R, Lampert PW (1982) Virus-induced alterations in homeostasis: alterations in differentiated functions of infected cells in vivo. Science 218:1125–1127

Traub E (1936) The epidemiology of lymphocytic choriomeningitis in white mice. J Exp Med 64:183–200

Volkert M, Lundstedt C (1971) Tolerance and immunity to the lymphocytic choriomeningitis virus. Ann N Y Acad Sci 181:183–195

Adrenal Necrosis Due to Besnoitiosis: Golden Hamster

J.K. Frenkel

Synonyms. Besnoitiosis, adrenal, hamster; *Besnoitia jellisoni* infection.

Gross Appearance

During late acute *Besnoitia* infection of hamsters necrotic foci of the adrenal cortex may be seen that are as small as 1 mm or less; these are irregular light brown areas which sometimes become confluent and may be accompanied by focal hemorrhage. During chronic *Besnoitia* infection the areas of discoloration are larger and may exceed the size of the normal hamster adrenal gland. Liver and spleen may become adherent to the adrenal (Fig. 519).

Microscopic Appearance

Besnoitia tachyzoites, resembling *Toxoplasma* in size and morphology, parasitize adrenocortical cells which undergo necrosis (Frenkel 1956). In advanced infections cell parasitization may extend into medulla and capsule. There may be compensatory hyperplasia of preserved adrenocortical cells (Figs. 520, 521).

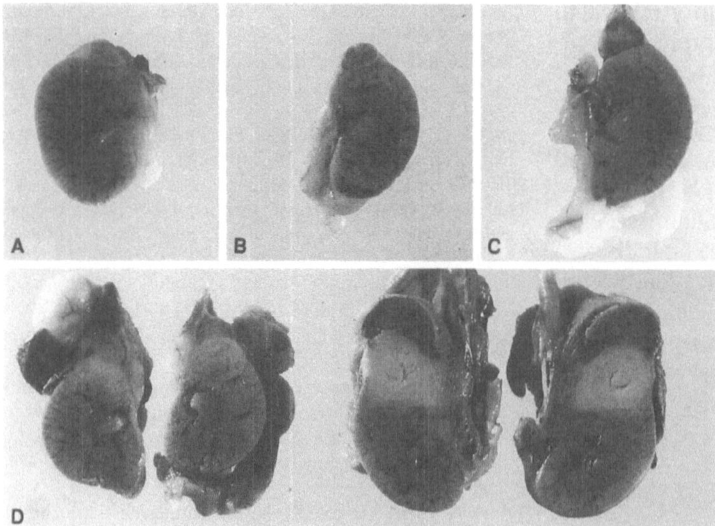

Fig. 519A–D. Kidneys with attached adrenal glands from hamsters with *Besnoitia* or *Toxoplasma* infection. **A** Normal hamster. **B** *Besnoitia* infection of 11 day's duration, showing foci of adrenocortical necrosis (*light*) accompanied by focal hemorrhage (*dark*) **C** *Toxoplasma* infection of 1 year's duration with infection necrosis of inner cortex and medulla and compensatory hyperplasia. **D** Hamster died with the equivalent of Addison's disease after *Besnoitia* infection of 175 days. Bisected right and left adrenals are enlarged because of progressive necrosis of adrenal cortical cells with compensatory hyperplasia of remaining cortical cells. The capsules of liver and spleen, above, have become adherent to the adrenal capsules in consequence of the chronic inflammatory reaction. 1.5×. (From Frenkel 1956)

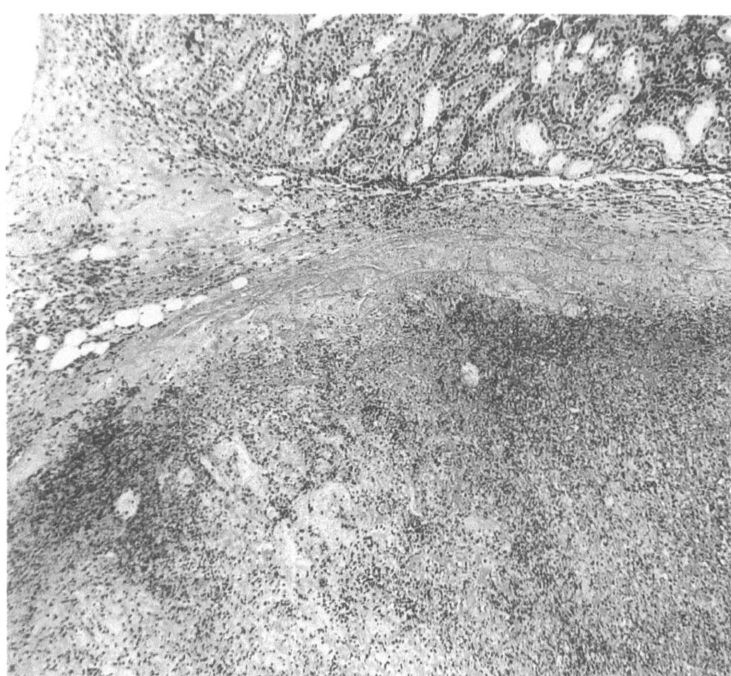

Fig. 520. Chronic *Besnoitia* infection of hamster. The infection is actively progressing in the adrenal, below, whereas the kidney, above, is unaffected. H&E, ×80. (From Frenkel 1987)

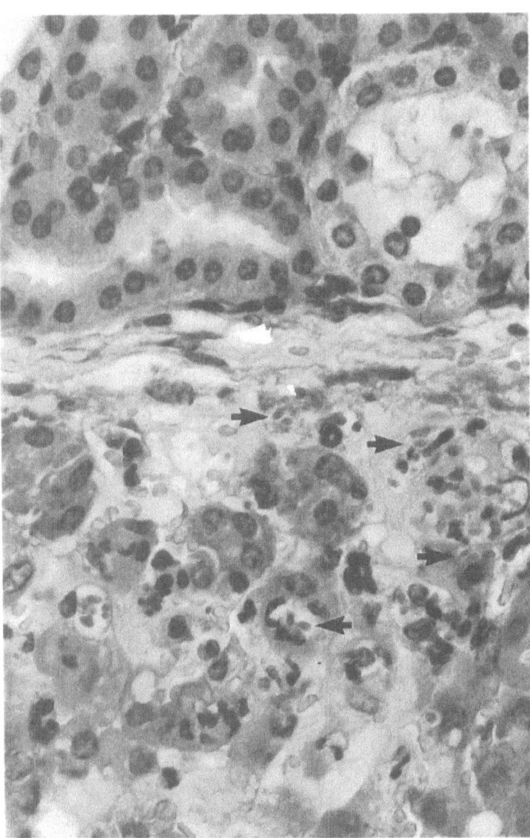

Fig. 521. Acute Besnoitia infection of 15 days' duration, showing adrenal involvement but sparing of the adjacent kidney (*top*). *Arrows*, intracellular and intercellular *Besnoitia* tachyzoites destroying cortical cells (*center, left*), whereas cortical cells are still well preserved *on extreme right*. H&E, ×560. (From Frenkel 1956)

Differential Diagnosis

The lesions have been studied in hamsters (*Mesocricetus auratus*) infected with *B. jellisoni*. The organism was originally isolated from *Peromyscus leucopus* in Idaho (Frenkel 1953). The actively multiplying forms, tachyzoites, are almost indistinguishable from those of *T. gondii*. The tissue cysts differ considerably in size; those of *Besnoitia* may exceed 1 mm, and those of *Toxoplasma* reach about 200 μm. The cyst wall of *Besnoitia* includes the host cell nucleus or nuclei, whereas the cyst wall of *Toxoplasma* is intracytoplasmic (Mehlhorn and Frenkel 1980). Spontaneous laboratory infection of hamsters may result from contamination of feed with oocysts, most likely from cats (Frenkel 1977).

Adrenal cortical necrosis in hamsters has been found associated also with chronic infections with *T. gondii*, *Mycobacterium kansasii*, and certain fungi, but irregularly so (Frenkel 1972, 1987).

Biologic Features

Natural History. Besnoitia administered subcutaneously gives rise to a generalized infection in hamsters, which for experimental studies has generally been treated with sulfadiazine or sulfamerazine-Na 60–120 mg% in drinking water. Depending on the dose of infection and adaptation of the organism, treatment for a few days delays death, and longer treatment permits immunity to develop which is associated with chronic infection (Frenkel 1956). In hamsters that die after 9 days adrenal infection can generally be diagnosed with the naked eye or a dissecting scope from the light staining necrotic foci. Histologically, adrenal cortical cells are focally or diffusely infected, accompanied by mononuclear inflammation and necrosis of infected cells. In hamsters surviving for weeks or months the adrenals may be markedly enlarged, with yellowish necrosis and hyperemic areas of regeneration.

Pathogenesis. The finding of progressive infection in the adrenals and retina of hamsters although other tissues appeared immune months after infection drew attention to these lesions. For the experimental analysis of the pathogenesis of this lesion hamsters were used that had been treated with sulfonamides sufficiently to delay their death until the 3rd week of infection. The adrenal lesions were found to depend on a functional adrenal cortex. *Besnoitia* lesions were absent in hypophysectomized hamsters, or animals whose cortex was inactive because of feedback inhibition with various glucocorticoids (Frenkel 1956). Besnoitia often proliferated around the subcutaneous deposits of relatively insoluble salts of corticosteroids. It was postulated that certain corticosteroids can so modify immunity mechanisms locally that general immunity becomes ineffective. This occurred in the adrenal cortex owing to endogenous corticoid production, at the sites of exogenous corticoid injection, and in the lungs when generalized hypercorticism is produced (Frenkel 1956). The pathogenesis of retinal infection was distinct (Frenkel 1961a).

At the time when this work was carried out, the nature of the hamster adrenal corticoid was still unknown. It was later shown that the adrenal secretory product of hamsters is cortisol (Schindler and Knigge 1959), similarly as in humans, whereas rats and mice secrete corticosterone, which has only a slight immunosuppressive effect. We compared the effects of stress, corticoid precursors, analogs, and blocking agents on hamster adrenal secretion (Frenkel et al. 1965) and compared it with the effects in humans. Cortisol levels in hamster adrenal vein blood were five- to tenfold higher than in peripheral venous blood (Frenkel et al. 1965). That the cortisol effect was not direct but by immunosuppression was evident in that it did not affect the proliferation of *Besnoitia* in cell culture or in nonimmune hamsters.

Recognition that local hypercorticism with immunosuppression was the basis of chronic adrenal infection in hamsters suggested application of this hypothesis to humans (Frenkel 1960, 1961b). Adrenal infection in man occurs with tuberculosis, histoplasmosis and other fungal infections, syphilis, cytomegalovirus infection, and possibly other agents. In humans and in hamsters the causative organisms are more numerous in the adrenals, granulomatous reaction, where present, is depressed, and the infection is progressive, leading to large lesions and sometimes adrenal insufficiency, even though immunity is evident in other tissues. Clarification of the pathogenesis of adrenal infection leading to Addison's disease in humans was based on the hamster *Besnoitia* model and an understanding of the immunity-depressing effects of corticosteroids.

Etiology. *B. jellisoni* is a tissue protozoan with a two-host cycle similar to *T. gondii*, *B. jellisoni* and other *Besnoitia* species have been found in white-footed mice (*Peromyscus*), kangaroo rats (*Dipodomys*), opossums (*Didelphis*), and muskrats among small mammals in North America, but also in reindeer and caribou in Canada and Alaska, and in Mexican burros. Besnoitia infections have been found in cattle in Spain and other Mediterranean countries, in impala, kudu, and blue wildebeest in South Africa, and rats from Hawaii. *Besnoitia* infections have also been found in various lizards in Central America, in opossums from the Amazon region in Brazil (Naiff and Arias 1983), and occasionally in snake in North America (Frenkel 1977).

Frequency. *Besnoitia* infection was prevalent for a time in a laboratory colony of *Peromyscus* from Utah. It is not otherwise known as a spontaneous laboratory infection.

Comparison with Other Species

In laboratory mice certain viral infections give rise to lesions in the adrenal cortex, apparently in the course of acute infection, but without evidence of productive infection continuing in chronically infected mice. The role of corticosterone secreted by the mouse adrenal cortex, and which has only slight immunosuppressive action compared to cortisol, has apparently not been investigated in detail.

References

Frenkel JK (1956) Effects of hormones on the adrenal necrosis produced by Besnoitia jellisoni in golden hamsters. J Exp Med 103:375–398

Frenkel JK (1960) Pathogenesis of infections of the adrenal gland, leading to Addison's disease in man: the role of corticoids in adrenal and generalized infection. Ann N Y Acad 84:391–440

Frenkel JK (1961a) Pathogenesis of toxoplasmosis with a consideration of cyst rupture in Besnoitia infection. Surv Ophthal 6:799–825

Frenkel JK (1961b) Infections involving the adrenal cortex. In: Moon HD (ed) The adrenal cortex. Hoeber, New York, pp 201–219

Frenkel JK (1972) Infection and immunity in hamsters. Prog Exp Tumor Res 16:326–367

Frenkel JK (1977) Besnoitia wallacei of cats and rodents: with a reclassification of other cyst-forming isosporoid coccidia. J Parasitol 63:611–628

Frenkel JK (1987) Experimental biology: use in infectious diseases research. In: Van Hoosier J, McPherson DW (eds) Laboratory hamsters. Academic, Orlando, pp 227–249

Frenkel JK, Cook K, Grady HJ, Pendleton SK (1965) Effects of hormones on adrenocortical secretion of golden hamsters. Lab Invest 14:142–156

Mehlhorn H, Frenkel JK (1980) Ultrastructural comparison of cysts and zoites of Toxoplasma gondii, Sarcocystis muris, and Hammondia hammondi in skeletal muscle of mice. J Parasitol 66:59–67

Naiff RD, Arias JR (1983) Besnoitia (Protozoa, Toxoplasmatinae) isolado de mucuras Didelphis marsupialis na região Amazônica. Brasil Mem Inst Oswaldo Cruz 78:431–435

Schindler WJ, Knigge KM (1959) Adrenal cortical secretion by the golden hamster. Endocrinology 65:739–747

Subject Index*

*Page numbers in **boldface** indicate the principal discussion; Figures are designated by the latter "f" following the page number; Tables are found on page numbers followed by the letter "t".

Springer-Verlag and the Environment